Haematology and Blood Transfusion
26 —————————————————
Hämatologie und Bluttransfusion

W0105805

Edited by
H. Heimpel, Ulm · D. Huhn, München
C. Mueller-Eckhardt, Gießen
G. Ruhenstroth-Bauer, München

Modern Trends in Human Leukemia IV

Latest Results
in Clinical and Biological Research
Including Pediatric Oncology

Organized on behalf of the Deutsche Gesellschaft für
Hämatologie und Onkologie and the Deutsches
Krebsforschungszentrum. Wilsede, June 16–19, 1980

Wilsede Joint Meeting on Pediatric Oncology I
Hamburg, June 20/21, 1980

Edited by
R. Neth, R. C. Gallo, T. Graf,
K. Mannweiler and K. Winkler

With 252 Figures and 118 Tables

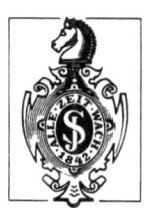

Springer-Verlag
Berlin Heidelberg New York 1981

Dr. Rolf Neth, Universitäts-Kinderklinik, Molekularbiologisch-hämato-logische Arbeitsgruppe, Martinistraße 52, D-2000 Hamburg 20, Federal Republic of Germany

Dr. Robert C. Gallo, National Cancer Institute, Laboratory of Tumor Cell Biology, Bethesda, Maryland 20014, USA

Dr. Thomas Graf, Institut für Virusforschung, Im Neuenheimer Feld 280, D-6900 Heidelberg 1, Federal Republic of Germany

Dr. Klaus Mannweiler, Heinrich-Pette-Institut für Experimentelle Viro-logie und Immunologie an der Universität Hamburg, Martinistraße 52, D-2000 Hamburg 20, Federal Republic of Germany

Dr. Kurt Winkler, Universitäts-Kinderklinik, Abteilung für Haematolo-gie und Onkologie, Martinistr. 52, D-2000 Hamburg 20, Federal Republic of Germany

Supplement to

BLUT – Journal Experimental and Clinical Hematology

Organ of the *Deutsche Gesellschaft für Hämatologie und Onkologie* der *Deutschen Gesellschaft für Bluttransfusion und Immunohämatologie* and of the *Österreichischen Gesellschaft für Hämatologie und Onkologie*

ISBN-13: 978-3-540-10622-7   e-ISBN-13: 978-3-642-67984-1
DOI:10.1007/ 978-3-642-67984-1

This work is subject to copyright. All rights are reserved, whether the whole or part of the material is concerned specifically those of translation, reprinting, re-use of illustrations, broadcasting, reproduction by photocopying machine or similar means, and storage in data banks. Under § 54 of the German Copyright Law where copies are made for other than private use a fee is payable to "Verwertungsgesellschaft Wort", Munich.

© Springer-Verlag Berlin Heidelberg 1981

The use of registered names, trademarks etc. in this publication does not imply even in the absence of a specific statement, that such names are exempt from the relevant protective laws and regulations and therefore free for general use.

2127/3321/543210

Scientific Organisation of the Sessions

Clinical Aspects

Frei, Emil III, Sidney Farber Cancer Institute, 44, Binney Street, Boston, MA 02115, USA
Lister, Andrew, Dept. Medical Oncology, St. Bartholomew's Hospital, West Smithfield, London EC1A7BE, U.K.

Cytogenetic and Lymphomas

Kaplan, Henry S., Dept. Radiology, Cancer Biology Research Laboratory, Stanford University Medical School, Stanford CA 94305, USA
Klein, George, Dept. Tumor Biology, Karolinska Institutet 104 Stockholm 60, Sweden

Cell Biology

Greaves, Mel F., Imperial Cancer Research Fund Laboratories P.O. Box 123, Lincoln's Inn Fields, London WC2A3PX, U.K.
Moore, Malcolm, Memorial Sloan-Kettering Cancer Center, 1275 York Avenue, New York, NY 10021, USA

Immunology

Eichmann, Klaus, Krebsforschungszentrum – Immunologie, Im Neuenheimer Feld 280, 6900 Heidelberg, West Germany
Mitchison, Nicholas Avrion, Tumor Immunology Unit, University College London, Gower Street, London WC1E6BT, U.K.

Virology and Molecular Biology

Duesberg, Peter, Dept. Molecular Biology, Wendell M. Stanley Hall, University of California, Berkeley, CA 94720, USA
Gallo, Robert C., National Cancer Institute, Bethesda, MD 20014, USA

Wilsede Joint Meeting on Pediatric Oncology I

Kabisch, Hartmut, Universitätskinderklinik, Abt. für Hämatologie und Onkologie, Martinistr. 52, 2000 Hamburg 20, West-Germany
Winkler, Kurt, Universitätskinderklinik, Abt. für Hämatologie und Onkologie, Martinistr. 52, 2000 Hamburg 20, West-Germany

Contents

Participants of the Meeting XV
Wilsede Scholarship Holders XIX
Preface XXI
Acknowledgement XXV

Frederick Stohlman Jr. Memorial Lecture

Klein, G.: The Relative Role of Viral Transformation and Specific
Cytogenetic Changes in the Development of Murine and Human
Lymphomas 3

Kaplan, H. S.: On the Biology and Immunology of Hodgkin's
Disease 11

Clinical Aspects

Rowley, J. D.: Chromosome Studies in Children and Adults with
Leukemia[1] 27

Georgii, A., Thiele, J., Vykoupil, K.-F.: Myeloid Dysplasia: the
Histopathology of Preleukemia 34

Lister, T. A., Johnson, S. A. N., Bell, R., Henry, G., Malpas, J. S.:
Progress in Acute Myelogenous Leukemia 38

Mayer, R. J., Weinstein, H. J., Rosenthal, D. S., Coral, F.'S.,
Nathan, D. G., Frei, E. III.: VAPA[10]: A Treatment Program for
Acute Myelocytic Leukemia 45

Preisler, H. D.: Rational Approaches to the Treatment of
Leukemia 53

Moloney, W. C., Rosenthal, D. S.: Treatment of Early Acute
Nonlymphatic Leukemia with Low Dose Cytosine Arabinoside .. 59

Rohatiner, A., Balkwill, F., Malpas, J.S., Lister, T.A.: A Phase I
Study of Human Lymphoblastoid Interferon in Patients with
Hematological Malignancies 63

Mertelsmann, R., Moore, M. A. S., Clarkson, B.: Methods and Clinical Relevance of Terminal Deoxynucleotidyl Transferase Determination in Leukemic Cells[2] 68

Hiddemann, W., Andreeff, M., Clarkson, B. D.: Quantitation of Chemotherapy-Induced Cytoreduction in Acute Leukemia[2] 73

Miller, D. R., Leikin, S., Albo, V., Sather, H., Karon, M., Hammond, D.: Intensive Therapy and Prognostic Factors in Acute Lymphoblastic Leukemia of Childhood: CCG 141. A Report from Childrens Cancer Study Group[2] 77

Henze, G., Langermann, H.-J., Ritter, J., Schellong, G., Riehm, H.: Treatment Strategy for Different Risk Groups in Childhood Acute Lymphoblastic Leukemia: A Report From the BFM Study Group[2] 87

Rivera, G.: Recurrent Childhood Lymphocytic Leukemia: Outcome of Marrow Relapses After Cessation of Therapy[2] 94

Sinks, L. F., Wang, J. J., Freeman, A. I.: The Treatment of Primary Childhood Acute Lymphocytic Leukemia with Intermediate Dose Methotrexate[2] 99

Chessells, J. M., Ninane, J., Tiedemann, K.: Present Problems in Management of Childhood Lymphoblastic Leukaemia: Experience from the Hospital for Sick Children, London[2] 108

Zintl, F., Plenert, W., Hermann, J.: Different Therapy Protocols for High Risk and Standard Risk ALL in Childhood 115

Sallan, S. E.: T-Cell Acute Lymphoblastic Leukemia in Children[2] 121

Rodt, H., Thierfelder, S., Kolb, H. J., Netzel, B., Haas, R. J., Wilms, K., Bender-Götze, C.: The Concept of GvHD-Suppression by In Vitro Treatment with Antisera[2] 124

Storb, R.: Bone Marrow Transplantation for the Treatment of Leukemia 136

Morgenstern, G. R., Powles, R. L.: Allogeneic Bone Marrow Transplantation for Acute Myeloid Leukemia in First Remission .. 139

Furusawa, M., Iino, T.: Use of Erythrocyte Ghosts for Therapy ... 143

Hardesty, B., Henderson, A. B., Kramer, G.: A Possible Biochemical Basis for the Use of Hyperthermia in the Treatment of Cancer and Virus Infection 146

Cytogenetic Aspects of Lymphomas

Rowley, J. D.: The Implications of Nonrandom Chromosome Changes for Malignant Transformation 151

Carrano, A. V., Lebo, R. V., Yu, L. C., Kan, Y. W.: Regional Gene
Mapping of Human Chromosomes Purified by Flow Sorting 156

Levan, G., Mitelman, F.: The Different Origin of Primary and
Secondary Chromosome Aberrations in Cancer 160

Cline, M. J., Stang, H. D., Mercola, K., Salser, W.: Insertion of
New Genes into Bone Marrow Cells of Mice 167

Scheer, D. I., Srimatkandada, S., Kamen, B. A., Dube, S., Bertino,
J. R.: Organization of the Methotrexate Resistant Mouse
L5178YR Dihydrofolate Reductase Gene and Transformation of
Human HCT-8 Cells by This Gene 171

Hauser, H., Graf, T., Beug, H., Greiser-Wilke, I., Lindenmaier,
W., Grez, M., Land, H., Giesecke, K., Schütz, G.: Structure of the
Lysozyme Gene and Expression in the Oviduct and Macropha-
ges 175

Zeuthen, J., Klein, G.: Some Recent Trends in Studies of Human
Lymphoid Cells: B-Cells, Epstein-Barr Virus, and Transformation 179

Wolf, H., Wilmes, E., Bayliss, G. J.: Epstein-Barr Virus: Its Site of
Persistence and Its Role in the Development of Carcinomas 191

Kaschka-Dierich, C., Bauer, I., Fleckenstein, B., Desrosiers, R.
C.: Episomal and Nonepisomal Herpesvirus DNA in Lymphoid
Tumor Cell Lines 197

Brade, L., Gissmann, L., Mueller-Lantzsch, N., zur Hausen, H.:
B-Lymphotropic Papovavirus (LPV) – Infections of Man? 204

Purtilo, D. T.: Immunopathology of the X-Linked Lymphoproliferative Syndrome 207

Nilsson, K., Forsbeck, K., Gidlund, M., Sundström, C., Tötterman,
T., Sällström, J., Venge, P.: Surface Characteristics of the U-937
Human Histiocytic Lymphoma Cell Line: Specific Changes
During Inducible Morphologic and Functional Differentiation In
Vitro 215

Radzun, H. J., Parwaresch, M. R., Lennert, K.: Enzyme Polymor-
phism as a Biochemical Cell Marker: Application to the Cellular
Origin and Homogeneity of Human Macrophages and to the
Classification of Malignant Lymphomas 222

Wielckens, K., Garbrecht, M., Schwoch, G., Hilz, H.: Human
Leukemic Lymphocytes – Biochemical Parameters of the Altered
Differentiation Status 225

Diehl, V., Kirchner, H. H., Schaadt, M., Fonatsch, C., Stein, H.:
Lymphoproliferation and Heterotransplantation in Nude Mice:
Tumor Cells in Hodgkin's Disease 229

Cell Biological and Immunological Aspects

Moore, M. A. S.: Genetic and Oncogenic Influences on Myelopoiesis 237

Broxmeyer, H. E., Bognacki, J., Dörner, M. H., deSousa, M., Lu,
L.: Acidic Isoferritins as Feedback Regulators in Normal and
Leukemic Myelopoiesis 243

Messner, H. A., Fauser, A. A., Buick, R., Chang, L. J.-A., Lepine,
J., Curtis, J. C., Senn, J., McCulloch, E. A.: Assessment of Human
Pluripotent Hemopoietic Progenitors and Leukemic Blast-For-
ming Cells in Culture 246

Afanasiev, B. V., Elstner, E., Saidali, M. A., Zabelina, T. S.:
Proliferation and Maturation of Hemopoietic Cells in Adult
Patients with Different Forms of Acute Leukemia and Chronic
Myeloid Leukemia in Agar and Liquid Cultures 251

Burk, E., Chennaoui-Antonio, L., Beiersdorf, H., Hellwege, H.
H., Winkler, K., Heinisch, B., Küstermann, G., Krause, U.,
Kitschke, H. J., Voigt, H., Neth, R.: Cytological and Cytochemical
Analysis of Plasma Clot Cultures and Peripheral Granulocytes
Related to Long Term Survival in Childhood ALL and Cancer
Patients Under Cytostatica Therapy 255

Hoelzer, D., Harriss, E. B., Carbonell, F.: Maturation of Blast
Cells in Acute Transformation of Chronic Myeloproliferative
Syndrome 261

Lau, B., Jäger, G., Thiel, E., Pachmann, K., Rodt, H., Thierfelder,
S., Dörmer, P.: Patterns of Cell Surface Differentiation of cALL
Positive Leukemic Blast Cells in Diffusion Chamber Culture 265

Forbes, P., Dobbie, D., Powles, R., Alexander, P.: Maturation of
Human Peripheral Blood Leukemic Cells in Short-Term Culture .. 268

Dexter, T. M.: Regulator-Dependent Hemopoiesis and Its Possible Relevance to Leukemogenesis 272

Gartner, S., Kaplan, H. S.: Long-Term Culture of Normal and
Leukemic Human Bone Marrow 276

Greenberg, H. M., Parker, L. M., Newburger, P. E., Said, J.,
Cohen, G. I., Greenberger, J. S.: Corticosteroid Dependence of
Continuous Hemopoiesis In Vitro with Murine or Human Bone
Marrow 289

Mitchison, N. A.: Cloning Cells of the Immune System 294

Greaves, M. F., Robinson, J. B., Delia, D., Ritz, J., Schlossman, S.,
Sieff, C., Goldstein, G., Kung, P., Bollum, F. J., Edwards, P. A. W.:
Comparative Antigenic Phenotypes of Normal and Leukemic
Hemopoietic Precursor Cells Analysed with a "Library" of
Monoclonal Antibodies[2] 296

van den Engh, G., Trask, B., Visser, J.: Surface Antigens of Pluripotent and Committed Haemopoietic Stem Cells 305

Beverley, P. C. L., Linch, D., Callard, R. E.: Human Leucocyte Antigens 309

Godal, T., Lindmo, T., Ruud, E., Heikkilä, R., Henriksen, A., Steen, H. B., Marton, P. F.: Immunologic Subsets in Human B-Cell Lymphomas in Relation to Normal B-Cell Development .. 314

Hengartner, H.: Clones of Murine Functional T Cells 320

Minowada, J.: Marker Profiles of Leukemia-Lymphoma Cell Lines[2] 323

Newman, R. A., Sutherland, D. R., Greaves, M. F.: Biochemical Characterization of an Antigen Associated with Acute Lymphoblastic Leukemia and Lymphocyte Precursors[2] 326

Becker, W.-M., Schmiegel, W.-H., Kabisch, H., Arndt, R., Thiele, H.-G.: Serologic Subtyping of cALL[2] 329

Baker, M. A., Roncari, D. A. K., Taub, R. N., Mohanakumar, T., Falk, J. A.: Acute Myeloblastic Leukemia-Associated Antigens: Detection and Clinical Importance[2] 332

Andersson, L. C., von Willebrand, E., Jokinen, M., Karhi, K. K., Gahmberg, C. G.: Glycophorin A as an Erythroid Marker in Normal and Malignant Hematopoiesis[2] 338

Eichmann, K.: The Network Concept and Leukemia 343

Klein, E.: Interpretation and In Vivo Relevance of Lymphocytotoxicity Assays 345

Milleck, J., Jantscheff, P., Thränhardt, H., Schöntube, M., Gürtler, R., Seifart, D., Pasternak, G.: Acute Leukemia and Nonspecific Killer Cells 351

Teodorescu, M., Hsu, C., Bratescu, A., DeBoer, K. P., Nelson, R., Kleinman, R., Wen, C. M.-J., Mayer, E. P., Pang, E. J.-M.: The Use of Bacteria as Markers of Leukemic Lymphocytes and for the Isolation of Natural Killer Cells 355

McGrath, M. S., Jerabek, L., Pillemer, E., Steinberg, R. A., Weissman, I. L.: Receptor Mediated Murine Leukemogenesis: Monoclonal Antibody Induced Lymphoma Cell Growth Arrest .. 360

Stoye, J. P., Moroni, C.: Effect of Bromodeoxyuridine on Endogenous Retrovirus Production in Differentiating Murine Lymphocytes 365

Schreiber, H., Flood, P. M., Kripke, M. L., Urban, J. L.: Modulation of Growth of Malignant Cells by Anti-Idiotypic Immunity 368

Kyewski, B., Hunsmann, G., Friedrich, R., Ketelsen, U.-P., Wekerle, H.: Thymic Nurse Cells: Intraepithelial Thymocyte Sojourn and Its Possible Relevance for the Pathogenesis of AKR Lymphomas 372

Schirrmacher, V., Bosslet, K.: Generation of Stable Antigen Loss Variants from Cloned Tumor Lines – An Example of Immuno-adaptation During Metastasis 377

Virological and Molecularbiological Aspects

Duesberg, P. H., Bister, K.: Transforming Genes of Retroviruses: Definition, Specificity, and Relation to Cellular DNA 383

Erikson, E., Erikson, R. L.: A Cellular Protein Phosphorylated by the Avian Sarcoma Virus Transforming Gene Product 397

Friis, R. R., Ziemiecki, A., Bosch, V., Boschek, C. B., Bauer, H.: Correlated Loss of the Transformed Phenotype and pp60^{src}-Associated Protein Kinase Activity 402

Moelling, K., Owada, M. K., Donner, P., Bunte, T.: The Transformation-Specific Protein pp60^{src} from an Avian Sarcoma Virus 405

Konze-Thomas, B., von der Helm, K.: Proteolytic Processing of Avian and Simian Sarcoma and Leukemia Viral Proteins 409

Kramer, G., Grankowski, N., Hardesty, B.: Control of Protein Synthesis. Phosphorylation and Dephosphorylation of Eukaryotic Peptide Initiation Factor 2 414

Graf, T., Royer-Pokora, B., Korzeniewska, E., Grieser, S., Beug, H.: Characterization of the Hematopoietic Target Cells of Defective Avian Leukemia Viruses by Velocity Sedimentation and Density Gradient Centrifugation Analyses 417

Vogt, P. K., Neil, J. C., Moscovici, C., Breitman, M. L.: PRCII, a Representative of a New Class of Avian Sarcoma Viruses 424

Souza, L. M., Bergmann, D. G., Baluda, M. A.: Identification of the Avian Myeloblastosis Virus Genome 429

Coffin, J. M., Tsichlis, P. N., Robinson, H. L.: Genetics of Leukemogenesis by Avian Leukosis Viruses 432

Hayward, W. S., Neel, B. G., Fang, J., Robinson, H. L., Astrin, S. M.: Avian Lymphoid Leukosis is Correlated with the Appearance of Discrete New RNAs Containing Viral and Cellular Genetic Information 439

Kung, H. J., Fung, Y. K., Crittenden, L. C., Fadly, A., Dube, S. K.: The Molecular Basis of Avian Retrovirus-Induced Leukemogenesis 445

Löliger, H.-C., von dem Hagen, D., Hartmann, W.: Studies of the Association of Leukemogenic and Oncogenic Properties in Avian Leukemia Viruses 452

Aaronson, S. A., Barbacid, M., Dunn, C. Y., Reddy, E. P.: Genetic Approaches Toward Elucidating the Mechanisms of Type-C Virus-Induced Leukemia 455

Blair, D. G., Oskarsson, M., McClements, W. L., Vande Woude, G. F.: The Long Terminal Repeat of Moloney Sarcoma Provirus Enhances Transformation 460

Waneck, G. L., Rosenberg, N.: Ontogeny of Abelson Murine Leukemia Virus Target Cells 467

Evans, L. H., Duesberg, P. H., Linemeyer, D. L., Ruscetti, S. K., Scolnick, E. M.: Structural and Functional Studies of the Friend Spleen Focus-Forming Virus: Structural Relationship of SFFV to Dualtropic Viruses and Molecular Cloning of a Biologically Active Subgenomic Fragment of SFFV DNA 472

van den Berg, K. J., Krump-Konvalinkova, V., Bentvelzen, P.: Enhancing Effect of Murine Leukemia Virus on Fibroblast Transformation by Normal BALB/C Mouse DNA Fragments ... 479

Essex, M., Grant, C. K., Cotter, S. M., Hardy, W. D. Jr.: Role of Viruses in the Etiology of Naturally Occuring Feline Leukemia ... 483

Snyder, H. W. Jr., Dutta-Choudhury, M., Hardy, W. D. Jr.: Relationship of the Feline Oncornavirus Associated Cell Membrane Antigen to a Feline Sarcoma Virus Encoded Polyprotein 488

Hardy, W. D. Jr., McClelland, A. J., Zuckerman, E. E., Snyder, H. W. Jr., MacEwen, E. G., Francis, D., Essex, M.: Feline Leukemia Virus Nonproducer Lymphosarcomas of Cats as a Model for the Etiology of Human Leukemias 492

Kettmann, R., Marbaix, G., Mammerickx, M., Burny, A.: Genomic Integration of Bovine Leukemia Provirus and Lack of Viral RNA Expression in the Target Cells of Cattle with Different Responses to BLV Infection 495

Portetelle, D., Bruck, C., Mammerickx, M., Burny, A.: Natural Antibodies to BLV gp51 Are Reactive Against the Carbohydrate Moiety of the Glycoprotein 498

Gallo, R. C., Poiesz, B. J., Ruscetti, F. W.: Regulation of Human T-Cell Proliferation: T-Cell Growth Factor and Isolation of a New Class of Type-C Retroviruses from Human T-Cells 502

Reitz, M. S. Jr., Poiesz, B. J., Ruscetti, E. W., Gallo, R. C.: Characterization by Nucleic Acid Hybridization of HTLV, a Novel Retrovirus from Human Neoplastic T-Lymphocytes 515

Torelli, U., Torelli, G., Narni, F., Donelli, A., Ferrari, S., Franchini, G., Calabretta, B.: Different Frequency Classes of Sequences in Heterogeneous Nuclear RNA of Normal Promyelocytes and Lymphoblasts and of Leukemic Blast Cells of Circulating Blood and of the HL60 Line 517

Thiel, H.-J., Matthews, T., Broughton, E., Butchko, A., Bolognesi, D.: Characterization of Antigens in SSV Nonproducer Cells 520

Bergholz, C. M.: Viral Gene Expression in Cells Transformed by Simian Sarcoma Virus, an Infectious Primate Type C Retrovirus .. 524

Jore, J., Dubbes, R., Coolen, J., Nooter, K.: Cell Fusion as a Tool for the Detection of Viral Footprints in Childhood Leukemia 527

Hehlmann, R., Schetters, H., Erfle, V.: ELISA for the Detection of Antigens Cross-Reacting with Primate C-Type Viral Proteins (p30, gp70) in Human Leukemic Sera 530

Erfle, V., Hehlmann, R., Schetters, H., Schmidt, J., Luz, A.: Radiation-Induced Murine Leukemias and Endogenous Retroviruses: The Time Course of Viral Expression 537

Löwer, J., Löwer, R., Stegmann, J., Frank, H., Kurth, R.: Retrovirus Particle Production in Three of Four Human Teratocarcinoma Cell Lines 541

General Summary

Deinhardt, F.: General Summary 547

Subject Index 551

---

[1] Special lecture for the Wilsede Joint Meeting on Pediatric Oncology I
[2] Were also presented in the Wilsede Joint Meeting on Pediatric Oncology I

Participants of the Meeting

Aaronson, A., Laboratory of RNA Tumor Viruses, National Cancer Institute, Bethesda, MD 20014, USA

Andersson, L., Transplantation Laboratory, University of Helsinki, Haartmaninkatu 3A, 00290 Helsinki 29, Finland

Andreeff, M., Memorial Sloan-Kettering Cancer Center, 1275 York Avenue, New York, NY 10021, USA

Baluda, M. A., UCLA Cancer Center, Dept. Microbiology and Immunolgy, 921 Westwood Boulevard, Los Angeles, CA 90024, USA

Barbacid, M., Laboratory of RNA Tumor Viruses, National Cancer Institute, Bethesda, MD 20014, USA

Beck, J. D., Memorial Sloan-Kettering Cancer Center, 1275 York Avenue, New York, NY 10021, USA

Bentvelzen, P., Radiobiological Institute, 151 Lange Kleiweg, Rijswijk, The Netherlands

Bertino, J., Yale University School of Medicine, 333 Cedar Street, New Haven, CT 06510, USA

Beverley, P. C. L., ICRF Human Tumour Immunology Group, University of London, University Street, London WC1E 6JJ, U.K.

Bister, K., Dept. Molecular Biology, Wendell M. Stanley Hall, University of California, Berkeley, CA 94720, USA

Brade, Lore, Institut für Virologie im Zentrum für Hygiene, Hermann-Herder-Straße 11, 7800 Freiburg i. Br., West-Germany

Burny, A., Faculté des Sciences Agronomiques de l'Etat, Chaire de Zootechnie, Gembloux, Belgium

Carrano, A., Biomedical Division, L-452, Lawrence Livermore Labs. Livermore, CA 94550, USA

Chermann, J.-C., Institut Pasteur, 25, Rue du Docteur Roux, 75724 Paris, Cédex 15, France

Cline, M., UCLA Center for Health Sciences, Dept. Medicine, Los Angeles, CA 90024, USA

Coffin, J. M., Dept. Molecular Biology, Tufts University, 136 Harrison Avenue, Boston, MA 02111, USA

Deinhardt, F., Max v. Pettenkofer-Institut, Pettenkoferstraße 9a, 8000 München 2, West-Germany

Dexter, T. M., Christie Hospital & Holt Radium Institute, Paterson Laboratories, Manchester M20 9BX, U.K.

Diehl, V., Medizinische Hochschule Hannover, Depàrtment für Innere Medizin, Karl-Wiechert-Allee 9, 3000 Hannover-Kleefeld, West-Germany

Duesberg, P., Dept. Molecular Biology, Wendell M. Stanley Hall, University of California, Berkeley, CA 94720, USA

Eichmann, K., Krebsforschungszentrum – Immunologie, Im Neuenheimer Feld 280, 6900 Heidelberg, West-Germany

Elstner, Elena, Abt. Zellkinetik, Zentralinstitut für Molekularbiologie, Lindenberger Weg 70, 1115 Berlin-Buch, GDR van den Engh, G., Radiobiological Institute 151 Lange Kleiweg, Rijswijk, The Netherlands

Erfle, V., Gesellschaft für Strahlen- und Umweltschäden, Ingolstädter Landstraße 1, 8042 Neuherberg, West-Germany

Erikson, Eleanor, Health Sciences Center, University of Colorado, 4200 East Ninth Avenue, Denver, CO 80262, USA

Essex, M., Dept. Microbiology, Harvard School of Public Health, 665 Huntington Avenue, Boston, MA 02115, USA

Evans, L., Dept. Molecular Biology, Wendell M. Stanley Hall, University of California, Berkeley, CA 92720, USA

Feldman, M., The Weizmann Institute of Science, P.O. Box 26, Rehovot 76 100, Israel

Fleckenstein, B., Institut für Klinische Virologie, Loschgestraße 7, 8520 Erlangen, West-Germany

Forbes, Penelope, Chester Beatty Research Institute, Clifton Avenue, Belmont, Sutton, Surrey SM2 5PX, U.K.

Frei III, E., Sidney Farber Cancer Institute, 44, Binney Street, Boston, MA 02115, USA

Friis, R. R., Institut für Virologie, Justus-Liebig-Universität, Frankfurter Straße 107, 6300 Gießen, West-Germany

Furusawa, M., Dept. Biology, Osaka City University, Sugimoto-Cho, Sumiyoshi-Ku, Osaka 558, Japan

Gallo, R. C., National Cancer Institute, Bethesda, MD 20014, USA

Gartner, Suzanne, Dept. Radiology, Cancer Biology Research Laboratory, Stanford University Medical Center, Stanford, CA 94305, USA

Georgii, A., Medizinische Hochschule Hannover, Pathologisches Institut, Karl-Wichert-Allee 9, 3000 Hannover-Kleefeld, West-Germany

Godal, T., Norsk Hydro's Institute for Cancer Research, Montebello, Oslo 3, Norway

Graf, T., Institut für Virusforschung, Im Neuenheimer Feld 280, 6900 Heidelberg 1, West-Germany

Greaves, M. F., Imperial Cancer Research Fund Laboratories, P.O. Box 123, Lincoln's Inn Fields, London WC2A 3PX, U.K.

Greenberger, J. S., Dept. Radiation Therapy, Harvard Medical School, 44, Binney Street, Boston, MA 02115, USA

Hardesty, B., Dept. Chemistry, The Clayton Foundation Biochemical Institute, University of Texas, Austin, TX 78712, USA

Hausen, H. zur, Institut für Virologie im Zentrum für Hygiene, Hermann-Herder-Straße 11, 7800 Freiburg i. Br., West-Germany

Hayward, W., Rockefeller University, 1230 York Avenue, New York, NY 10021, USA

Hehlmann, R., Institut für Biologie, Ingolstädter Landstraße 1, 8042 Neuherberg, West-Germany

Helm, K. von der, Max v. Pettenkofer-Institut, Pettenkoferstraße 9a, 8000 München 2, West-Germany

Hengartner, H., Experimentelle Pathologie, Universität Zürich, Schmelzbergstraße 12, 8091 Zürich, Switzerland

Hölzer, D., Zentrum für Innere Medizin und Kinderheilkunde, Universität Ulm, Steinhövelstraße 9, 7900 Ulm, West-Germany

Kabisch, H., Universitäts-Kinderklinik, Abt. für Hämatologie und Onkologie, Martinistr. 52, 2000 Hamburg 20, West-Germany

Kaplan, H. S., Dept. Radiology, Cancer Biology Research Laboratory, Stanford University Medical School, Stanford, CA 94305, USA

Kettmann, R., Faculté des Sciences Agronomiques de l'Etat, Chaire de Zootechnie, Gembloux, Belgium

Klein, Eva, Dept. Tumor Biology, Karolinska Institutet, 104 Stockholm 60, Sweden

Klein, G., Dept. Tumor Biology, Karolinska Institutet, 104 Stockholm 60, Sweden

Kirsten, W. H., Dept. Pathology, University of Chicago, 950 East 50th Street, Chicago, IL 60637, USA

Kramer, Gisela, Dept. Chemistry, The Clayton Foundation Biochemical Institute, University of Texas, Austin, TX 78712, USA

Kurth, R., Friedrich-Miescher-Laboratorium der Max-Planck-Gesellschaft, Spemannstraße 37–39, 7400 Tübingen, West-Germany

Lajtha, L. G., Christie Hospital & Holt Radium Institute, Paterson Laboratories, Manchester M20 9BX, U.K.

Lau, Barbara, Gesellschaft für Strahlen- und Umweltforschung mbH, Abteilung Experimentelle Hämatologie und Immunologie, Landwehrstraße 61, 8000 München 15, West-Germany

Levan, G., Genetiska Institutionen, Göteborgs Universitet, Stigbergsliden 14, 41463 Göteborg, Sweden

Linemeyer, D. L., National Cancer Institute, Bethesda, MD 20014, USA

Lister, A., Dept. Medical Oncology, St. Bartholomew's Hospital, West Smithfield, London EC1A 7BE, U.K.

Löliger, H.-Ch., Institut für Kleintierzucht, Dörnbergstraße 25–27, 3100 Celle, West-Germany

Mannweiler, K., Heinrich-Pette-Institut für Experimentelle Virologie und Immunologie an der Universität Hamburg, Martinistraße 52, 2000 Hamburg 20, West-Germany

Mayer, R., Sidney Farber Cancer Institute, 44, Binney Street, Boston, MA 02115, USA

McCredie, K. B., Leukemia Service, M. D. Anderson Hospital, 6723 Bertner Avenue, Houston, TX 77030, USA

McGrath, M., Dept. Pathology, Stanford University Medical Center, Stanford, CA 94305, USA

Mercola, Karen, Dept. Medicine, University of California, Los Angeles, CA 90024, USA

Mertelsmann, R., Memorial Sloan-Kettering Cancer Center, 1275 York Avenue, New York, NY 10021, USA

Messner, H., The Ontario Cancer Institute, 5000 Sherbourne Street, Toronto, Ontario M4X, 1K9, Canada

Milleck, J., Zentralinstitut für Krebsforschung, Lindenbergerweg 80, 115 Berlin-Buch, GDR

Miller, D. R., Memorial Sloan-Kettering Cancer Center, 1275 York Avenue, New York, NY 10021, USA

Minowada, J., Roswell Park Memorial Institute, 666 Elm Street, Buffalo, NY 14263, USA

Mitchison, N. A., Tumor Immunolgy Unit, University College London, Gower Street, London WC1E 6BT, U.K.

Mölling, Karin, Max-Planck-Institut für Molekulare Genetik, Ihnestraße 63–73, 1000 Berlin 33, West-Germany

Moloney, W. C., Peter Bent Brigham Hospital, Hematology Division, 721 Huntington Avenue, Boston, MA 02115, USA

Moore, M. A. S., Memorial Sloan-Kettering Cancer Center, 1275 York Avenue, New York, NY 10021, USA

Munk, K., Deutsches Krebsforschungszentrum, Im Neuenheimer Feld 280, 6900 Heidelberg, West-Germany

Neth, R., Universitäts-Kinderklinik Hamburg-Eppendorf, Martinistraße 52, 2000 Hamburg 20, West-Germany

Newman, R., Imperial Cancer Research Fund Laboratories, P.O. Box 123, Lincoln's Inn Fields, London WC2A 3PX, U.K.

Nilsson, K., The Wallenberg Laboratory, Box 562, University of Uppsala, 75122 Uppsala, Sweden

Nooter, K., Radiobiological Institute, 151 Lange Kleiweg, Rijswijk, The Netherlands

Pragnell, I., Beaton Institute for Cancer Research, Switchback Road, Bearsden, Glasgow G61 1BD, Scotland

Preisler, H., Roswell Park Memorial Institute, 666 Elm Street, Buffalo, NY 14263, USA

Purtilo, D. T., Dept. Pathology, University of Massachusetts Medical Center, Worcester, MA 01605, USA

Radzun, H. J., Klinikum der Christian-Albrechts-Universität Kiel, Institut für Pathologie, Hospitalstraße 42, 2300 Kiel, West-Germany

Reitz, M., National Cancer Institute, Bethesda, MD 20014, USA

Riehm, H. J., Kinderklinik der Freien Universität Berlin, Heubnerweg 6, 1000 Berlin 19, West-Germany

Rivera, G., St. Jude Children's Research Hospital, 332 North Lauderdale, P.O. Box 318, Memphis, TN 38101, USA

Rodt, H., Institut für Hämatologie, Abteilung Immunologie, Landwehrstraße 61, 8000 München 2, West-Germany

Rohatiner, A., Dept. Medical Oncology, St. Bartholomew's Hospital, West Smithfield, London EC1A 7BE, U.K.

Rosenberg, Naomi E., Cancer Research Center, Tufts University School of Medicine, 136 Huntington Avenue, Boston, MA 02111, USA

Rowley, Janet D., Dept. Medicine, Section of Hematology/Oncology, Box 420, 950 East 59th Street, Chicago, IL 60637, USA

Sallan, S. E., Sidney Farber Cancer Institute, 44, Binney Street, Boston, MA 02115, USA

Scherrer, K., Institut de Recherche Biologie-Moléculaire, F-75221 Paris Cédex 5, France

Schirrmacher, V., Institut für Virusforschung, Im Neuenheimer Feld 280, 6900 Heidelberg 1, West-Germany

Schreiber, H., Dept. Pathology, La Rabida Children's Hospital and Research Center, East 65th Street at Lake Michigan, Chicago, IL 60649, USA

Simon, M. M., Krebsforschungszentrum – Immunologie, Im Neuenheimer Feld 280, 6900 Heidelberg, West-Germany

Stegmann, J., Friedrich-Miescher-Laboratorium der Max-Planck-Gesellschaft, Spemannstraße 37–39, 7400 Tübingen 1, West-Germany

Stehelin, D., Institut Pasteur de Lille, 15 rue Camille Guérin, B. P. 3415, 59019 Lille, France

Storb, R., Division of Oncology, Providence Hospital, 500 17th Avenue, Seattle, WA 98122, USA

Stoye, J., Friedrich-Miescher-Institut, Grenzacherstraße 487, 4002 Basel, Switzerland

Stuhlmann, Heidi, Heinrich-Pette-Institut für Experimentelle Virologie und Immunologie an der Universität Hamburg, Martinistraße 52, 2000 Hamburg 20, West-Germany

Teich, Natalie M., Imperial Cancer Research Fund Laboratories, Lincoln's Inn Fields, London WC2A 3PX, U.K.

Teodorescu, M., Dept. Microbiology, Medical Center, University of Illinois, Chicago, IL 60612, USA

Thiel, J., Medical Center, Dept. Surgery, Duke University, Durham, NC 27710, USA

Torelli, U., Instituto di Patologia Speciale Medica e Metodologia Clinica, Via del Pozzo, 71, 41100 Modena, Italy

Van de Woude, G., National Institutes of Health, 9000 Rockville Pike, Bethesda, MD 20014, USA

Vogt, P. K., Dept. Microbiology, USC Medical Center, 2025 Zonal Avenue, Los Angeles, CA 90034, USA

Wernet, P., Medizinische Klinik, Abteilung Innere Medizin, Otfried-Müller-Straße, 7400 Tübingen, West-Germany

Wielckens, K., Physiologisch-Chemisches Institut, Martinistraße 52, 2000 Hamburg 20, West-Germany

Wekerle, H., Max-Planck-Institut für Immunbiologie, Stübeweg 51, 7800 Freiburg-Zähringen, West-Germany

Witz, I. P., Faculty of Life Science, Dept. Microbiology, Tel-Aviv University, Tel Aviv, Israel

Wolf, H., Max v. Pettenkofer-Institut, Pettenkoferstraße 9a, 8000 München 2, West-Germany

Yohn, D. S., OSU Comprehensive Cancer Center, McCampbell Hall, Columbus, OH 4310, USA

Zeuthen, J., Institute for Human Genetics, Bartholin Byggningen, Aarhus University, 8000 Aarhus C, Denmark

Zintl, F., Universitäts-Kinderklinik, Kochstraße 2, 69 Jena, GDR

Wilsede Scholarship Holders
(Granted by the Deutsche Krebshilfe
and the Leukemia Society of America)

Andreesen, Reinhard, Medizinische Univ.-Klinik, Hugstetter Straße 55, D-7800 Freiburg

Barnekow, Angelika, Institut für Virologie der Justus-Liebig Universität Gießen, Fachbereich Humanmedizin, Frankfurter Straße 107, D-6300 Gießen

Bergholz, Carolyn, Dept. Microbiology, Medical Sciences Building, University of Illinois, Urbana, IL 61801, USA

Berhold, Rosemarie, Univ.-Kinderpoliklinik Gießen, Feulgenstraße 12, D-6300 Gießen

Breu, Herbert, Kinderklinik der Westfälischen Wilhelms-Universität, Abteilung für Hämatologie und Onkologie, Robert-Koch-Str. 31, D-4400 Münster

Broxmeyer, Hal. E., Memorial Sloan-Kettering Cancer Center, 1275 York Avenue, New York, NY 10021, USA

Carbonell, Felix, Abt. für klinische Physiologie, Universität Ulm, Oberer Eselsberg, D-7900 Ulm

Dölken, Gottfried, Klinikum der Albert-Ludwigs-Universität, Med. Univ.-Klinik, Hugstetter Straße 55, D-7800 Freiburg

Dube, Shyam, Dept. Epidemiology, Yale University, 60 College Street, New Haven, CT 06510, USA

Freudenstein, Christa, Deutsches Krebsforschungszentrum – Institut für Virusforschung, Im Neuenheimer Feld 280, D-6900 Heidelberg

Gaedicke, Gerhard, Zentrum für Kinderheilkunde, Abt. Hämatologie II, Prittwitzstr. 43, D-7900 Ulm

Hagner, Gerhard, Freie Universität Berlin, Universitätsklinikum Charlottenburg, Abt. Innere Medizin m.S. Hämatologie und Onkologie, Spandauer Damm 130, D-1000 Berlin 19

Harbers, Klaus, Heinrich-Pette-Institut für Experimentelle Viorologie und Immunologie an der Universität Hamburg, Martinistr. 52, D-2000 Hamburg 20

Hardy, William Jr., Memorial Sloan-Kettering Cancer Center, Laboratory of Veterinary Oncology, 1275 York Avenue, New York, NY 10021, USA

Henze, Günter, Universitätskinderklinik, Heubnerweg 6, D-1000 Berlin 19

Heilbronn, Regine, Stadtstraße 4, D-7800 Freiburg

Issels, Rudolf, Ludwig-Maximilians-Universität München, Klinikum Großhadern, Med. Klinik III, Marchionistr. 15, D-8000 München 70

Janka, Gritta, Abt. f. Hämatologie und Onkologie, Kinderklinik der Universität München im Dr. von Haunerschen, Kinderspital, Lindwurmstr. 4, D-8000 München

Koeppen, Klaus-Michael, Krankenhaus Neukölln, II. Innere Abteilung, Rudower Str. 56, D-1000 Berlin 47

Konze-Thomas, Beate, Max v. Pettenkofer-Institut für Hygiene und Med. Mikrobiologie der Ludwig-Maximilians-Universität, Pettenkoferstr. 9a, D-8000 München 2

Meier, Claus Richard, Gesellschaft für Strahlen- und Umweltforschung mbH, Landwehrstr. 61, D-8000 München

Meyer, Peter, Eberhard-Karls-Universität, Abt. Innere Med. II, Otfried-Müller-Str. 25, D-7400 Tübingen

Müller, Stephan, Universitätskinderklinik, Heubnerweg 6, D-1000 Berlin 19

Nerl, Christoph, Straßberger Str. 20, D-8000 München 40

Ritter, Jörg, Universitäts-Kinderklinik, Abt. für Hämatologie und Onkologie und der Poliklinik, Robert-Koch-Str. 31, D-4400 Münster

Schmitz, N., Zentrum für Innere Medizin am Klinikum der Justus-Liebig-Universität, D-6300 Gießen

Seelis, Rudolfo E. A., Abt. Innere Medizin II der Med. Fakultät an der Rhein-Westf.-Techn. Hochschule Aachen, Goethestr. 27–29, D-5100 Aachen

Siegert, Wolfgang, Med. Klinik III, Klinikum Großhadern, Marchionistr. 15, D-8000 München

Snyder, Harry, Memorial Sloan-Kettering Cancer Center, 1275 York Avenue, New York, NY 10021, USA

Stünkel, Klaus, Gesellschaft für Strahlen- und Umweltforschung mbH, Landwehrstr. 61, D-8000 München

Wernicke, Dorothee, Friedrich-Miescher-Laboratorium der Max-Planck-Gesellschaft, Spemannstr. 37–39, D-7400 Tübingen

Weh, Hans-Josef, Akazienstr. 13, D-6501 Klein-Winternheim

Ziegler, Andreas, Med. Klinik, Innere Abteilung, Eberhard-Karls-Universität, Otfried-Müller-Str., D-7400 Tübingen

Preface

Gut ist eine Lehrart, wo man vom Bekannten zum Unbekannten fortschreitet; schön ist sie, wenn sie sokratisch ist, d.i. wenn sie dieselben Wahrheiten aus dem Kopf und Herzen des Zuhörers herausfragt. Bei der ersten werden dem Verstand seine Überzeugungen in Form abgefordert, bei der zweiten sie ihm abgelockt.

> Professor Friederich Schiller Jena, in a letter written on 23 February 1793 to his friend and supporter Körner, father of the poet Theodor Körner.

Established clinicians and scientists as well as students again tried the Wilsede experiment for three days and nights and learned from each other. In our fourth Wilsede meeting on "Modern Trends in Human Leukemia" we concentrated once again on questions regarding the practical application of research and its benefits to the patient.

The main emphasis of leukemia research has changed since the first Wilsede meeting in 1973. Virology is no longer the sole interest. Advances in immunology and cell genetics and a better understanding of

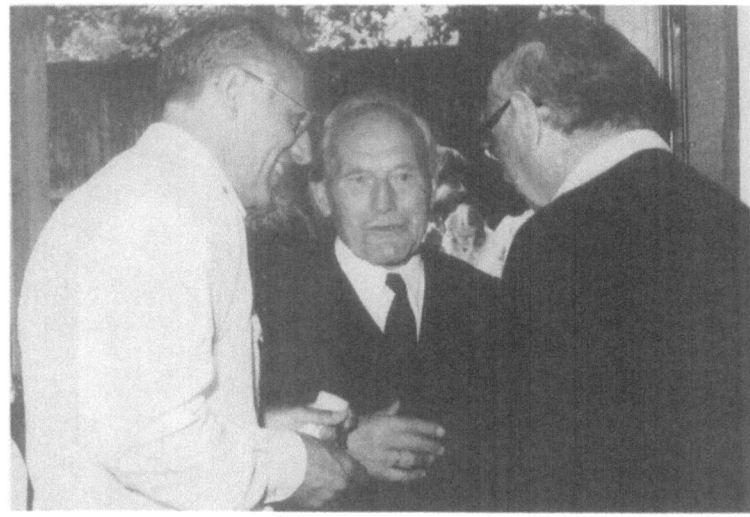

Dr. h. c. Alfred Toepfer speaking with participants of the meeting in Wilsede

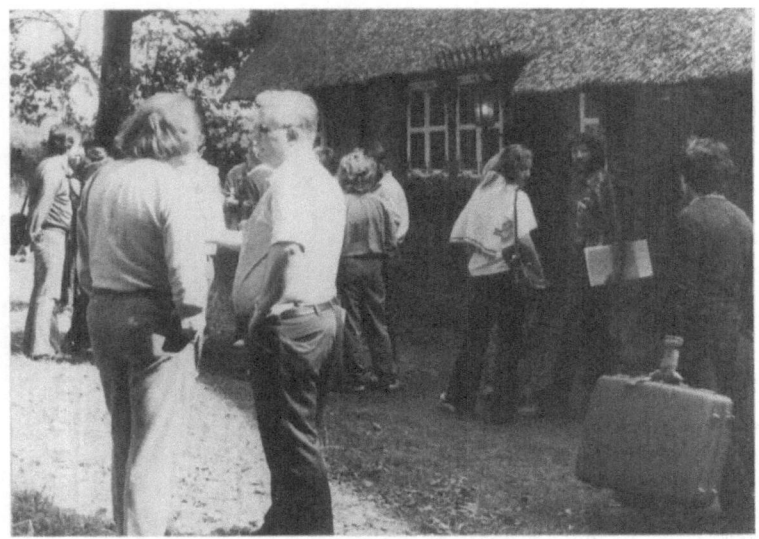

Arrival and discussion of participants in front of the meeting place "De Emmenhoff"

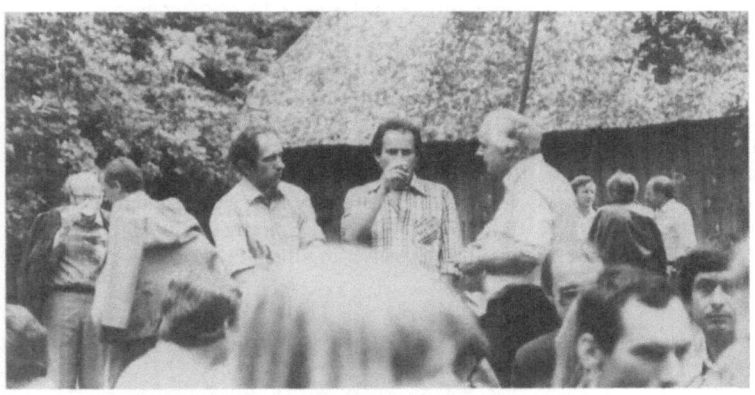

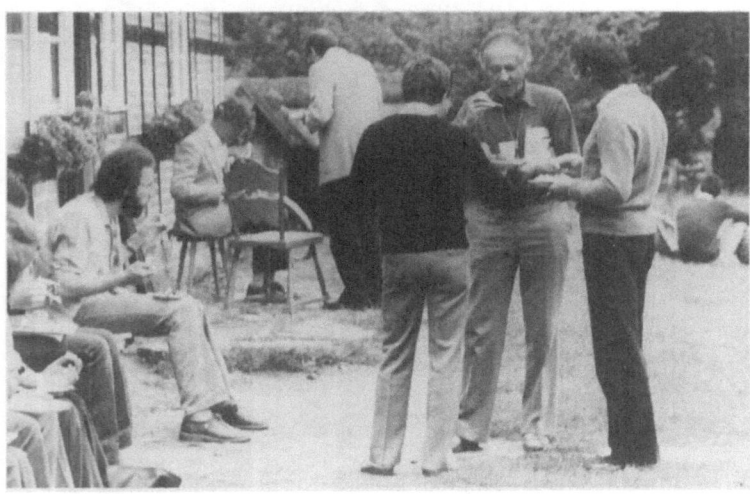

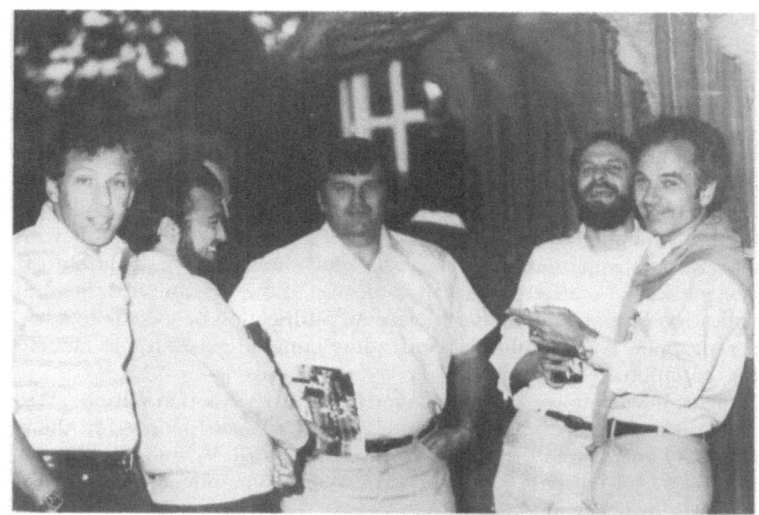

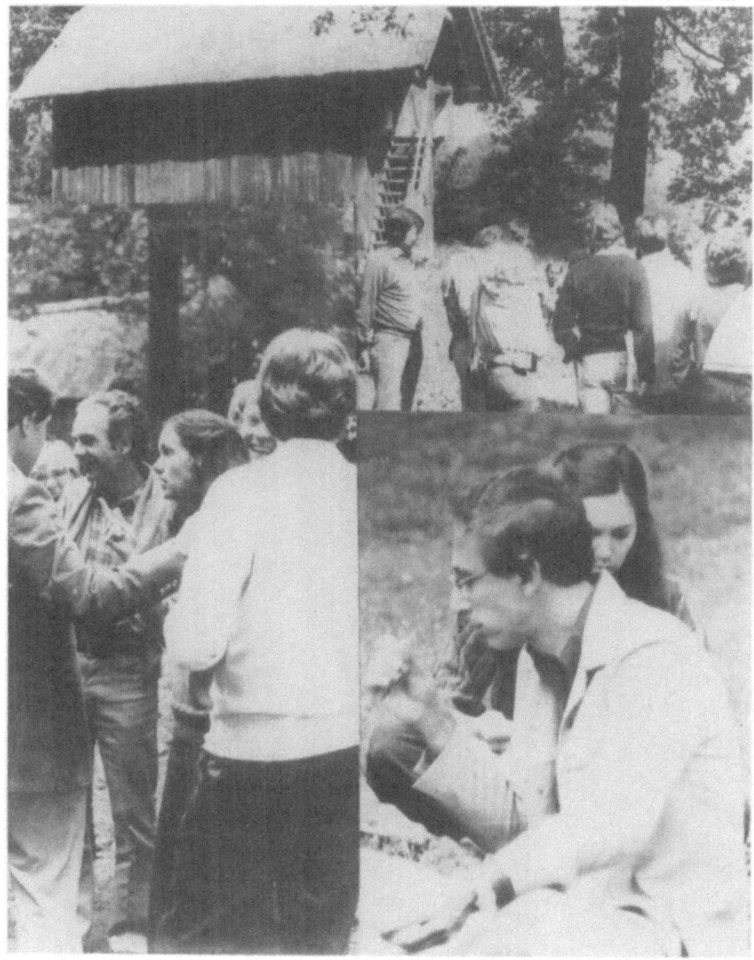

Personal and scientific discussion in Wilsede June 1980

Fotos: R. Völs

the mechanisms regulating normal and pathological blood cell differentiation have had a considerable impact on the direction of leukemia research.

I would like to thank all chairmen for their efforts in organizing a program which included most of the important results and also future aspects of human leukemia. We have learned at the Wilsede meeting that the individual fields of interest raise similar cell biological questions, the solution of which require increasing efforts for multidisciplinary collaboration. At the next Wilsede meeting in 1982 new insights certainly will have become apparent through additional knowledge in the field of cytogenetics of cancer cells and through new possibilities in the application of monoclonal antibodies and purification of specific regulatory proteins with inhibitory and stimulating effects on blood cell differentiation.

During the meeting we usually stayed in De Emmenhoff in Wilsede. We would like to express our gratitude to all Wilsede people for their hospitality and also to the Verein Naturschutzpark e.V., and last but not least to Dr. Alfred Toepfer and his associates for their idealistic efforts to preserve this peaceful place for us.

Hamburg, April 1981   Rolf Neth

Acknowledgement

We should like to thank all who made this workshop possible:

Deutsche Forschungsgemeinschaft*
Deutsche Krebshilfe
Deutsches Krebsforschungszentrum Heidelberg
Freie und Hansestadt Hamburg
Hamburger Landesverband für Krebsbekämpfung und Krebsforschung e.V.
Hamburgische Wissenschaftliche Stiftung
Internationale Union Against Cancer (UICC)**
Leukemia Society of America
Paul Martini Stiftung
Niedersächsisches Sozialministerium
Universität Hamburg (Hertha-Grober-Stiftung)

For generous hospitality we thank the Stiftung F. V. S. zu Hamburg, the Amerikahaus in Hamburg, the Freie and Hansestadt Hamburg, the Hamburger Staatsoper and the HADAG Seetouristik und Fährdienst AG

---

* Contract No. 4851/10/79
** National Cancer Institute, National Institutes of Health, Contract No. N01-CO-65341

**Frederick Stohlman Jr.
Memorial Lecture**

Wilsede, June 21 1978

Memorial Tribute to Dr. Frederick Stohlman
Presented by William C. Moloney

Gallo, Robert C.: Cellular and Virological
Studies Directed to the Pathogenesis of the
Human Myelogenous Leukemias

Pinkel, Donald: Treatment of Childhood
Acute Lymphocytic Leukemia

Wilsede, June 18 1980

Klein, George: The Relative Role of Viral
Transformation and Specific Cytogenetic
Changes in the Development of Murine and
Human Lymphomas

Kaplan, Henry S.: On the Biology and Immunology of Hodgkin's Disease

Haematology and Blood Transfusion Vol. 26
Modern Trends in Human Leukemia IV
Edited by Neth, Gallo, Graf, Mannweiler, Winkler
© Springer-Verlag Berlin Heidelberg 1981

The Relative Role of Viral Transformation and Specific Cytogenetic Changes in the Development of Murine and Human Lymphomas

G. Klein

This talk will be limited to a consideration of lymphoma and leukemia development (or certain types) in mice and men where there is extensive evidence for the role of the specific genetic changes recognizable at the chromosomal level. To start with the conclusion, it is clear that lymphoma development can be initiated by a variety of agents. In all probability, the initiation process creates long-lived preneoplastic cells, which are frozen in their state of differentiation and capable of continued division. These cells constitute the raw material for the subsequent cytogenetic evolution that converges towards a common, distinctive pattern. The nature of this pattern as it appears in the overt lymphomas depends on the subclass of the target lymphocyte rather than on the initiating ("etiologic") agent.

A. Human Lymphomas

The most extensive evidence concerns Burkitt lymphoma (BL). About 97% of the BLs tested that arose in the high endemic regions of Africa were monoclonal proliferations of Epstein-Barr virus(EBV)-carrying cell clones of B lymphocyte origin (Klein 1975; Klein 1978; Zur Hausen et al. 1970). BL tumor cells in vivo and derived cell lines are similar in carrying multiple copies of the EBV genome and often carry around 30–40 per cell. Some of the EBV genome copies are integrated with the cellular DNA, while the majority are present as free plasmids (Kaschka-Dierich et al. 1976; Falk et al. 1977). BL cells show no detectable viral expression in vivo except the EBV-determined nuclear antigen, EBNA (Reedman and Klein 1973), which is a DNA-binding protein that is present in all cells carrying EBV DNA. Super-

ficially at least the properties of EBNA resemble those of the tumor (T) antigens induced by the oncogenic papovarivurses (Klein et al., to be published; Luka et al. 1978). In the majority of the cases, BL-derived cell lines arise by the growth in vitro of the same clone that is tumorigenic in vivo (Fialkow et al. 1971; Fialkow et al. 1973). These cell lines are also similar to the tumor in vivo with regard to EBNA expression. In addition, many lines (termed producers) also contain a small number of cells that switch on viral production; other lines are nonproducers (Nadkarni et al. 1969).

The EBV-carrying lymphoid cell lines with an essentially similar EBV DNA status and viral gene expression can also be derived from the peripheral blood (Diehl et al. 1968) or the lymph nodes (Nilsson et al. 1971) of normal seropositive donors; they are referred to as lymphoblastoid cell lines (LCLs). LCLs differ from BL lines in a number of phenotypic characteristics (Nilsson and Pontén 1975). On the basis of the limited information now available it has not been possible to attribute this to differences in the viral genome or the virus-cell relationship (for review see Adams and Lindah 1974). The cytogenetic differences between LCLs and BL lines discussed below suggest, on the other hand, that the differences may be determined by the cellular genome rather than by the viral genome.

There is firm evidence that EBV is a transforming virus in vitro (Gerber and Hoyer 1971; Henle et al. 1967; Miller 1971; Moss and Pope 1972) and induces lethal lymphoproliferative disease in certain nonhuman primates in vivo (Frank et al. 1976). In humans, primary infection of adolescents or young adults causes infectious mononucleosis, a self-limiting benign lymphoproliferative disease (for review see Henle and Henle 1972). During mononucleosis a relatively small number of EBV-carrying B blasts appear in the peripheral circulation; they disappear again during convalescence (Klein et al. 1976). They are probably reduced in number by the EBV-specific killer T cells that appear in parallel. The killer cells can lyse autologous and allogeneic EBV-carrying (but not EBV-negative) target cells without any apparent syngeneic restriction (Bakacs et al. 1978; Jondal et al. 1975; Svedmyr & Jondal 1975; Svedmyr et al. 1978). In fatal cases of mononucleosis the lymphoid tissues are usually infiltrated with EBNA-positive cells (Britton et al. 1978; Miller, personal communication). In some acute cases of infectious mononucleosis EBV DNA could be demonstrated in the bone marrow during the acute phase of the disease (Zur Hausen 1975). Infectious mononucleosis is thus accompanied by, and probably due to, an extensive but usually temporary proliferation of EBV-carrying cells. Moreover, it has been postulated that a number of chronic mononucleosis like conditions, which border on lymphoma and are often familiar and X-linked, are due to polyclonal proliferation of EBV-carrying cells which is not properly immunoregulated (Purtilo et al. 1978).

As already mentioned, experimental oncogenicity of EBV is restricted to a few New World monkey species (Frank et al. 1976). Large apes and Old World monkeys are resistant. This is understandable, because they carry EBV-related herpesviruses that induce cross-neutralizing antibodies. The EBV-like chimpanzee, baboon, and orangoutan viruses were studied in some detail (Falk et al. 1977; Gerberg et al. 1976; Ohno et al. 1977; Rabin et al. 1978). They can immortalize B lymphocytes. Their DNA sequences are partially homologous with EBV and their antigens are crossreactive but not identical.

New World monkeys tested carried no EBV-related virus and had no cross-neutralizing antibodies. Some of them have lymphotropic herpesviruses of their own (reviewed by Deinhardt et al. 1974), but these are quite different from the EBV family and will not be discussed here.

The nature of the EBV-induced malignant lymphoproliferative disease in susceptible New World monkeys (e.g., marmosets) has not been analyzed in detail. It is not yet clearly established whether it is due to the polyclonal growth of virally transformed cells like the rare fatal cases of human mononucleosis or is a monoclonal tumor like BL.

Parallel cytogenetic and nude mouse inoculation studies (Nilsson et al. 1977; Zech et al. 1976) have recently dispelled the earlier notion that all EBV-transformed human lines are tumorigenic irrespective of origin. Virally immortalized normal B lymphocytes remained purely diploid during several months of cultivation in vitro, failed to grow subcutaneously in nude mice, and had a low (1%–3%) cloning efficiency in agarose. After prolonged passage in vitro they became aneuploid as a rule and acquired the ability to grow in nude mice and in agarose. In contrast, BL biopsy cells and derived lines were aneuploid and tumorigenic from the beginning and had a high clonability in agarose. In immunologically privileged sites such as the nude mouse brain or the subcutaneous tissue of the newborn nude mouse, both diploid LCL and aneuploid BL lines could grow progressively, however (Giovanella et al. 1979). Growth in these immunologically privileged sites did not enable the diploid LCL to grow subsequently in the subcutaneous tissue of the adult nude mouse, however.

The chromosomal changes of the long-passaged LCLs showd no apparent specific features. In contrast, most BL cells contain the same highly specific marker. The marker was first identified as 14q+, with an extra band at the distal end of the long arm of one chromosome 14 (Manolov and Manolova 1972). 14q+ markers were subsequently described in a variety of other lymphoreticular noeplasias (Fleischman and Prigogina 1977; Fukuhuara and Rowley 1978; Mark et al. 1977; McCaw et al. 1977; Mitelman and Levan 1973; Yamada et al. 1977; Zech et al. 1976). Closer scrutiny revealed important differences between the 14q+ marker of BL and non-BL lymphomas. In BL the extra band is derived from chromosome 8 (Zech et al. 1976) and represents a reciprocl translocation between 8 and 14 with precisely identical breaking points in different cases (Manolova et al. 1979). In non-BL with a 14q+ marker the donor chromosome was variable; pieces could be derived from chromosomes 1, 4, 10, 11, 14, 15 or 18 in addition to 8 (reviewed by Fukuhara and Rowley 1978).

The BL-associated reciprocal 8;14 translocation is not limited to EBV-carrying African

BL. It was also found in EBV-negative American BL (McCaw et al. 1977; Zech et al. 1976) and in the rare B-cell form of acute lymphocytic leukemia (Mitelman et al. 1979) believed to represent the neoplastic growth of the same cell type as BL. This, together with the fact that EBV-transformed LCLs of non-BL origin do not carry the 8;14 translocation, suggests that EBV is not involved in causing the translocation.

We have suggested (Klein 1978) that African BL develops in at least three steps. The *first step* is the EBV-induced immortalization of some B lymphocytes upon primary infection. This does not differ from the seroconversion of normal EBV carriers, except perhaps in one respect. The prospective study in the high endemic West Nile district has suggested that pre-BL patients may carry a higher load of EBV-harboring cells than normal controls (de Thé et al. 1978). The *second step* is brought about by an environment-dependent factor, perhaps chronic holoendemic malaria (Burkitt 1969; O'Connor 1961), that would urge the latent EBV-carrying cells frozen at a particular stage of B-cell differentiation to chronic proliferation and could further facilitate this process by a relative immunosuppression. In a way this would resemble the promotion step in experimental two-phase carcinogenesis. By forcing the long-lived preneoplastic cells to repeated division, the environmental cofactor would provide the scenario for cytogenetic diversification. The *third and final step* would occur when the "right" reciprocal 8;14 translocation occurred; this would lead to the outgrowth of an autonomous monoclonal tumor.

The reciprocal translocation could arise by a purely random Darwinian process or by more specific mechanisms as suggested by Fukuhara and Rowley (1978). The ubiquity of EBV, the high virus load carried by the African populations at risk, and the large number of cell divisions that must occur in the chronically hyperplastic lymphoreticular system of the parasite-loaded children makes a purely random process perfectly conceivable, particularly when contrasted against the relative rarity of the disease even in the high endemic regions.

The majority of the sporadic cases in nonendemic areas (Andersson et al. 1976), which show no evidence of clustering, are constituted by EBV negative BLs. The identical 8;14 translocation suggests that their development

is triggered by the same final cytogenetic event, while the earlier initiating and promoting steps are probably quite different. Initiation may be due to another viral or nonviral agent or could reflect a spontaneous (mutation-like?) change.

The frequent involvement of chromosome 14 in the genesis of human neoplasia of largely, if not exclusively, B-cell origin suggests that some determinant(s) on this chromosome is (are) closely involved with the normal responsiveness of the B lymphocyte to growth-controlling mechanisms. It is interesting to note that chromosome 14 anomalies were found in a high frequency in ataxia teleangiectasia, a condition noted for a marekdly increased incidence of lymphoreticular neoplasia (McCaw et al. 1975). It must be noted, however, that the most frequent breakpoint in chromosomes of patients with ataxia telangiectasia is in band 14q12, whereas the BL-associated breakpoint is in band 14q32.

B. Murine T Cell Leukemia

Dofuko et al. (1975) reported that the cells involved in "spontaneous" T cell leukemias of the AKR mouse frequently contain 41 chromosomes insted of 40, with trisomy of chromosome 15 as the most common change. We found a similar predominance of trisomy 15 in T cell leukemias induced in C57BL mice by two different substrains of the radiation leukemia virus (Wiener et al. 1978a,b) and by the chemical carcinogen dimethylbenz(a)anthrancene (Wiener et al. 1978c). Trisomy 17 was the second most common anomaly, much less frequent than trisomy 15, and never found without the latter. Trisomy 15 was also identified as the main cytogenetic change in X-ray-induced mouse lymphomas (Chang et al. 1977). In contrast, lymphoreticular neoplasias of non-T cell origin, induced by the Rauscher, Friend, Graffi, and Duplan viruses, some B lymphomas of spontaneous origin, and a series of mineral oilinduced plasmacytomas showed no trisomy 15 (Wiener et al., unpublished data). The question whether they have other types of distinctive chromosomal changes has not yet been answered.

It is sometimes postulated that all murine T cell lymphomas are due to the activation of latent type C viruses. Careful examination of the pathogenesis of these lymphomas makes this most unlikely, however (for review see Haran-Ghera and Peled 1979). It is more likely that X-rays and chemical and viral carcinogens can all play the role of initiating agents that can create long-lived preleukemic cells. The development of overt leukemia depends on additional changes that occur during the prolonged latency of the preleukemic cells in their host. It is very likely that the duplication of certain gene(s), reflected by the trisomy 15, plays a key role in this process.

The trisomy of the spontaneous AKR leukemia is particularly remarkable in this context. The high leukemia incidence of this strains stems from prolonged inbreeding and selection for leukemia. As already mentioned in the first part of this article, AKR mice carry at least four different genetic systems that favor leukemia development by independent mechanims (for review see Lilly and Pincus 1973). In spite of this high genetic preneness for leukemia, the disease fails to appear until 6–8 months after birth. This long latency period, together with the appearance of trisomy 15 in overt leukemia, supports the notion that the leukemogenic virus is not self-sufficient in changing normal T lymphocytes to autonomous leukemia cells.

Is there a specific region on chromosome 15 that needs to be duplicated for the development of leukemia? We have also examined the karyotype of dimethylbenz(a)anthracene-induced T cell leukemias in CBAT6T6 mice (Wiener et al. 1978a,b). The T6 marker has arisen by a breakage of chromosome 15 not far from the centromere and translocation of the distal part of the long arm to chromosome 14. Six independently induced leukemias showed trisomy of the 14;15 translocation, while the small T6 marker was present in only two copies. This suggests the involvement of specific region(s) in leukemogenesis localized in the distal part of the long arm of chromosome 15. Additional translocations will be helpful in defining the region more precisely.

C. Is Trisomy a Cause or a Consequence of a Murine T-Cell Leukemia?

It is conceivable that trisomy 15 is merely a consequence of leukemogenesis. It could be imagined, for example, that it is only one among many different trisomies that can arise but that the others are incompatible with continued life and proliferation of the murine T-lymphocytes. We have recently excluded this possibility by inducing leukemias in mice that carry Robertsonian translocation (Spira et al., to be published). T-cell leukemias were induced by the chemical carcinogen DMBA and by Moloney virus, respectively, in mice carrying 1;15, 5;16, and 6;15 Rb translocations. In the resulting leukemias the entire translocation chromosome was present in three copies. This proves that trisomy of even the longest chromosome (No. 1) must be tolerated by the cell if it is fused with the crucially important chromosome 15. This strongly supports the idea that trisomy of chromosome No. 15 is essential for T-cell leukemogenesis.

Our most recent studies (Wiener et al., to be published) have focused on the induction of T-cell leukemias in F_1 hybrids derived from crosses between mouse strains with cytogenetically distinguishable 15-chromosomes. The CBAT6T6 strain that carries the characteristic 14;15 translocation was crossed with strains AKR, C57Bl, and C3H, all of which have cytogenetically normal 15-chromosomes. T-cell leukemias were induced in the resulting F_1 hybrids by DMBA and Moloney virus, respectively. Duplication of chromosome 15 was nonrandom, depending on the genetic content of the chromosome. In the crosses between T6T6 and AKR, the AKR-derived normal 15 chromosome was duplicated preferentially. Both the C57Bl×T6T6 and C3H×T6T6 F_1 hybrids showed the opposite behavior, with preferential duplication of the T6-derived 14;15 translocation chromosome. Since the chances for duplication must be approximately equal for the 15 chromosomes derived from one or the other parental strain, this must mean that the selective advantage of the two alternative 15-duplications must be unequal in the course of leukemia development. These findings suggest a certain "hierarchy" among what is probably an allelic series of genes located on chromosome 15. Apparently, the genes are unequal with regard to the selective advantage they convey on the preleukemic cell in relation to its transition to turning into overt leukemia.

D. Is Abelson Virus a Transducer or Cellular Gene?

In contrast to all other known mouse leukemia viruses, Abelson virus transforms (immortalizes) lymphocytes in vitro and induces leukemia after short latency periods in vivo. It has been shown (Klein 1975) that the viral genome contains a large cellular insert that occupies the most of the middle portion of the viral genome. It specifies a large polyprotein that is probably associated with the cell membrane and is endowed with protein kinase activity.

We have recently examined the karyotype of Abelsonvirus induced leukemias (Klein al. 1980) and found it to be purely diploid with no demonstrable anomalies by banding analysis. Moreover, the Abelson virus transformed lines remained diploid over long periods of time.

Is it conceivable that the change in gene dosage that is achieved by the duplication of a whole chromosome in leukemias that arise after long latency periods is directly achieved by the viral transduction of a corresponding piece of crucial genetic information? If this is correct, it would follow that directly transforming viruses that carry pieces of normal genetic information and induce tumors with short latency periods would tend to induce diploid tumors.

Clearly, changes in gene dosage, whether achieved by chromosome duplication or viral transduction, must play an important role in the emancipation of tumor cells from host control.

E. Some Conclusions

The following points can be made on the basis of these findings and related findings of others.

I. Transformation In Vitro Is Not Synonymous with Tumorigenicity In Vivo

This point has been made many times before, but it can hardly be overemphasized. To mention only a few examples, Dulbecco and Vogt (1960) showed in their pioneering studies that foci of cells transformed in vitro by polyoma virus were not necessarily tumorigenic; at least one additional step was required for growth in vivo. Stiles et al. (1975) reported that human lines transformed by simian virus 40 failed to grow in nude mice in contrast to the regular takes of culture lines derived from tumors in vivo. Diploid lymphoblastoid cell lines transformed in vitro by EBV are clearly "immortal" but nontumorigenic in nude mice as already mentioned (Nilsson et al. 1977).

Transformation in vitro may merely reflect a relative emancipation of the cell from its earlier dependence on exogenous mitogenic signals. Most and perhaps all normal cells have a limited lifespan in vitro. Lymphocytes will not grow, not even temporarily, unless supplied with appropriate mitogenic factors. Transformation in vitro abolishes this requirement. It also "freezes" differentiation at a given level.

It is noteworthy that transformed fibroblasts and lymphocytes show certain common changes associated with immortalization in spite of their very different phenotypes – namely, increased resistance to saturation density, decreased serum requirements, and altered lectiyn agglutination and capping patterns (Steinitz and Klein 1975; Steinitz and Klein 1977; Yefenof and Klein 1976; Yefenof et al. 1977).

Most DNA viruses that transform in vitro induce DNA synthesis and mitosis in their target cells (Einhorn and Ernberg 1978; Gerber and Hoyer 1971; Gershon et al. 1965; Martin et al. 1977; Robinson and Miller 1975). For the oncogenic papovavirus systems it has been shown that the virally determined T-antigen or one from of it plays a direct role in initiating host cell DNA synthesis (Martin et al. 1977).

If transformation in vitro reflects a "built-in" ability to grow in the absence of exogenous stimulation, tumorigenicity in vivo must imply in addition, resistance to negative feedback regulations of the host. The latter may be brought out by appropriate cytogenetic changes. Trisomy, as observed in the murine T cell leukemias, may tilt the balance of the long-lived preoplastic cells towards definite disobedience through gene dose effects. Reciprocal translocations that give rise to the Philadelphia chromosome and the 8;14 translocation associated with BL may also work through gene dosage – e.g., by position effects that stop the function of important regulatory genes when they are dislocated from their natural surroundings. Similar position effects may be responsible for the action of src, the extra genetic information carried by the transforming avian sarcoma viruses. Conceivably, this originally cell-derived information may become integrated, together with the rest of the proviral DNA, into new regions where it is no longer subject to the same control as in the original location (Stehelin et al. 1976; Varmus et al. 1976). In this connection, our recent finding on the Abelson virus induced leukemia system may be of interest. This virus, as the only one among the known murine leukemia viruses, transforms in vitro and induces leukemia after only a short latency period in vivo. It is a highly defective virus, with a large cellular insert in its middle (Rosenberg and Baltimore 1980). Sequences homologous with the cellular insert and proteins identical or immunologically cross reactive with its product are present in normal mouse cells.

We have recently examined a series of Abelson virus induced leukemias and found them to be purely diploid (Klein et al. 1980). It is intriguing to speculate that transformation is compatible with diploidy in this case, since the provirus-mediated integration of the cell-derived sequences may alter gene dosage in a way appropriate to generate leukemia.

The apparently tissue-specific involvement of different chromosomes in tumor-associated nonrandom karyotype changes suggests that genes that are of crucial importance for the responsiveness of different cell types to growth control are located on different chromosomes. Some determinant on human chromosome 14 thus appears to be involved with the normal responsiveness of the B lymphocyte; determinants on chromosome 22 or 9 (or both) appear to influence myeloid differentiation; the dosage of some determinant on murine chromosome 15 seems to influence the balance between the restrained proliferation of the preleukemic cell and overt leukemia.

II. Host Cell Controls Can Modify the Expression of Transformation In Vitro

The successful isolation of phenotypic revertants from both chemically and virally transformed cell lines demonstrates the importance of host cell controls for the expression of transformation-associated characteristics. Sachs and his group (Yamamoto et al. 1973) have shown that specific chromosomal changes must play an important role in transformation and reversion. As a rule transformation was accompanied by the duplication of some chromosomes. On reversion, the same chromosomes often decreased in number, whereas others increased (Benedict et al. 1975; Yamamoto et al. 1973). Sachs speaks about expressor and

suppressor elements and stresses the importance of their balance for the control of the normal vs the transformed phenotype. The temperature-sensitive host control mutants, isolated from virally transformed cell lines by Basilico (1977), are another important demonstration of cellular forces that can counteract the transforming function of an integrated viral genome.

III. Host Cell Controls Can Reverse Tumorigenic to Nontumorigenic Phenotypes

Tumorigenicity in vivo can be counteracted experimentally by two fundamentally different types of control, i.e., genetic and epigenetic. The former was demonstrated by somatic hybridization experiments. Fusion of tumorigenic cells with low or nontumorigenic normal or transformed partners has regularly led to a suppression of tumorigenicity as long as the hybrid has maintained a nearly complete karyotype (Harris 1971; Harris et al. 1969; Klein et al. 1971; Wiener et al. 1971). High tumorigenicity reappeared after the loss of specific chromosomes derived from the nontumorigenic partner (Jonasson et al. 1977; Wiener et al. 1971).

Suppression of tumorigenicity by normal cells was equally effective with tumors of viral, chemical, and spontaneous origin. Different types of normal cells were effective, including fibroblasts, lymphocytes, and macrophages. It is not known whether the normal karyotype compensates a deficiency of the malignant cell by genetic complementation or acts by imposing normal responsiveness to its own superimposed growth control. The latter possibility appears more likely. It could be explored by determining whether the reappearance of high tumorigenicity is linked to the loss of different chromosomes, depending on the type of normal cell used for the original suppressive hybridization.

A fundamentally different, nongenetic mechanism of malignancy suppression was discovered by Mintz, who demonstrated the normalization of diploid teratocarcinoma cells after their implantation into the early blastocyte (Mintz and Illmensee 1975). It is not yet clear whether this is a special case, dependent on the pluripotentiality of the teratocarcinoma cell and its normal karyotype, or is of more general significance. The well-documented abilities of certain tumor cells to respond to differentiation-inducing stimuli represent more limited examples of the same or similar phenomena (Azumi and Sachs 1977; Rossi and Friend 1967).

IV. Concept of Convergence in Tumor Evolution

This concept is not new. In essence, it corresponds to one of the rules of tumor progression as formulated by Foulds (1958). He stated that the "multiple reassortment of unit characteristics" that formed the basis of the progression concept "could follow one of several alternative pathways of development." Some aspects of this process were stated here in a more specific way. They are as follows:

1. Like chemical or physical carcinogens, *viruses* play essentially the role of *initiators* in tumor progression. Their major effect is the establishment of *long-lived* preneo*plastic* cells.

2. *Specific genetic changes* are responsible for the transition of preneoplastic to frankly malignant cells. In some systems they are expressed as cytogenetically detectable chromosomal anomalies which are characteristic for the majority of the tumors that originate from the same target cell. The changes may arise by random mechanisms. They are selectively fixed due to the increased growth advantage of the clone that carries them. This advantage is based on a decreased responsiveness to growth-controlling or differentiation-inducing host singals. This selection process, rather than any specific induction mechanism, is responsible for the "cytogenetic convergence" of preneoplastic cell lineages initiated ("caused") by widely diverse agents towards the same nonrandom chromosomal change.

3. The cytogenetic changes act by shifting the balance between genes that favor progressive growth in vivo and genes that counteract it. Changes in effective gene dosage are brought about by nonrandom duplication of a whole chromosome, as in trisomy, or by reciprocal translocation that may effect gene expression on the donor or the recipient chromosome.

Acknowledgements

This work was supported by Grant Nr. 2 R01 CA 14054-06 awarded by the National Cancer Institute, U.S. Department of Health, Education, and Welfare.

References

Adams A, Lindahl T (1974) In: De Thé G, Epstein MA, zur Hausen H (eds) Oncogenesis and Herpesviruses. II. Proceedings of a Symposium, Nuremberg, West Germany, part I. International Agency for Research on Cancer, Lyon, pp 125–132 – Andersson M, Klein G, Ziegler JL, Henle W (1976) Nature 260:357–359 – Azumi J-I, Sachs L (1977) Proc Natl Acad Sci USA 74:253–257 – Bakacs T, Svedmyr E, Klein E, Rombo L, Weiland D (1978) Cancer Lett 4:185–189 – Basilico C (1977) Adv Cancer Res 24:223–266 – Benedict WF, Rucker N, Mark C, Kouri RE (1975) J Natl Cancer Inst 54:157–162 – Britton S, Andersson-Anvret M, Gergely P, Henle W, Jondal M, Klein G, Sandstedt B, Svedmyr E (1978) N Engl J Med 298:89–92 – Burkitt DP (1969) J Natl Cancer Inst 42:19–28 – Chang TD, Biedler JL, Stocker E, Old LJ (1977) Proc Am Assoc Cancer Res 18:225 – Deinhardt FW, Falk LA, Wolfe LG (1974) Adv Cancer Res 19:167–205 – Diehl V, Henle G, Henle W, Kohn G (1968) J Virol 2:663–666 – Dofuko R, Biedler JL, Spengler BA, Old LJ (1975) Proc Natl Acad Sci USA 72:1515–1517 – Dulbecco R, Vogt M (1960) Proc Natl Acad Sci USA 46:1617–1623 – Einhorn L, Ernberg I (1977) Int J Cancer 21:157–160 – Falk L, Henle G, Henle W, Deinhardt F, Schudel A (1977) Int J Cancer 20:219–226 – Fialkow PJ, Klein G, Giblett ER, Gothoskar B, Clifford P (1971) Lancet i: 883–886 – Fialkow PJ, Klein E, Klein G, Clifford P, Singh S (1973) J Exp Med 138:89–102 – Fleischman EW, Prigogina EL (1977) Hum Genet 35:269–279 – Foulds I (1958) J Chronic Dis 8:2–37 – Frank A, Andeman WA, Miller G (1976) Adv Cancer Res 23:171–201 – Fukuhara S, and Rowley JD (1978) Int J Cancer 22:14–21 – Gerber P, Hoyer BH (1971) Nature 231:46–47 – Gerber P, Pritchett RF, Kieff ED (1976) J Virol 19:1090–1093 – Gershon D, Hausen P, Sachs L, Winocour E (1965) Proc Natl Acad Sci USA 54:1584–1592 – Giovanella B, Nilsson K, Zech L, Yim O, Klein G, – Stehlin JS (1979) Int J Cancer 24:103–113 – Haran-Ghera N, Peled A (1979) Adv Cancer Res 30:45–88 – Harris H (1971) Proc R Soc Lond [Biol] 179:1–20 – Harris H, Miller OJ, Klein G, Worst P, Tachibana T (1969) Nature 223:363–368 – Henle W, Diehl V̇, Kohn G, zur Hausen H, Henle Ġ (1967) Science 157:1064–1065 – Henle W, Henle G (1972) In: Biggs PM, De Thé G, Payne LN (eds) Oncogenesis and herpesviruses. International Agency for Research on Cancer, Lyon, pp 269–274 – Jonasson J, Povey S, Harris H (1977) J Cell Sci 24:217–254 – Jondal M, Svedmyr E, Klein E, Singh S (1975) Nature 255:405–47 – Kaschka-Dierich C, Adams A, Lindahl T, Bornkamm GW, Bjursell G, Giovanella B, Singh S (1976) Nature 260:302–306 – Klein G (1975) Cold Spring Harbor Symp Quant Biol 39:783–790 – Klein G (1978) In: Kurstak E, Maramorosch K (eds) Viruses and environment. Academic Press, New York, pp 1–12 – Klein G,

Bregula U, Wiener F, Harris H (1971) J Cell Sci 8:659–672 – Klein G, Svedmyr E, Jondal M, Persson PO (1976) Int J Cancer 17:21–26 – Klein G, Ohno S, Rosenberg N, Wiener F, Spira J, Baltimore D (1980) Int J. Cancer 25:805–811 – Klein G, Luka J, Zeuthen J (to be published) Cold Spring Harbor Symp Quant Biol – Lilly F, Pincus T (1973) Adv Cancer Res 17:231–277 – Luka J, Lindahl T, Klein G (1978) J Virol 27:604–611 – Manolov G, Monolova Y (1972) Nature 237:33–34 – Manolova Y, Manolov G, Kieler J, Levan A, Klein G (1979) Hereditas 90:5–10 – Mark J, Ekedahl C, Hagman A (1977) Hum Genet 36:277–282 – Martin RG, Persico-Dilauro M, Edwards CAF, Oppenheim A (1977) In: Schultz, J, Brada Z (eds) Genetic manipulation as it affects the cancer problem. Academic, New York, pp 87–102 – McCaw BK, Kaiser B, Hecht F, Harnden DG, Teplitz RL (1975) Proc Natl Acad Sci USA 72:2071–2075 – McCaw BK, Epstein AL, Kaplan HS, Hecht F (1977) Int J Cancer 19:482–486 – Miller G (1971) Yale J Biol Med 43:358–361 – Mintz B, Illmensee K (1975) Proc Natl Acad Sci USA 72:3585–3589 – Mitelman F, Levan G (1973) Hereditas 89:207–232 – Mitelman F, Andersson-Anvret M, Brandt L, Catovsky D, Klein G, Manolov G, Manolova Y, Mark-Vendel E, Nilsson PG (1979) Int J Cancer 24:27–33 – Moss DJ, Pope JH (1972) J Gen Virol 17:233–236 – Nadkarni JS, Nadkarni JJ, Clifford P, Manolov G, Fenyö EM, Klein E (1969) Cancer 23:64–79 – Nilsson K, Pontén J (1975) Int J Cancer 15:321–341 – Nilsson K, Klein G, Henle W, Henle G (1971) Int J Cancer 8:443–450 – Nilsson K, Giovanella BC, Stehlin JS, Klein G (1977) Int J Cancer 19:337–344 – O'Connor GT (1961) Cancer 14:270–283 – Ohno S, Luka J, Falk L, Klein G (1977) Int J Cancer 20:941–946 – Purtilo DT, Bhawan J, Hutt LM, De Nicola L, Szymanski I, Yang JPS, Boto W, Maier R, Thorley-Lawson D (1978) Lancet 15:798–801 – Rabin H, Neubauer RH, Hopkins RF III, Nonoyma M (1978) Int J Cancer 21:762–767 – Reedman BM, Klein G (1973) Int J Cancer 11:499–520 – Robinson J, Miller G (1975) J Virol 15:1065–1072 – Rosenberg N, Baltimore D (1980) Isolation of Abelson murine leukemia virus. In: Klein G (ed) Viral oncology. Raven, New York, pp 187–203 – Rossi GB, Friend C (1976) Proc Natl Acad Sci USA 58:1373–1380 – Spira J, Wiener F, Ohno S, Klein G (to be published) Proc Natl Acad Sci USA – Stehelin D, Varmus HE, Bishop JM, Vogt PK (1976) Nature 260:170–173 – Steinitz M, Klein G (1975) Proc Natl Acad Sci USA 72:3518–3520 – Steinitz M, Klein G (1977) Eur J Cancer 13:1269–1275 – Stiles GD, Desmond W Jr, Sato G, Saier MH (1975) Proc Natl Acad Sci USA 72:4971–4975 – Svedmyr E, Jondal M Proc Natl Acad Sci USA 72:1622–1626 – Svedmyr E, Jondal M, Henle W, Weiland O, Rombo L, Klein G (1978) Clin Lab Immunol 1:225–232 – de Thé G, Geser A, Day NE, Tukei PN, Williams EH, Beri DP, Smith PG, Dean AG, Bornkamm GW, Feorino P, Henle W (1978) Nature 274:756–761 – Varmus HE, Stehelin DS, Spector D, Tal J, Fjuita D, Padgett T, Roulland-Dussoix D, Kung HJ, Bishop JM (1976): Baltimore D, Huang AS, Fox CF (eds) Animal virology. Academic, New York, pp 339–358 – Wiener F, Klein G, Harris H (1971) J Cell Sci 8:681–692 – W ener F, Ohno S, Spira J, Haran-Ghera N, Klein G (1978a) J Natl Cancer Inst 61:227–238 – Wiener F, Ohno S, Spira J, Haran-Ghera N, Klein G (1978b) Nature 275:658–660 – Wiener F, Spira J, Ohno S, Haran-Ghera N, Klein G (1978c) Int J Cancer 22:447–453 – Wiener F, Spira J, Babonits M, Haran-Ghera N, Klein G (to be published) – Yamada K, Yoshioka M, Oami H (1977) J Natl Cancer Inst 59:1193–1195 – Yamamoto T, Hayashi M, Rabinowitz Z, Sachs L (1973) Int J Cancer 11:555–566 – Yefenof E, Klein G (1976) Exp Cell Res 99:175–178 – Yefenof E, Klein G, Ben-Bassat H, Lundin L (1977) Exp Cell Res 108:185–190 – Zech L, Haglund U, Nilsson K, Klein G (1976) Int J Cancer 17:47–56 – Zur Hausen H (1975) Biochim Biophys Acta 417:25–53 – Zur Hausen H, Schulte-Holthausen H, Klein G, Henle W, Henle G, Clifford P, Santesson L (1970) Nature 228:1056–1068

10

Haematology and Blood Transfusion Vol. 26
Modern Trends in Human Leukemia IV
Edited by Neth, Gallo, Graf, Mannweiler, Winkler
© Springer-Verlag Berlin Heidelberg 1981

On The Biology and Immunology of Hodgkin's Disease*

H. S. Kaplan

A. Neoplastic Nature of Hodgkin's Disease

The nature of Hodgkin's disease has been the subject of more than 100 years of intense debate. The occurrence of massive lymphadenopathy, with later spread to the lungs, liver, bone marrow, and other tissues, and the inevitably fatal course of the disease suggested to many scholars that it was a form of malignant neoplasm. Others, however, impressed with its frequently febrile course, with the occasional waxing and waning in size of enlarged lymph nodes, and with the frequent coexistence of tuberculosis or other infectious diseases at autopsy, considered it some form of granulomatous infection or inflammation. Finally, as awareness has grown concerning the curious defect of immune responsiveness which occurs so often in Hodgkin's disease, a third hypothesis has been put forward suggesting that it may stem from a chronic immunologic disorder. Certain similarities to the histologic features seen in immunologic reactions of the graft-vs-host type led Kaplan and Smithers (1959) to suggest that Hodgkin's disease might represent an autoimmune process involving an interaction between neoplastic and normal lymphoid cells, a hypothesis later extended and developed by others (De Vita 1973; Green et al. 1960; Order and

Hellman 1972). Definitive evidence that Hodgkin's disease is indeed a malignant neoplasm, albeit a remarkably atypical one, finally emerged during the last two decades from cytogenetic and cell culture studies which demonstrated that the giant cells of Hodgkin's disease satisfy two of the most fundamental attributes of neoplasia: aneuploidy and clonal derivation.

B. Origin and Characteristics of the Giant Cell Population

It was once considered that the giant binucleate or multinucleate Reed-Sternberg cells most closely resembled and were therefore probably derived from the histiocyte (Rappaport 1966). However, histochemical studies (Dorfman 1961) failed to reveal the presence of nonspecific esterase, an enzyme characteristically present in cells of the monocyte-histiocyte-macrophage series. Meanwhile, growing awareness of the remarkable changes in size and morphology which small lymphocytes may undergo during the process of lymphoblastoid transformation in response to lectins and specific antigens led to the hypothesis that the Reed-Sternberg cell might be an unusual form of transformed lymphocyte (Dorfman et al. 1973; Taylor 1976).

There has also been disagreement as to whether Reed-Sternberg cells are capable of DNA synthesis and mitosis. Although giant mitotic figures have been observed by some investigators, cells arrested in mitosis by treatment with vinblastine appeared to be limited to the mononuclear cell population in other studies (Marmont and Damasio 1967). After short-term incubation of cell suspensions of

* Clinical investigations at Stanford University Medical Center described in this article were supported by research grant CA-05838 from the National Cancer Institute, National Institutes of Health, U.S. Department of Health, Education, and Welfare. The collaborative assistance of a multidisciplinary team of colleagues is gratefully acknowledged

fresh lymph node biopsies from ten patients with Hodgkin's disease, autoradiographic evidence of incorporation of tritiated thymidine into DNA was seen only in mononuclear cells (Peckham and Cooper 1969), suggesting that the mononuclear Hodgkin's cells are the actively proliferating neoplastic cells and that the Reed-Sternberg cells are nonproliferating, end-stage, degenerative forms. Later studies, however, were more successful in revealing labeling in Reed-Sternberg cells, as were cell culture studies by Kadin and Asbury (1973) and by Kaplan and Gartner (1977). In the last-cited report, it was observed that 17 (20.7%) of 82 binucleate or multinucleate giant cells were labeled (Fig. 1), a proportion only moderately less than that observed among the mononuclear cell population (334 of 918, or 36.5%). Moreover, binucleate mitotic figures could be seen in some cells of the same culture. Accordingly, it is now clear that Reed-Sternberg cells are indeed capable of DNA synthesis and mitotic division and may thus be considered, together with their mononuclear counterparts, to be the neoplastic cells of Hodgkin's disease.

Chromosome studies have been carried out by the direct method or following short-term incubation of tissues involved by Hodgkin's disease in at least 100 cases from 1962 through

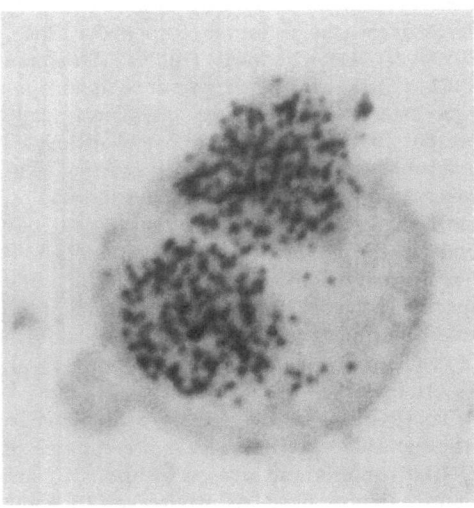

Fig. 1. Autoradiograph of cells from a long-term culture of involved spleen tissue from a patient with Hodgkin's disease. Both nuclei of a binucleate Reed-Sternberg cell are labeled with tritiated thymidine

1978 (for review, cf. Kaplan 1980). In addition to cells having a modal chromosome number of 46, believed to represent normal lymphoid cells, another cell population with pseudodiploid or aneuploid chromosome numbers, often in the hypotetraploid range, was detected in 68 cases. For example, Whitelaw (1969) observed near-tetraploids in 31 (16%) of 193 scorable mitoses from four cases of Hodgkin's disease. Aneuploid cells have been detected not only in the more aggressive histopathologic forms but in the paragranuloma or lymphocyte predominance types as well, confirming that even these indolent forms are neoplastic in nature. Marker chromosomes have been observed in 40 of 100 cases, although no single characteristic abnormality has been consistently encountered.

Perhaps the most compelling evidence of the neoplastic character of Hodgkin's disease stems from observations indicating the clonal derivation of these aneuploid cells. One of the most remarkable clones of aneuploid Hodgkin's cells encountered to date is that described by Seif and Spriggs (1967). Of 63 cells 18 had chromosome numbers between 77 and 86. There were two unusually long marker chromosomes (M_1 and M_2); both were present in ten cells, and M_2 alone in an eleventh cell. Clonal distributions of marker chromosomes have been documented in at least half of the 40 instances in which marker chromosomes have been detected to date (cf. Kaplan 1980).

Controversy concerning the cell of origin of the Reed-Sternberg cell has not been resolved by electron micrographic or cytochemical studies. Some investigators (Dorfman et al. 1973) have been impressed by the resemblance of the nuclei of mononuclear and hyperlobated Hodgkin's cells to those of transformed lymphocytes. However, Carr (1975) placed greater emphasis on the presence of elaborate cytoplasmic processes, actin-like cytoplasmic microfibrils, and small lysosomes, some closely resembling those present in macrophages, and concluded that "the ultrastructure of the malignant reticulum cell is such as to make it likely that it is of macrophage lineage". Several investigators have found nonspecific esterase activity to be absent or only very weakly positive in the giant cells of Hodgkin's disease, whereas others have described distinct granular activity in such cells. Using fluoresceinated antisera to human immunoglobins, some investigators have detected surface and/or cytoplasmic IgG in a varying proportion of Hodgkin's giant cells. Immunohistochemical staining procedures have revealed both lambda and kappa light chains in the cytoplasm of many of these cells (Garvin et al. 1974; Taylor 1976). Since an individual B-lymphocyte is not capable of synthesizing both types of light chains (Gearhart et al. 1975), the presence of both lambda and kappa suggests that cytoplasmic immunoglobulin was not endogenously synthesized by these cells.

Long-term cultures of the giant cells of Hodgkin's disease were studied by Kadin and Asbury (1973) and by Kaplan and Gartner (1977). Permanent cell lines derived from tissues or pleural effusions involved by Hodgkin's disease have been successfully established by several groups (Gallmeier et al. 1977; Long et al. 1977; Roberts et al. 1978; Schaadt et al. 1979; H. S. Kaplan et al., unpublished

work). However, all such efforts confront the dilemma that no definitive criteria exist for the unambiguous identification of Reed-Sternberg cells in vitro. Kaplan and Gartner (1977) observed that the giant cells from involved spleens grew in culture as round or oval adherent cells with diameters ranging from 20 to more than 75 μ, often exhibiting a strong tendency to adhere not only to the surface of the culture vessel but also to each other, leading to the formation of irregular clusters (Fig. 2). When fixed and stained, cells from such cultures exhibited morphologic features entirely consistent with those of Hodgkin's or Reed-Sternberg cells; most were mononuclear, but from 10 to 20% were binucleate, and 1%–2% contained three or more nuclei. In one such culture established from the spleen of a patient with Hodgkin's disease, analysis of 70 countable mitotic figures revealed that all were

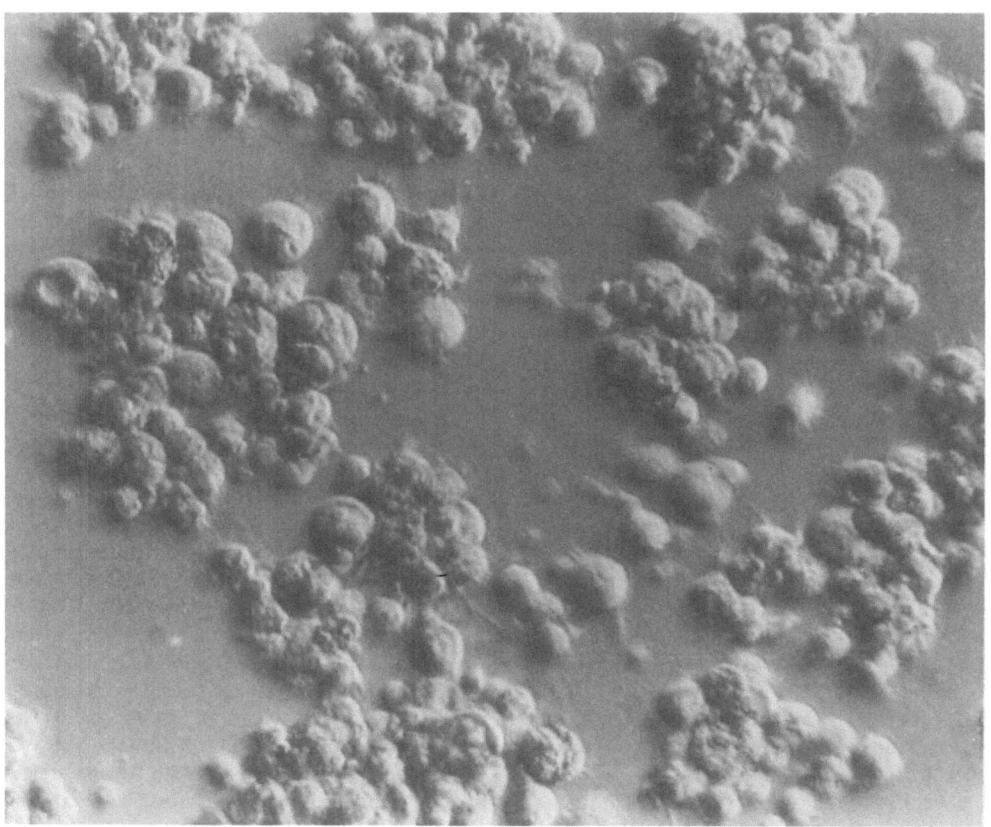

Fig. 2. Long-term culture of cells from the involved spleen of a patient with Hodgkin's disease. Note the clusters of adherent giant cells. The huge size of these cells may be appreciated by comparison with that of the occasional lymphocytes still persisting

13

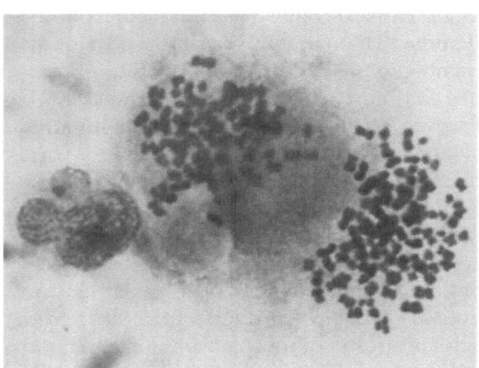

Fig. 3. Binucleate mitosis in an obviously aneuploid giant cell from the involved spleen of a patient with Hodgkin's disease after several weeks in culture

aneuploid; of these 63 were hyperdiploid with a mode of 53 chromosomes, 6 were hypotetraploid with chromosome numbers of approximately 77–91, and one was hyperoctoploid with over 190 chromosomes (Fig. 3).

These cells satisfied another criterion of neoplasia, heterotransplantability, after intracerebral inoculation into congenitally athymic nude mice. The giant cells possessed both Fc and complement receptors as revealed by their capacity for the formation of IgG-EA and IgM-EAC$_{3b}$ rosettes, respectively. In contrast, they lacked T- and B-lymphocyte markers: they failed to form E rosettes and revealed no evidence of surface membrane immunoglobulin. The cultured giant cells exhibited sluggish but definite phagocytic activity for India ink, heat-killed *Candida,* and antibody-coated sheep erythrocytes. Culture supernatants from several cases consistently revealed the presence of elevated concentrations of lysozyme, and in some instances, the cultured giant cells were clearly positive when stained for nonspecific esterase (Kaplan and Gartner 1977).

Kadin et al. (1978), using immunofluorescent reagents for surface and intracellular gamma, alpha, and mu heavy chains and kappa and lambda light chains, examined suspensions of viable Reed-Sternberg cells from 12 patients with Hodgkin's disease. IgG, kappa, and lambda were often detected on the cell surface, whereas IgM and IgA were absent. Whenever surface immunoglobulin (SIg) was detected, cytoplasmic immunoglobulin (CIg) of the same type was also present within the same cell; conversely, CIg was often present in the absence of SIg. Every giant cell that contained CIg contained both kappa and lambda light chains. When viable cells were incubated in medium containing fluorescein-conjugated aggregated human IgG, evidence of both cell surface binding and intracellular uptake of fluorescent aggregates was observed. They concluded that the immunoglobulin found in Reed-Sternberg cells is not synthesized by these cells; instead, it appears to be ingested by them from the extracellular environment.

Collectively, these cell culture and immunofluorescence studies may have resolved the controversy concerning the origin and nature of the Reed-Sternberg and Hodgkin's giant cells. Their capacity for sustained proliferation in vitro, aneuploidy, and heterotransplantability establishes their neoplastic character, whereas the cell marker studies, phagocytic activity, positive staining reactions for nonspecific esterase, and capacity to excrete lysozyme strongly suggest that they are derived from the macrophage or other closely related cells of the mononuclear phagocyte system rather than from the lymphocyte.

C. Natural History and Mode of Spread

Lymphangiography swept away earlier misconceptions concerning the unpredictable, capricious distribution of lymph node involvement in patients with Hodgkin's disease and made possible systematic attempts to map sites of disease. Rosenberg and Kaplan (1966), in a study of 100 consecutive, previously untreated patients with Hodgkin's disease, found that involvement of various chains of lymph nodes was distinctly nonrandom; when a given chain of lymph nodes was affected, other chains known to be directly connected with it via lymphatic channels were likely also to be involved, either concurrently or at the time of first relapse. Even extralymphatic sites such as the lung, liver, and bone marrow were more likely to be involved in association with certain predictable patterns of lymph node and/or spleen involvement. These studies were subsequently extended (Kaplan 1970, 1980) to overlapping series of 340 and 426 consecutive previously untreated cases, with results which strongly confirmed and reinforced the initial conclusions. Similar analyses have been presented by other groups of investigators (Banfi et al. 1969; Han and Stutzman 1967), again with generally similar conclusions.

Two distinctively different theories, the "contiguity" theory of Rosenberg and Kaplan (1966) and the "susceptibility" theory of Smithers (1970, 1973), have been proposed to account for the patterns of spread observed in Hodgkin's disease. The contiguity theory postulates that Hodgkin's disease is a monoclonal neoplasm of unifocal origin which spreads secondarily by metastasis of pre-existing tumor cells, much like other neoplasms, except that the spread is predominantly via lymphatic rather than blood vascular channels. The term *contiguity* refers to the existence of direct connections between pairs of lymph node chains by way of lymphatic channels which do not have to pass through and be filtered by intervening lymph node or other lymphatic tissue barriers.

Smithers (1973) suggested that the giant cells of Hodgkin's disease may move in and out of lymph nodes from the blood stream, following a traffic pattern similar to that known to occur with normal lymphocytes. Emphasis was placed on the concept that Hodgkin's disease is a systemic disorder of the entire lymphatic system. Thus, the possibility was suggested that the disease may have a multifocal origin, perhaps by spread of a causative agent with de novo reinduction in different sites rather than the spread of pre-existing tumor cells. After an initial site had become involved, the theory predicted that each of the remaining lymph node chains would have an independent probability of next becoming involved which was assumed to be proportional to the probabilities of initial involvement of the corresponding lymph node chains in patients with Stage I disease.

Careful mapping of the initial sites of involvement in consecutive, previously untreated patients revealed the occurrence of non-contiguous patterns in only 4 (2%) of 185 patients with Stage II disease (Kaplan 1970). Hutchison (1972) compared the observed distributions in 158 of our Rye Stage II cases whose calculated frequencies were based on the random association of two or more sites with the probabilities given by their respective frequencies in 53 observed Stage I cases. The observed patterns for two or three involved sites departed significantly from random expectation. In particular, there was an apparent deficiency of bilateral cervical node involvement in the absence of associated mediastinal lymphadenopathy, an excess frequency of

association between cervical and mediastinal node involvement, and a marked deficiency of all noncontiguous contralateral distributions.

Lillicrap (1973) compared the predictions of the Smithers susceptibility hypothesis with the observed patterns of spread in three different series of patients with Hodgkin's disease. Bilateral cervical lymph node disease was observed significantly less often than predicted, whereas involvement of the neck and mediastinum was more frequent than predicted. There were 46 instances of homolateral cervical-axillary involvement and only two contralateral cases, whereas equal numbers of each would have been predicted by susceptibility theory. Conversely, the observed patterns were consistent with the contiguity theory in all but 8 (4%) of 212 cases. Modifications of the susceptibility theory were subsequently proposed by Smithers et al. (1974) in an attempt to make the theory more consistent with observed distribution frequencies. These modifications, which accept the concept of spread via lymphatic channels, exhibit appreciably better agreement with observed patterns of two and three sites of involvement.

The contiguity theory has also been tested with respect to the sites of first relapse in patients with regionally localized disease treated with limited field radiotherapy. Rosenberg and Kaplan (1966) found that 22 of 26 extensions of disease were to contiguous lymph node chains. Similar findings have been reported by others (Banfi et al. 1969; Han and Stutzman 1967). The most controversial issue is the association between involvement of the lower cervical-supraclavicular lymph nodes and the subsequent occurrence of relapse in the upper lumbar para-aortic nodes. Among 80 such cases at risk, Kaplan (1970) observed para-aortic node extensions in 29 (36%). This was the single most prevalent site of extension in patients treated initially with local or limited field, supradiaphragmatic radiotherapy. Transdiaphragmatic extension was also the first manifestation of relapse in 33 (40%) of 83 patients with clinical Stage I and II disease studied by Rubin et al. (1974). Many para-aortic lymph node relapses occurred several years after initial treatment and frequently involved lymph nodes which were well visualized and appeared normal on the original lymphangiogram. It was suggested (Kaplan 1970; Rosenberg and Kaplan 1966) that spread in these instances had occurred in the retrograde direc-

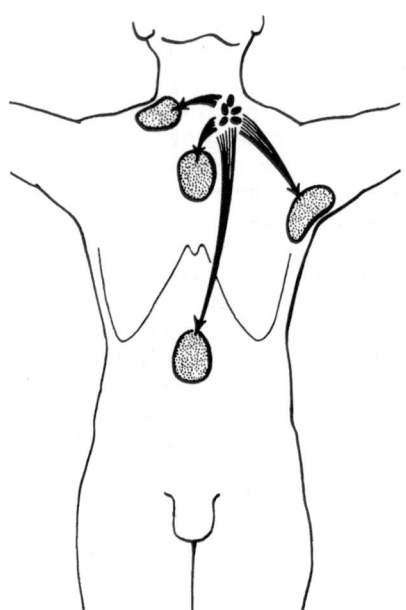

Fig. 4. Schematic diagram of postulated retrograde spread of Hodgkin's disease from low cervical-supraclavicular to para-aortic/celiac nodes via the thoracic duct and of contiguous spread to the mediastinal, ipsilateral axillary, and contralateral cervical-supraclavicular nodes. Reproduced, by permission, from the paper by Kaplan (1970)

tion from the supraclavicular fossa downward along the thoracic duct into the lumbar para-aortic nodes (Fig. 4).

The occasional presence of Reed-Sternberg and Hodgkin's giant cells in the thoracic duct lymph has been documented by Engeset et al. (1968). There is little dispute that these cells may enter the thoracic duct from involved lymph nodes below the diaphragm and travel upward to involve the cervical-supraclavicular lymph nodes. The possibility of retrograde spread from one peripheral lymph node chain to other, more distal chains by way of lymphatic channels lacking valves is also widely accepted. However, the concept of retrograde spread along the thoracic duct has been much more controversial because the duct is equipped with valves which should prevent retrograde flow. Yet, the pressure in the duct is only a few millimeters of water and reversal of flow was readily observed following chronic ligation of the thoracic duct in dogs (Neyazaki et al. 1965). Pressure gradients along the canine thoracic duct were often opposite to those

required for antegrade flow (Browse et al. 1971). However, Dumont and Martelli (1973) were able to demonstrate radiopaque material in the para-aortic lymph nodes of only 1 of 16 dogs after ligation and cannulation of the thoracic duct and injection of opaque contrast material in the retrograde direction. Retrograde flow might well occur more often in the thoracic duct of man, which is usually vertical, than in that of dogs, which is horizontal. Rouvière (1932) noted that although the human thoracic duct usually has two competent valves at its upper end, a not infrequent normal variation involves the presence of a single incompetent valve, which is usually compensated by oblique insertion of the duct through the vein wall. Conceivably, prolonged compression and partial occlusion of the duct by enlarged lymph nodes near its insertion into the subclavian vein may cause dilatation of the duct with secondary valvular incompetence and reversal of flow.

The role of vascular invasion (Rappaport and Strum 1970) in the spread of Hodgkin's disease is not fully understood. In a careful review of the original biopsy material in 11 patients with regionally localized Hodgkin's disease who developed extranodal dissemination following primary radiotherapy, Lamoureux et al. (1973) failed to find evidence of vascular invasion. Kirschner et al. (1974) noted that vascular invasion was present in 7 (16%) of 44 spleens involved by Hodgkin's disease and was associated with hepatic and bone marrow metastasis, early relapse, and decreased survival, whereas vascular invasion detected in 4 of 91 lymph node biopsies was not attended by an increased frequency of extranodal dissemination or a decreased survival rate. In a series of patients whose lymph node biopsies showed vascular invasion, Naeim et al. (1974) observed an average survival time of only 21.8 months, significantly less than the 65.8 month average survival of those patients in whom vascular invasion was not demonstrable in the original lymph node biopsies.

D. Nature of the Immunologic Defect

Unresponsiveness to tuberculin was the first immunologic abnormality observed in patients with Hodgkin's disease. Dorothy Reed (1902 reported that tuberculin was given in five cases but without reaction." However, the immunologic deficiency is not specifically restricted to tuberculosis. Schier et al. (1956) tested the capacity of patients with Hodgkin's disease to mount delayed hypersensitivity reactions to a diversified battery of natural antigens and found that most were unresponsive to all of the antigens tested. Unfortunately, the significance of the early studies cannot be assessed because many patients had been treated, and none had been staged by modern methods.

A series of 50 previously untreated patients with Hodgkin's disease, all staged with the aid of lymphangiography and other modern diagnostic procedures, was studied at the National Cancer Institute by Brown et al. (1967). Responsiveness to the five antigens tested was impaired relative to controls. However, reactions in eight patients with clinical Stage I Hodgkin's disease appeared to be comparable with those of normal controls. With increasing clinical stage, responsiveness decreased sharply. Positive responses to one or more intradermal antigens were noted in seven of eight patients with Stage I disease, 13 of 24 in Stage II, three of seven in Stage III, and 5 of 11 in Stage IV. These studies were later extended to a total of 103 patients with previously untreated disease with generally similar results (Young et al. 1972). Only seven patients, all of whom had constitutional symptoms, were completely anergic (unresponsive to all tests).

Among a total of 185 patients studied at Stanford University Medical Center from 1964 through 1968 there were 28 patients with previously untreated Stage I disease, of whom only 12 (43%) responded to mumps antigen and few responded to any other cutaneous antigen (Kaplan 1970). A second study initiated in 1969 accrued 154 previously untreated patients, all staged with the aid of lymphangiography and laparotomy with splenectomy (Eltringham and Kaplan 1973). Only 51 of 151 evaluable patients (34%) responded to one or more intradermal antigens, and a positive reaction to mumps antigen was observed in only 40 (25%) of 151 patients. There was no significant influence of clinical stage on response to mumps antigen. In contrast to the observations of the Bethesda group, unresponsiveness did not occur more frequently among patients with constitutional symptoms. In tests with streptokinase-streptodornase (SK–SD), only 6 (10%) of 58 untreated patients with Hodgkin's disease reacted to 5 units, whereas 93% of age – and sex-matched controls were known to respond to the same dose level (Eltringham and Kaplan 1973).

Clinical investigations using chemical agents known to have the property of inducing delayed cutaneous hypersensitivity reactions essentially indistinguishable from those induced by tuberculin have the advantage that the fact of exposure to the agent and the timing of that exposure are both under the control of the investigator. The most extensively used of these chemicals is 2,4-dinitrochlorobenzene (DNCB). In a series of 50 untreated patients, Brown et al. (1967) observed positive responses in 35 (70%) to sensitization with DNCB at a concentration of 2.0%. Impressed by the fact that all eight of their patients with Stage I disease reacted positively to DNCB and that seven of the eight reacted to at least one intradermal antigen, the Bethesda group concluded that the development of anergy is probably a secondarily acquired manifestation associated with advancing anatomic extent of involvement rather than an intrinsic component of the pathogenesis of Hodgkin's disease.

In an initial study involving 185 previously untreated patients sensitized with 2.0% DNCB at Stanford University Medical Center from 1964 through 1968, an extremely high incidence of anergy was observed, even in patients with Stage I disease (Kaplan 1970). De Gast et al. (1975) also observed negative reactions to challenge after sensitization with the same concentration of DNCB in 20 of 30 patients (67%), including two of five with Stage I disease, and Case et al. (1976) reported negative reactions in 24 of 50 patients (48%), including three of eight with Stage I disease.

In a subsequent Stanford study involving untreated patients staged routinely with lymphangiography and laparotomy with splenectomy, three different sensitizing concentrations of DNCB (0.1, 0.5, and 2.0%) were used (Eltringham and Kaplan 1973). Sensitization and challenge with DNCB occurred prior to the initiation of treatment. At a sensitizing concentration of 0.5%, only 10 (26%) of 39 patients responded as compared with 83% of normal controls. This study was ultimately extended to encompass a total of 531 previously untreated patients of all stages (Kaplan 1980). There were 113 positive responses (36.3%) among 311 patients with Stage I and II disease, a response rate only slightly greater than that among patients with Stage III and IV disease (56 of 220, or 25.5%). Of a total of 355 asymptomatic patients, 128 (36.1%) responded, a significantly higher response rate than that of patients with constitutional symptoms (41 of 176, or 23.3%). These data support the conclusion that cell-mediated immune reactivity is indeed impaired in patients with Hodgkin's disease. However, the impairment is not an all-or-none phenomenon but a more subtle continuous gradient of immunologic deficit which is present in some degree even in patients with the earliest manifestations of the disease.

A number of in vitro tests are considered analogs of cell-mediated immune responses. These include the capacity of lymphocytes to: (1) undergo lymphoblastoid transformation after stimulation by lectins or antigens and to respond in the mixed lymphocyte reaction, (2) to bind sheep erythrocytes to their surface membranes (E-rosette formation), and (3) to bind and become agglutinated by certain lectins and to mediate the polar migration (capping) and shedding of the bound lectins from the cell membrane. Brown et al. (1967) noted a mean lymphocyte response to phytohemagglutinin (PHA) of 49% in 43 patients with untreated Hodgkin's disease, a highly significant decrease from the 72% mean value observed in their controls. However, responses in patients with Stage I disease were within the normal range. Very similar responses to PHA were noted by De Gast et al. (1975) in a series of 30 patients with Hodgkin's disease. However, these investigators noted that lymphocyte stimulation by α-hemocyanin was impaired in 11 of 15 patients and that the DNCB skin test reaction was also negative in 10 of the 11 nonresponsive individuals. Lymphoblastoid responses to another antigen, tetanus toxoid, were negative in six of nine patients studied by Fuks et al. (1976a). Gaines et al. (1973) observed that lymphocytes from three patients with positive *Toxoplasma* dye test titers as well as those of 20 with negative titers failed to respond to *Toxoplasma* antigen in vitro. Responses to SK-SD were also negative in 22 of 23 untreated patients. Holm et al. (1976) in a study of 31 patients with Hodgkin's disease noted that only 1 of 12 skin test positive patients had an impaired lymphocyte response to the antigen in vitro; conversely, only 1 of 19 patients with a negative skin test reaction had a normal lymphoblastoid response to tubercu-

lin (PPD) in vitro. Deficient responses to PPD were observed in 7 (47%) of 15 patients with Stage I or II disease and in 11 (55%) of 20 patients with Stage III or IV disease.

Modifications of technique succeeded in revealing unambiguous abnormalities of the PHA stimulation response even in patients with Stage I disease. Matchett et al. (1973) noted good initial responses during the first 2 days in patients with localized disease, but these responses were not sustained at 4 or 5 days. When the daily uptake of tritiated thymidine (^{3}H-TdR) by limiting concentrations of cells was used as the index of response, all of 26 patients, including those with localized disease and no symptoms, showed a striking degree of abnormality. Levy and Kaplan (1974) measured the uptake of tritiated leucine (^{3}H-Leu) into protein in peripheral blood lymphocytes stimulated with a range of PHA concentrations. This assay requires only 20 h for completion, so that cell viability can be preserved in the absence of serum, thus enhancing precision and reproducibility. They studied 37 normal subjects and 44 consecutive untreated patients with Hodgkin's disease, all staged with lymphangiography, bone marrow biopsy, and in those with negative marrow biopsies, laparotomy with splenectomy. The peak response of normal donor lymphocytes was noted at a PHA concentration of 1 μg/ml. The response of lymphocytes from patients was very significantly below normal at all but the highest PHA concentrations tested. The impairment of response was observed both in patients with limited (Stage I and II) as well as those with advanced (Stage III and IV) disease. These results remained essentially unchanged after this study had been extended (Fuks et al. 1976a) to include 132 patients with untreated Hodgkin's disease (Fig. 5). Stimulation by another lectin, concanavalin A (Con A), revealed impaired responses in a series of 18 patients. Concentration-dependent defects in lymphocyte response to PHA were also observed by Ziegler et al. (1975) and by Faguet (1975) in untreated patients with various stages of Hodgkin's disease.

Negative mixed lymphocyte reactions (MLR) were observed by Lang et al. (1972) in 7 (22%) of 32 patients with untreated Hodgkin's disease. In a study of 30 patients, Rühl et al. (1975) found that the capacity of lymphocytes from patients with Hodgkin's disease to respond to allogeneic cells was significantly

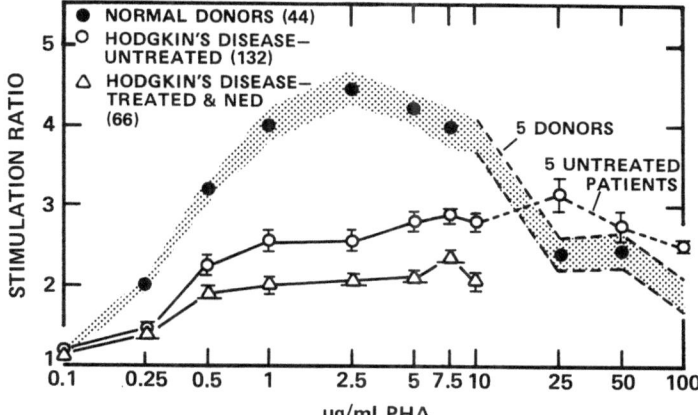

Fig. 5. Impaired lymphoblastoid response to a range of concentrations of phytohemagglutinin (PHA), as measured by a tritiated leucine uptake assay (Levy and Kaplan 1974), by peripheral blood lymphocytes from 132 untreated patients with Hodgkin's disease and 66 other patients in remission following radiotherapy. Reproduced, by permission of the *Journal of Clinical Investigation*, from the paper by Fuks et al. (1976a)

impaired, whereas their capacity to stimulate responses by normal lymphocytes was essentially intact, a result diametrically opposed to that observed by Björkholm et al. (1975) in a study of 39 previously untreated patients. Fuks et al. (1976a) observed positive responses in eight of nine untreated patients whose lymphocytes were used as stimulator cells in one-way allogeneic MLR tests; however, five of these responses were only weakly positive. The lymphocytes of these patients were found to respond adequately to stimulation either by normal donor cells or by cells from other patients with Hodgkin's disease, positive reactions being observed in 20 (95%) of 21 such combinations. A somewhat different test, the autologous mixed lymphocyte reaction, was employed in a recent study (Engleman et al. 1980); the capacity of peripheral blood T-lymphocytes from patients with untreated Hodgkin's disease as well as those previously treated with radiotherapy and in long-term remission to respond was found to be profoundly impaired.

The capacity to form spontaneous E-rosettes with uncoated sheep erythrocytes, a specific property of human T-lymphocytes, was observed by Bobrove et al. (1975) to be impaired in 13 of 15 untreated patients with Hodgkin's disease, whereas the percentage of T-lymphocytes detected by cytotoxic antibody assay was normal. In contrast, the levels of active rosette-forming cells (a subpopulation of T-lymphocytes with high affinity receptors for sheep erythrocytes) were within normal limits in two series of patients with untreated Hodgkin's disease (D.P. King and H.S. Kaplan, cited in Kaplan 1980; Lang et al. 1977).

Significant progress has been made in elucidating the mechanisms underlying the selective impairment of cell-mediated immune responses in Hodgkin's disease. It is now well established that cells capable of specific suppression of immune responses exist in the lymphoid system. Twomey et al. (1975) observed that peripheral blood mononuclear cells from 16 of 30 patients with Hodgkin's disease had an impaired capacity to stimulate responses by lymphocytes from normal donors in the one-way MLR test. Of these 16 patients, all but one had Stage III or IV disease and two had been previously treated. Stimulation was markedly increased when adherent cells were removed by passage through glass wool as well as by preincubation of the cells in a protein synthesis inhibitor, cycloheximide. Similar results were subsequently reported by Goodwin et al. (1977) who found in addition that the inhibitory activity could be counteracted by indomethacin, a known prostaglandin synthetase inhibitor, suggesting that a suppressor cell producing prostaglandin E_2 might be responsible for the hyporesponsiveness to PHA of peripheral blood cells from patients with Hodgkin's disease. This group (Sibbitt et al. 1978) later reported that the PHA response of lymphocytes in patients with Hodgkin's disease could be restored to normal by removal of glass wool adherent suppressor cells and again inhibited by restoration of such cells to the cultures. Suppressor responses have also been reported in a high percentage of patients with Hodgkin's disease by Engleman et al. (1979) and by Hillinger and Herzig (1978). However, the specificity of these suppressor effects remains to be established.

Tests of binding affinity, agglutinability, and capacity for cap formation with lectins such as Con A have provided important new approaches to the study of lymphocyte surface membranes. Ben-Bassat and Goldblum (1975) found that cap formation by peripheral blood lymphocytes from patients with Hodgkin's disease was markedly reduced. Mintz and Sachs (1975) noted a mean of only 2.1% of cap forming cells among 15 patients with active Hodgkin's disease and 10.6% in patients with remission versus 24.9% in normal individuals. Both groups noted an increased agglutinability of patients' peripheral blood lymphocytes by Con A. Aisenberg et al. (1978) found that cap forming cell levels were below normal in 9 of 13 patients with untreated Stage I-A and II-A disease, six of eight in Stage III-A, and eight of eight in Stages III-B and IV. Thus, a subpopulation of lymphocytes in patients with Hodgkin's disease appears to have membrane alterations reflected in enhanced lectin agglutinability and diminished cap formation.

Humoral factors in serum may alter the T-lymphocyte surface membrane, perhaps by masking specific receptors, and thus inhibit or abrogate cell-mediated immune functions. Grifoni et al. (1970) reported that cytotoxic antilymphocyte antibodies are present in the sera of patients with Hodgkin's disease and that such antibodies can inhibit the PHA stimulation response of normal lymphocytes in vitro. Fuks et al. (1976c) discovered that impaired E-rosette formation and PHA responses by lymphocytes from patients with Hodgkin's disease could be consistently restored to normal levels by short-term incubation in fetal calf serum. In a search for direct evidence of an E-rosette inhibitor in the sera of patients with Hodgkin's disease, Fuks et al. (1976b) noted that when lymphocytes were first restored to normal E-rosette forming cell (E-RFC) levels by incubation in fetal calf serum and then reincubated in medium containing 20% Hodgkin's disease serum, E-rosette levels were again significantly reduced in 22 (85%) of 25 patients. In contrast, Hodgkin's disease serum significantly depressed the response of only 1 of 12 patients with non-Hodgkin's lymphomas and failed to depress the E-rosette levels of lymphocytes from any of 34 normal subjects or of 12 patients with various types of carcinomas.

Since the spleen seemed a likely tissue of origin for the serum E-rosette inhibitor, Bieber et al. (1975) prepared extracts from the involved spleens of eight patients with Hodgkin's disease. These extracts consistently showed marked E-rosette inhibiting activity, whereas similarly prepared extracts from the spleens of most patients with non-Hodgkin's lymphomas and from normal spleens of acute trauma victims were devoid of such activity. Rosette levels depressed by the Hodgkin's disease spleen extract could again be restored to normal levels by incubation in fetal calf serum. Lymphocytes from patients with Hodgkin's disease were susceptible to the spleen extracts after they had first been restored to normal responsiveness by incubation in fetal calf serum. Analysis of the active fraction initially indicated the presence of β-lipoprotein, C-reactive protein, and the Clq component of complement. Subsequently, Bieber et al. (1979) fractionated the sera of patients with Hodgkin's disease on sucrose gradients and then on potassium bromide isopyknic gradients, followed by thin-layer chromatography. The active material proved to be a glycolipid, the further chemical characterization of which is still in progress. Similarly fractionated normal sera were devoid of detectable amounts of this inhibitory substance.

By radioiodination of the surface proteins of peripheral blood mononuclear cells from four patients with Hodgkin's disease, Moroz et al. (1977) demonstrated the presence of a blocking protein which could be released from the cell surface by incubation with levamisole, an antihelminthic drug. The blocking protein reacted with antibody to human spleen ferritin but contained no detectable iron and could be dissociated into 18 000-dalton subunits, suggesting that it is an apoferritin rather than ferritin. After release of the blocking protein by treatment with levamisole, the E-rosette response of peripheral blood lymphocytes from patients with Hodgkin's disease rose to normal levels. It is of course possible that apoferritin is merely acting as a carrier for a low molecular weight E-rosette inhibitory substance, perhaps the glycolipid material identified by Bieber et al. (1979).

There is thus abundant evidence that virtually all patients with Hodgkin's disease, including those with localized involvement, suffer from a selective, often subtile, impairment of cell-mediated immunity. In vivo this deficit is expressed by an increased susceptibility to certain types of bacterial, fungal, and viral infections and by a decreased capacity for delayed hypersensitivity reactions to recall antigens or chemical allergens. A spectrum of in vitro test responses, including lymphoblastoid transformation by lectins and specific antigens, the capacity to form E-rosettes, and the capacity for cap formation after lectin binding, are also impaired. These alterations appear to be due to functional alterations of T-lymphocytes rather than to quantitative depletion of either T- or B-lymphocytes. Humoral inhibitors in the sera of patients with Hodgkin's disease and suppressor cell effects have been implicated.

References

Aisenberg AD, Weitzman S, Wilkes B (1978) Lymphocyte receptors for concanavalin A in Hodgkin's disease. Blood 51:439–443 – Banfi A, Bonadonna G, Carnevali G, Fossati-Bellani F (1969) Malignant lymphomas: further studies on their preferential sites of involvement and possible mode of spread. Lymphology 2:130–138 – Ben-Bassat H, Goldblum N (1975) Concanavalin A receptors on the surface membrane of lymphocytes from patients with Hodgkin's disease and other malignant lymphomas. Proc Natl Acad Sci USA 72:1046–1049 – Bieber MM, Fuks Z, Kaplan HS (1975) E-rosette inhibiting substance in Hodgkin's disease spleen extracts. Clin Exp Immunol 29:369–375 – Bieber MM, King DP, Strober S, Kaplan HS (1979) Characterization of an E-rosette inhibitor (ERI) in the serum of patients with Hodgkin's disease as a glycolipid. Clin Res 27:81A – Björkholm M, Holm G, Mellstedt H, Pettersson D (1975) Immunological capacity of lymphocytes from untreated patients with Hodgkin's disease evaluated in mixed lymphocyte culture. Clin Exp Immunol 22:373–377 – Bobrove AM, Fuks Z, Strober S, Kaplan HS (1975) Quantitation of T- and B-lymphocytes and cellular immune function in Hodgkin's disease. Cancer 36:169–179 – Brown RS, Haynes HA, Foley HT, Godwin HA, Berard CW, Carbone PP: Immunologic, clinical and histologic features of 50 untreated patients. Ann Intern Med 67:291–302 – Browse NL, Lord RSA, Taylor A (1971) Pressure waves and gradients in the canine thoracic duct. J physiol (Lond) 213:507–524 – Carr I (1975) The ultrastructure of the abnormal reticulum cells in Hodgkin's disease. J Pathol 115:45–50 – Case DC Jr, Hansen JA, Corrales E, Young CW, DuPont B, Pinsky CM, Good RA (1976) Comparison of multiple in vivo and in vitro parameters in untreated patients with Hodgkin's disease. Cancer 38:1807–1815 – De Gast GC, Halie MR, Nieweg HO (1975) Immunological responsiveness against two primary antigens in untreated patients with Hodgkin's disease. Eur J Cancer 11:217–224 – De Vita VT (1973) Lymphocyte reactivity in Hodgkin's disease: a lymphocyte civil war. N Engl J Med 289: 801–802 – Dorfman RF (1961) Enzyme histochemistry of the cells in Hodgkin's disease and allied disorders. Nature 190:925–926 – Dorfman RF, Rice DF, Mitchell AD, Kempson RI, Levine G (1973) Ultrastructural studies of Hodgkin's disease. Natl Cancer Inst Monogr 36:221–238 – Dumont AE, Martelli AB (1973) Experimental studies bearing on the question of retrograde spread of Hodgkin's disease via the thoracic duct. Cancer Res 33:3195–3202 – Eltringham JR, Kaplan HS (1973) Impaired delayed hypersensitivity responses in 154 patients with untreated Hodgkin's disease. Natl Cancer Inst Monogr 36:107–115 – Engeset A, Brennhovd IO, Christensen I, Hagen S, Høst H, Liverud K, Nesheim A (1968) Sternberg-Reed cells in the throacic duct lymph of patients with Hodgkin's disease. A preliminary report. Cytologic studies in connection with lymphography. Blood 31:99–103 – Engleman EG, Benike C, Hoppe R, Kaplan HS (1979) Suppressor cells of the mixed lymphocyte reaction in patients with Hodgkin's disease. Transplant Proc 11:1827–1829 – Engleman EG, Benike C, Hoppe RT, Kaplan HS, Berberich RT (1980) Autologous mixed lymphocyte reaction in patients with Hodgkin's disease: evidence for a T cell defect J Clin Invest 66:149–158 – Faguet GB (1975) Quantitation of immunocompetence in Hodgkin's disease. J Clin Invest 56:951–957 – Fuks Z, Strober S, Bobrove AM, Sasazuki T, McMichael A, Kaplan HS (1976a) Long-term effects of radiation on T- and B-lymphocytes in peripheral blood of patients with Hodgkin's disease. J Clin Invest 58:803–814 – Fuks Z, Strober S, Kaplan HS (1976b) Interaction between serum factors and T-lymphocytes in Hodgkin's disease. N Engl J. Med 295:1273–1278 – Fuks Z, Strober S, King DP, Kaplan HS (1976c) Reversal of cell surface abnormalities of T-lymphocytes in Hodgkin's disease after in vitro incubation in fetal sera. J Immunol 117:1331–1335 – Gaines JD, Gilmer MA, Remington JS (1973) Deficiency of lymphocyte antigen recognition in Hodgkin's disease. Natl Cancer Inst Monogr 36:117–121 – Gallmeier WM, Boecker WR, Bruntsch U, Hossfeld DK, Schmidt CG (1977) Characterization of a human Hodgkin cell line and a lymphoblastic EBNA-negative cell line derived from a non-Hodgkin's lymphoma patient. Haemotol Bluttransfus. 20:277–281 – Garvin AJ, Spicer SS, Parmley RT, Munster AM (1974) Immunohistochemical demonstration of IgG in Reed-Sternberg and other cells in Hodgkin's disease. J Exp Med 139:1077–1083 – Gearhart PJ, Sigal NH, Klinman NR (1975) Production of antibodies of identical idiotype but diverse immunoglobulin classes by cells derived from a single stimulated B cell. Proc Natl Acad Sci USA 72:1707–1711 – Goodwin JS, Messner RP, Bankhurst AD, Peake GT, Saiki JH, Williams RC Jr (1977) Prostaglandin-producing suppressor cells in Hodgkin's disease.

N Engl J Med 297:963–968 – Green I, Inkelas M, Allen LB (1960) Hodgkin's disease: a maternal-to-foetal lymphocyte chimaera? Lancet 1:30–32 – Grifoni V, Del Giacco GS, Tognella S, Manconi PE, Mantovani G (1970) Lymphocytotoxins in Hodgkin's disease. Ital J Immunol Immunopathol 1:21–31 – Han T, Stutzman L (1967) Mode of spread in patients with localized malignant lymphomas. Arch Intern Med 120:1–7 – Hillinger SM, Herzig GP (1978) Impaired cell-mediated immunity in Hodgkin's disease mediated by suppressor lymphocytes and monocytes. J Clin Invest 61:1620–1627 – Holm G, Mellstedt H, Björkholm M, Johansson B, Killander D, Sundblad R, Söderberg G (1976) Lymphocyte abnormalities in untreated patients with Hodgkin's disease. Cancer 37:751–762 – Hutchison GB (1972) Anatomic patterns by histologic type of localized Hodgkin's disease of the upper torso. Lymphology 5:1–14 – Kadin ME, Asbury AK (1973) Long-term cultures of Hodgkin's tissue. A morphologic and radioautographic study. Lab Invest 28:181–184 – Kadin ME, Stites DP, Levy R, Warnke R (1978) Exogenous origin of immunoglobulin in Reed-Sternberg cells of Hodgkin's disease. N Engl J Med 299:1208–1214 – Kaplan HS (1970) On the natural history, treatment, and prognosis of Hodgkin's disease. Harvey Lectures, 1968–1969, Academic Press New York pp 215–259 – Kaplan HS (1980) Hodgkin's Disease, 2nd ed. Harvard University Press, Cambridge, MA – Kaplan HS, Gartner S (1977) "Sternberg-Reed" giant cells of Hodgkin's disease: cultivation in vitro, heterotransplantation, and characterization as neoplastic macrophages. Int J Cancer 19:511–525 – Kaplan HS, Smithers DW (1959) Auto-immunity in man and homologous disease in mice in relation to the malignant lymphomas. Lancet 2:1–4 – Kirschner RH, Abt AB, O'Connell MJ, Sklansky BD, Greene WH, Wiernik PH (1974) Vascular invasion and hematogenous dissemination of Hodgkin's disease. Cancer 34:1159–1162 – Lamoureux KB, Jaffe ES, Berard CW, Johnson RE (1973) Lack of identifiable vascular invasion in patients with extranodal dissemination of Hodgkin's disease. Cancer 31:824–825 – Lang JM, Oberling F, Tongio M, Mayer S, Waitz R (1972) Mixed lymphocyte reaction as assay for immunological competence of lymphocytes from patients with Hodgkin's disease. Lancet 1:1261–1263 – Lang JM, Bigel P, Oberling F, Mayer S (1977) Normal active rosette-forming cells in untreated patients with Hodgkin's disease. Biomedicine 27:322–324 – Levy RA, Kaplan HS (1974) Impaired lymphocyte function in untreated Hodgkin's disease. N Engl J Med 290:181–186 – Lillicrap SC (1973) Modes of spread of Hodgkin's disease. Br J Radiol 46:18–23 – Long JC, Zamecnik PC, Aisenberg AC, Atkins L (1977) Tissue culture studies in Hodgkin's disease. Morphologic, cytogenetic, cell surface and enzymatic properties of cultures derived from splenic tumors. J Exp Med 145:1481–1500 – Marmont AM, Damasio EE (1967) The effects of two alkaloids derived from Vinca Rosea on the malignant cells in Hodgkin's disease, lymphosarcoma and acute leukemia in vivo. Blood 29:1–21 – Matchett KM, Huang AT, Kremer WB (1973) Impaired lymphocyte transformation in Hodgkin's disease. Evidence for depletion of circulating T-lymphocytes. J Clin Invest 52:1908–1917 – Mintz U, Sachs L (1975) Membrane differences in peripheral blood lymphocytes from patients with chronic lymphocytic leukemia and Hodgkin's disease. Proc Natl Acad Sci USA 72:2428–2432 – Moroz C, Lahat M, Biniaminov M, Ramot B (1977) Ferritin on the surface of lymphocytes in Hodgkin's disease patients. A possible blocking substance removed by levamisole. Clin Exp Immunol 29:30–35 – Naeim F, Waisman J, Coulson WF (1974) Hodgkin's disease: the significance of vascular invasion. Cancer 34:655–662 – Neyazaki T, Kupic EA, Marshall WJ, Abrams HL (1965) Collateral lymphatico-venous communication after experimental obstruction of the thoracic duct. Radiology 85:423–431 – Order SE, Hellman S (1972) Pathogenesis of Hodgkin's disease. Lancet 1:571–573 – Peckham MJ, Cooper EH (1969) Proliferation characteristics of the various classes of cells in Hodgkin's disease. Cancer 24:135–146 – Rappaport H (1966) Tumors of the hematopoietic system. Atlas of tumor pathology, Sect III, Fasc 8. Armed Forces Institute of Pathology, Washington, DC – Rappaport H, Strum SB (1970) Vascular invasion in Hodgkin's disease: its incidence and relationship to the spread of the disease. Cancer 25:1304–1313 – Reed DM (1902) On the pathological changes in Hodgkin's disease, with especial reference to its relation to tuberculosis. Johns Hopkins Med J 10:133–196 – Roberts AM, Smith KL, Dowell BL, Hubbard AK (1978) Cultural, morphological, cell membrane enzymatic, and neoplastic properties of cell lines derived from a Hodgkin's disease lymph node. Cancer Res 38:3033–3043 – Rosenberg SA, Kaplan HS (1966) Evidence for an orderly progression in the spread of Hodgkin's disease. Cancer Res 26:1225–1231 – Rouvière H (1932) Anatomie des lymphatiques de l'homme. Masson, Paris – Rubin P, Keys H, Mayer E, Antemann R (1974) Nodal recurrences following radical radiation therapy in Hodgkin's disease. AJR 120:536–548 – Rühl H, Vogt W, Borchert G, Schmidt S, Moelle R, Schaoua H (1975) Mixed lymphocyte culture stimulatory and responding capacity of lymphocytes from patients with lymphoproliferative diseases. Clin Exp Immunol 19:55–65 – Schaadt M, Fonatsch C, Kirchner H, Diehl V (1979) Establishment of a malignant, Epstein-Barr virus (EBV)-negative cell line from the pleura effusion of a patient with Hodgkin's disease. Blut 38:185–190 – Schier WW, Roth A, Ostroff G, Schrift MH (1956) Hodgkin's disease and immunity. Am J Med 20:94–99 – Seif GSF, Spriggs AL (1967) Chromosome changes in Hodgkin's disease. J Natl Cancer Inst 39:557–570 – Sibbitt WL, Bankhurst AD, Williams RC (1978) Studies of cell subpopulations mediating mitogen hyporesponsiveness in patients with Hodgkin's disease. J Clin Invest 61:55–63 – Smithers DW (1970) Spread of Hodgkin's disease. Lancet 1:1261–1267 – Smithers DW (1973) Modes of spread. In: Smithers DW (ed) Hodgkin's Disease. Churchill-Livingstone, Edinburgh London pp 107–117 – Smithers DW, Lillicrap SC, Barnes A (1974) Patterns of lymph node involvement in relation to hypotheses about the modes of spread of Hodgkin's disease. Cancer 34:1779–1786 – Taylor CR (1976) An immunohistological study of follicular lymphoma, reticulum cell sarcoma and Hodgkin's disease. Eur J Cancer 12:61–75 – Twomey JJ, Laughter AH, Farrow S, Douglass CC (1975) Hodgkin's disease. An immunodepleting and immunosuppressive disorder. J Clin Invest 56:467–475 – Whitelaw DM (1969) Chromosome complement of lymph node cells in Hodgkin's disease. Can Med Assoc J 101:74–81 – Young RC, Corder MP, Haynes HA, De Vita VT (1972) Delayed hypersensitivity in Hodgkin's disease. A study of 103 untreated patients. Am J Med 52:63–72 – Ziegler JB, Hansen P, Penny R (1975) Intrinsic lymphocyte defect in Hodgkin's disease: analysis of the phytohemagglutinin dose-response. Cell Immunol Immunopathol 3:451–460

Clinical Aspects

Haematology and Blood Transfusion Vol. 26
Modern Trends in Human Leukemia IV
Edited by Neth, Gallo, Graf, Mannweiler, Winkler
© Springer-Verlag Berlin Heidelberg 1981

Chromosome Studies in Children and Adults with Leukemia*

J. D. Rowley

A. Introduction

The study of the chromosome pattern (karyotype) of human leukemic cells is one of the most rapidly progressing areas of clinical research. As more patients are examined, we are now able to correlate the karyotype with the type of leukemia and with the patient's response to therapy. Chromosome analysis of leukemic cells thus can provide information of both diagnostic and prognostic significance. The clinical usefulness is largely the result of new technical advances in staining procedures that allow us to identify each chromosome precisely with banding techniques.

Many fewer patients with lymphoid leukemias have been studied than those with myeloid leukemia; only two unselected series of patients with acute lymphocytic leukemia (ALL) whose cells have been examined with the new banding techniques have been reported, and thus correlations between the karyotype and the type of leukemia and response to therapy are generally inconclusive. Chromosome abnormalities will be described in various myeloid leukemias including chronic myeloid leukemia, Ph[1]-positive acute leukemia, and acute nonlymphocytic leukemia. Within each category, the data that have been collected will be correlated with clinical information.

* This work was supported in part by The University of Chicago Cancer Research Foundation and by Grant Numbers CA-16910 and CA-19266 awarded by the National Cancer Institute, U.S. Dept. of Health, Education, and Welfare. The Franklin McLean Memorial Research Institute was operated by The University of Chicago for The U.S. Department of Energy under Contract No. EY 76-C-02-0069

B. Methods

An analysis of chromosomal patterns, to be relevant to a malignant disease, must be based on a study of the karyotype of the tumor cells themselves. In the case of leukemia the specimen is usually a bone marrow aspirate that is processed immediately or cultured for a short time (Testa and Rowley, to be published). In patients with a white blood cell count higher than 14,500 and with about 10% immature myeloid cells, it is possible to culture a sample of peripheral blood for 24 or 48 h without adding phytohemagglutinin (PHA). In most instances cells from unaffected tissues will have a normal karyotype. The chromosome abnormalities observed in the leukemic cells thus represent somatic mutations in an otherwise normal individual.

Chromosomes obtained from bone marrow cells, particularly from patients with leukemia, frequently are very fuzzy, and the bands may be indistinct. The observation of at least two "pseudodiploid" or hyperdiploid cells or three hypodiploid cells, each showing the same abnormality, is considered evidence for the presence of an abnormal clone; a clone is defined as a group of cells all of which have arisen from a single cell. Patients with such clones are classified as abnormal; those whose cells show no alterations or in whom the alterations involve different chromosomes in different cells are considered to be normal. Isolated changes may be due to technical artifacts or to random mitotic errors.

In the following discussion the chromosomes are identified according to the Paris Nomenclature (Paris Conference 1972), and the karyotypes are expressed as recommended under this system. The total chromosome number is indicated first, followed by the sex chromosomes, and then by the gains, losses, or rearrangements of the autosomes. A "+" sign or "−" sign before a number indicates a gain or loss, respectively, of a whole chromosome; a "+" or "−" after a number indicates a gain or loss of part of a chromosome. The letters "p" and "q" refer to the short and long arms of the chromosome, respectively; "i" and "r" stand for "isochromosome" and "ring chromosome". "Mar" is marker, "del" is deletion, "ins" is insertion, and "inv" is inversion. Translocations are identified by "t" followed by the chromosomes involved in the first set of brackets; the chromosome bands in which the breaks occurred are indicated in the second brackets. Uncertainty about the chromosome or band involved is signified by "?".

C. Ph[1]-Positive Myelogenous Leukemia

Cytogenetic studies on patients with chronic myelogenous leukemia (CML) have been the keystone for karyotype analysis of other human malignancies. New discoveries that have resulted from examination of CML have subsequently been confirmed in other hematologic malignancies and in many solid tumors as well.

I. Chromosome Studies of Chronic Myelogenous Leukemia

Nowell and Hungerford in 1960 reported the first consistent chromosome abnormality in human cancer; they observed an unusually small G-group chromosome which appeared to have lost about one-half of its long arm in leukemic cells from patients with CML (Nowell and Hungerford 1960). The question whether the deleted portion of the long arm of the Ph[1] chromosome was missing from the cell or whether it was translocated to another chromosome could not be answered at that time, because it was impossible to identify each human chromosome precisely with the techniques then available. Furthermore, the identity of this chromosome as either a No. 21 or No. 22 could not be established. Despite this uncertainty, the Ph[1] chromosome was a very useful marker in the study of patients with CML.

Bone marrow cells from approximately 85% of patients who have clinically typical CML contain the Ph[1] chromosome (Ph[1]+) (Sandberg 1979; Whang-Peng et al. 1968); the other 15% of the patients usually have a normal karyotype (Ph[1]−). A perplexing observation, still not explained, was that patients with Ph[1]+ CML had a much better prognosis than those with Ph[1]− CML (42− vs 15-month survival). However, as was shown by Whang-Peng et al. (1968) a change in the karyotype was a grave prognostic sign; the

median survival after such a change was about 2 months.

Chromosome banding techniques were first used in the cytogenetic study of leukemia for identification of the Ph[1] chromosome as a deletion of No. 22 (22q−) (Caspersson et al. 1970; O'Riordan et al. 1971). Since quinacrine fluorescence revealed that the chromosome present in triplicate in Down's syndrome was No. 21, the abnormalities in Down's syndrome and CML were shown to affect different pairs of chromosomes.

The question of the origin of the Ph[1] (22q−) chromosome was answered in 1973, when Rowley reported that the Ph[1] chromosome results from a translocation rather than a deletion as many investigators had previously assumed (Rowley 1973a). Additional chromosome material was observed at the end of the long arm of one. No. 9 (9q+) and was approximately equal in length to that missing from the Ph[1] chromosome; it had staining characteristics similar to those of the distal portion of the long arm of No. 22. It was proposed, therefore, that the abnormality of CML was an apparently balanced reciprocal translocation t(9;22)(q34;q11). Karyotypes of 802 Ph[1]+ patients with CML have been examined with banding techniques by a number of investigators, and the 9;22 translocation has been identified in 739 (92%). It is now recognized that variant translocations may occur (Rowley 1980a; Sandberg 1979); one is a simple translocation involving No. 22 and some chromosome other than No. 9, which has been seen in 29 patients. The other is a complex translocation involving three or more different chromosomes; except in two cases, two of the chromosomes involved were found to be No. 9 and No. 22. This type of translocation has been observed in 31 patients. The great specificity of the translocation involving Nos. 9 and 22 remains an enigma. The survival curves for patients with variant translocations appeared to be the same as those for patients with the standard t(9;22).

When patients with CML enter the terminal acute phase, about 20% appear to retain the 46,Ph[1]+ cell line; additional abnormalities are superimposed on the Ph[1]+ line in 80% of patients (Rowley 1980a; Sandberg 1979). In a number of cases the change in the karyotype preceded the clinical signs of blast crisis by 2 to 4 months. Bone marrow chromosomes from 242 patients with Ph[1]+ CML who were in acute phase have been analyzed with banding techniques (Rowley 1980a). Forty showed no change in their karyotype, whereas 202 patients had additional chromosome abnormalities. The most common changes frequently occur in combination to produce modal numbers of 47 to 52. The chromosome aberrations observed most often are a gain of No. 8, a duplication of the Ph^1, an isochromosome for the long arm of No. 17, and a gain of No. 19.

Only two reports have been published relating specific chromosome changes in the acute phase to survival of patients, and the results are conflicting. Thus, Prigogina et al. (1978) found that patients who did not shown additional abnormalities in the acute phase had a longer survival than those whose karyotypes showed such changes. Sonta and Sandberg (1978), however, found no difference in survival between these two groups.

II. Ph^1-Positive Acute Leukemia

Our interpretation of the biologic significance of the Philadelphia chromosome has been modified over the course of the last nine years as our clinical experience with this marker has widened. Thus, earlier it was proposed that cases of acute myeloblastic leukemia (AML) in which the Ph^1 chromosome was present should be reclassified as cases of chronic myeloid leukemia in blast transformation. This notion, which was broadened to include the cases that appeared to be ALL at diagnosis, was generally accepted until about 1977. More recently, however the tendency has been to refer to patients who have no prior history suggestive of CML as having Ph^1-positive leukemia (Rowley 1980a). It is becoming increasingly evident that the observed interrelations of $Ph^1 +$ leukemias are complex indeed. Thus,

some patients have a high percentage of lymphoblasts, others have a high percentage of myeloblasts, and still others have a mixture of myeloblasts and lymphoblasts. In the future the use of cell surface markers will help to define these groups of patients further.

D. Acute Nonlymphocytic Leukemia

The use of chromosome banding techniques has markedly increased our understanding of the types and frequency of chromosome abnormalities in acute nonlymphocytic leukemia (ANLL), including AML, erythroleukemia, and acute monocytic leukemia. Extra, missing, or rearranged chromosomes previously described on the basis of morphology alone can now be identified precisely in terms of the particular chromosomes or chromosome bands involved. We and others have also shown that the karyotype pattern of the leukemic cells is correlated with survival. Patients with a normal karyotype have a significantly longer median survival (10 months) than do patients with an abnormal karyotype (4 months) (Golomb et al. 1978). As illustrated in Fig. 1, this difference in survival is more pronounced for AML than for acute myelomonocytic leukemia (AMMo1). Leukemic patients who are alive at 1 year are much more likely to have only normal metaphases.

Approximately 50% of the patients studied with banding have detectable karyotypic changes; these abnormalities are present prior to therapy and usually disappear when the patient enters remission. The same aberrations reappear in relapse, sometimes showing evidence of further karyotypic change superimposed on the original abnormal clone. Although the karyotypes of patients with ANLL may be variable, the chromosome changes in

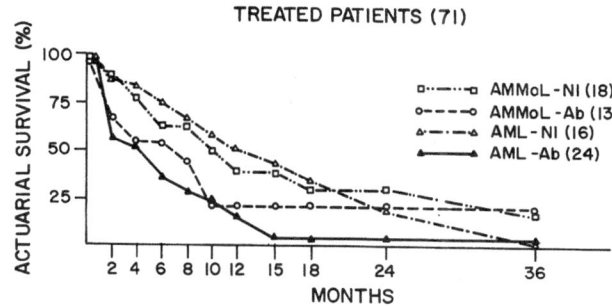

Fig. 1. Actuarial survival of treated patients versus time in months according to cytologic diagnosis (AML, AMMoL) and normal (Nl) or abnormal (Ab) karyotype. Reproduced from Golomb et al. (1978), with permission

191 chromosomally abnormal patients are available for analysis (Testa and Rowley 1980). Roughly one-third of the patients have 46 chromosomes but with an abnormal pattern, one-fourth have fewer than 46 chromosomes, and the remainder have 47 or more chromosomes. The nonrandom distribution of chromosome losses and gains is particularly evident in patients with 45–47 chromosomes. A gain of No. 8 is the most common abnormality in ANLL and loss of one No. 7 is the next most frequent change (Fig. 2). Gains or losses of some chromosomes occurred only in patients with more complex karyotypes; they are likely to represent secondary changes occurring in clonal evolution rather than primary events.

Two structural rearrangements seen in ANLL appear to have special significance. The more common of these was described as the complex pattern, $-C, +D, +E, -G$. The precise nature of the abnormality was resolved by Rowley (Rowley 1973b) who used the Q-banding technique to determine that it is a balanced translocation between Nos. 8 and 21 $[t(8;21)(q22;q22)]$. This translocation is frequently associated with loss of a sex chromosome, about one-third of males with the 8; 21 translocation are $-Y$, and one-third of the females are missing an X (Rowley 1973b; Second International Workshop on Chromosomes in Leukemia, 1980). This association is especially noteworthy, since sex chromosome abnormalities are otherwise rarely seen in ANLL. The translocation appears to be restricted to patients with acute myeloblastic leukemia (M_2 in the FAB classification). According to data collected at the Second International Workshop (Second International Workshop on Chromosomes in

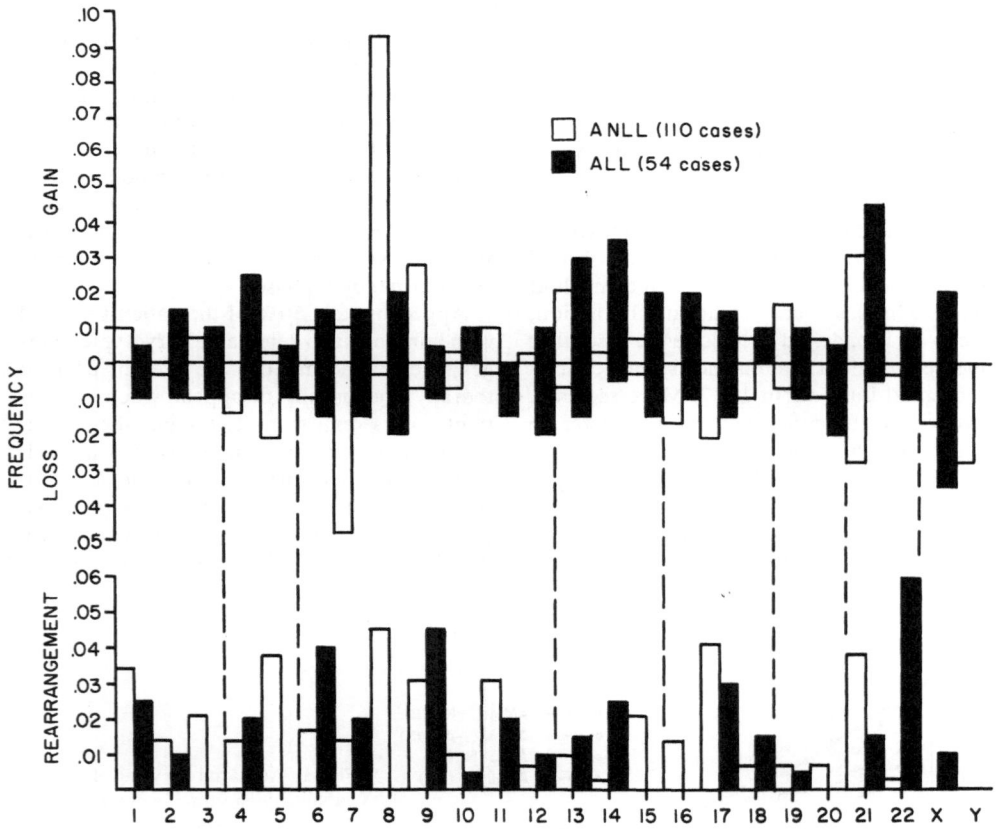

Fig. 2. Histogram of chromosome abnormalities (gains, losses, and rearrangements) in 110 cases of ANLL and in 54 cases of ALL, excluding documented cases of secondary karyotypic evolution. The frequency of each abnormality is calculated as a proportion of all abnormalities. Reproduced from Cimino et al. (1979), with permission

Leukemia, 1980), the median survival of patients with the t(8;21) was 11.5 months, with some subgroups having a median survival as long as 15 months.

Another significant structural rearrangement is that observed in acute promyelocytic leukemia (APL), which is a unique form of acute leukemia characterized by hemorrhagic episodes, disseminated intravascular coagulation (DIC), and infiltration of the marrow with atypical "hypergranular" promyelocytes. The FAB cooperative study group recently recognized that not all patients have coarse granules, and therefore it added a category called the M_3 variant. The variant category was identified largely on the basis of the clinical features and a specific chromosome abnormality, namely, a translocation involving the long arms of Nos. 15 and 17 [t(15;17)(q25;q22)] (Rowley et al. 1977; Second International Workshop on Chromosomes in Leukemia, 1980). It is important to make a correct early diagnosis because the initial therapy, which includes the use of heparin for control of bleeding, is associated with a significant improvement in survival. Whereas the correct diagnosis should not be difficult in typical cases, the M_3 variant, in which granules may be lacking or reduced in number, may cause confusion. Every one of our M_3, variant patients also had the typical translocation.

E. Acute Lymphoblastic Leukemia

Chromosome abnormalities have been observed in about one-half of the patients with ALL (Sandberg 1979). It has long been recognized that aneuploid patients with ALL have higher modal chromosome numbers than do patients with ANLL. Many fewer data are available on the types and frequency of chromosome changes in ALL than in ANLL.

Only two unselected series of patients with ALL, each studied with banding, have been reported; Oshimura et al. (1977) described results in 31 patients, and Cimino et al. (1979) described the results in 16 patients. There have been a number of other reports on one or a few patients, all selected for some unusual cytogenetic abnormalities, most frequently the presence of a Philadelphia (Ph¹) chromosome (Rowley 1980a). The small number of patients and the complexity of the karyotypes make the identification of nonrandom patterns in ALL

very difficult at present. Despite these handicaps, at least one karyotypic abnormality seems to be relatively specifically associated with one type of ALL classified with the use of immunologic markers. It seems reasonable to assume that other associations will become apparent in the future as we gain additional information about both the karyotypic pattern and the cell surface markers of subpopulations of lymphoid cells that will be defined with more sophisticated immunologic techniques.

The chromosome pattern in 53 patients with ALL has recently been reviewed (Rowley 1980b). The most frequent single change in this group is a gain of one No. 21; the second most frequent change is a gain of one No. 14, and the next most frequent is a gain of one No. 13 (Fig. 2). The only chromosome lost with any frequency is one X chromosome. Abnormalities of the Y chromosome have not been described. The most common deletion is that involving the long arm of No. 6; the break point in 6q appears to be somewhat variable, involving the region from 6q11 to 6q25.

Patients with B-cell ALL constitute a small percentage (about 4%) of those with ALL, and they are identified because their cells express surface immunoglobulin. With rare exceptions, every ALL patient whose leukemic cells have been identified as B-cells had an abnormality of No. 14 which was the result of a translocation of material from another chromosome to the end of the long arm (14q+) (Rowley 1980b). The 8;14 translocation was regularly seen in patients who also had a solid tumor phase of Burkitt's lymphoma (Berger et al. 1979; Slater et al. 1979). Other abnormalities in addition to the 14q+ chromosome have been trisomy for part or all of the long arm of No. 1, structural rearrangements involving both the long and short arms of No. 6, and an additional No. 7. Cells from some patients were examined for Epstein-Barr virus (EBV) and were found to be negative (Slater et al. 1979). In one patient the cells had a characteristically low level of adenosine deaminase (Cimino et al. 1979).

A 14q+ chromosome is a frequent occurence in other malignant lymphoproliferative diseases, particularly, though not exclusively, in those of B-cell origin. The translocation was first discovered in Burkitt lymphoma. A translocation involving the long arms of No. 8 and No. 14 has been detected in almost all Burkitt tumors of both African and non-African origin, independent of whether they are EBV-positive or -negative (Kaiser-McCaw et al. 1977; Zech et al. 1976). A 14q+ abnormality is rarely observed in myeloid disorders, and therefore the proposal that No. 14 may carry genes that are important in lymphocyte proliferation has been supported by all recent data (Kaiser-McCaw et al. 1977).

The data on chromosome patterns in ALL are only preliminary; however, some differences between the types of abnormalities seen in ANLL and ALL are apparent (Fig. 2). In ANLL the most common single change is a gain of one No. 8, followed by loss of No. 7 and rearrangements of No. 8 and No. 21 (Testa and Rowley 1980). Gain or loss of No. 21 is frequent, and loss of a sex chromosome, X or Y, usually occurs in association with structural aberrations of No. 8 or No. 21, or both. In ALL, the most common change is gain of one or two No. 21s, followed by gains of Nos. 13 or 14 and then gain of one No. 15 or an X, usually in males (Cimino et al. 1979). Two ALL patients showed the gain of one No. 8 initially, and evolution of the karyotype in three others involved the gain of one No. 8. The most frequent structural change in ALL is a deletion of No. 6, usually affecting the long arm. Rearrangements of No. 17 are often observed in both leukemias. In ANLL, gains of Nos. 6, 14, and 15 are rare and are seen only in patients with complex patterns; gain of the X has not been seen.

As described earlier, the presence of an abnormal clone of cells in patients with ANLL has a significant association with response to therapy and, therefore, with patient survival (Golomb et al. 1978). The lack of a sufficient number of ALL patients studied with banding makes such a correlation in patients with ALL difficult at the present time. Whang-Peng et al. (1976) related the unbanded karyotypic patterns to survival in 331 patients with ALL and concluded that "the appearance of aneuploid cells in the bone marrow at the onset or later in the disease is of no prognostic significance but persistence of these lines and the development of total aneuploidy signals a poor prognosis".

There are very few data relating the survival time of patients with ALL to the presence at diagnosis of clonal chromosome abnormalities identified with banding. Thus, in the series reported by Oshimura et al. (1977), length of

survival was listed only for patients with an abnormal karyotype, and one-half of these were treated prior to the chromosome analysis. The median survival of the eight abnormal patients whom they studied prior to treatment was 13 months. In our limited series at The University of Chicago (Cimino et al. 1979) the median survival of eight patients with an abnormal karyotype was 10+ months (range, 2 to 33 months), as compared with 23+ months (11 to 56+ months) for eight patients with an initially normal karyotype. The duration of the initial remission differed considerably, being only 1 month (0 to 18+ months) in chromosomally abnormal patients, whereas it was 12+ months (1.5 to 46+ months) in chromosomally normal patients.

However, in a recent report, Secker Walker et al. (1978) concluded that the presence of an abnormal clone was not an adverse factor. Of six patients who had only abnormal cells at diagnosis, one relapsed after 4 years and the others remained in first remission for a longer period than this. These data are relevant to the observations of Bloomfield et al. (1978) and Chessells et al. (1979) that the survival of patients with Ph^1-positive ALL is very short. The range is 2 to 24 months, with a median for both children and adults of about 12 months. This contrasts with a median survival of more than 2 years in adult Ph^1-negative ALL (Bloomfield et al. 1978). However, if one compares the median survival of patients with Ph^1+ ALL (12 months) with that of other ALL patients who have aneuploidy (10–13 months), the survival times are the same.

F. Conclusions

The primary focus in this review has been on the identification of nonrandom chromosome changes in various myeloproliferative and lymphoproliferative disorders. Although the data available for these disorders are quite variable both with regard to the number of patients studied and the quality of banding, patterns of chromosome changes can be discerned that differ among the various groups. Wherever possible these patterns have been related to structural and functional characteristics of these cells as determined by others as well as to the clinical correlations of particular chromosome changes. In the future these correlations must be extended to relate specific chromosome aberrations, particularly translocations and deletions, to alterations of the function of genes located at these sites.

References

Berger R, Bernheim A, Brouet JC, Daniel MT, Flandrin G (1979) t(8;14) translocation in a Burkitt's type of lymphoblastic leukaemia (L3). Br J Haematol 43:87–90 – Bloomfield CD, Lindquist LL, Brunning RD, Yunis JJ, Coccia PF (1978) The Philadelphia chromosome in acute leukemia. Virchows Archiv [Cell Pathol] 28:81–92 – Caspersson T, Gahrton G, Lindsten J, Zech L (1970) Identification of the Philadelphia chromosome as a number 22 by quinacrine mustard fluorescence analysis. Exp Cell Res 63:238–244 – Chessells JM, Janossy, G, Lawler SD, Secker Walker LM (1979) The Ph^1 chromosome in childhood leukaemia. Br J Haematol 41:25–41 – Cimino MC, Rowley JD, Kinnealey A, Variakojis D, Golomb HM (1979) Banding studies of chromosomal abnormalities in patients with acute lymphocytic leukemia. Cancer Res 39:227–238 – Golomb HM, Vardiman JW, Rowley JD, Testa JR, Mintz U (1978) Correlation of clinical findings with quinacrine-banded chromosomes in 90 adults with acute nonlymphocytic leukemia. N Engl J Med 299:613–619 – Kaiser-McCaw B, Epstein AL, Kaplan AL, Hecht F (1977) Chromosome 14 translocation in African and North American Burkitt's lymphoma. Int J Cancer 19:482–486 – Nowell PC, Hungerford DA (1960) A minute chromosome in human chronic granulocytic leukemia. Science 132:1197 – O'Riordan ML, Robinson JA, Buckton KE, Evans HJ (1971) Distinguishing between the chromosomes involved in Down's syndrome (trisomy 21 and chronic myeloid leukemia (Ph^1) by fluorescence. Nature 230:167–168 – Oshimura M, Freeman AI, Sandberg AA (1977) Chromosomes and causation of human cancer and leukemia. XXVI. Banding studies in acute lymphoblastic leukemia (ALL). Cancer 40:1161–1172 – Paris Conference (1972) Standardization in human cytogenetics. Birth Defects 8/7: – Prigogina EL, Fleischman EW, Volkova MA, Frenkel MA (1978) Chromosome abnormalities and clinical and morphologic manifestations of chronic myeloid leukemia. Hum Genet 41:143–156 – Rowley JD (1973a) A new consistent chromosomal abnormality in chronic myelogenous leukemia identified by quinacrine fluorescence and Giemsa staining. Nature 243:290–293 – Rowley JD (1973b) Identification of a translocation with quinacrine fluorescence in a patient with acute leukemia. Ann Genet (Paris) 16:109–111 – Rowley JD (1980a) Ph^1 positive leukaemia, including chronic myelogenous leukaemia. Clin Haematol 9:55–86 – Rowley JD (1980b) Chromosome abnormalities in acute lymphoblastic leukemia. Cancer Genet Cytogenet 1:263–271 – Rowley JD, Golomb HM, Vardiman J, Fukuhara S, Dougherty C, Potter D (1977) Further evidence for a non-random chromosomal abnormality in acute promyelocytic leukemia. Int J Cancer 20:869–872 – Sandberg AA (1979) Chromosomes in Human Cancer and Leukemia. Elsevier/North-Holland, New York – Secker Walker LM, Lawler SD, Hardisty RM (1978) Prognostic implications of chromosomal findings in acute lymphoblastic leukaemia at diagnosis. Br J Med 2:1529–1530 – Second International Workshop on Chromosoms in Leukemia. Cancer Genet Cytogenet (1980) 2: 89–113 – Slager RM, Philip P, Badsberg E, Behrendt H, Hansen NE, Heerde PV (1979) A 14q+ chromosome in a B-cell acute lymphocytic leukemia and in a leukemic non-endemic Burkitt lymphoma. Int J Cancer 23:639–647 – Sonta S, Sandberg AA (1978) Chromosomes and causation of human cancer and leukemia. XXIX. Further studies on karyotypic progression in CML. Cancer 41:153–163 – Testa JR, Rowley JD (1980) Chromosomal banding patterns in patients with acute nonlymphocytic leukemia. Cancer Genet Cytogenet 1:239–247 – Testa JR, Rowley JD (to be published) Chromosomes in leukemia and lymphoma with special emphasis on methodology. In: Catovsky D (ed) The leukemic cell. Churchill-Livingston, Edinburgh – Whang-Peng J, Canellos GP, Carbone PP, Tjio HH (1968) Clinical implications of cytogenetic variants in chronic myelocytic leukemia (CML). Blood 32:755–766 – Whang-Peng J, Knutsen T, Ziegler J, Leventhal B (1976) Cytogenetic studies in acute lymphocytic leukemia: Special emphasis in longterm survival. Med Pediatr Oncol 2:333–351 – Zech L, Hoglund U, Nilsson K, Klein G (1976) Characteristic chromosomal abnormalities in biopsies and lymphoid-cell lines from patients with Burkitt and non-Burkitt lymphomas. Int J Cancer 17:47–56

Haematology and Blood Transfusion Vol. 26
Modern Trends in Human Leukemia IV
Edited by Neth, Gallo, Graf, Mannweiler, Winkler
© Springer-Verlag Berlin Heidelberg 1981

Myeloid Dysplasia: the Histopathology of Preleukemia*

A. Georgii, J. Thiele, and K.-F. Vykoupil

The clinical term "preleukemia" is understood as an alteration of the bone marrow and peripheral blood preceding overt acute myeloid leukemia (AML, review by Saarni and Linman 1973). However, in the majority of cases the diagnosis is only a retrospective one, derived from many mostly clinical and cytogenetic investigations (Fisher et al 1973; Dreyfus 1976; Linman and Bagby 1978; Pierre 1978). The aim of our study was to determine whether there are characteristic lesions of the bone marrow preceding obvious leukemia and if wether those lesions are similar in cases evolving AML or CML later on.

Among more than 15,000 biopsies of the bone marrow which were performed during the last 10 years 195 patients were selected whose examination of the bone marrow was initiated by the clinical assumption of a possible preleukemic state. This selection following the suggested clinical diagnosis of so-called preleukemia inherits a problem: there may be no clear cut separation between a preleukemic state of leukemia and a myeloproliferative disorder or CML in early stage or chronic megakaryocytic-granulocytic myelosis (CMGM, see Georgii 1979).

A re-evaluation of the semithin sections of these bone cylinders displayed two different categories of disorders: 62 patients had either nonneoplastic lesions (leukemoid reaction, 12; hyperergic myelitis (mostly rheumatic), 23; pernicious anemia, 11; panmyelophthisis, 3 and other diseases 13 or early stage CML 35 and oligoblastic leukemia 5. The remaining second category of 93 patients showed distinc-

tive and identical morphological features of the bone marrow which probably correspond to hemopoietic dysplasia of Linman and Bagby (1978), but should be rather called myeloid dysplasia, MD, (Thiele et al. 1980a): Histopathology is characterized by a hypercellularity (Fig 1a) in most of the cases, a frequently occurring megaloblastoid and at least macrocytic differentiation of erythropoiesis (Figs. 1b, 2a). There are many sideroblasts of the granular type and a shift to the left of the neutrophilic granulopoiesis which displays the so called pseudo-Pelger-Huët anomaly of maturation (Figs. 2a,b). It should be emphasized that there is no increase in blasts along the peritrabecular generation zones of granulopoiesis. Megakaryocytes are not only increased but exhibit abnormal cells such as frequent naked nuclei, micromegakaryocytes, and too many immature forms (Figs. 1a, 2b). The myeloid stroma contains a patchy edema and often a remarkable perivascular plasmacytosis (Figs. 1a, 2c). Electron microscopy of these cell confirms these findings and extends our results of an abnormal cellular differentiation in MD (for details see Thiele et al. to be published a).

Of these 93 patients with the histomorphology of MD at the time of their first and initial biopsy, sequential corings of the iliac crest (up to five times in periods ranging from 2 months to 3½ years) as well as review of the clinical records revealed that 26 cases evolved obvious leukemia and the remaining 67 did not show apparent leukemia until now (Table 1).

Initial main clinical symptoms were mostly unspecific, ranging from fatigue, loss of weight, easy bleeding, and pallor to physical findings such as dermal hemorrhage, slight to moderate hepatomegaly, and minimal splenomegaly.

* Supported by the Deutsche Forschungsgemeinschaft (DFG Ge 121/19)

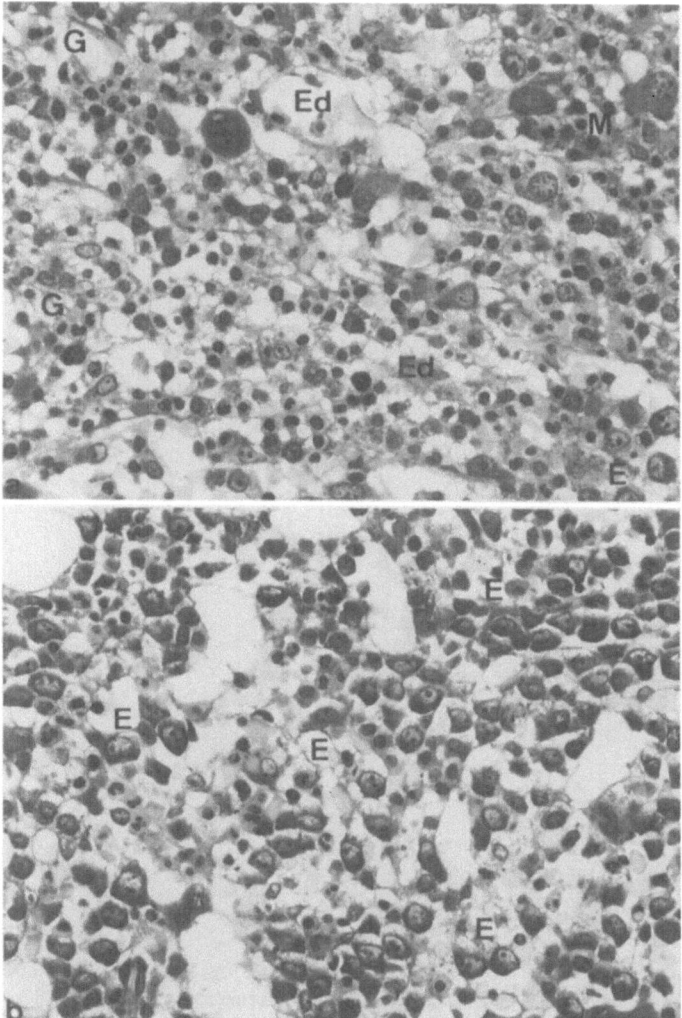

Fig. 1a,b. Survey of myeloid dysplasia in semithin sections of plastic embedded trephine biopsies. **a** Low magnification with patchy edema of the stroma *(Ed)*, a macrocytic/megaloblastoid erythropoiesis *(E)*, abnormal megakaryopoiesis *(M)* and dispersed neutrophilic granulopoesis *(G)*. **b** The higher magnification shows the prominent megaloblastoid differentiation of erythropoiesis *(E)*. a×234, b×256

Statistical evaluation of principle hematological data showed that median values of the retrospective group – regardless wether AML or CML was the evolving disease – and the prospective group showed no significant differences (for details see Thiele et al., to be published b). Median values of these data accompanying MD of 75 patients (retrospective and prospective group) are listed in Table 2.

Our results demonstrate that common morphological alterations exist in the bone marrow before onset of AML and CML and that they are associated with a normochromic anemia and a slight to moderate pancytopenia of the peripheral blood count. The clinical as well as statistical evaluation of our retrospective and prospective groups of patients confirms this statement (Thiele et al., to be published b). The term "preleukemia" should therefore be replaced by MD, which does not necessarily imply evolution towards leukemia in every case but refers also to CML. Hemopoietic dysplasia as proposed by Linman and Bagby (1978) only pertains to the hematopoietic cells and does not include the changes of the mesenchymal cells and stroma nor the development of chronic myeloproliferative disorders such as CML. The maturation defects of erythro- and granulopoiesis are in agreement with the megaloblastoid differention observed in aplastic or so-called iron refractory anemia or preleukemia (Saarni and Linman 1973;

Retrospective group		Prospective group
26/93 evolved leukemia with the following histological categories:		0 / 67
		Deadline of this study was 1 February 1980; no leukemia among the 67 patients observed so far –
AML	11	
CML	9	
CML with blastic crisis	6	
	26	

Table 1. 93 patients who showed myeloid dysplasia (MD) in the first and initial biopsy of the bone marrow

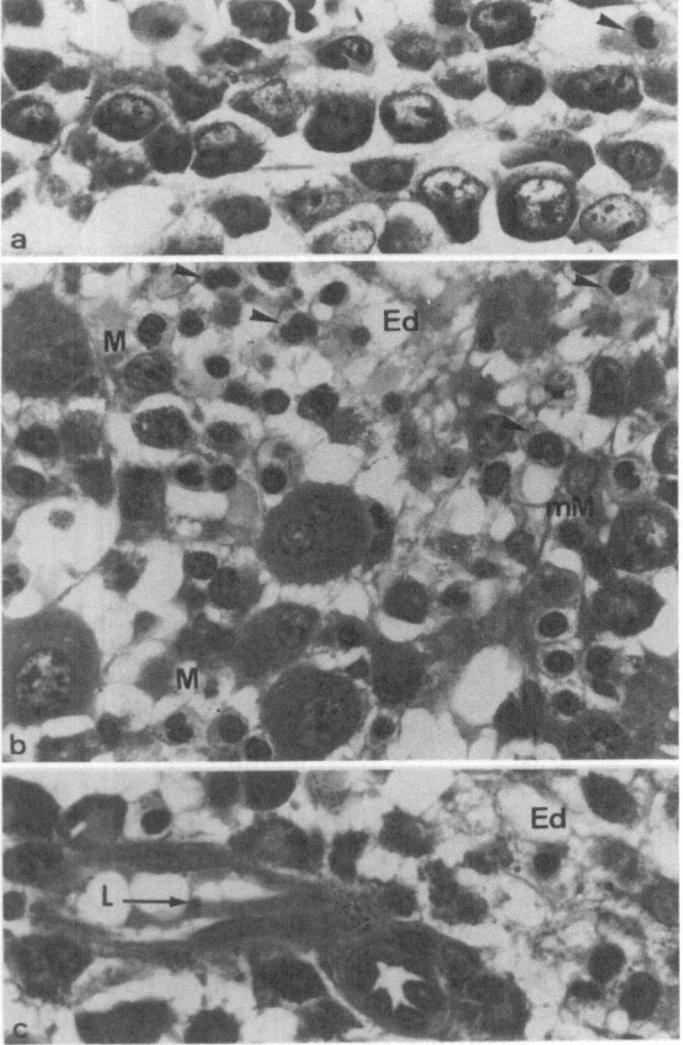

Fig. 2a–c. Conspicuous abnormalities in myeloid dysplasia. **a** Megaloblasts with linear deployment along a sinus wall and a so-called Pelger form of neutrophils *(arrow head,* see below). **b** Atypia of neutrophilic granulopoesis with hyposegmentation of nuclei associated with mature cytoplasm (pseudo-Pelgerforms, *arrow heads).* Megakaryopoiesis *(M)* with immature forms and micromegakaryocytes *(mM).* There is also also a patchy edema of the stroma *(Ed).* **c** Perivascular plasmacytosis along a marrow capillary with lumen *(L)* and prominent endothelial cells surrounded by edema *(Ed).* a–c×792

Total	75		Hb$_E$	30.3 pg
Sex	33M/42F		Leukocytes	3.9×10^3 µl
age	66 years		Neutrophils	47%
ESR	28/89 (Westergren)		Monocytes	3%
Erythrocytes	$3.0 \times 10^6/\mu l$		Platelets	141×10^3 µl
Hemoglobin	9.1g/dl			

Table 2. Clinical findings in 75 patients with myeloid dysplasia (MD) at the time of their first biopsy (median values)

Maldonado et al. 1976) as well as the frequent pseudo-Pelger forms (Linman and Bagby 1978), results which in the majority are derived from aspirates of the bone marrow. These morphological atypia account for the functional disturbances of colony formation and iron metabolism as demonstrated in "preleukemic" states by several authors (Golde and Gline 1973; Senn et al. 1976; Hast and Reizenstein 1977; Koeffler 1978). Cytogenetic studies may be of a major value to establish or confirm the diagnosis of a possible preleukemic condition as shown by Pierre (1978) and our findings of a Philadelphia-chromosome occurring before obvious CML in four cases (Thiele et al., 1979).

References

Dreyfus B (1976) Preleukemic states. I. Definition and classification. II. Refractory anemia with a excess of myeloblasts in the bone marrow (smoldering acute leukemia). Blood Cells 2:33–55 – Fisher WB, Armentrout SA, Weisman R, Graham RC (1973) "Preleukemia" A myelodysplastic syndrome often terminating in acute leukemia. Arch Intern Med 132:226–232 – Georgii A (1979) Histopathology of bone marrow in human chronic leukemias. In: Neth, R (eds) Modern trends in human leukemias III. Berlin Heidelberg New York, Springer, pp 60–70 – Golde DW, Cline MJ (1973) Human preleukemia.

Identification of a maturation defect in vitro. N Engl J Med 28821:1083–1086 – Hast R, Reizenstein P (1977) Studies on human preleukaemia. I. Erythroblast and iron kinetics in aregenerative anaemia with hypercellular bone marrow. Scand J Haematol 19:347–354 – Koeffler HP, Golde DW (1978) Cellular maturation in human preleukemia. Blood 52:355–361 – Linman JW, Bagby GC (1978) Preleukemic syndrome (hemopoietic dysplasia). Cancer 42:854–864 – Maldonado JE, Maigne J, Lecoq D (1976) Comparative electronmicroscopic study of the erythrocytic line in refractory anemia (preuleukemia) and myelomonocytic leukemia. Blood Cells 2:167–185 – Pierre RV (1978) Preleukemic syndromes Virchows Arch [Cell Pathol] 29:29–37 – Saarni, MI, Linman, JW (1973) Preleukemia. The hematologic syndrome preceding acute leukemia. Am J Med 55:38–48 – Senn JS, Price GB, Mak TW, McCulloch EA (1976) An approach to human preleukemia using cell culture studies. Blood Cells 2:161–166 – Thiele J, Vykoupil KF, Georgii A (1979) Präleukämien: Knochenmarks- und Chromosomenbefunde zum Versuch einer Definition. Verh. Dtsch Ges Path f 63:372–379 – Thiele J, Vykoupil KF, Georgii A (1980a) Myeloid dysplasia (MD): A hematological disorder preceding acute and chronic myeloid leukemia. A morphological study on sequential core biopsies of the bone marrow in 27 patients. Virchows Arch, A, [Pathol Anat] 389:343–367 – Thiele J,.Vykoupil KF, Perschke B, Babilas J, Török M, Krmpotic E, Bodenstein H, Georgii A (to be published b) Preleukaemic lesions of the bone marrow or myeloid dysplasia (MD): Morphological and clinical features in a combined retro- and prospective study of 93 patients.

Haematology and Blood Transfusion Vol. 26
Modern Trends in Human Leukemia IV
Edited by Neth, Gallo, Graf, Mannweiler, Winkler
© Springer-Verlag Berlin Heidelberg 1981

Progress in Acute Myeologenous Leukemia

T. A. Lister, S. A. N. Johnson, R. Bell, G. Henry, and J. S. Malpas

A. Introduction

Experimental and potentially life threatening combination chemotherapy has been used for the induction of remission of acute myelogenous leukaemia (AML) for a little over 10 years. During that time the proportion of patients entering remission has risen from less than a quarter to approaching three-quarters. Furthermore, there is now evidence to suggest that about one-fifth of those now entering remission will remain disease free for more than 3 years and be "at risk for cure".

Between 1969 and 1980 588 consecutive adults with AML were treated at St. Bartholomew's Hospital, 443 of them in prospective trials. Selected data from these studies, which have been reported in part elsewhere (Crowther et al. 1973; Powles et al. 1977; Lister et al. 1980) are presented to illustrate what has been learnt during the last decade and to provide a new base line, instead of the natural history of the disease, with which to compare future studies.

B. Materials and Methods

I. Patients

Five hundred and eighty-eight consecutive adults were treated for AML at St. Bartholomew's Hospital between June 1969 and July 1980. Four hundred and forty-three were treated on prospective trials of combination chemotherapy. Exclusions from the trials were made because of advanced age and extensive prior chemotherapy. No patient under the age of 60 years who had not received therapy was excluded. Clinical details of the patients entered in to the different trials are shown in Tables 1–3.

II. Treatment Programmes

Three generations of combination chemotherapy experiments have been undertaken since 1969: in each of them cytosine arabinoside and an anthracycline antibiotic have been the central component of the treatment. At the outset, adults of all ages were treated the same (Trials I, II, III). For the duration of Trials IVA–VIII patients of more than 60 years of age were treated in a separate programme (Trial IVB). This policy was reversed in 1978 at the beginning of Trial IX, since which time adults of all ages have received the same initial therapy. Antibio-

Table 1. Patient details. n = 443; Sex M:F = 243:200

Age	Range	14–77 years
	Mean	49 years
	Median	53 years
Platelet count	Range	5–704
	Mean	69.89
	Median	45
Blast count	Range	0–495.0
	Mean	29.76
	Median	3.8

Table 2. Morphological variants

FAB classification	No. of patients
M1	108
M2	109
M3	27
M4	138
M5	39
M6	22
Total	443

Table 3. Patient entry and exclusions

Date	Trial	No.	Non-trial		Total
			Prior chemotherapy	Transfusion only	
June 1969–July 1970	Barts I	41	6	7	54
August 1970–February 1971	Barts II	20	0	2	22
February 1971–July 1972	Barts III	55	5	10	70
July 1972–April 1973	Barts IVA	37	0	0	37
May 1973–June 1974	Barts V	36	10	9	55
July 1974–November 1974	Barts VII	18	4	3	25
November 1974–February 1978	Barts VIII	86	0	0	86
August 1974–February 1978	Barts IVB	59	31	57	147
March 1978–July 1980	Barts IX, X	91	1	0	92
Total		443	57	88	588

tic and blood component therapy have changed gradually during the decade and are outlined in Table 4.

C. Results

I. Response to Initial Therapy

Complete remission was achieved in 187 out of 443 (42%). The two most important factors correlating with the response to therapy were the age of the patient at presentation and the initial treatment received (Table 5). The complete remission rate was significantly higher for patients under the age of 60 than those of 60 years and older ($P=0.003$). It was also significantly highest for patients receiving intensive chemotherapy comprising adriamycin, cytosine arabinoside and 6-thioguanine (ACT II), especially in the under 60 age group.

Thrombocytopenia at presentation was

Table 4. Initial therapy

Trial	Remission induction	Programme name	Continuation therapy	Antibiotics		Platelet support
				Prophylactic	Therapeutic	
I, II, IVA, V	Daunorubicin[a] cytosine arabinoside[b]	DR+Ara-C	CT[d]±IT	–	Ampicillin+ Flucloxicillin	Fresh blood
II, III	Kinetic modification of DR+Ara-C	DR+ Ara-C(KM)	CT±IT	–	Ampicillin+ Flucloxicillin	Pooled platelets
IVB	Intensification of DR+Ara-C	DR+Ara-C(I)	CT±IT	–	Ampicillin+ Flucloxicillin	
VIII	Adriamycin, vincristine prednisolone, cytosine arabinoside[e]	AD-OAP	CT+IT	FRACON[e]	Aminoglycoside +Carbenicillin or Cephazolin	Single donor
X[f]	Adriamycin, cytosine arabinoside, thioguanine[a]	ACT I	None	None	Aminoglycoside +Cephazolin	Single donor
IX[f]	Adriamycin, cytosine arabinoside, thioguanine[a]	ACT II	None	FRACON[e]		Single donor

[a] Bell et al. (to be published)
[b] Crowther et al. (1973)
[c] Lister et al. (1980)
[d] CT=Chemotherapy; II=Immunotherapy
[e] Schimpff et al. (1975)
[f] ACT I more intensive than ACT II

39

Treatment		<60	≥60	Total	
DR+Ara-C	I III IVA V	69/148 (47%)	5/21 (24%)	74/169	(44%)
DR+Ara-C modifications	II	5/13 (39%)	2/7 (29%)	7/20	(35%)
	VII	3/18 (17%)	–	3/18	(17%)
	IVB	–	19/59 (29%)	15/59	(29%)
AD-OAP	VIII	39/86 (45%)	–	39/86	(45%)
ACT I	X	11/27 (40%)	4/14 (29%)	15/41	(37%)
ACT II	IX	29/36 (80%)	5/14 (36%)	34/50	(68%)
Total		156/328 (48%)	31/115 (27%)	187/443	(42%)

Table 5. Response to initial treatment. ACT II vs DR+Ara-C: $P=<0.02$; ACT II vs ACT I: $P=<0.05$; and ACT II vs AD-OAP: $P=<0.05$

a poor prognostic factor overall, with complete remission only being achieved in 29 out of 96 patients in whom the platelet count was less than $20 \times 10^9/l$ compared with 158 out of 347 ($P=0.05$) in whom it was more. However, since the introduction of the routine use of platelet concentrates in Trial VIII this prognostic difference has disappeared, with complete remission being achieved in 18 out of 42 patients in whom the platelet count was less than $20 \times 10^9/l$ compared with 70 out of 135 in whom it was more ($P=$n.s) in Trials VIII, IX and X bombined.

II. Duration of First Complete Remission

Out of 187 patients in whom complete remission was achieved 50 are alive without relapse and three died in complete remission, one of coliform septicaemia during consolidation, one (aged 70) of myocardial infarction and one

in a car accident (Fig. 1). No patient has relapsed so far after 5 years.

D. Possible Factors Influencing Duration of First Complete Remission

I. Intensity of the Initial Therapy

Comparison of the duration of first remission in patients receiving Daunorubicin and cytosine arabinoside (Trials I, III, IVA and V) with those receiving AD-OAP (Trial VIII), ACT I (Trial X) and ACT II (Trial IX) show a significant advantage over those receiving ACT I and all the rest and a significant advantage of AD-OAP over those receiving daunorubicin and cytosine arabinoside (Fig. 2). The intensity of treatment had increased with each change of chemotherapy (see Table 4).

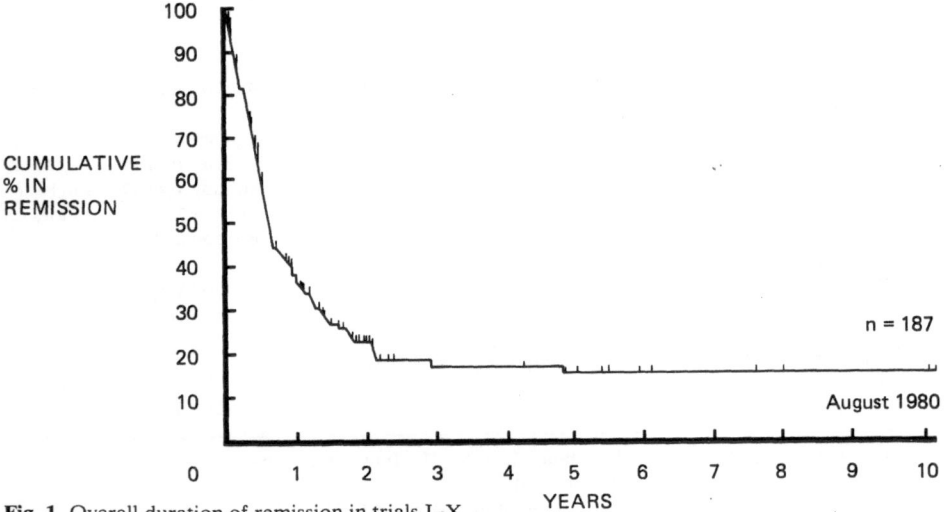

CUMULATIVE % IN REMISSION

n = 187

August 1980

YEARS

Fig. 1. Overall duration of remission in trials I–X

40

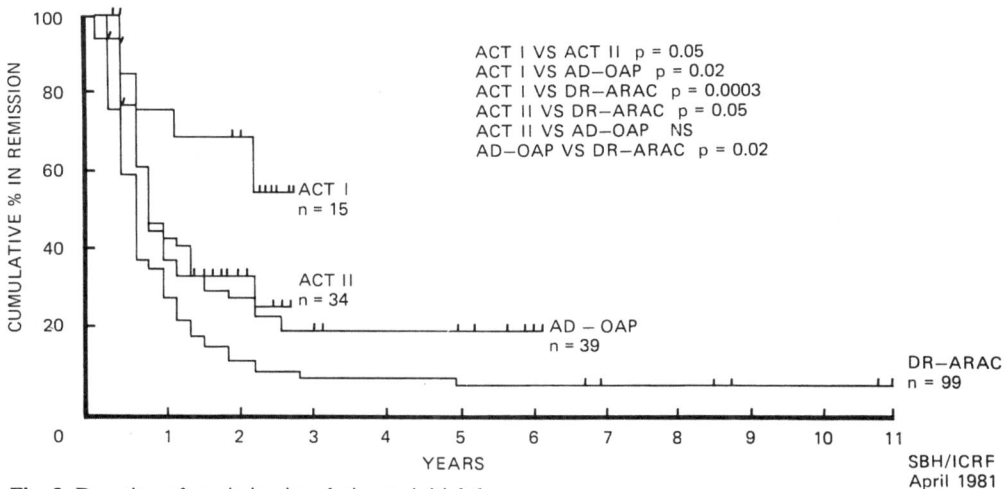

Fig. 2. Duration of remission in relation to initial therapy

SBH/ICRF
April 1981

II. Continuation Therapy

Four different types of continuation therapy were used: –

1. None (Trials IX and X);
2. Chemotherapy alone [Trials II, III and IVA (randomised study)];
3. Chemotherapy and "immunotherapy" comprising BCG and allogeneic blast cells: Trials II, III, IVA (randomised study), Trial V (all patients), and Trial VIII (randomised study); and
4. Chemotherapy and immunotherapy with BCG [Trial VIII (randomised study)].

Comparison of the duration of remission of these four groups demonstrates no advantage for continuation of therapy after consolidation (Fig. 3). The group with the best duration of remission was in fact that receiving no continuation therapy but the most intensive initial (remission induction and consolidation) treatment. There are not, however, comparisons between concurrently randomised groups of patients and the follow up is shortest in the group with the most favourable result.

The different "immunizing" manœuvres, with the addition of either BCG alone or BCG and allogeneic blast cells, did not confer any

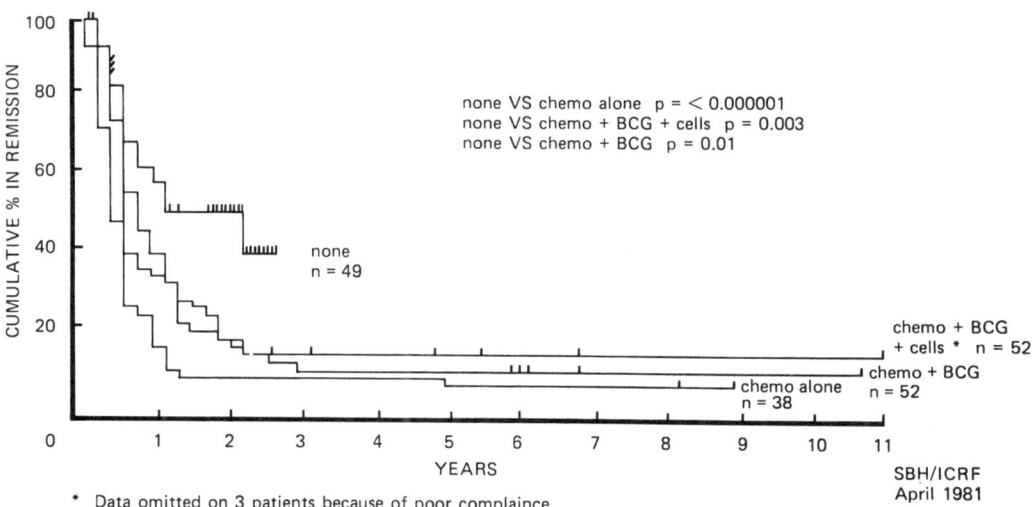

* Data omitted on 3 patients because of poor complaince

SBH/ICRF
April 1981

Fig. 3. Duration of remission influence of continuation therapy

advantage in terms of duration of first complete remission.

None of the other factors analysed, particularly age (or inital physical findings, blast count, platelet count, blast cell morphology) correlated with the duration of first complete remission.

E. Survival

The most important factor determining survival was the outcome of initial therapy (Fig. 4). Sixty-two patients remain alive between 3 months and 11 years.

F. Long Survival

Thirty-six patients have lived more than 3 years. Only 2 out of 13 cases who were in first complete remission at that time have subsequently relapsed, the latter at 4.5 years. An additional four patients recurred within 6 months of the first remission, entered second remission and have remained disease free subsequently for a minimum of 4 years. Detailed analysis of the presentation features of these patients reveals them to be a heterogenous group with no specific factors in common other than long survival.

G. Discussion

The results of combination chemotherapy for adults with AML at St. Bartholomew's Hospital have been presented. They confirm the trend reported by others (Keating et al., to be published; Priester et al. 1980; Gale and Cline 1977; Rees et al. 1977; Mayer et al. see this volume) that intensification of early therapy can result in complete remission being achieved in the majority of adults under the age of 60. It is important to qualify this with the rider that intensification of the cytotoxic chemotherapy without adequate supportive care is valueless. This is clear from the results of Trial VIII, in which the initial treatment was intensified. The routine use of platelet concentrates and powerful antibiotic combinations obliterated the prognostic disadvantage of thrombocytopenia and infectious complications at presentation. However, the management of infection during the neutrophil nadir was not adequate with a high incidence of fatal gram negative infection, especially in patients not receiving gastrointestinal tract decontamination. The apparent advantage of this was not appreciated until a similar high incidence of fatal gram negative infection was observed in Trials IX and X (Rohatiner et al. 1981). The high complete remission rate for patients under 60 in Trial IX (ACT II) was achieved against a background of more intensive sup-

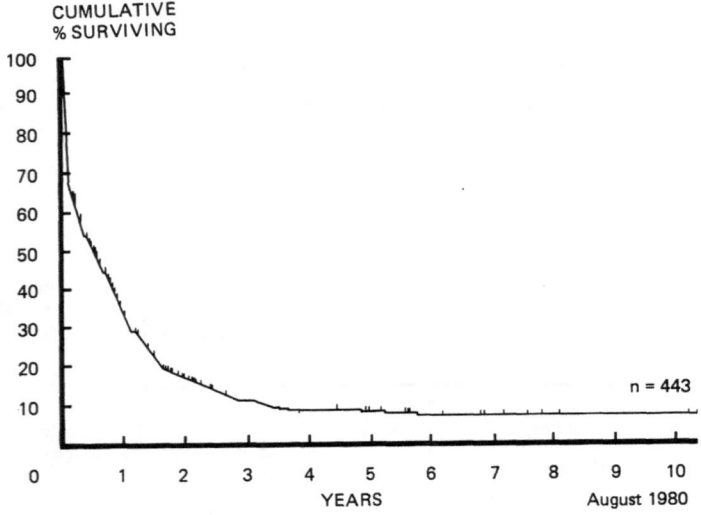

Fig. 4. Overall survival in trials in 1–10

portive care, including the use of gastro intestinal tract decontamination, aggressive antibiotic therapy for fever as before, and scrupulous attention to the increased incidence of pneumonia. The use of transtracheal aspiration has made it possible to obtain bacterial isolates and thus potentially influence antibiotic therapy in approximately 50% of the patients with suspected chest infection from whom sputum could not be obtained (Slevin et al.1981).

Early analysis of the most recent Trials (IX, X) suggest that the intensity of the very early therapy is critical to the duration of remission. It is not possible to comment yet on the relevance of "consolidation" therapy, although there is some evidence to support the contention that "early intensification" improves the duration of remission (Bell et al., to be published). The role of maintenance or continuation (philosophically more attractive) therapy has certainly not been established. However, the comparisons made have not all been concurrent nor has identical early therapy been used in all the studies analysed.

As in all other reported series, a very close correlation between the response to initial therapy and survival has been observed. The obvious corollary of this, namely that overall survival in all studies must now be better than previously since the complete remission rate is so much higher, has yet to be established. There is, however, no doubt that long survival has never been seen in patients in whom the bone marrow is not returned to normal. Extensive analysis of those patients surviving more than 3 years has revealed a wealth of negative correlations between presentation features and survival with only a suspicion that the intensity of the early therapy is important. This is based solely on the fact that a high proportion of the long survivors were treated in the Trial VIII study and must be tempered by the fact that this is the most recent study, by definition, in which long survivors have occurred. Further long follow up is obviously required.

In spite of all these reservations, we believe that these results should be viewed with optimism. Ten years ago the major publications on this subject were only able to record, with justifiable optimism, that it was possible to achieve remission in AML and that it should be treated with curative intent. The data presented here in complete concordance with that of others (Ellison and Glidewell 1979;

Keating et al., to be published) show that a significant proportion will live at least 3 years. Exciting experiments with bone marrow transplantation, both in terms of eradication of leukaemia and mismatched grafting, further manipulation of chemotherapy and the design of good clinical experiments may lead to the speculation of the seventies becoming the reality of the eighties.

Acknowledgments

The authors are pleased to acknowledge the contribution of the technical and clerical staff of the Departments of Medical Oncology and Haematology and the expert care provided by the nursing and medical staff of Dalziel and Annie Zunz Wards. The manuscript was typed by Miss Jill Davey.

References

Bell R, Rohatiner AZS, Ford J, Slevin ML, Amess J, Malpas JS, Lister TA (to be published) Short term therapy for acute myelogenous leukaemia – Crowther D, Powles RL, Bateman CJT, Beard MEJ, Gauci CL, Wrigley PFM, Malpas JS, Hamilton Fairley G, Bodley Scott R (1973) Management of adult acute myelogenous leukaemia. Br Med J 1:131–137 – Ellison RR, Glidewell 0 (1979) Improved survival in adults with acute myelocytic leukaemia. Proc Am Assoc Cancer Res 20:651 – Gale RP, Cline MJ (1977) High remission-induction rate in acute myeloid leukaemia. Lancet 1:497–499 – Keating MJ, Smith TC, McCredie KB (to be published) A four year experience with Anthracycline, Cytosine Arabinoside, Vincristine and Prednisone combination chemotherapy in 325 adults with acute leukaemia. Cancer – Lister TA, Whitehouse JMA, Oliver RTD, Bell R, Johnson SAN, Wrigley PFM, Ford JM, Cullen MH, Gregory W, Paxton AM, Malpas JS (1980) Chemotherapy and immunotherapy for acute myelogenous leukaemia. Cancer 46:2142–2148 – Powles RL, Russell J, Lister TA, Oliver RTD, Whitehouse JMA, Malpas JS, Chapuis B, Crowther D, Alexander P (1977) Immunotherapy for acute myelogenous leukaemia. A controlled clinical study 2½ years after entry of last patient. Br J Cancer 35:265–275 – Priesler H, Browman G, Henderson E, Hryniuk W, Freeman A (1980) Treatment of acute myelocytic leukaemia. Effects of early intensive consolidation. Proc. ASCO 21:C-493 – Rees JKH, Sandler RM, Challender J, Hayhoe FGJ (1977) Treatment of acute myeloid leukaemia with a triple cytotoxic regime: DAT. Br J Cancer 36:770–776 – Rohatiner AZS, Lowes LA, Lister TA (1981) Infection in acute myelogenous leukaemia. An analysis of 168 patients. Journal of Hospital Infection, in press – Slevin ML, Lowes A, Bell R, Catto-Smith A, Ford JM, Malpas JS, Lister TA (1981) The role of transtracheal aspiration in the diagnosis of respiratory infection in neutropenic patients with acute leukaemia. Leukemia Research 5:165–168 – Schimpff SC, Green WH, Young VM, Fratner CC, Jepson J, Cusack N (1975) Infection prevention in acute non-lymphocytic leukaemia. Laminar air flow room reverse isolation with oral non-absorbable antibiotic prophylaxis. Ann Intern Med 82:351–358

Haematology and Blood Transfusion Vol. 26
Modern Trends in Human Leukemia IV
Edited by Neth, Gallo, Graf, Mannweiler, Winkler
© Springer-Verlag Berlin Heidelberg 1981

VAPA[10]: A Treatment Program for Acute Myelocytic Leukemia*

R. J. Mayer, H. J. Weinstein, D. S. Rosenthal, F. S. Coral, D. G. Nathan and E. Frei, III

A. Introduction

During the past decade, the combination of an anthracycline and continuous infusion cytosine arabinoside chemotherapy has been associated with an increase in the complete response rate of patients under age 60 having acute myelocytic leukemia (AML) from 35%–55% (Carey et al. 1975; Clarkson et al. 1975) to approximately 75% (Evans et al. 1975; Gale 1979; Haghbin et al. 1977; Preisler et al. 1979; Rees and Hayhoe 1978; Yates et al. 1973). This encouraging advance, however, has not led to prolonged periods of remission and indefinite survival as seen in childhood acute lymphocytic leukemia. The median duration of complete remission in most recent studies in AML is in the range of 12–14 months (Armitage and Burns 1976; Evans et al. 1975; Haghbin et al. 1977; Moreno et al. 1977; Peterson and Bloomfield 1977; Preisler et al. 1979; Rees and Hayhoe 1978; Spiers et al. 1977). In early 1976 a therapeutic program (VAPA[10] protocol) was initiated in an attempt to overcome the causes of relapse in patients with AML. It was postulated that the high failure rate in AML patients in complete remission might be the result of inadequate cytoreduction during the maintenance period, the development of drug resistance, the presence of "sanctuaries" into which effective chemotherapy could not penetrate, and the presence of a mutant myeloid progenitor cell which over a period of time would progressively replace or even suppress the growth of the differentiated product of normal hematopoiesis. It was appreciated that if the latter possibility were true, it would be unlikely that intensive chemotherapy would have any long-term beneficial effect in patients with AML and that the only rational therapeutic option would be replacement of these progenitor cells through a maneuver such as bone marrow transplantion. Others are presently testing the utility of marrow transplantation in patients with AML shortly after complete remission is obtained (Blume et al. 1980; Powles et al. 1980; Thomas et al. 1979).

This report reviews the status of the VAPA[10] protocol at the time of an 1 April 1980 analysis. The protocol, designed with curative intent, has resulted in a complete remission rate of 70%. Among the complete responders, it is projected that $71\% \pm 13\%$ of the patients will be alive 24 months after diagnosis was made. and $49\% \pm 17\%$ will continue disease free 24 months after their initial complete remission was documented.

B. Materials and Methods

I. Patients

One hundred and six consecutive previously untreated patients less than 50 years of age with AML were evaluated and entered onto this study between February 1976 and 1 April 1980. The diagnosis of AML was based on examination of bone marrow aspirate morphology and histochemical stains. When such a diagnosis was confirmed, patients were entered onto the program and all patients receiving any amount of protocol drug therapy, regardless of their clinical condition, were considered evaluable for analysis.

* Supported in part by Grants CA 22719, CA 17700, and CA 17979, National Institutes of Health, Bethesda, Maryland 20014

II. Treatment Program

Chemotherapy consisted of two phases: a remission induction phase followed by an intensive sequential combination chemotherapy phase. The remission induction program (Fig. 1) was similar to the treatment plan of others, administering 3 days of an anthracycline (adriamycin) and 7 days of continuous infusion cytosine arabinoside with the addition of vincristine and prednisolone. Marrow status was assessed on the 14th day of the treatment program with another 5 days of therapy instituted at that time if the bone marrow was hypercellular or if leukemic blasts were still readily identifiable. Patients were removed from study and considered induction therapy failures if they did not achieve complete remission following these two courses of therapy.

Patients who achieved complete remission were treated with intensive sequential combination chemotherapy during a 14-month "maintenance" period (Fig. 2). This period of treatment was subdivided into four sequences of drug combinations. Sequence I, designated as "early intensification", consisted of 5-day courses of adriamycin and cytosine arabinoside given every 3–4 weeks for four courses. Treatment was resumed after each course when the circulating granulocyte count had reached 500/mm^3 and the platelet count was greater than 100,000/mm^3. Sequence II consisted of adriamycin and azacytidine given as 5-day courses every 4 weeks for four courses. This was followed by Sequence III, which included 6-mercaptopurine, vincristine, methotrexate, and methyl prednisolone (POMP) given in 5-day courses every 3 weeks on four occasions. Sequence IV was designated as "late intensification" and consisted of 5-day courses of cytosine arabinoside given every 3–4 weeks on four occasions. Treatment was discontinued after the completion of Sequence IV, approximately 15 months after the onset of "maintenance" therapy.

Central nervous system prophylaxis was not included per se in the protocol design. Intensification courses with continuous infusions of cytosine arabinoside were given in part to provide therapeutic concentrations of cytosine arabinoside in the central nervous system, thereby potentially eradicating microscopic disease at that site.

III. Criteria for Response

Patients were considered to be in complete remission if they were asymptomatic, had no physical findings suggestive of leukemia, and had normal bone marrow examinations and normal peripheral counts. Relapse was defined as the presence of 5% marrow blasts or the documentation of any extramedullary sites of leukemia. Bone marrow aspirations were performed every 8 weeks during the intensive sequential phase and every 3 months for the 1st year after the discontinuation of chemotherapy. Surveillance lumbar punctures were performed initially at the time complete bone marrow remission was documented and subsequently every 2–3 months during the intensive therapy phase.

IV. Statistical Analysis

The duration of survival was measured from the time of diagnosis, while the duration of remission extended from the date complete bone marrow remission was confirmed. Kaplan-Meier analyses of survival and continuous complete remission intervals were plotted on a semilogarithmic scale so as to compare the failure rates during successive monthly intervals. Deaths during remission were treated as failures, while withdrawals were considered evaluable up until the time they were electively removed from the protocol.

C. Results

One hundred and six patients were entered onto this study over a 4-year period. At the time of an 1 April 1980 review (Table 1), 105

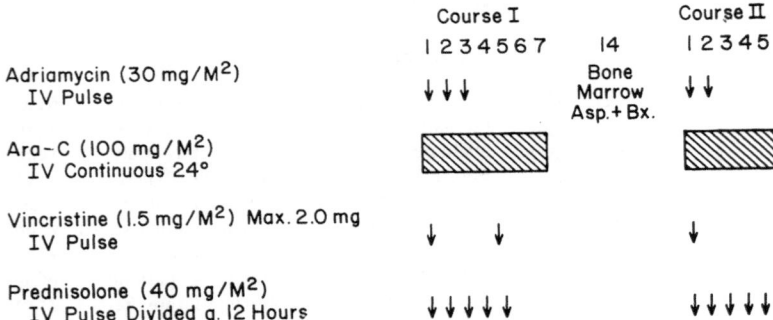

Fig. 1. VAPA[10]: remission-induction schema

Sequence I	Sequence II
Adriamycin 45mg/M²/d Day I IV Pulse	Adriamycin 30mg/M²/d Day I IV Pulse
Ara-C 200mg/M²/d Days I-5 Continuous Infusion	Azacytidine 150mg/M²/d Days I-5 Continuous Infusion
q 3-4 weeks X 4	q 4 weeks X 4

Sequence III	Sequence IV
Vincristine 2.0mg/M²/d Day I IV Pulse	Ara-C 200mg/M²/d Days I-5 Continuous Infusion
Methyl Prednisolone 800mg/M²/d Days I-5 IV Pulse	q 3 weeks X 4
6-Mercaptopurine 500mg/M²/d Days I-5 IV Pulse	
Methotrexate 7.5mg/M²/d Days I-5 IV Pulse	
q 3 weeks X 4	

Fig. 2. VAPA[10]: intensive sequential maintenance schema

were evaluable for analysis, with 61 being 17 years of age or younger and 44 being between ages 18–50. The median age for the entire group of 105 evaluable patients was 14.5 years. This unusual age distribution for AML patients reflects the referral patterns of the Longwood Avenue area hospitals and the fact that most pediatricians throughout New England send their children with this disease to a tertiary care facility such as the Sidney Farber Cancer Institute-Children's Hospital Medical Center. Complete remissions have been achieved in 74/105 (70%) of evaluable patients with younger patients having a slightly increased chance of achieving a complete remission (74%) than their older counterparts (66%). These data are similar to the reports of others

(Evans et al. 1975; Gale 1979; Haghbin et al. 1977; Preisler et al. 1979; Rees and Hayhoe 1978; Yates et al. 1973).

I. Remission Duration and Survival

Among the 74 complete responders there have been eight (11.0%) withdrawals for reasons including cardiomyopathy, bone marrow transplantation, and physician-patient desire to discontinue therapy. Of these eight patients, seven remain in their initial complete remission. There have been two remission deaths, one occurring in a 33-year-old woman who developed a fatal pneumonia at the time of drug-induced myelosuppression and another in a 31-year-old woman who expired from

Table 1. VAPA update as of 1 April 1980

	AGE 0–50	AGE 0–17	AGE 18–50
# Entered	106	61	45
Too early	1	0	1
Inevaluable	0	0	0
# Evaluable	105	61	44
# Complete remissions	74 (70%)	45 (74%)	29 (66%)
Withdrawals	8	5	3
Remission deaths	2	0	2
Relapses	24	16	8
Bone marrow	14	7	7
CNS	8	8	0
Myeloblastoma	2	1	1
# Continuous complete remission	40	24	16
Completed therapy	22	15	7
Relapses off therapy	4	3	1

47

refractory congestive heart failure presumably induced by adriamycin. Among the remaining 64 patients who entered complete remission, 40 remain disease free, while 24 have relapsed. All relapses in the adult age group have occurred in bone marrow, with one patient showing his first sign of recurrence by the development of a pleural myeloblastoma but with myeloblasts detected shortly thereafter in the bone marrow. In contrast, one-half of the 16 pediatric age relapses have occurred in the central nervous system. Six of these recurrences were detected through surveillance lumbar punctures. The median time to central nervous system relapse after documentation of complete bone marrow and spinal fluid remission was 4.5 months (range: 1.5–13.5). Six of the eight central nervous system relapses were followed within 0.5 months to 7.0 months by the reappearance of leukemic cells in bone marrow.

Figure 3 presents a Kaplan-Meier plot of the probability of remaining in complete remission among the complete responders. The median followup for these 74 patients is 9 months (range: 1 + to 48 + months) following the date they achieved complete remission. As previously noted, treatment was discontinued at approximately 15 months. The median duration of complete remission in 22.4 months. Utilizing two standard deviation confidence limits, the probability for complete responding patients to remain in remission at 12 months and 24 months is 67% ± 13% and 49% ± 17% respectively. Figure 4 presents a Kaplan-Meier

plot of the same data comparing the pediatric and adult age groups. There is no significant difference in remission duration based on age.

Twenty-two patients have completed the VAPA[10] program. Of these 22, four have relapsed "off therapy", while 18 remain in unmaintained complete remission. The median duration of time following the completion of therapy for this group of 22 patients is 11 + months. Three of the four late recurrences were noted in the bone marrow, while the other patient developed a nasopharyngeal myeloblastoma. All three patients who developed a bone marrow relapse entered a second remission following a single course of the VAPA[10] induction regimen and remain alive and disease free.

As seen in Fig. 5, the median survival for the entire group of 105 patients is 26.1 months. The 31 nonresponders had a median survival of only 0.5 months, while the median time to death among the complete responders has not yet been reached with a Kaplan-Meier plot suggesting a plateau in the 65%–70% range. Two standard deviation confidence limits indicate the probability of survival among complete responding patients to be 85% ± 9%, 71% ± 13%, and 66% ± 15% at 12, 24, and 36 months respectively.

II. Toxicity

The major toxicity during VAPA[10] remission induction in essentially all patients has been fever, necessitating the use of broad-spectrum

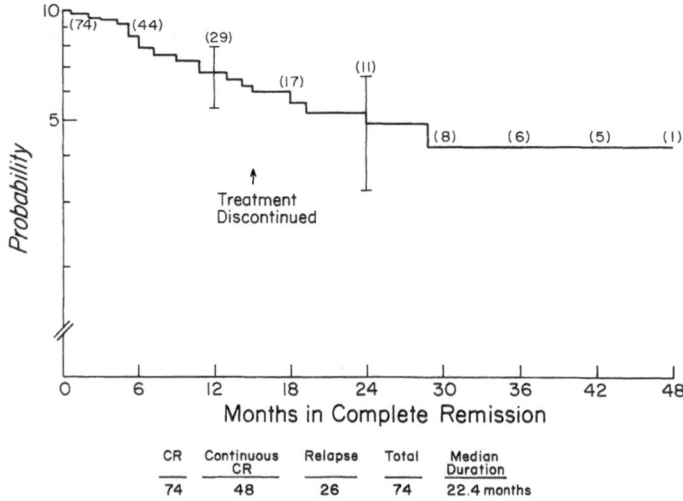

CR	Continuous CR	Relapse	Total	Median Duration
74	48	26	74	22.4 months

Fig. 3. VAPA[10]: Kaplan-Meier plot of probability of remaining in complete remission among all complete responders. The *vertical bars* at the 12 and 24 month points represent two standard deviation confidence limits

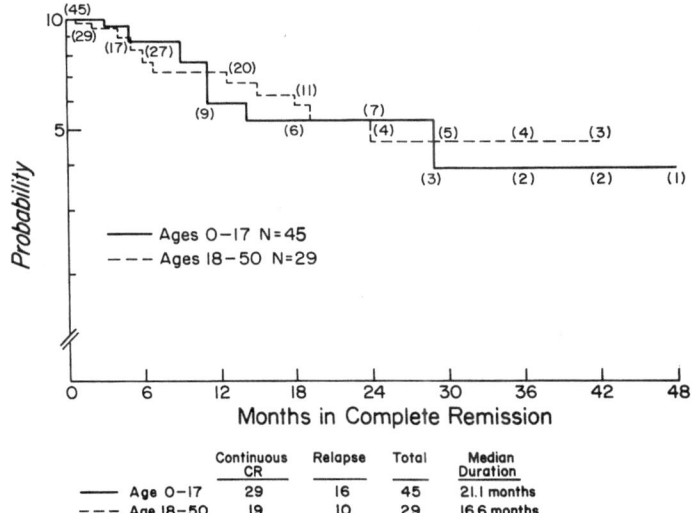

Fig. 4. VAPA[10]: Kaplan-Meier plot of probability of remaining in complete remission comparing pediatric and adult age groups

	Continuous CR	Relapse	Total	Median Duration
— Age 0-17	29	16	45	21.1 months
- - - Age 18-50	19	10	29	16.6 months

antibiotics. Culture-documented bacteremias have been present in about 20% of patients. In addition, approximately 25% of the pediatric patients under age 10 have experienced life-threatening gastrointestinal difficulties characterized by bloody diarrhea, esophagitis, ileus, bowel distension, and the development of signs of peritoneal irritation. These episodes of typhlitis resolved when bone marrow function recovered.

The early intensification phase of the maintenance program (Sequence I) was associated with severe thrombocytopenia requiring plate-let transfusions in 70% of courses and neutropenia to the point of agranulocytosis. The drug-induced myelosuppression was most severe between the 12th and 17th day of each treatment cycle and usually resolved by the 21st day. Fevers occurring at times of granulocytopenia necessitated short-term hospitalizations and the use of broad-spectrum antibiotics in 30% of the courses, but a culture-documented infection was only present in 17% of these febrile episodes.

The use of azacytidine and adriamycin in the second 5-day cycle phase of the maintenance

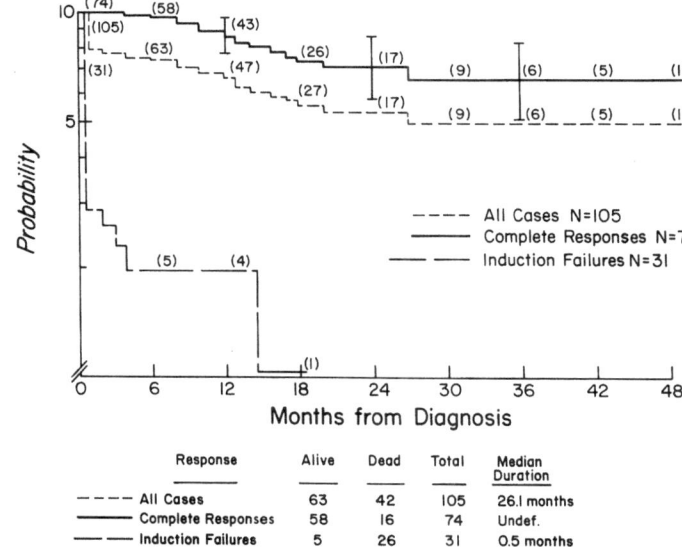

Fig. 5. VAPA[10]: Kaplan-Meier plot of probability of survival. The *vertical bars* at the 12, 24, and 36 month points in the curve representing complete responders represent two standard deviation confidence limits

Response	Alive	Dead	Total	Median Duration
- - - - All Cases	63	42	105	26.1 months
—— Complete Responses	58	16	74	Undef.
— — Induction Failures	5	26	31	0.5 months

period (Sequence II) was generally well tolerated with the extreme nausea and vomiting associated with "bolus" azacytidine administration rarely present. Severe thrombocytopenia and granulocytopenia induced by this drug combination were rare, but in about 10% of courses the myelosuppression did not resolve by the 28th day of a given treatment cycle as was expected but was occasionally prolonged, lasting as long as 7 weeks. This lengthy bone marrow depression necessitated the delay of chemotherapy in several instances, but such patients were able to tolerate further azacytidine-adriamycin without difficulty and have enjoyed similar remission durations as have other patients.

There have been no major toxicities associated with "POMP" (Sequence III) except for a rare case of cholestatic jaundice thought to be related to the 6-mercaptopurine. The late intensification treatments (Sequence IV) with cytosine arabinoside led to severe myelosuppression, but only 12% of the courses have been associated with fever necessitating hospitalization.

The length of the treatment period including remission induction and the sequential chemotherapy phase averaged 450 days. Initially, 120 of these days were spent in the hospital for the administration of intravenous chemotherapy or for systemic antibiotics. During this study, the pharmacokinetics of continuous intravenous and continuous subcutaneous infusions of cytosine arabinoside were evaluated (Weinstein et al. 1978). The results indicated comparable drug levels and myelosuppression with both routes of administration. Because of these data, patients were no longer admitted to the hospital for 5-day intravenous infusions of cytosine arabinoside, but instead received outpatient subcutaneous infusions via a portable infusion pump (Auto Syringe, Inc., Hooksett, New Hampshire). Time of hospitalization was thereby reduced from 120 to 80 days.

D. Discussion

The major thrust of the VAPA[10] program was directed not at remission induction where a 65%–75% complete response rate was anticipated, but rather at the "maintenance" period where it was hoped that intensive therapy might lead to a significant prolongation in remission duration and survival. Protocol design was specifically directed at circumventing major potential obstacles to long-term remission. These include:

1. *Inadequate cytoreduction during the maintenance period.* The VAPA[10] program offered intensive therapy at drug doses higher than the remission induction levels at the beginning (Sequence I) and at the conclusion (Sequence IV) of the 15-month maintenance period. As seen in Figure 1, four cycles of cytosine arabinoside given by continuous infusion for 5 days at a dose of 200 mg/m²/day were administered at the start and at the end of "maintenance". The initial four cycles were accompanied by a single administration of adriamycin. Each of these treatment cycles was administered on a 21–28 day schedule with no dose de-escalation made for myelosuppression or infection. The rationale for early and late intensification was data from experimental murine models demonstrating a steep dose response curve for cytosine arabinoside (Skipper 1978). Clinical data to support this concept comes from a recent AML study in which patients received only a single cycle of intensive induction chemotherapy which resulted in a median, unmaintained remission of 10 months (Vaughn et al. 1980).

2. *The development of drug resistance.* In experimental in vitro and in vivo leukemia models, there is evidence that relapse results from the selection and overgrowth of drug resistant cell lines (Skipper 1978). Initially, during treatment with a given program the majority of chemotherapeutically-sensitive cells are progressively eliminated, but at some point ("nadir") further leukemic cell kill is counterbalanced by the overgrowth of resistant cells which eventually results in clinical relapse. By back extrapolation from the kinetics of remission induction and relapse in patients with AML, this "nadir" was estimated to occur at approximately 3–4 months of treatment with a given regimen. Hence, two different drug programs (Sequences II and III) of non-cross-resistant agents were interposed between the early and late intensification periods. In the first of these, azacytidine, an active agent in the treatment of AML which has been reported to be non-cross-resistant with cytosine arabinoside (Van Hoff et al. 1976), was given at induction level doses in combination with adriamycin. In the second of these two drug programs, 6-mercaptopurine and methotrexate, each having some degree of

activity in AML (Ho and Frei 1971), were introduced along with vincristine and prednisone.

3. *The presence of pharmacologic "sanctuaries"*. While meningeal leukemia has been reported in patients with AML (Pippard et al. 1979; Wolk et al. 1974; Zachariah et al. 1978), it is far less common than in acute lymphocytic leukemia. The central nervous system is the initial site of recurrence in only 10%–15% of relapsing AML patients and is far more often seen in pediatric than in adult age groups (Chard et al. 1978; Pizzo et al. 1976). It was thought conceivable, however, that prolonging survival of patients with AML might yet be associated with an increased incidence of meningeal leukemia (Wolk et al. 1974). The VAPA[10] program did not include treatment directed solely at the central nervous system. Cytosine arabinoside, however, when administered by continuous infusion, has been shown to pass readily through the blood brain barrier, reaching cytotoxic concentrations when administered in doses such as those employed in the early and late intensification plans (Ho and Frei 1971). This approach, especially in the pediatric age group, will require re-examination in the future, since 8 of the 16 relapses in patients under age 18 have occurred in the central nervous system.

A preliminary analysis of the VAPA[10] experience suggests that age at presentation, sex, or height of the initial white blood count up to 200,000/mm^3 does not have prognostic significance in terms of either remission induction rate or remission duration. The duration of complete remission was further uninfluenced by the number of courses (i.e., whether a second induction treatment was begun on day 14) required to achieve a complete remission. The remission induction rate may be slightly reduced among patients having the acute promyelocytic leukemia subtype (8/15), while the relapse potential seems higher in patients having acute monocytic leukemia (5/10).

These data are extremely encouraging and indicate that intensive, sequential combination chemotherapy given to patients with AML who have achieved complete remission can extend the median duration of that remission for 2 years, prolong survival in these individuals for an indefinite period of time, and allow a subsequent period of unmaintained remission in excess of an additional year. The Kaplan-Meier plots (Figs. 3–5) furthermore suggest that a plateau has been achieved among patients who have remained in complete remission for greater than 24 months, making the likelihood of late relapse less and raising the possibility of cure in a significant number of such individuals. The only other therapeutic modality that appears to achieve a similar result for patients with AML is intensive chemotherapy and total body irradiation followed by allogeneic bone marrow transplantation when performed early during the initial remission (Blume et al. 1980; Powles et al. 1980; Thomas et al. 1979). This approach, however, is limited to patients who not only achieve a complete remission, but also have a histocompatible sibling.

The VAPA[10] experience suggests that AML, even if it is a disease caused by an abnormal bone marrow clone, can be suppressed for extended periods of time by chemotherapy alone in at least 33% of patients under age 50. It will now be possible to examine factors affecting durations of remission and to design specific therapeutic strategies based on these findings.

References

Armitage JD, Burns CP (1976) Maintenance of remission in adult acute nonlymphoblastic leukemia using intermittent courses of cytosine arabinoside (NSC-63878) and 6-thioguanine (NSC-752). Cancer Treat Rep 60:585–589 – Blume KG et al. (1980) Bone marrow ablation and allogeneic marrow transplantation in acute leukemia. N Engl J Med 302:1041–1046 – Bodey GP et al. (1976) Late intensification therapy for acute leukemia in remission: Chemotherapy and immunotherapy. JAMA 235:1021–1025 – Carey RW et al. (1975) Comparative study of cytosine arabinoside therapy alone and combined with thioguanine, mercaptopurine or daunorubicin in acute myelocytic leukemia. Cancer 36:1560–1566 – Chard RL et al. (1978) Increased survival in childhood acute nonlymphocytic leukemia after treatment with prednisone, cytosine arabinoside, 6-thioguanine, cyclophosphamide, and oncovin (PATCO) combination chemotherapy. Med Pediatr Oncol 4:263–273 – Clarkson BD et al. (1975) Treatment of acute leukemia in adults. Cancer 36:775–795 – Evans DIK et al. (1975) Treatment of acute myeloid leukemia of childhood with cytosine arabinoside, daunorubicin, prednisone, and mercaptopurine or thioguanine. Cancer 36:1547–1551 – Gale RPL (1979) Advances in the treatment of acute myeologenous leukemia. N Engl J Med 300:1189–1199 – Haghbin M et al. (1977) Treatment of acute nonlymphoblastic leukemia in children with a multiple drug protocol. Cancer 49:1417–1421 – Henderson ES (1969) Treatment of acute leukemia. Semin Hemat 6:271–319 – Ho DHW, Frei E III (1971) Clinical pharmacology of 1-B-D-arabinosylcytosine. Clin Pharmacol Therap 12:944–954 – Moreno H et al. (1977) Cytosine arabinoside and 6-thioguanine in the treatment of childhood acute myeloblastic leukemia. Cancer 40:998–1004 – Peterson BA, Bloomfield CD (1977) Prolonged maintained remission of adult acute nonlymphocytic leukemia. Lancet 2:158–160 – Pippard MJ et al. (1979) Infiltration of central nervous system in adult acute myeloid leukaemia. Br Med J 1:227–229 – Pizzo PA et al. (1976) Acute myelogenous leukemia in children: A preliminary report of combination chemotherapy. J Pediatr 88:125–130 – Powles RL et al. (1980) The place of bone marrow transplantation in acute myelogenous leukaemia. Lancet 1:1047–1050 – Preisler HD et al. (1979) Treatment of acute nonlymphocytic leukemia: Use of anthracycline-cytosine arabinoside induction therapy and comparison of two maintenance regimens. Blood 53:455–464 – Rees JKH, Hayhoe FGJ (1978) DAT (daunorubicin, cytarabine, 6-thioguanine) in acute myeloid leukaemia. Lancet 1:1360–1361 – Skipper HE (1978) Reasons for success and failure in treatment of murine leukemias with drugs now employed in treating human leukemias. In: Cancer Chemotherapy, Volume I. University Microfilms International: Southern Research Institute – Spiers ASD et al. (1977) Prolonged remission maintenance in acute myeloid leukaemia. Br J Med 2:544–547 – Thomas ED et al. (1979) Marrow transplantation for acute nonlymphoblastic leukemia in first remission. N Eng J Med 301:597–599 – Van Hoff DD et al. (1976) 5-azacytidene: A new anticancer drug with effectiveness in acute myelogenous leukemia. Ann Int Med 82:237–245 – Vaughn WP et al. (1980) Long chemotherapy-free remissions after single-cycle timed sequential chemotherapy for acute myelocytic leukemia. Cancer 45:859–865 – Weinstein H et al. (1978) Pharmacology of cytosine arabinoside (a-C). Proc Am Assoc Cancer Res 19:157 – Wolk RW et al. (1974) The incidence of central nervous system leukemia in adults with acute leukemia. Cancer 33:863–869 – Yates JW et al. (1973) Cytosine arabinoside (NSC-63878) and daunorubicin (NSC-83142) therapy in acute nonlymphocytic leukemia. Cancer Chemother Rep 57:485–487 – Zachariah C et al. (1978) Prolonged meningeal leukemia: Occurrence during hematologic remission of acute myeloblastic leukemia. JAMA 239:1423–1424.

Haematology and Blood Transfusion Vol. 26
Modern Trends in Human Leukemia IV
Edited by Neth, Gallo, Graf, Mannweiler, Winkler
© Springer-Verlag Berlin Heidelberg 1981

Rational Approaches to the Treatment of Leukemia*

H. D. Preisler

A. Introduction

Advances in the treatment of acute myelocytic leukemia (AML) have largely resulted from empirical drug trials in man. Such trials have led to the recognition of drug combinations which produce remissions in more than one-half of the patients who are under 70 years of age (Yates et al. 1973; Preisler et al. 1977; Rees et al. 1977; Jacquillat et al. 1976). While intensive remission induction therapy will produce complete hematologic remissions in as many as 75% of the patients, large numbers of leukemic cells must persist in the patients who enter remission, since the disease recurs in the majority of patients less than 1½ years after remission is induced. The selection of a treatment regimen on the basis of the regimen having produced a high remission rate in a majority of patients (75%, for example) also mandates that this particular regimen is not appropriate for the patients who do not enter remission (25%–45% of patients). Clearly, for this group of individuals the use of a different treatment regimen would have been preferable.

In the Department of Medical Oncology at Roswellj Park Memorial Institute we have been approaching these problems on a two-track basis. On the one hand we have continued to treat patients empirically using our clinical observations to dictate our therapeutic approach. To this end 3 years ago we initiated a treatment program designed to deliver intensive chemotherapy to patients already in remission to reduce and perhaps ablate the leukemic cells remaining in patients who entered complete remission (Preisler et al. 1980, to be published a). At the same time we began to study the factors which determined response to therapy, so that we would be able to determine in advance the appropriate chemotherapeutic regimen for individual patients (Rustum and Preisler 1979a; Preisler, to be published; Preisler et al. 1979b). This paper represents a progress report on our studies.

B. Empirical Clinical Studies

The therapeutic regimen (P970701) illustrated in Fig. la has been used to treat all patients of less than 70 years of age with AML since June 1977 (Preisler et al., to be published a). The regimen illustrated in Fig. 1b (P950501) was used to treat patients between 1975 and 1977 (Preisler et al. 1979b). Table 1 compares the remission induction efficacy of the two regimens. Given the number of patients studied, there is no significant difference in the overall induction efficacy of the two regimens. Figure 2 compares the duration of remission for three groups of patients: those treated with P950501, those treated with P970701, and a subgroup of patients induced into remission on P970701 but who did not receive the consolidation or maintenance portions of P970701 because their private physicians felt that intensive postremission therapy was not indicated. Comparison of the life table plots for remission duration of the three groups of patients demonstrates a highly statistically significant ($P<0.01$) difference in remission duration between patients induced and maintained on P970701 and those patients who received the same remission induction regimen

* This study was supported by U.S.P.H.S. Grants CA-5834, CA-24162 and ACS Grant CH-168

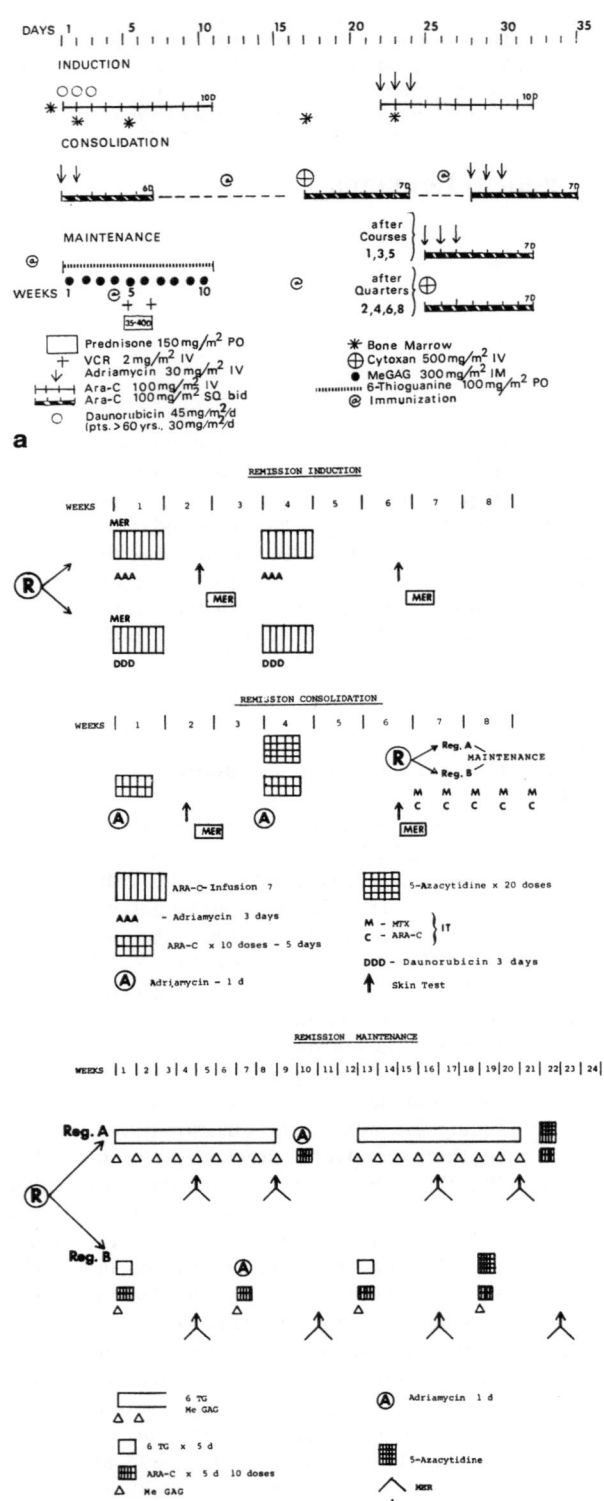

Fig. 1. a Schema for protocol 970701.
b Schema for protocol 950501

		Total	≤50	>50≤70
CR/TOT.	P950501	24/36 (66%)	16/20 (80%)	8/16 (50%)
	P970701	52/73 (71%)	29/35 (83%)	24/38 (63%)

Table 1. Outcome of remission induction therapy

but who recieved more gentle maintenance therapy (generally monthly 5-day courses of cytosine arabinoside (ara C) and 6-thioguanine, with or without BCG).

Comparison of remission durations of patients on P970701 and P950501 suggest that the more intensive post-remission induction regimen employed in P970701 resulted in: a reduction in the number of early relapses and a longer median duration of remission with a higher proportion of patients in remission beyond the second year. These observations suggest that early intensive consolidation chemotherapy prolongs remission durations by reducing the number of leukemic cells remaining after remission induction therapy is administered.

It should be noted that P970701 produced severe toxicity with significant thrombocytopenia and granulocytopenia lasting for more than one week's time occurring after each course of intensive chemotherapy administered to patients in remission. The administration of cotrimoxazole to patients has prevented the occurrence of infectious complications (Preisler et al., to be published) and the administration of platelet transfusions every other day to patients whose platelet counts were less than 20,000/µl has prevented hemorrhagic complications.

C. Prediction of Response to Therapy

The outcome of remission induction therapy is determined by both the patients ability to survive remission induction therapy (biological fitness) and by the drug sensitivity of a patient's leukemic cells. Table 2 illustrates the outcome of remission induction therapy given different combinations of biological fitness and drug sensitivity. Needless to say, this construction presumes that adequate serum levels of drug for an adequate duration are achieved during therapy.

To evaluate the ability of an in vitro drug sensitivity assay to predict in vivo drug responsiveness one must be careful to use the outcome of remission induction therapy of only those patients for whom one can assess the in vivo response of leukemic cells to therapy. Hence, patients who die early in the course of therapy or who die during a period of marrow hypoplasia must be considered to be inevaluable, since in both cases it is not possible to determine whether the patient would have entered remission or whether leukemic cells would have persisted or regrown shortly after marrow hypoplasia was induced (Preisler 1978). For these reasons, we consider complete remission to be indicative of in vivo drug sensitivity and either persistence

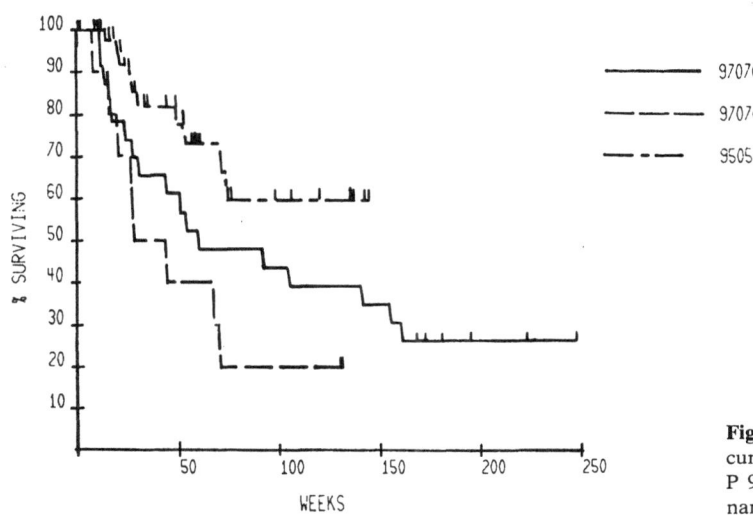

Fig. 2. Remission duration curves. *NC*, same induction as P 970701 but gentle maintenance therapy

Biologically fit[a]	Drug sensitivity	Outcome
yes	yes	Complete remission
yes	no	Persistent leukemia
no	yes	Death early in therapy or while hypoplastic
no	no	Death early in therapy with persistent leukemia

Table 2. The outcome of remission induction therapy given different combinations of biological fitness and drug sensitivity

[a] Ability to survive the effects of intensive remission induction therapy.

of leukemia despite therapy or the regrowth of leukemic cells subsequent to a period of marrow hypoplasia to be indicative operationally of drug resistant disease.

Figure 3 illustrates the method we have employed to determine the sensitivity of leukemic cells to ara C and daunorubicin, and 4 illustrates the relationship between in vitro sensitivity and the outcome of remission induction therapy with these two agents. There is a clear-cut and highly statistically significant relationship between the percent age of clonogenic leukemic cells killed by ara C and DNR and in vivo response to therapy (Preisler 1980, to be published).

D. Comments

Despite recent significant increases in the percentage of complete remissions induced by aggressive remission induction therapy, a significant proportion of patients still fail to enter remission and the majority of patients fail to survive for prolonged periods of time. Empirical approaches to this problem will include the administration of still more intensive remission induction regimens so that patients with disease resistant to currently employed regimens might be induced into remission. More aggressive regimens will, however, result in greater toxicity and in more toxic deaths, deaths which

CRITERIA FOR EVALUATION OF PTS. FOR RELATIONSHIP IN IN VITRO vs. IN VIVO TREATMENT

ESTIMATION OF IN VIVO DRUG SENSITIVITY

1. DRUG SENSITIVE DISEASE = COMPLETE REMISSION

2. RESISTANT DISEASE

    A. PERSISTANT MARROW LEUKEMIA DESPITE CHEMO RX

    B. RX PRODUCES MARROW HYPOCELL. BUT ON REGEN. LEUK. CELLS RETURN

3. INEVALUABLE

    A. PATIENTS WHO DIE EARLY IN COURSE OF RX

    B. PATIENTS WHO DIE WHILE APLASTIC

CLONAL EST. IN VITRO DRUG SENSITIVITY

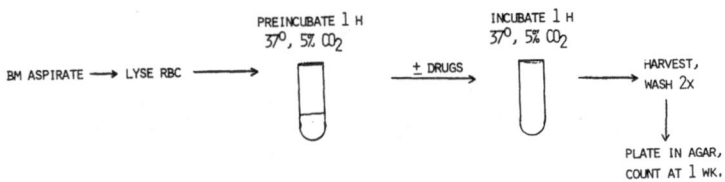

Fig. 3. Drug sensitivity assay

RELATIONSHIP BETWEEN SENSITIVITY OF LCFUc TO ARA C + DNR

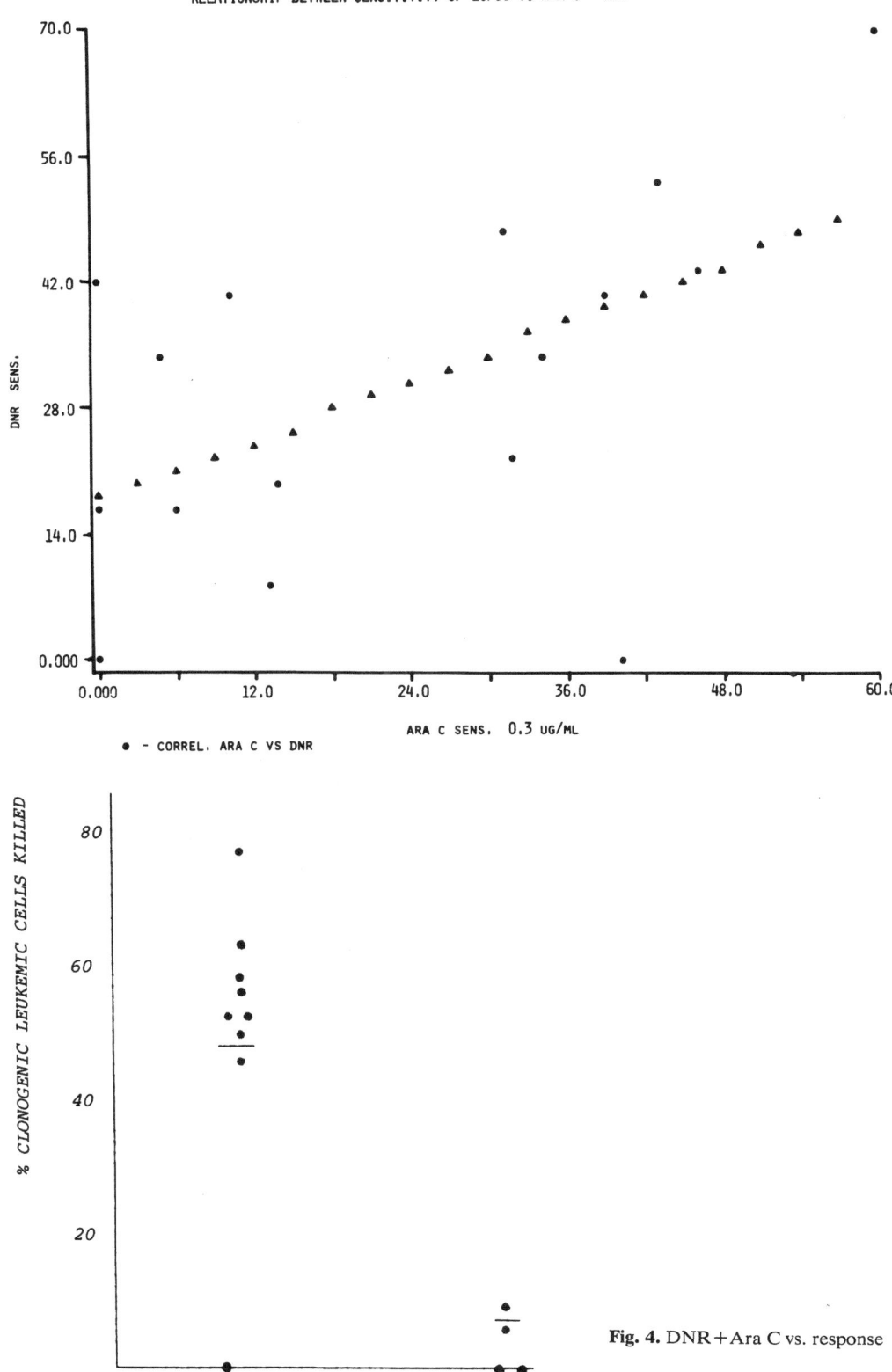

● - CORREL. ARA C VS DNR

Fig. 4. DNR+Ara C vs. response

57

may counterbalance the potential benefits of the more aggressive regimens. The development of reliable in vitro drug sensitivity assays would permit the use of remission induction regimens tailored to each patient and, hence, will simplify remission induction therapy, since ineffective drugs will be recognized and will not be administered on the chance basis that they will be therapeutically efficacious.

Until the reliability of in vitro drug sensitivity tests in confirmed, treatment regimens based upon empirical clinical observations will continue to be the main vehicle for improvement in the outlook for patients with AML. It is intuitively clear that intensive remission consolidation regimens appear to be the next step in the evolution of clinical protocols. Since our P970701 appears to have produced promising results, the next phase in our studies will be the administration of a greater number of courses of intensive consolidation therapy employing a greater variety of drugs.

References

Jacquillat C, Weil M, Gemon-Auderc MF, (1976) Clinical study of rubidizone (22050 R.P.), a new daunorubicin-derived compound, in 170 patients with acute leukemias and other malignancies. Cancer 37:653–659 – Preisler HD (1978) Failure of remission induction in acute myelocytic leukemia. Med Pediatr Oncol 4:275–276 – Preisler HD (1980) Prediction of response to remission induction therapy in AML. In: Proc. of Amer. Assoc. Cancer Res., 71st Ann. Meeting, May 28–31, 1980, San Diego, California, Abstract #616 – Preisler HD (to be published) Prediction of response to chemotherapy in acute myelocytic leukemia. Blood – Preisler HD, Bjornsson S, Henderson ES (1977) Adriamycin-cytosine arabinoside therapy for adult acute myelocytic leukemia. Cancer Treat Rep 61:89–92 – Preisler HD, Rustum YM, Epstein J (1979a) Therapy of acute nonlymphocytic leukemia. II. Biological characteristics and prediction of response. NY State J Med 79:884–499 – Preisler HD, Bjornsson S, Henderson ES, (1979b) Treatment of acute nonlymphocytic leukemia: Use of anthracycline-cytosine arabinoside induction therapy and a comparison of two maintenance regimens. Blood 53:455–464 – Preisler H, Browman G, Henderson ES, (1980) Treatment of acute myelocytic leukemia: Effects of early intensive consolidation. In: Proc. Amer. Assoc. Clin. Oncol., 16th Annual Meeting, May 26–27, 1980, San Diego, California, Abstract #C-493 – Preisler HD, Bjornsson S, Henderson ES, (to be published a) Remission induction in acute nonlymphocytic leukemia: Comparison of a 7-day and 10-day infusion of cytosine arabinoside in combination with adriamycin. Med Pediatr Oncol – Preisler HD, Early A, Hryniuk (to be published b) Prevention of infection in leukemic patients receiving intensive remission maintenance therapy. Blood – Rees JKH, Sandler RM, Challener J, (1977) Treatment of acute myeloid leukaemia with a triple cytotoxic regimen: DAT. Br J Cancer 36:770–776 – Rustum YM, Preisler HD (1979) Correlation between leukemic cell retention of 1-β-D-arabinosylcytosine-5'-triphosphate and response to therapy. Cancer Res 39:42–49 (1979). – Yates JP, Wallace HJ, Ellison RR, (1973) Cytosine arabinoside and daunorubicin therapy in acute nonlymphocytic leukemia. Cancer Chemother Rep 57:485–487

Haematology and Blood Transfusion Vol. 26
Modern Trends in Human Leukemia IV
Edited by Neth, Gallo, Graf, Mannweiler, Winkler
© Springer-Verlag Berlin Heidelberg 1981

Treatment of Early Acute Nonlymphatic Leukemia with Low Dose Cytosine Arabinoside

W. C. Moloney and D. S. Rosenthal

Successful induction of remissions in adults with acute nonlymphatic leukemia (ANLL) requires the use of high dose aggressive chemotherapy which is not well tolerated by older adults and few remissions are obtained in patients with ANLL secondary to refractory anemia and other disorders (Moloney and Rosenthal, to be published) For years investigators have attempted to discover methods of producing remissions by inducing leukemic cells to differentiate and recently Sachs (1978) has pointed out that a number of agents were capable of inducing maturation in leukemic mouse myeloblasts. Among the chemical compounds investigated was cytosine arabinoside (Ara-C) an antimetabolite extensively used in high dosage for treatment of ANLL. Based on these experimental findings Baccarani and Tura (1979) treated a patient with refractory anemia and excess myeloblasts in the marrow with a short course of low dose Ara-C and obtained an excellent clinical and hematological improvement with partial bone marrow remission. Encouraged by this report we have treated two patients with early ANLL and seven patients with RDA-ANLL with low dose Ara-C. Observations on these cases and preliminary findings on the effect of low dose Ara-C on leukemic cells cultured in diffusion chambers are presented in this paper.

A. Methods and Materials

Patients were followed and laboratory studies carried out in the Hematology Division of Peter Bent Brigham Hospital. Bone marrow biopsies and aspirates were carried out initially and repeated during the course of the disease. Blood and marrow smears were stained with Wright Giemsa and histochemical methods included those for leucocyte alkaline phosphatase and peroxidase activity; iron stains were carried out routinely on all marrow specimens. Bone marrow cells were cultured in diffusion chambers (DC) implanted in the abdominal cavities of previously irradiated rats. Details of this method have previously been published (Greenberger et al. 1977, 1978). For studies on the effect of low dose Ara-C, host animals were treated by subcutaneous injections daily for 21 days with 0.1 mg Ara-C per kilogram.

B. Clinical Results

Two patients with early de novo ANLL were treated with low dose Ara-C and achieved complete remission.

Case 1 (E.E.): This 78-year-old male had a 6 month history of myalgia and developed progressively severe fever, night sweats, and pain in the back, and chest. There was no hepatosplenomegaly and blood studies were within normal limits except for a rapid E.S.R. As part of a diagnostic work-up a bone marrow biopsy and aspirate were carried out and revealed a hypercellular but variable cell population; some areas were relatively normal but elsewhere sheets of myeloblasts, some containing Auer rods, were present. Treatment with Ara-C 0.8 mg per kilogram (50 mg) s.c. was carried out for 20 days. After one week the patient improved, fever, night sweats and pain ceased and after an initial moderate fall the platelets, WBC, and hematocrit rose to normal levels (Fig. 1). He has been maintained for over 6 months in hematological remission with monthly 5 day courses of Ara-C 0.4 mg daily s.c. Following remission bone marrow aspirations have revealed M1 marrows.

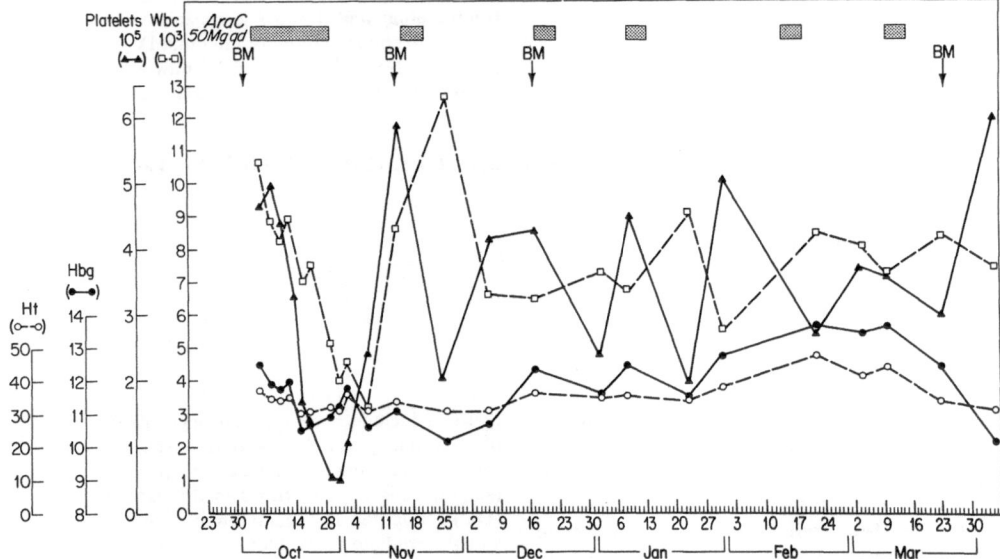

Fig. 1. Treatment of early AML with low dose Ara-C (Patient E.E.)

Case 2 (F.A.): This 43-year-old, previously well female developed over a 4 week period progressive weight loss, fever, and severe generalized intermittent bone pain. There were no positive physical findings except marked sternal tenderness. Blood studies were unremarkable except for a mild degree of anemia and a rapid E.S.R. A bone scan, carried out to detect possible metastatic cancer, showed abnormal uptake in the ribs, pelvis, and long bones. Marrow aspirate and biopsy were performed and revealed hypercellularity with a variable picture. In some areas there were sheets of myeloblasts with Auer rods noted in some cells; elsewhere the marrow was hypercellular with a shift to the left, but myeloblasts were absent. The patient experienced increased bone pain which required narcotics for relief. She was started on Ara-C 1 mg per kilogram (50 mg) daily s.c. and

this was continued for 21 days. Bone pain markedly decreased after the first week of therapy and she gained weight and strength. A moderate fall in hematocrit, WBC, and platelets developed after 21 days of therapy, but following cessation of Ara-C there was a rapid rise in platelets followed by a slower increase in WBC and hematocrit to normal levels. A marrow aspirate taken two months after Ara-C was started showed an M1 marrow. The patient has regained full activities, gained 20 pounds, and is now in her 4th month of remission. Maintenance therapy consists of Ara-C 50 mg daily s.c. for five days each month (Fig. 2).

In addition to the cases of early ANLL seven other patients have been treated; three sideroblastic RDA-ANLL cases failed to respond to several courses of low dose Ara-C and four patients with RDA-ANLL have been started

Category	Total Cases	Complete remission	Failure	Early	Alive	Dead
Early ANLL Sideroblastic	2	2	0	0	2	0
RDA-ANLL Nonsideroblastic	5	0	3	2	4	1
RDA-ANLL	2	0	0	2	2	0
Total	9	2	3	4	8	1

Table 1. Results of Low Dose Ara-C Therapy

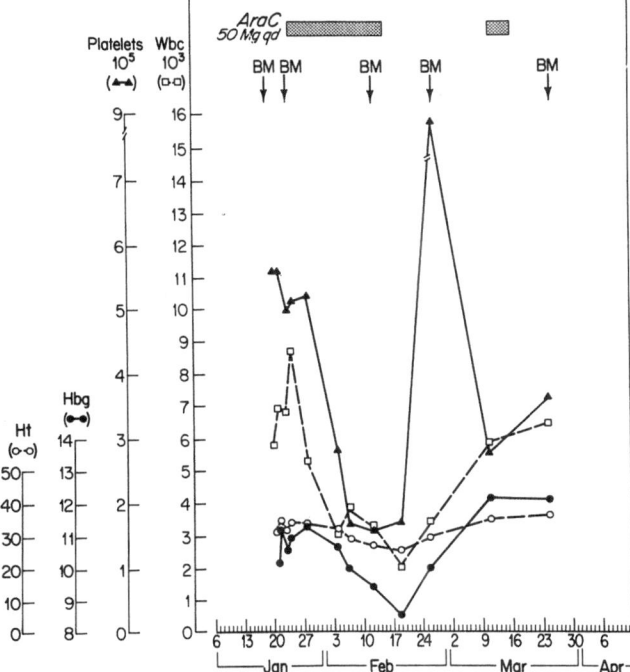

Fig. 2. Treatment of early AML with low dose Ara-C (Patient F.A.)

on therapy but it is too early to evaluate results in these cases. (See Table 1).

C. Results of diffusion Chamber Studies

Studies have been carried out over the past 5 years on the proliferation and maturation of marrow cells from patients with RDA, leukemia, and other disorders. Cells from young normal marrow donors mature and fail to proliferate; in older patients cells mature and frequently a marked lymphocytosis develops (Fig. 3). Studies on patients with RDA, early ANLL, and de novo ANLL showed that cells (1) failed to proliferate or (2) grew and matured at least to promyelocytes in all but 9% of 117 cases.

Observations of the effect of low dose Ara-C on growth and maturation of marrow cells were carried out by treating host rats with 0.1 mg per kilogram Ara-C daily s.c. for 21 days. The pretreatment marrow cells of patient F.A. with early ANLL showed a striking neutrophilocytosis on day 5 followed by an intense lymphocytosis from days 8–14. In the untreated control cultures a similar but less intense cellular response occurred (Fig. 4). In

four cases of RDA-ANLL and one nonleukemic RDA an effect on maturation by low dose Ara-C was noted in two instances but was equivocal in three other patients. In one case of de novo ANLL myeloblasts proliferated actively and neither growth nor maturation was influenced by Ara-C.

D. Discussion

The successful results of low dose Ara-C therapy in two cases of early ANLL may be unique since in both cases the disease was discovered incidentally and the marrows were only partially replaced with blasts. The early stage of ANLL is more commonly encountered in cases of RDA "going over" to ANLL. Since these elderly patients have little hope of achieving remissions with present day aggressive chemotherapy, low dose Ara-C might offer an alternative form of therapy at least in some cases. Unfortunately our first three patients with sideroblastic RDA-ANLL failed to obtain remissions with low dose Ara-C and the results in four additional cases, recently started on therapy, are unavailable. However, further clinical trials should be carried out not

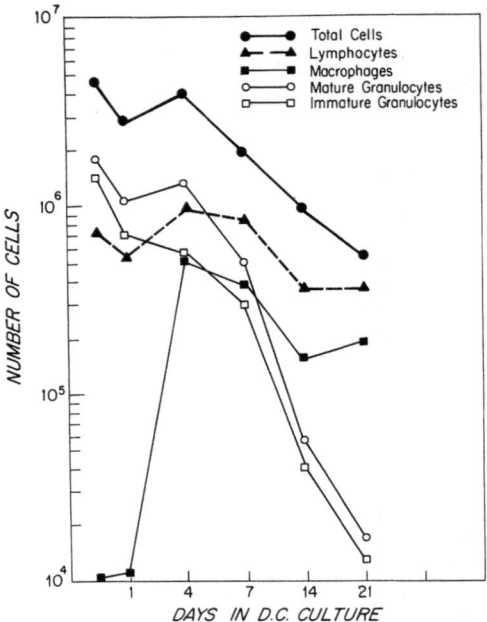

Fig. 3. Diffusion culture of bone marrow cells from 11 older adults

DC culture studies may prove useful in selecting candidates for low dose Ara-C therapy and more importantly may provide a method of investigating the fundamental problems of growth and differentiation of leukemic myeloblasts in man.

References

Baccarini M, Tura S (1979) The differentiation of myeloid leukemic cells: New possibilities for therapy. Br Haematol 42:485–487 – Greenberger JS, Hassen LR, Karpas A, France DS, Moloney WC (1977) Leukocyte alkaline phosphatase elevation in human acute leukemia derived cells cultured in diffusion chambers. Scand J Haematol 19:224–254 – Greenberger JS, Gans PJ, King V, Muse MB, Karpas A, Moloney WC (1978) Diffusion chamber culture in irradiated rats of myeloblasts and promyelocytes from 84 untreated patients with myeloid leukemias or refractory dysmyelopoietic anemia: Comparison to continuous tissue culture lines. In: Benvelzen (eds) Advances in comparative leukemia research 1977. Elsevier/North Holland Biomedical Press – Hoelzer D, Harriss EB, Kurrle E, Schmucker H, Hellriegal KP (1979) Differentiation ability of peripheral blood cells from patients with acute leukemia or blast crisis in chronic myelogenous leukemia. In: Neth R, Gallo RC, Hofschneider PH, Mannweiler K (eds) Modern trends in human leukemia III. Springer, Berlin–Heidelberg–New York, pp 217–222 – Moloney WC, Rosenthal DS (to be published) Secondary acute myelogenous leukemia. Top Hematol – Sachs L (1978) The differentiation of myeloid leukemic cells: New possibilities for therapy. Br J Haematol 40:509–517

only with low dose Ara-C but with other antileukemic agents investigated by Sachs (1978).

It is well established that leukemic cells will differentiate in DC cultures (Hoelzer et al. 1979). Our preliminary experiments indicate that low dose Ara-C may enhance differentiation of leukemic cells in some cases of ANLL.

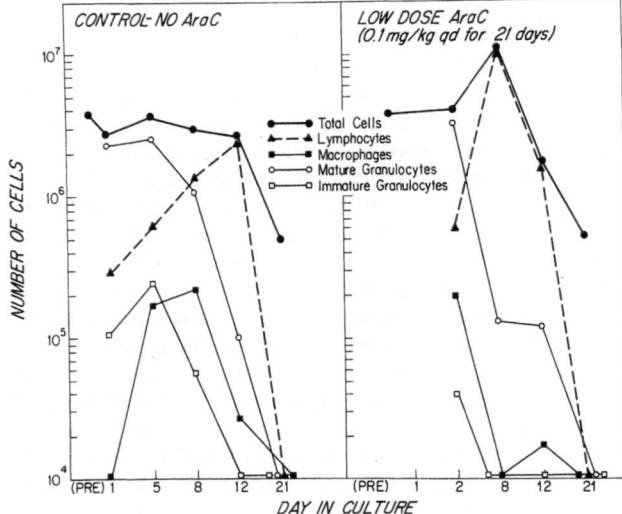

Fig. 4. Bone marrow cells in D.C. culture (Patient F.A.)

Haematology and Blood Transfusion Vol. 26
Modern Trends in Human Leukemia IV
Edited by Neth, Gallo, Graf, Mannweiler, Winkler
© Springer-Verlag Berlin Heidelberg 1981

A Phase I Study of Human Lymphoblastoid Interferon in Patients with Hematological Malignancies

A. Rohatiner, F. Balkwill, J. S. Malpas, and T. A. Lister

A. Introduction

Objective responses to leukocyte Interferon have now been demonstrated in acute lymphoblastic leukaemia (Hill et al. 1980), chronic lymphocytic leukaemia (Gutterman et al. 1979), myeloma (Mellsted et al. 1979; Idestrom et al. 1979; Osserman and Sherman 1980) and non-Hodgkin's lymphoma (NHL) (Gutterman et al. 1979; Merigan et al. 1978). In 1977 Balkwill and Oliver demonstrated an in vitro cytostatic effect on myeloblasts using human lymphoblastoid interferon (HLBI) (Balkwill and Oliver 1977). This prompted us to undertake a Phase I study of HLBI in patients with acute myeloblastic leukaemia (AML), which is currently in progress. The preliminary results form the basis of this report.

B. Aims

The aims of the study are the following:
1. To determine the maximum tolerated dose of HLBI when given by continuous intravenous infusion;
2. To establish the toxic effects of HLBI given by infusion;
3. To study the pharmacokinetics of HLBI given by intravenous infusion; and
4. To compare the in vitro and in vivo effects of known levels of HLBI in patients with AML.

C. Patients and Methods

Details of the patients studied and the doses administered are shown in Tables 1 and 2.

Table 1. Phase I study of HLBI. Clinical details of 13 patients

Diagnosis	No. of patients
AML	10
NHL – Follicular	1
Myeloma	1
CLL	1
Total	13

Table 2. Phase I study of HLBI. Dosage and scheduling

Patient	HLBI dose (Megaunits/m²)	No. of days
1	5	Intravenous bolus × 1
2	5	Intravenous bolus × 2
3	3.7	Infusion × 5
4–7	5	Infusion × 5
8–10	7.5	Infusion × 5
11–13	10	Infusion × 5

D. Results

I. Clinical Toxicity

All patients complained of general malaise and anorexia, and all became pyrexial between 2 and 24 h after administration of HLBI. Four patients complained of rigors, 3 of headaches and 1 of joint pains. Patient 2 experienced a hypotensive episode after the second injection of HLBI.

II. Haematological and Biochemical Toxicity

All patients had bone marrow infiltration rendering interpretation of the blood count extremely difficult. In patients with AML, there was a fall in haemoglobin and platelet counts compatible with advancing disease. There was no evidence of renal impairment and liver function tests remained normal throughout.

D. Pharmacokinetic Study

I. Interferon Assay

Interferon activity in serum was measured by reduction of RNA synthesis in V3 cells challenged with Semliki forest virus. Background levels of 10 units/ml were found in pre-treatment sera. Serum interferon levels attained by intravenous injection and infusion are shown in Figures 1, 2 and 3.

E. In Vitro Study

In patients with AML, bone marrow blasts and, where possible, peripheral blood myeloblasts were cultured using a microculture technique with HLBI at concentrations of 10, 10^2, 10^3 and 10^4 units/ml. Growth was assessed by uptake of tritiated thymidine and viable cell counts after 3 days of culture. The degree of growth inhibition with various concentrations of HLBI is shown in Table 3.

Interferon decreased cell survival and inhibited uptake of tritiated thymidine at concentrations greater than 10 units/ml. Growth inhibition was dose dependant. There was no difference in sensitivity between bone marrow and peripheral blood blasts.

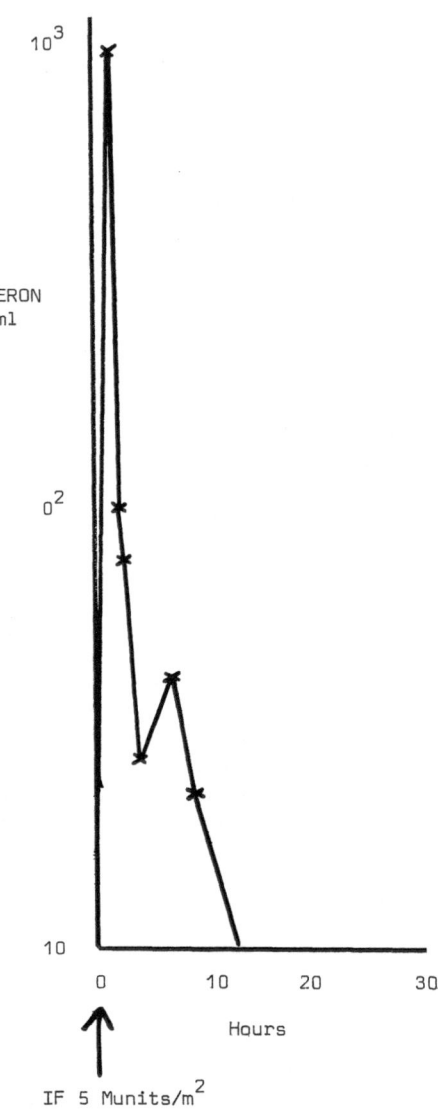

Fig. 1. Interferon levels after injection of 5 Megaunits/m^2 intravenously

F. Conclusions

The symptoms observed are similar to those reported with leukocyte interferon when given intramuscularly. Up to 10×10^6 units/m^2 daily can be given intravenously, but to avoid toxicity and in order to achieve consistent levels intravenous HLBI should be given by continuous infusion.

After intravenous injection of HLBI, high peak levels are achieved at 30 min, but interferon is rapidly cleared in the first h after injection. When given by continuous intravenous infusion, interferon levels increase over 72 h and then remain elevated. Continuous infusion is therefore an appropriate mode of administration for thrombocytopenic patients.

The results of the in vitro study confirm the cell growth inhibitory affects of HLBI on human myeloblasts. The degree of growth inhibition is dose dependant. However, the

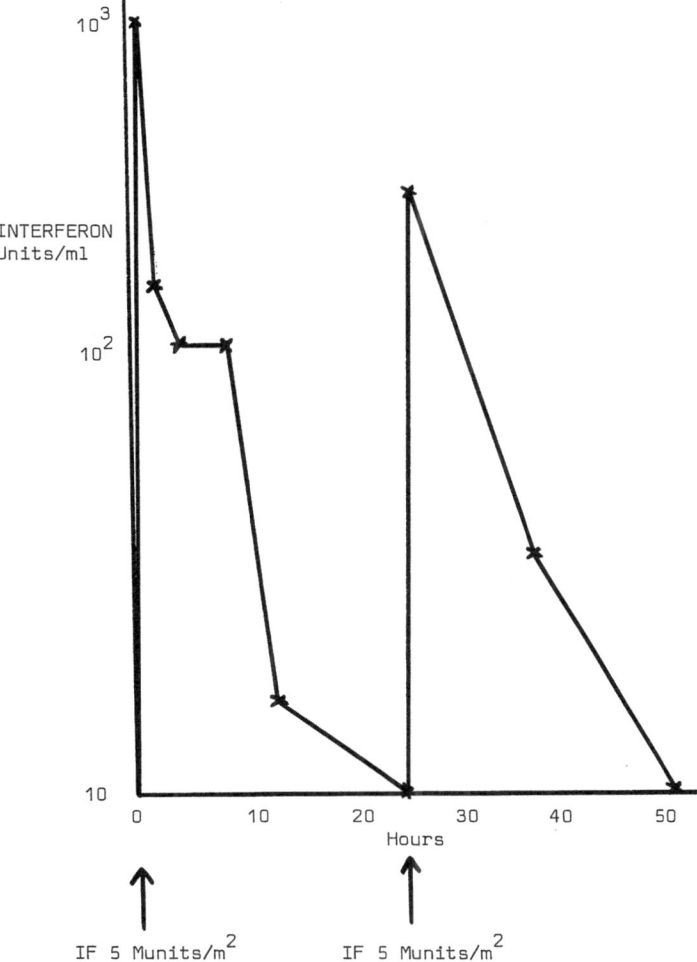

INTERFERON
Units/ml

Hours

IF 5 Munits/m^2 IF 5 Munits/m^2

Fig. 2. Interferon levels after injection 5 Megaunits/m^2 intravenously

concentrations of interferon that resulted in 50% inhibiton of growth in vitro were 3–10 times higher than the serum levels attained. With possible further escalation of the dose, levels of 10^3 units/ml may be attainable.

The study continues – it is planned to further escalate the daily dose and duration of infusions up to a maximum of 30 days. Administration of HLBI by subcutaneous injection will also be investigated.

Interferon concentrations (units/ml)				
	10	10^2	10^3	10^4
% Reduction of control cell numbers				
Median	5.7	19.1	41.5	61.6
Range	0–18.3	2.5–38.0	8.4–60.3	28.2–84
% Reduction of thymidine incorporation				
Median	10.4	22.8	39.8	51.3
Range	0–33.2	2.4–38.1	12.9–59.1	28.8–69

Table 3. The effect of interferon on cell growth and thymidine uptake in bone marrow and peripheral blood myeloblasts

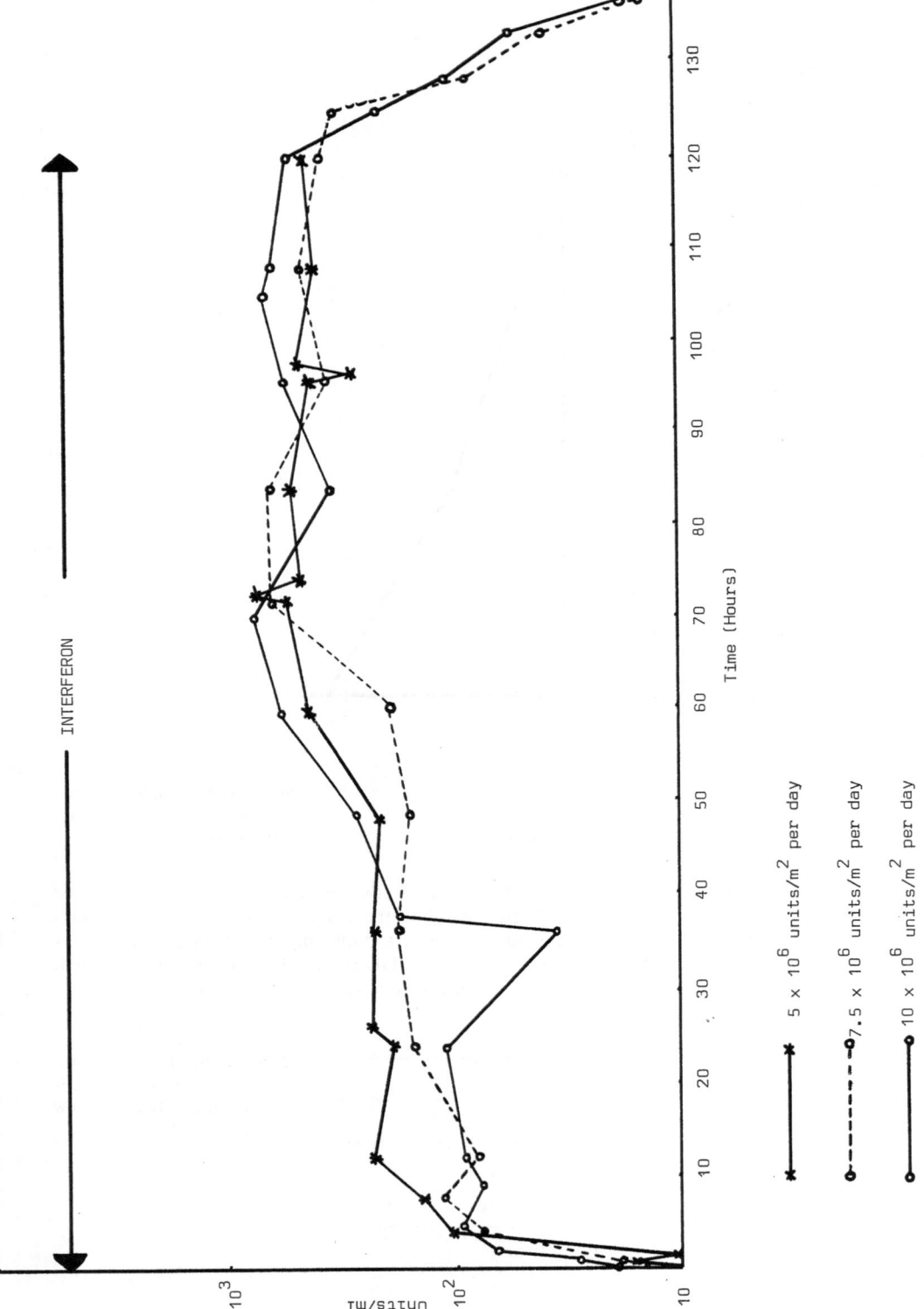

Fig. 3. Interferon levels with continuous infusions of HLBI at different doses

5×10^6 units/m^2 per day

7.5×10^6 units/m^2 per day

10×10^6 units/m^2 per day

INTERFERON

Units/ml

Time (Hours)

References

Balkwill FR, Oliver RTD (1977) Growth inhibitory effects of Interferon on normal and malignant human haemopoietic cells. Int J Cancer 20:500–505 – Gutterman J, Yap Y, Buzdar A, Alexanian R, Hersh E, Cabanillas F (1979) Leukocyte Interferon (IF) induced tumor regression in patients (PTS) with breast cancer and B cell neoplasms. AACR 674 – Hill NO, Leob E, Khan A, Pardue A, Hill JM, Aleman C, Dorn G (1980) Phase I human leukocyte interferon trials in leukaemia and cancer. AACR C-167 – Idestrom G, Cantell K, Killander D, Nilson K, Strander H, Willems J (1979) Interferon therapy in multiple myeloma. Acta Med Scand 105:149–154 – Mellstedt H, Bjorkholm M, Johansson B, Ahre A, Holm G, Strander H (1979) Interferon therapy in myelomatosis. Lancet I:245–247 – Merigan TC, Sikora K, Bredden JH, Levy R, Rosenberg S (1978) Preliminary observations on the effect of human leukocyte interferon in non-Hodgkin's lymphoma. N Engl J Med 29:1458–1453 – Osserman EF, Sherman WH (1980) Preliminary results of the American Cancer Society (ACS) – sponsored trial of human leukocyte Interferon (FI) in multiple myeloma (MM). AACR 643

Haematology and Blood Transfusion Vol. 26
Modern Trends in Human Leukemia IV
Edited by Neth, Gallo, Graf, Mannweiler, Winkler
© Springer-Verlag Berlin Heidelberg 1981

Methods and Clinical Relevance of Terminal Deoxynucleotidyl Transferase Determination in Leukemic Cells*

R. Mertelsmann, M. A. S. Moore and B. Clarkson

A. Summary

Terminal deoxynucleotidyl transferase (TdT) is a unique DNA polymerase which is only found in immature cells of lymphoid lineage (pre-T/pre-B). Because of this restricted distribution of TdT, biochemical and immunofluorescence techniques have been employed to determine the distribution of TdT phenotypes in human leukemias and lymphomas, showing high levels of TdT in ∼95% of acute lymphoblastic leukemia (ALL) and lymphoblastic lymphoma (LBL), ∼50% of patients with acute undifferentiated leukemia (AUL), ∼10% of patients with acute nonlymphoblastic leukemia (ANLL), and ∼30% of patients with chronic myeloid leukemia (CML) and other myeloproliferative (MPS) or myelodysplastic (MDS) syndromes in blast crisis. High levels of TdT activity are associated with a clinical response to remission inducing therapy with vincristine and prednisone in a high proportion of patients (50%–90%), irrespective of clinical and morphologic diagnosis. Preliminary studies furthermore suggest that TdT might serve as a sensitive indicator of subclinical disease in ALL in complete remission.

B. Introduction

Terminal deoxynucleotidyl transferase is a unique DNA polymerase which adds deoyribonucleotides onto an appropriate primer mole-cule in the absence of any directing template polynucleotide (Bollum 1979). Under physiologic conditions TdT is restricted to thymocytes and to a subpopulation of bone marrow lymphocytes which exhibit characteristics of immature T (Incefy et al. 1980; Silverstone et al. 1976) or B cells (Janossy et al. 1979, 1980; Vogler et al. 1978). All other cell types, including myeloid, erythroid, and putative pluripotent stem cells, do not exhibit detectable TdT activity (Mertelsmann et al. 1979a). Because of the restricted distribution to early developmental stages of lymphocytes, which loose TdT activity during final maturation into circulating cells, it has been speculated that TdT might play a role in the generation of immunologic diversity (Bollum 1979). Figure 1 depicts a schematic model of human hematopoiesis and the cell types to which TdT appears restricted under physiologic conditions.

Since the first report by Kung et al. (1978) about high levels of TdT in ALL, this enzyme has been widely employed in the phenotypic analysis of hemopoietic neoplasias (Bollum 1979; Donlon et al. 1977; Gordon et al. 1978; Janossy et al. 1980; Kung et al. 1978; Mertelsmann et al. 1978a,b, 1979a,b, 1981; Modak et al. 1980; Sarin et al. 1976; Vogler et al. 1978). This report reviews current technologies for demonstration of TdT and its significance in the clinical and pathophysiologic evaluation of human leukemias and lymphomas.

C. Techniques for Demonstration of TdT

Several biochemical methods have been developed to quantitate TdT activity in human tissues, yielding qualitatively similar results. In order to be able to study routinely obtained

* Supported by Grant Number CA-20194 awarded by the National Cancer Institute, U.S. Dept. of Health, Education, and Welfare, and by the Gar Reichman Foundation

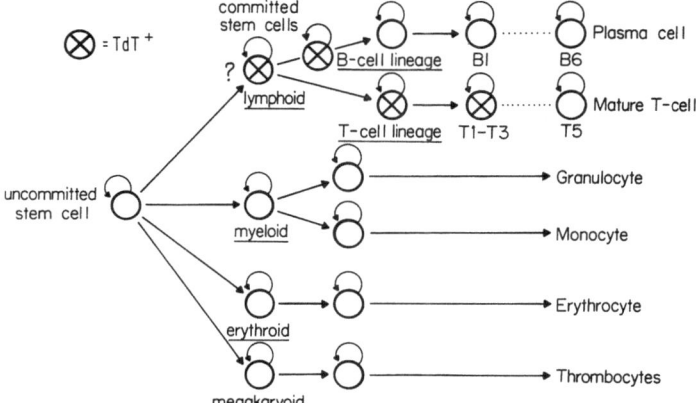

Fig. 1. Schematic model of human hematopoiesis

blood ($\sim$5 ml) and marrow specimen ($\sim$1 ml), we have recently developed a biochemical microassay which is highly sensitive and specific for TdT in human blood cells (Modak et al. 1980).

Bollum (1979) and Kung et al. (1978) reported the successful preparation of specific antisera against homogeneous calf thymus TdT, which recently also have become commercially available, including a monoclonal anti-calf thymus TdT antibody (BRL Biochemicals, Bethesda, Md). Using anti-TdT antibody and indirect immunofluorescence, TdT

Table 1. TDT activities in acute leukemias and in lymphomas. Total No. studied: 1000

Clinical diagnosis	% TdT +
Acute leukemias	
ALL	
non-T, non-B	94
T	85
pre-B	80
B	0
ANLL	9
AUL	55
Lymphomas	
LBL	96
Burkitt's	0
DPDL	0
DHL, DML	8
NPDL, NML, NHL	0
DWDL (CLL)	0
Hodgkin's	0
IBLA	0

in bone marrow cells appears predominantly in the nucleus, while thymocytes reveal predominantly cytoplasmic fluorescence (Bollum 1979). However, more sophisticated fixation techniques preserving cellular ultrastructure are required for the definitive subcellular localization of TdT (Steinmann et al. 1981). Newer techniques for analysis of TdT distribution in human blood cells include application of flow cytometry (unpublished work) and of metabolic labeling techniques for quantitation of newly synthesized TdT molecules in a given cell suspension (unpublished work). All techniques for demonstration of TdT have yielded almost identical results regarding the distribution of TdT in hemopoietic tissues and neoplasias. All observations will therefore be reviewed together, without further reference to the particular techniques employed.

D. Distribution of TdT in Human Leukemias and Lymphomas

I. Acute Leukemias

In acute leukemias (Table 1) the highest levels of TdT activity are found in $\sim$95% of "non-T, non-B" and T cell ALL. ALL of the TdT negative [TdT($-$)] T cell type probably represents leukemic or lymphomatous proliferation of a more mature T cell, while the exact phenotype and physiologic equivalent of TdT-negative non-T, non-B ALL remains to be determined (Mertelsmann et al. 1979a). Recently, a previously unrecognized ALL phenotype exhibiting intracytoplasmic μ chains ("pre-B" phenotype) has been described which was found to be associated with high levels of TdT in ~80% (Janossy et al. 1980; Vogler et al. 1978). The absolute level of TdT in ALL lymphoblasts has not been found to correlate with clinical features or prognosis. Most leukemias exhibiting high levels of TdT activity appear to be sensitive to vincristine and prednisone, including the TdT(+) "non-B, non-T", "T", and the "pre-B" phenotypes (Janossy et al. 1980; Vogler et al. 1978).

Elevated levels of TdT have also been observed in some patients with ANLL (Bollum 1979; Gordon et al. 1978; Mertelsmann et al. 1978a, 1979a). In our own cases with 10% overall incidence of TdT(+) phenotypes in 300 cases of ANLL (unpublished), more extensive phenotypic analysis revealed evidence of involvement of more than one cell lineage in the leukemic process in approximately one-half of these TdT(+) ANLL cases, leading to the concept of bi- or polyphenotypic leukemias (Mertelsmann et al. 1978a, 1979a) (Fig. 2). In other TdT(+) cases mostly carrying a diagnosis of AUL with equivocal morphology and cytochemistry only the TdT assay allowed cell type identification (Gordon et al. 1978). The exact phenotype can sometimes not be determined even when employing multiple marker techniques including TdT assays and could represent "nonlymphoid, nonmyeloid" stem cells, e.g., early megakaryoblasts and erythroblasts, which require even more sophisticated techniques for diagnosis (Mertelsmann et al. 1979a,b). Recently, we have been able to show correlation between

elevated TdT activity and production of T cell growth factor (TCGF, Interleukin 2), suggesting a specific common regulatory abnormality in all TdT(+) human leukemias irrespective of clinical diagnosis (Mertelsmann et al.1981).

II. Myelodysplastic and Myeloproliferative Syndromes

All myeloproliferative syndromes (MPS: P. vera, CML) and myelodysplastic syndromes (MDS: RAEB, CMMOL) were found to be TdT(−) during the chronic phase of their disease, while approximately 30% of blast phase CML and 15% of other MDS and MPS terminating in acute leukemia were found to exhibit high levels of TdT activity (Table 2). It is of clinical significance that the majority of TdT(+) acute leukemias preceded by MPS or MDS have also responded to therapy with vincristine and prednisone (data not shown, see Mertelsmann et al. 1979b).

The phenotype in MDS and MPS in blast phase appears to be labile with changes in the

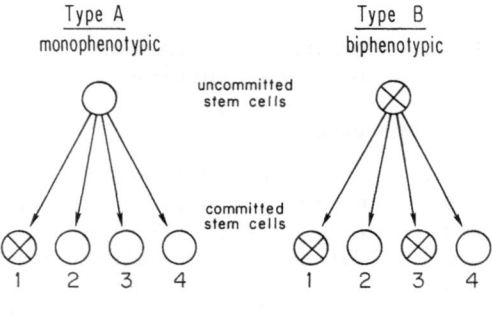

Type A
monophenotypic

Type B
biphenotypic

uncommitted stem cells

committed stem cells

1 2 3 4   1 2 3 4

⊗ leukemic cell compartment

1,2,3,4 = anyone of the 4 major hematopoietic cell lineages

Fig. 2. Hypothetical pathogenetic types of human leukemia

Table 2. TdT activities in myeloproliferative (MPS), myelodysplastic (MDS), and lymphoproliferative (LPS) syndromes. Total No. studies: 300

Clinical diagnosis	% TdT +
MDS/MPS chronic phase	
CML	0
CMMOL	0
RAEB	0
Aplastic anemia	0
MDS/MPS acute phase	
CML	30
CMMOL	10
RAEB	10
P. vera	30
Aplastic anemia	10
LPS	
CLL	
– B	0
– T	10
Prolymphocytic leukemia	0
Hairy cell leukemia	0
LSA-leukemia	0
Mycosis f., Sezary's s.	5
Multiple myeloma	0
Waldenstroem's mg	0
Cold agglutinin s.	0

predominant cell type occurring either spontaneously or after therapy, while this appears to be more unusual in de novo ALL or ANLL (unpublished work).

III. Lymphoproliferative Disorders

Recent studies by Donlon et al. (1977), Kung et al. (1978), and ourselves (Mertelsmann et al. 1978b, 1979a) have demonstrated the clinical significance of TdT determinations in patients with non-Hodgkin's lymphoma (Table 1). In patients with lymphoblastic lymphomas of the T and "null" cell type high levels of TdT were observed as seen in ALL. Because a definitive histologic diagnosis is sometimes difficult to make in this group of patients we have often found TdT determinations providing important diagnostic information. Lymphoproliferative diseases of the mature T and B cell type have been found to be TdT(−) (Table 1). Although diffuse histiocytic lymphomas, which are diagnosed on the basis of the presence of large cells resembling histiocytes, generally represent B-cell proliferations, a few cases of "true" histiocytic lymphomas with cells exhibiting phagocytic properties and more recently lymphomas of the null cell type have been described which exhibited high levels of TdT in involved tissue (Gordon et al. 1978; Mertelsmann et al. 1978b). Although it is too early to determine the significance of these marker studies for the response to therapy and long-term prognosis in this group of patients, all patients with lymphoid neoplasias with high levels of TdT studied by us had a characteristic clinical course resembling that of ALL.

IV. TdT Determinations in the Monitoring of Disease Activity in TdT + Neoplasia

We have reported significantly elevated TdT levels in ALL bone marrow in complete remission on and off therapy as compared to normal controls (Mertelsmann et al. 1978b). The TdT levels characteristically fluctuated, which could not be explained by technical problems or chemotherapy. A preliminary analysis of our own data suggests an increased risk of relapse in patients with persistently elevated TdT values in CR. The clinical and biologic significance of elevated TdT levels in ALL in patients in long-term remission off chemotherapy remains to be analyzed; if indicative of residual disease, this observation would be important for the understanding of the pathophysiology of leukemias and for the design of therapeutic strategies.

E. Conclusion

From our own studies and work by published others it appears that determination of TdT activity and definition of cell phenotypes in hematopoietic malignancies are useful tools for the classification of these disorders and have significant prognostic, clinical, and pathogenetic implications. Although several questions still remain unsolved, this comprehensive approach, when correlated with clinical presentation and conventional morphology, might help the physician by providing objective diagnostic criteria for prognostic subgroups unidentifiable by conventional methods. Furthermore, this approach will help to understand the underlying pathogenetic processes leading to the clinical syndromes of human leukemias and lymphomas.

Acknowledgments

The skillful technical assistance of Ms. Lorna Barnett und Ms. Sa An Hu is greatly appreciated. We would like to thank Ms. Cynthia Garcia for typing the manuscript.

References

(Representative references were selected, which list further literature regarding specific aspects of TdT.) – Bollum FJ (1979) Terminal deoxynucleotidyl transferase as a hematopoietic cell marker. Blood 54:1203–1215 – Donlon JA, Jaffe ES, Braylon RC (1977) Terminal deoxynucleotidyl transferase activity in malignant lymphomas. N Engl J Med 297:461–464 – Gordon SD, Hutton JJ, Smalley RV, Meyer ML, Vogler WR (1978) Terminal deoxynucleotidyl transferase (TdT), cytochemistry, and membrane receptors in adult acute leukemia. Blood 52:1079–1088 – Incefy GS, Mertelsmann R, Yata K, Dardenne M, Bach JF, Good RA (1980) Induction of differentiation in human marrow T-cell precursors by the synthetic serum thymic factor, FTS. Clin Exp Immunol 40:396–406 – Janossy G, Bollum FJ, Bradstock KF, McMichael A, Rapson N, Greaves MF (1979) Terminal transferase-positive human bone marrow cells exhibit the antigenic phenotype of common acute lymphoblastic leukemia. J Immunol 124:1525–1529 – Janossy G, Hoffbrand AV, Greaves MF, Ganeshaguru K, Pain C, Bradstock KF, Prentice HG, Kay HEM, Lister TA (1980) Terminal transferase enzyme assay and immunological membrane markers in the diagnosis of leukaemia: a multiparameter analysis of 300 cases. Br J Hematol 44:221–234 – Kung PC, Long JC, McCaffrey RP, Ratlif RL, Harrison TA, Baltimore D (1978) Terminal deoxynucleotidyl transferase in the diagnosis of leukemia and malignant lymphoma. Am J Med 64:788–794 – Mertelsmann R, Koziner B, Ralph P, Filippa D, McKenzie S, Arlin ZA, Gee TS, Moore MAS, Clarkson BD (1978a) Evidence for distinct lymphocytic and monocytic populations in a patient with terminal transferase positive acute leukemia. Blood 51:1051–1056 – Mertelsmann R, Mertelsmann I, Koziner B, Moore MAS, Clarkson BD (1978b) Improved biochemical assay for terminal deoxynucleotidyl transferase in human blood cells: Results in 89 adult patients with lymphoid leukemias and malignant lymphomas in leukemic phase. Leuk Res 2:57–69 – Mertelsmann R, Koziner B, Filippa DA, Grossbard E, Incefy G, Moore MAS, Clarkson BD (1979a) Clinical significance of TdT, cell surface markers and CFU-c in 297 patients with hematopoietic neoplasias. In: Neth R, Gallo RC, Hofschneider P-H, Mannweiler K (eds), Modern trends in human leukemia III, Springer, Berlin Heidelberg New York p 131 – Mertelsmann R, Moore MAS, Clarkson BD (1979b) Sequential marrow culture studies and terminal deoxynucleotidyl transferase activities in myelodysplastic syndromes. In: Schmalzl R, Hellriegel KP (ed) Preleukemia, Springer, Berlin Heidelberg New York, p 106 – Mertelsmann R, Gillis S, Moore MAS, Koziner B (1981) Abnormal TCGF response pattern in human leukemias exhibiting high TdT activity. In: Moore, MAS (ed) Differentiation factors in cancer, Raven Press, New York – Modak MJ, Mertelsmann R, Koziner B, Pahwa R, Moore MAS, Clarkson BD, Good RA (1980) A micromethod for determination of terminal deoxynucleotidyl transferase (TdT) in the diagnostic evaluation of acute leukemias. Cancer Res Clin Oncol 98:91–104 – Sarin PS, Anderson PN, Gallo RC (1976) Terminal deoxynucleotidyl transferase activities in human blood leukocytes and lymphoblast cell lines: High levels in lymphoblast cell lines and in blast cells of some patients with chronic myelogenous leukemia in acute phase. Blood 47:11–20 – Silverstone AE, Cantor H, Goldstein G, Baltimore D (1976) Terminal deoxynucleotidyl transferase is found in prothymocytes. J Exp Med 144:543–548 – Steinmann G, Mertelsmann R, de Harven E, Moore MAS (1981) Ultrastructural demonstration of terminal deoxynucleotidyl transferase (TdT). Blood 57:368–371 – Vogler LB, Crist WM, Bockman DE, Pearl ER, Lawton AR, Cooper MD (1978) Pre-B cell leukemia. A new phenotype of childhood lymphoblastic leukemia. N Engl J Med 298:872–878

Haematology and Blood Transfusion Vol. 26
Modern Trends in Human Leukemia IV
Edited by Neth, Gallo, Graf, Mannweiler, Winkler
© Springer-Verlag Berlin Heidelberg 1981

Quantitation of Chemotherapy-Induced Cytoreduction in Acute Leukemia*

W. Hiddemann, M. Andreeff, and B. D. Clarkson

A. Introduction

In acute leukemia response to chemotherapy is usually assessed by relative changes of the percentage of leukemic blasts on bone marrow smears. In contrast to quantitative evaluations of cell numbers in peripheral blood which yield a high accuracy, especially since the introduction of electronic equipment, similar approaches have not been available for bone marrow aspirates due to its variable cell and volume composition of blood and bone marrow (bm).

We here report first results of a newly developed technique which allows one to accurately quantify the absolute number of cells per mm³ bm. This parameter was used to measure treatment-induced cytoreduction rates during induction therapy of acute non-lymphocytic leukemia (ANLL) and was also applied to a phase II study of high dose thymidine (TdR) therapy in end stage acute leukemias and lymphomas.

B. Materials and Methods

The principle of the method is as follows: Cell kinetic differences between pure bm obtained by Jamshidi biopsy and bm aspirate and blood as measured by flow cytometry (Andreeff et al. 1980; Traganos et al. 1977) are used to identify the proportion of contaminating blood *cells* in bm aspirates, which subsequently permits one to calculate the remaining proportion of pure bm cells per mm³ aspirate. Blood *volume* contamination is determined by the ratio of red cell hematocrits in aspirate and blood, as distribution studies of radioactive labeled erythrocytes have shown that mature red cells circulate exclusively

intravascularly and are not present in pure bm tissue (Fauci 1975; Donohue et al. 1958; Holdrinet et al. 1980). The red cell hematocrit in bm aspirates, therefore, represents the admixed peripheral blood volume. Combining the two described procedures, pure bm volume and bm cell number are determined from bm aspirates, and thus the absolute number of bm cells per mm³ bm volume becomes quantifiable. The additional evaluation of the proportion of leukemic cells on biopsy cytospin preparations provides the means to determine the number of leukemic bm cells per mm³ bm (Hiddemann et al. 1980).

Leukemic cell number per mm³ bm was measured prior to and at the 2nd and 5th day of induction therapy for ANLL in ten previously untreated patients. The induction regimen consisted of daunorubicin 60 mg/m² per day on days 1, 2, and 3 and cytosine arabinoside started with an initial loading dose of 25 mg IV, followed by a 5 day infusion of 200 mg/m² per day and 6-thioguanine 200 mg/m² per day orally administered from days 1 to 5 (Arlin et al. 1979). In four patients with end stage acute leukemias and non-Hodgkin lymphomas, therapy induced cytoreduction was monitored during clinical phase II evaluation of high dose TdR. TdR was administered by continuous infusion over 18 to 28 days in a dose of 140 to 240 g/m² per day (Blumenreich et al. 1980).

C. Results

I. Induction therapy of ANLL

In nine of the ten patients a total cell kill of 2.0 to 3.9 $\log^{10}$ of leukemic bm cells was measured during the 5 days of therapy as shown by the examples in Fig. 1. In all nine patients less than 5% blasts were found on bm examinations 1 week after completion of chemotherapy. Six of the nine patients subsequently went into complete remission (CR), two died in bm aplasia, and one developed an early relapse

* Supported by grants DFG Hi 288/I, ACS-CH 154, NCI-CAO5826

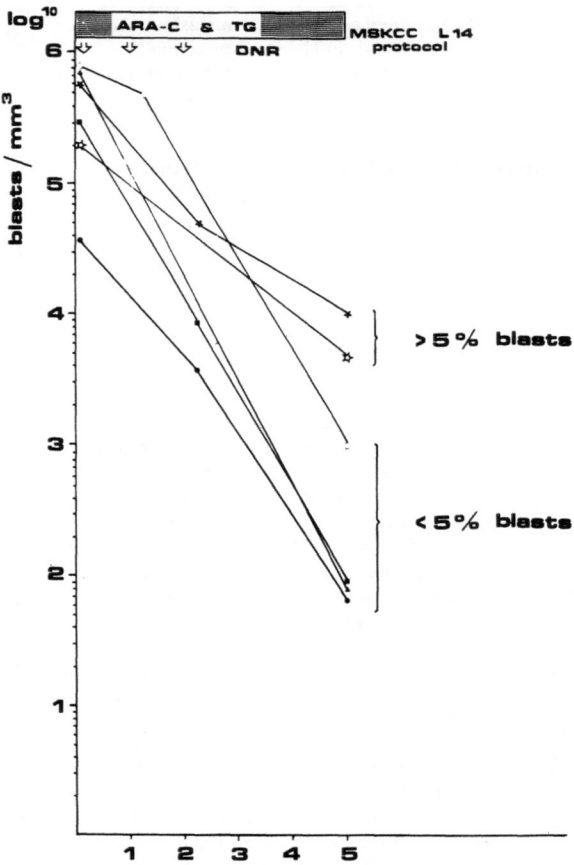

Fig. 1. Treatment-induced blast cell reduction in the bone marrow during induction therapy in five patients with ANLL. *Open* and *solid stars* represent cytoreduction rates in one patient who received two identical courses of the induction regimen

4 weeks after completion of the first induction course. In one patient leukemic cell mass in the bm was only reduced by 1.4 $\log^{10}$ during induction therapy and posttreatment bm examination still showed 60% leukemic blasts. A second course of the identical regimen resulted in a similar cytoreduction of 1.7 $\log^{10}$ and 40% blasts were found on posttreatment bm examination. The cytoreduction rates of this patient are represented by the two upper curves in Fig. 1.

II. High Dose TdR

For three of the four patients cell kill rates of 0.17, 0.13, and 0.13 $\log^{10}$ per day were measured and all three achieved bm aplasia as documented by bm biopsy. The one patient who was treated over a period of 28 days achieved a total reduction in the leukemic bm cell mass of 3.6 $\log^{10}$ and went into CR. The fourth patient did not respond to TdR as judged by morphologic examination of bm aspirates and biopsies, and a total blast cell reduction of only 0.9 $\log^{10}$ (0.05 $\log^{10}$/d) was found after 25 days of TdR therapy.

D. Discussion

Quantitation of chemotherapy-induced cytoreduction by monitoring the absolute number of leukemic cells per mm³ bm provides a new quantitative determinant to evaluate treatment efficacy in acute leukemia. This parameter complements and facilitates clinical trials with new drugs such as high dose TdR, as the sensitivity of leukemic cells to the applied therapy is quantifiable in vivo and after short periods of drug exposure, which allows one to detect response or nonresponse at an early stage of treatment.

For induction therapy of ANLL quantitation of therapeutic response not only permits

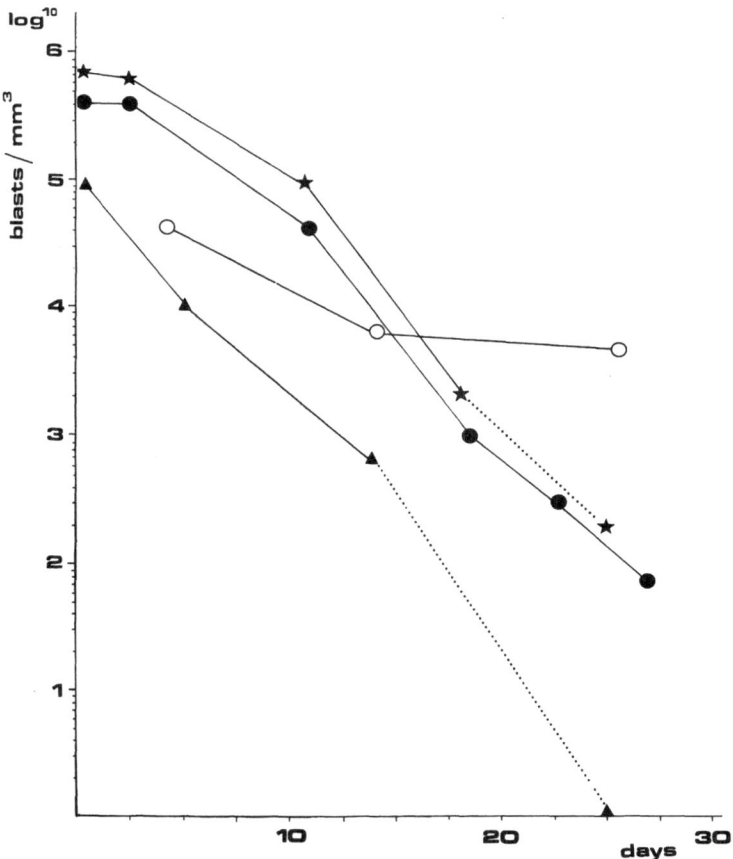

Fig. 2. Treatment-induced blast cell reduction in the bone marrow during high dose Thymidine therapy. *Dotted lines* represent cytoreduction rates after the end of TdR infusion

one to discriminate responders and nonresponders. The present data indicate that even in the group of responders different blast cell reduction rates were achieved. They ranged from a total of 2.0 to 3.9 log[10] during the 5 day treatment period, suggesting that different amounts of residual leukemic cells may remain after therapy within a group of patients who all fulfill the hematologic criteria for a complete bm response. Quantitation of therapeutic response may therefore result in a quantitative assessment of remission status which may become a determining prognostic factor for remission duration, especially since increasing evidence suggests that maintenance chemotherapy has a minor or even no effect on the duration of complete remission (Lewis et al. 1976; Omura et al. 1977; Sauter et al. 1980; Vaughan et al. 1980).

References

Andreeff M, Darzynkiewicz Z, Sharpless TK, Clarkson BD, Melamed MR (1980) Discrimination of human leukemia subtypes by flow cytometric analysis of cellular DNA and RNA. Blood 55:282–293 – Arlin Z, Gee T, Fried J, Koenigsberg E, Wolmark N, Clarkson BD (1979) Rapid induction of remission in acute nonlymphocytic leukemia (ANLL). Am Assoc Cancer Res 29:112 – Blumenreich M, Andreeff M, Murphy ML, Young C, Clarkson B (1980) Phase II study of mM thymidine in acute leukemia with flow microfluorometric analysis of drug induced kinetic alterations in the bone marrow. Am Assoc Cancer Res 21:179 – Donohue DM, Gabrio BW, Finch CA (1958) Quantitative measurements of hematopoietic cells of the marrow. J Clin Invest 37:1564–1570 – Fauci AS (1975) Human bone marrow lymphocytes. I. Distribution of lymphocyte subpopulations in the bone marrow of normal individuals. J Clin Invest 56:98–111 – Hiddemann W, Büchner T, Arlin Z, Gee T, Burchenal JH, Clarkson BD (1980) Acute non-lymphocytic leukemia-early determinants for response to chemotherapy. Am Soc Clin Oncol 21:438 – Holdrinet RSG, Egmond JV, Wessels JMC, Haanen C (1980) A method for quantification of peripheral blood admixture in bone marrow aspirates. Exp Hematol 8:103–117 – Lewis JP, Linman JW, Rajak TF, Bateman JR (1976) Effect of "maintenance" chemotherapy on survival in adults with acute nonlymphocytic leukemia. Clin Res 24:158A – Omura GA, Vogler WR, Lynn MJ (1977) A controlled clinical trial of chemotherapy vs. BCG vs. no further therapy in remission maintenance of acute myelogenous leukemia. Am Soc Clin Oncol 18:272 – Sauter C, Alberto P, Berchtold W, Cavalli F, Fopp M, Tschopp L (1980) Three to five months remission induction treatment (IT) of acute myelogenous leukemia (AML) followed by maintenance treatment (MT) or no MT. Am Soc Clin Oncol 21:433 – Traganos F, Darzynkiewicz Z, Sharpless T, Melamed MR (1977) Simultaneous staining of ribonucleic and deoxyribonucleic acids in unfixed cells using acridine orange in a flow cytofluorometric system. J Histochem Cytochem 25:46–56 – Vaughan WP, Karp EJ, Burke PJ (1980) Long chemotherapyfree remissions after single-cycle timed-sequential chemotherapy for acute myelocytic leukemia. Cancer 45:859–865

Haematology and Blood Transfusion Vol. 26
Modern Trends in Human Leukemia IV
Edited by Neth, Gallo, Graf, Mannweiler, Winkler
© Springer-Verlag Berlin Heidelberg 1981

Intensive Therapy and Prognostic Factors in Acute Lymphoblastic Leukemia of Childhood: CCG 141

A report from Childrens Cancer Study Group*

D. R. Miller, S. Leikin, V. Albo, H. Sather, M. Karon, and D. Hammond

A. Introduction

Studies reported by CCSG (Miller et al. 1974; Robison et al. 1980), other cooperative groups (George et al. 1973), and independent pediatric cancer centers (Simone 1976) have clearly indicated that front-end prognostic factors can be as important, or more important, than the therapy itself in determining the results of a modern clinical trial in previously untreated children with acute lymphoblastic leukemia (ALL). This effect becomes even more pronounced as the majority of patients are surviving free of disease for 5 or more years. Definitive results of clinical trials may require 5 to 7 years of follow up to determine the optimal duration of therapy or even longer to determine the rate of long-term survival.

Treatment strategies using multiple-drug induction and maintenance therapy, central nervous system (CNS) prophylaxis, and intensive supportive care have resulted in complete remission rates of 90%–95% or greater and disease-free survival of 5 years or more in 50%–60% of all patients. Because treatment interacts with host and disease, this study, CCG 141, was launched in 1975 to evaluate prognostic factors that influence induction rate, duration of complete continuous remission (CCR), and survival and to identify subsets of patients with a high risk of early failure or with a particularly favorable prognosis. The efficacy of more intensive induction and maintenance therapy was evaluated in patients with a poor prognosis based upon initial white blood cell (WBC) count.

The purpose of this report is to present the results of the treatment regimens and to redefine prognostic groups based upon the prospective evaluation of front-end factors.

B. Materials and Methods

I. Patients

Previously untreated children under 20 years of age were eligible for this study. Informed consent in accordance with institutional policies approved by the U.S. Department of Health, Education, and Welfare was obtained prior to entry on study. Criteria for response to therapy and status of disease were those used by the Childrens Cancer Study Group (CCSG). Remission status of the bone marrow was determined by the per cent of blasts ($<5\% = M_1$, $6\% - 25\% = M_2$, $>25\% = M_3$). The prognostic groups, i.e., "low risk," "average risk," and "poor risk," are defined by age and WBC at diagnosis as presented by Nesbit et al. (1979) and currently in use by CCSG.

II. Special Determinations

Stained and unstained bone marrow slides or cover slips were evaluated using a modification of the FAB classification (Bennett et al. 1976; Miller et al., to be published). Quantitative immunoglobulins G, A, and M were performed by the methods of Fahey and McKelvey (1965).

III. Therapy Regimens

The study schema is presented in Fig. 1, and the dosage schedule in the treatment regimens is listed in Table 1. Patients were assigned to two treatment groups i.e. the "low" (initial institutional WBC less than 20×10^9/l) (LR$_1$) or "high" group (initial WBC equal to or greater than 20×10^9/l, and/or mediastinal widening on chest PA; and lateral, Bucky films

* Principal investigators of CCSG and their grant support are listed in the acknowledgments

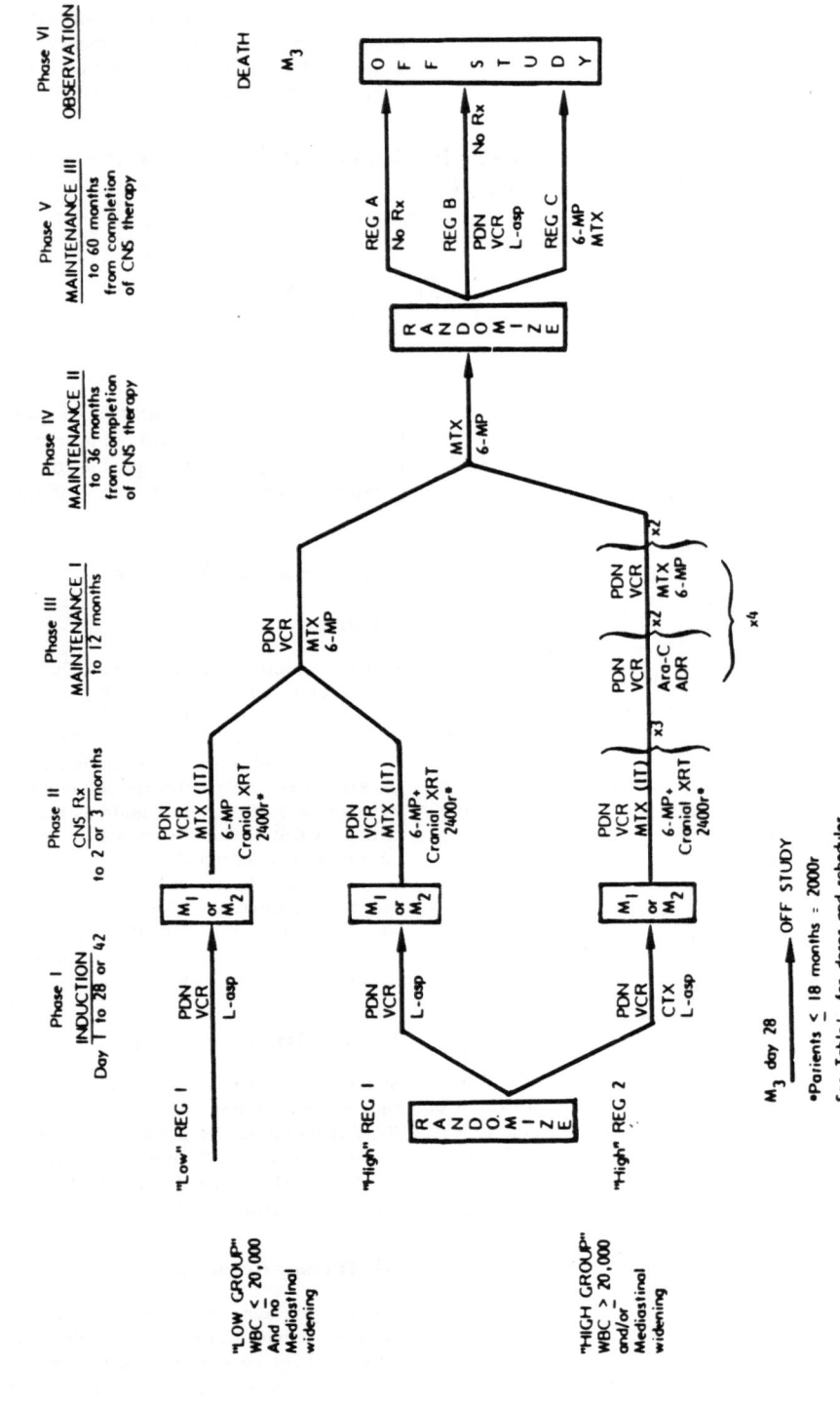

Fig. 1 Schema of CCG 141

Table 1. Dosage schedule of treatment regimens

Group	Induction	CNS-RX	Maintenance I	Maintenance II AND III
"Low" "High"	Reg. 1[a] PDN 40mg/m^2 q d p.o. VCR 1.5mg/m^2 q wk IV L-Asp 6000 IU/m^2 IM tiw (9 doses)	Reg. 1[a] PDN 40mg/m^2 q d × 5 q mo p.o. VCR 1.5mg/m^2 q mo IV IT MTX 12mg/m^2 q wk × 6 6-MP 75mg/m^2 q d p.o. + 2400r Cranial XRT[b]	Reg. 1[a] PDN 40mg/m^2 q d × 5 mo p.o. VCR 1.5mg/m^2 q mo IV MTX 20mg/m^2 q wk p.o. 6-MP 75mg/m^2 q d p.o.	MTX 20mg/m^2 q wk p.o. 6-MP 75mg/m^2 q d p.o. for 2 yrs. (4 yrs in Maint. III, Reg. C)
"High"	Reg. 2[a] Same as Regimen 1, plus Cytoxan 100mg/m^2 q d p.o.	Reg. 2[a] POMP-I PDN 40mg/m^2 q d × 4 p.o. VCR 1.5mg/m^2 q mo IV)q IT-MTX 12mg/m^2 d-1&4) 14d 6-MP 500mg/m^2 p.o. q d 4) × 3 + 2400r Cranial XRT[b] After 42 days, Mainte- nance I therapy is begun.	Reg. 2[a] POCA PDN 40mg/m^2 q d × 4 p.o. VCR 1.5mg/m^2 q 21 d IV ADR 40mg/m^2 q 21 d IV Ara-C 100 mg/m^2 q d × 4 IV, IM, SQ, q 21 d twice POMP PDN 40mg/m^2 q d p.o. VCR 1.5mg/m^2 q mo IV MTX 5 mg/m^2 q d × 4 p.o. 6-MP 500mg/m^2 q d × 4 p.o. every 14 days twice.	MTX 20mg/m^2 q wk p.o. 6-MP 75mg/m^2 q d p.o. for 2 yrs. (4 yrs in Maint. III, Reg. C)

[a] Refer to Schema (Fig. 1) for group, phase, and regimen
[b] Patients ≤ months of age receive 2000r

and/or tomography). "High" patients were random-ly assigned to either "High Regimen 1" (HR$_1$) or "Regimen 2" (R$_2$).

In May 1976 after the results of CCG 101 indicated that mediastinal mass was not an indepen-dent prognostic factor, patients were no longer stratified on the basis of presence or absence of mediastinal mass. At that time five patients with initial WBC <20 × 10^9/l had been randomized to either HR$_1$ or R$_2$. Patients with M$_1$ marrow on day 28 or M$_1$ or M$_2$ marrow on day 42 advanced to CNS prophylaxis which consisted of 2400 rads to the cranium and intrathecal (IT) methotrexate (MTX) as 12 mg/m^2 weekly for 6 weeks (HR$_1$) or twice weekly for 3 weeks (R$_2$). Pulses of vincristine (VCR) and prednisone (PDN) were dropped during Main-tenance II. At 36 months from completion of CNS therapy, patients in complete continuous remission were randomized to receive either no further thera-py (Reg. A), a 4-week reinduction with PDN, VCR, and L-asparaginase (LASP) (Reg. B), or continued maintenance therapy with 6-mercaptopurine (6-MP) and MTX for 2 more years (Reg. C). All

males underwent bilateral testicular open-wedge biopsies prior to randomization to Maintenance III.

Patients were considered off study for the follo-wing reasons: M$_3$ marrow on day 28 or any time during CNS or maintenance phases, death, severe toxicity, major protocol violation, or loss to follow-up. Patients experiencing an extramedullary relapse were reinduced with PDN, VCR, LASP, and IT MTX and were restarted on maintenance at the point of relapse. CNS relapse was treated with IT MTX and an additional 2400 rads of cranial and 1200 rads spinal irradiation. Testicular relapse was treated with 2000 rads bilateral testicular irradia-tion.

C. Biostatistical Considerations

The log rank method of life table analysis (Peto et al. 1977) was used to evaluate the relative relapse rates or death rates for the treatment regimens and to determine the importance of prognostic characteristics under investigation. The Cox regression model (1972) for life table data was used in the multivariate analysis of prognostic factors determined to be of significance in the univariate analysis.

Complete data required to redefine prognostic groups were available on 360 (40.8%) of the 882 eligible patients. The age and WBC characteristics of the patients with incomplete data (59.2%) are similar to those for whom complete data were available.

D. Results

I. Progress

A total of 911 patients were registered on study, of whom 29 were ineligible (wrong diagnosis-ANLL, prior antileukemic therapy, clinical data and flow sheets never submitted). Of the 882 eligible patients, 576 were entered oni LR_1, 151 on HR_1, and 155 on R_2. The clinical characteristics of the patients entered on study are presented in Table 2. The median followup is over 36 months for all patients entered on study.

II. Inductions

The rates of complete remission (M_1 marrow) for all eligible patients entered on LR_1, HR_1, and R_2 were 95%, 93%, and 91%, respectively. A total of 827 patients (93.8%) completed induction with an M_1 marrow by day 28 or 42, and 832 (94.3%) were entered on the CNS therapy phase, five of whom had M_2 bone marrow ratings. Significant unfavorable factors of response to induction therapy, as determined by univariate analysis, were age >10 years, initial WBC $>20 \times 10^9$/l, presence of CNS disease at diagnosis, L_2 and L_3 morphology, decreased IgG, Down's syndrome, and <30% PAS positive lymphoblasts. Marrow status on day 14 of induction was also a significant predictor in that 99.7% (454/455) of children with an M_1 bone marrow on day 14 were M_1 at completion of induction, and only 81.4% (57/70) with M_3 marrow on day 14 were M_1 on day 28 or 42 of induction. Children over 10 years of age with initial WBC $>20 \times 10^9$/l and depressed IgG had a complete remission rate of only 55%.

Using multivariate regression analysis in a subset of 319 patients in whom complete data

Characteristic	%		%
Age, years		*FAB Morphology*	
<1.5	6	L_1 (>75% L_1)	84
1.5–3	18	L_2 (>25% L_2)	15
>3–10	54	L_3	1
>10	22		
WBC ($\times 10^{-9}$/liter)		*Immunoglobulins*	
<10	53	Normal	82
10–49	30	Depressed (1 or more)	18
≥50	17		
Low Risk[a]	22.2	*Hemoglobin (gm/dl)*	
Average risk	60.0	<7	43
High risk	17.8	7–10	45
		>10	12
Sex			
Male	57	Massive hepatomegaly	13
Female	43	Massive splenomegaly	14
		Massive adenopathy	7
Race		Lymphoma syndrome	5
White	89		
Non-white	11	Down's syndrome	2
CNS disease at diagnosis	4	M_3 BM, d14	10
Mediastinal mass	7		

Table 2. Clinical characteristics of eligible patients entered on CCG-141

[a] As defined by Nesbit et al. (1979)

on all the selected prognostic variables were available, age > 10 years ($P=0.0008$), CNS disease at diagnosis ($P=0.0007$), and depressed IgG ($P=0.004$) were the strongest predictors of induction failure.

III. Duration of CCR

Duration of CCR and hematologic remission is longer and relative relapse rate is lower in children entered on LR_1 than in patients entered on HR_1 and R_2 in which no significant differences are noted (Fig. 2). At 48 months, 65.2%, 48.1%, and 39.1% of patients on LR_1, HR_1, and R_2, respectively, remain in CCR. When HR_1 and R_2 are analyzed by average and high risk prognostic groups as defined by Nesbit (1979) no superiority of either regimen is observed. Of the patients completing induction, 57.6% remain in CCR.

IV. Maintenance II

During Maintenance II pulses of monthly PDN and VCR were deleted. No significant differences in relative relapse rates in the three regimens were observed (0/E 0.91, 1.14, 1.35 in LR_1, HR_1, and R_2, respectively, $P=0.16$). When compared to the previous CCG trial (CCG 101/143) in which monthly pulses of PDN and VCR were given throughout maintenance, no significant differences are apparent when data in comparable prognostic groups are compared (Fig. 3).

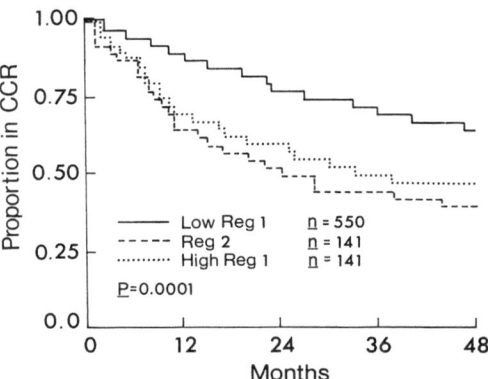

Fig. 2. Duration of complete continuous remission from start of CNS therapy by treatment regimen. First events include bone marrow or extramedullary relapses or death

V. CNS Relapse

The incidence of isolated CNS relapse in LR_1, HR_1, and R_2 is 4.7%, 8.5%, and 12.8%, respectively. These differences are significant (0/e=0.66, 1.46, 2.36, $P=0.001$). In all patients successfully completing induction, the overal CNS relapse rate is 6.7%.

VI. Testicular Relapse

During maintenance therapy, testicular relapse has occurred in 44 boys, or 9.6% of 459 patients at risk. The testicular relapse is

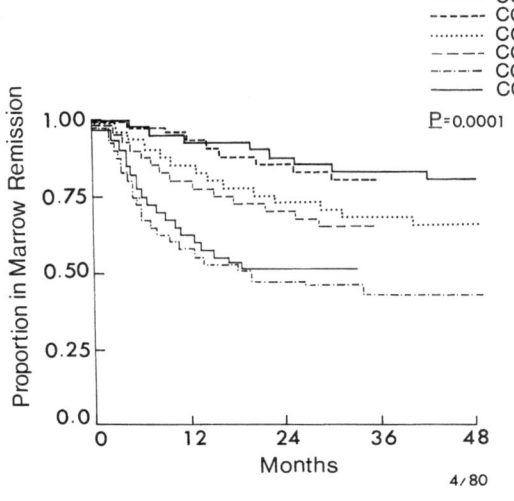

Fig. 3. Rate of bone marrow relapse by prognostic groups in CCG 101/143 and CCG 141. The differences within risk groups between the two studies are not statistically significant. The differences between the risk groups are highly significant ($P=0.0001$)

significantly higher in HR_1 (14.5%, 0/E 1.84) than in R_2 (7.4%, 0/E 0.98) or LR_1 (8.9%, 0/E = 0.85) (P = 0.047).

VII. Survival After First Isolated Relapse

Isolated bone marrow, CNS, and testicular relapses have occurred in 204, 57, and 34 patients, respectively. Despite reinduction therapy and prophylactic IT MTX in patients experiencing extramedullary relapses, the median survival after isolated testicular and CNS relapse was 19 months and 22 months, respectively. Median survival after first bone marrow relapse occurring predominantly in high risk patients during the first 24 months of therapy was only 10 months (Fig. 4).

VIII. Prognostic Factors

1. Disease-Free Survival (CCR)

Using the Cox regression model for life table data, significant variables for predicting disease-free survival were identified (Table 3). In rank order these are:
1. Log WBC
2. Hemoglobin
3. IgM
4. Splenomegaly
5. Age and age^2
6. Day 14 bone marrow and
7. Sex

IgG and FAB morphology were of borderline significance (P = 0.07 and 0.09). Platelet count, CNS disease at diagnosis,

Table 3. Significant variables for predicting disease-free survival in CCG-141[a]

Rank	Variable	Significance Level (P-Value)
1	log WBC	0.002
2	Hemoglobin	0.005
3	IgM	0.005
4	Splenomegaly	0.007
5	Age and Age^2	0.040 & 0.014
6	Day 14 marrow	0.029
7	Sex	0.036
8	IgG	0.070
9	Morphology	0.090

[a] Platelet count, CNS disease at diagnosis, nodal enlargement, mediastinal mass status, race, IgA, and hepatomegaly were not significant predictors of outcome in a multivariate context

lymph node enlargement, mediastinal mass, race, IgA, and hepatomegaly were not significant predictors of disease-free survival. Using this multivariate analysis, we established new definitions of good, average, and poor prognosis (risk) groups (Table 4). Good prognosis patients have all favorable factors; poor prognosis patients have one or more unfavorable characteristics. Average prognosis patients comprised the remainder. Using these criteria, good, average, and poor prognosis groups comprised 28.1%, 50.8%, and 21.1%, respectively, of the entire patient population. The 48-month CCR rates in the three groups, excluding infants <1 year, are 92.1%, 55.4%, and 45.7%, respectively (Fig. 5). The 48-month survival rates for the three groups are 93.9%, 61.6%, and 20.8% (not shown).

2. Survival

A different rank order of factors predicting survival from entry on study was determined. Log WBC, IgG, age (age^2), and FAB morphology were significant predictors (P = <0.05), and IgM, CNS disease at diagnosis, and hemoglobin were of borderline significance (P 0.06–0.159) as predictors of survival (Table 5).

E. Discussion

Generally, the outlook in "high risk" or poor prognosis ALL associated with early relapse

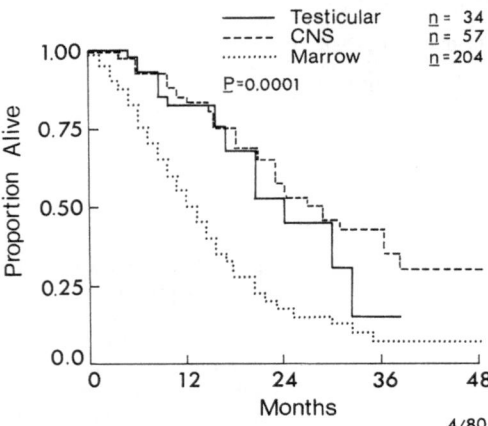

Fig. 4. Survival after first isolated relapse by type of first relapse

Table 4. Favorable and unfavorable characteristics

Factor	Prognostic group		
	Good	Average	Poor
WBC $\times 10^9$/l	<20	20–100	>100
Age, yrs.	2–10	>10	<1
Lymphoma syndrome	(0)	(<3)	(3 or more)
Hgb, gm/d1	<10		>10
L,S,N	Not markedly enlarged		Markedly enlarged
Mediastinal mass	Absent		Present
CNS disease at Dx	Absent	Absent	Present
FAB morphology	≥75% L_1	≥75% L_1	≥25% L_2
Ig, depressed	0–1	0–3	
BM d14	M_1 or M_2	$M_{1,2,3}$	

and death remains bleak despite efforts to improve the duration of disease-free and overall survival in this subset of patients accounting for approximately 20%–25% of childhood ALL. During the past 8 years the duration of disease-free and long-term survival has not changed significantly despite efforts to increase the intensity and perforce the toxicity of therapy. In this study more intensive induction, CNS, and maintenance therapy in poor prognosis patients, defined by initial WBC alone, was no better than standard and much less toxic therapy. Others have observed that intensification of therapy did not achieve better results in patients variously defined as having a poor prognosis (Haghbin et al. 1974, to be published; Aur et al. 1978; Sallan et al.

1980). Future directions in the treatment of childhood ALL will be aimed at decreasing morbidity and late effects of cancer therapy through maximally effective and minimally toxic regimens. This study has identified a subset of patients, comprising 28% of the total, with a projected five-year disease-free survival of >90% (Table 4).

In addition to the important contribution of leukemic thrust or burden as measured by the degree of organomegaly and lymphadenopathy, the hemoglobin level, and the presence of mediastinal (thymic) mass and CNS disease at diagnosis, this study also identified three additional statistically significant favorable prognostic factors–L_1 lymphoblast morphology using a modification of the FAB classification,

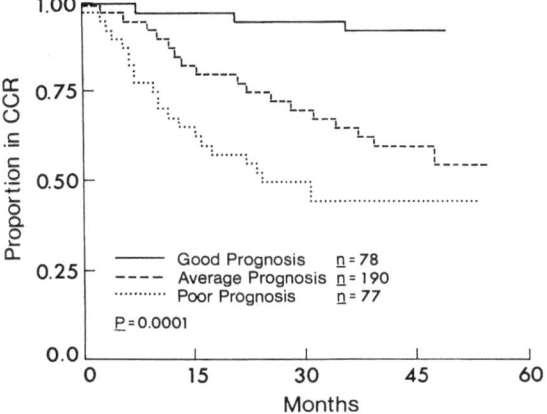

Fig. 5. Complete continuous remission by newly defined prognostic groups (see text). The differences are highly significant ($P = 0.0001$)

Table 5. Significant variables for predicting survival from on study in CCG-141[a]

Rank	Variable	Significance Level (P-Value)
1	Log WBC	0.001
2	IgG	0.009
3	Age and age^2	0.038 & .003
4	Morphology	0.048
5	IgM	0.067
6	CNS disease at diagnosis	0.089
7	Hemoglobin	0.159

[a] Platelet count, nodal enlargement, splenomegaly, hepatomegaly, sex, mediastinal mass status, and race were not significant predictors of outcome in a multivariate context

normal or elevated immunoglobulin levels, and M_1 bone marrow status on day 14 of induction therapy. Detailed accounts of the prognostic significance of FAB morphology (Miller et al., to be published) and immunologic factors (Leikin et al., to be published) are presented in companion papers. Others (Jacquillat et al. 1974; Frei and Sallan 1978) have found that rapid lysis of bone marrow blasts and restoration of normal hematopoiesis are associated with a good prognosis. Failure to respond promptly to induction therapy implies the rapid emergence of drug resistant cells, misdiagnosis, or inadequate therapy. Monitoring of the initial response to induction therapy appears warranted so that modification of induction therapy can be introduced early in treatment and assure the best possible chance of complete remission. Despite the excellent remission rates achievable with current therapy, the relapses occurring early in maintenance suggest that the accepted definition of complete remission requires revision and that more accurate and quantitative methods to determine the residual leukemic population are needed. Techniques such as terminal deoxynucleotidyl transferase, cytofluorometry, use of monoclonal antibodies, and cytogenetic markers may be helpful.

Immunoglobulin G ($P=0.009$) and lymphoblast morphology ($P=0.048$) were significant for survival but only marginally for disease-free survival ($P=0.07$ and $P=0.09$, respectively). This is probably because decreased IgG and L_2 lymphoblast morphology were associated with a higher probability of induction failure and subsequent death. A similar explanation could account for CNS disease at diagnosis being a stronger predictor of survival than of disease-free survival.

The beneficial role of monthly pulses of PDN and VCR during maintenance therapy has never been determined in a prospective trial. Simone et al. (1975) suggested that monthly pulses of PDN and VCR contributed to immunosuppression and more infectious disease complications without improving the overall therapeutic results. In CCG 141 pulses of PDN and VCR were discontinued after 12 months in all patients. When the data in CCG-141 were compared to those obtained in the two previous CCSG studies (CCG 101,143) no statistically significant differences in duration of hematologic remission (Fig. 3), disease-free survival or overall survival are noted, suggesting that VCR-PDN pulses may not be required during maintenance.

Patients experiencing an isolated bone marrow, testicular, or CNS relapse were at high risk of early death with median survivals after the first relapse of 10, 19, and 22 months, respectively. The relatively short survival after isolated extramedullary relapse occurred despite reinduction with PDN, VCR, and LASP and prophylactic or specific retreatment to the CNS. These results suggest that more intensive reinduction and maintenance programs are required in patients experiencing isolated extramedullary relapses. Bone marrow transplantation is an alternative approach for patients sustaining an early bone marrow relapse and is now being studied by CCSG.

The data generated by this study have defined new prognostic groups based upon clinical, morphologic, and immunologic features and will be used to design the new generation of ALL protocols. A key feature of the new studies will be to reduce further the acute and late toxic effects of therapy in patients with a good prognosis and to improve upon the 45% disease-free survival of children with a poor prognosis.

Acknowledgments

Institutions and Principal Investigators of CCSG Participating in CCG 141

Institution	Investigator	Grant No.
Group Operations Office	D. Hammond	CA 13539
University of Southern California	J. Weiner	
Comprehensive Cancer Center	R. Honour	
Los Angeles, California	H. Sather	
University of Michigan Medical Center	R. Heyn	CA 02971
Ann Arbor, Michigan		

Children's Hospital National Medical Center
  George Washington University,
  Washington, D.C.
	S. Leikin	CA 03888

Memorial Sloan-Kettering Cancer Center
  Cornell University,
  New York, N.Y.
	D. R. Miller	CA 23742

Childrens Hospital of Los Angeles
  University of Southern California,
  Los Angeles, California
	G. Higgins	CA 02649

Babies Hospital
  Columbia University,
  New York, N.Y.
	J. Wolff	CA 03526

Children's Hospital of Pittsburgh
  University of Pittsburgh,
  Pittsburgh, Pennsylavania
	V. Albo	CA 07439

Children's Hospital of Columbus
  Ohio State University,
  Columbus, Ohio
	W. Newton	CA 03750

Children's Orthopedic Hospital and Medical
  Center,
  University of Washington
  Seattle, Washington
	R. Chard	CA 10382

University of Wisconsin Hospitals Madison, Wisconsin	N. Shahidi	CA 05436
University of Minnesota Health Sciences Center, Minneapolis, Minnesota	M. Nesbit	CA 97306

Children's Memorial Hospital
  Northwestern University
  Chicago, Illinois
	G. Honig	CA 07431

University of Utah Medical Center Salt Lake City. Utah	E. Lahey	CA 10198

Strong Memorial Hospital
  University of Rochester
  Rochester, New York
	M. Klemperer	CA 11174

Children's Hospital
  University of Louisville,
  Louisville, Kentucky
	D. R. Kmetz	–

University of British Columbia, Vancouver, British Columbia	M. Teasdale	Vancouver

Children's Hospital of Philadelphia
  University of Pennsylvania,
  Philadelphia, Pennsylvania
	A. Evans	CA 11796

James Whitcomb Riley Hospital for Children
  Indiana University,
  Indianapolis, Indiana
	R. Baehner	CA 14809

New Jersey College of Medicine and
  Dentistry,
  Newark, New Jersey
	L. Vitale	CA 12637

Harbor General Hospital
  University of California Los Angeles,
  Torrance, California
	J. Finklestein	CA 14560

University of California Medical Center San Francisco, California	A. Ablin	CA 17829

Rainbow Babies and Childrens Hospital
  Case Western Reserve University
  Cleveland, Ohio
	S. Gross	CA 203020

University of Texas Health
  Sciences Center
  San Antonio, Texas
	T. Williams	–

References

Andreeff M, Darzynkiewicz Z, Sharpless TK, Clarkson BD, Melamed MR (1980) Discrimination of heman leukemia subtypes by flow cytometric analysis of cellular DNA and RNA. Blood 55:282–293 – Aur RJA, Simone JV, Verzoza MS, Hustu HD, Barker LF, Pinkel DP, Rivera G, Dahl GV, Wood A, Stagner S, Mason C (1978) Childhood acute lymphocytic leukemia. Study VIII. Cancer 42:2123–2134 – Bennett JM, Catovsky D, Daniel MT, Flandrin G, Galton DAG, Gralnick NR, Sultan D (French-American-British [FAB] Cooperative Group) (1976) Proposal for the classification of the acute leukemias. Br J Haematol 33:451–458 – Cox DR Regression models and liefe tables. J R Stat Soc [Br] 34:187–220 – Fahey J, McKelvey EM (1965) Quantitative determination of serum immunoglobulins in antibody agar plates. J Immunol 94:84–90 – Frei EJ, Sallan SE (1978) Acute lymphoblastic leukemia treatment. Cancer 42:828–838 – George S, Fernbach K, Vietti T, Sullivan MP, Lane DM, Haggard ME, Berry DH, Lonsdale D, Komp D (1973) Factors influencing survival in pediatric acute leukemia. Cancer 32:1542–1553 – Haghbin M, Tan CT, Clarkson BD, Mike V, Burchenal J, Murphy ML (1974) Intensive chemotherapy in children with acute lymphoblastic leukemia (L-2 protocol). Cancer 33:1491–1498 – Haghbin M, Murphy ML, Tan CTC, Clarkson BD, Thaler H, Passe S, Burchenal J (1981) A long-term clinical follow-up of children with acute lymphoblastic leukemia treated with intensive chemotherapy regimens. Cancer 46:241–252 – Jacquillat C, Weil M, German MF (1974) Combination therapy in 130 patients with acute lymphocytic leukemia. Cancer Res 33:3284–3289 – Leikin S, Miller DR, Sather H, Albo V, Esber E, Johnson A, Rogentine N, Hammond D (to be published) Immunologic evaluation in the prognosis of acute lymphoblastic leukemia. Blood – Miller DR, Sonley M, Karon M, Breslow N, Hammond D (1974) Additive therapy in the maintenance of remission in acute lymphoblastic leukemia of childhood: the effect of the initial leukocyte count. Cancer 34:508–517 – Miller DR, Leikin S, Albo V, Sather H, Hammond D (to be published) Prognostic significance of lymphoblast morphology (FAB classification) in childhood acute lymphoblastic leukemia. Br J Haematol – Nesbit ME, Coccia PF, Sather HN, Robison LL, Hammond GD (1979) Staging in pediatric malignancies. In: Proceedings of american cancer society national conference on the care of the child with cancer. American Cancer Society, New York, pp 31–38 – Peto R, Pike MC, Armitage P, Breslow NE, Cox DR, Howard SV, Mantel N, McPherson K, Peto J, Smith PG (1977) Design and analysis of randomized clinical trials requiring prolonged observation of each patient. II. Analysis and examples. Br J Cancer 35:1–39 – Robison LL, Sather HN, Coccia PF, Nesbit ME, Hammond GD (1980) Assessment of the interrelationship of prognostic factors in childhood acute lymphoblastic leukemia: A report from Childrens Cancer Study Group. Am J Pediatr Hematol Oncol 2:5–14 – Sallan SE, Ritz J, Pesando J, Geiber R, O'Brien C, Hitchcock S, Coral F, Schlossman SF (1980) Cell surface antigens: Prognostic implications in childhood acute lymphoblastic leukemia. Blood 55: 395–402 – Simone JV, Aur RJA, Hustu HO, Verzosa M, Pinkel D (1975) Combined modality therapy of acute lymphocytic leukemia. Cancer 35:25–35 – Simone JV (1976) Factors that influence haematological remission duration in acute lymphocytic leukaemia. Br J Haematol 32:465–472

Haematology and Blood Transfusion Vol. 26
Modern Trends in Human Leukemia IV
Edited by Neth, Gallo, Graf, Mannweiler, Winkler
© Springer-Verlag Berlin Heidelberg 1981

Treatment Strategy for Different Risk Groups in Childhood Acute Lymphoblastic Leukemia: A Report From the BFM Study Group*

G. Henze, H.-J. Langermann, J. Ritter, G. Schellong, and H. Riehm

A. Introduction

Development of effective treatment programs for childhood acute lymphoblastic leukemia (ALL) has led to marked improvement of prognosis. The proportion of patients remaining in first remission for at least 5 years is generally estimated to be in the range of 50% once remission is achieved (Frei and Sallan 1978; Riehm et al. 1980; Robison et al. 1980). Since remission rates have been shown to be 90%–95% with currently used induction therapy, successful induction of remission is no longer an essential problem. Nevertheless, the quality of remission is apparently unsatisfactory in about one-half of the patients, eventually resulting in recurrence of the disease. Predictors of outcome have been defined and include white blood count (WBC), sex, thymic involvement, central nervous system disease at diagnosis, immunologic markers, unfavorable age, and blast cell morphology (Dow et al. 1977; Henze et al. 1979; Mathé et al. 1971; Sallan et al. 1978; Simone et al. 1975; Wagner and Baehner 1979; Working Party on leukemia in Childhood 1978); but attempts to adapt the therapeutic strategy to the presence of factors associated with a poor prognosis have not been able to enhance significantly therapeutic results. The approach of the BFM study group with the concept of intensive multidrug remission induction gives hope for an overall 75% relapse-free survival in childhood ALL.

B. Patients and Methods

Between October 1970 and March 1979, 277 children and adolescents were enrolled in sequence in two BFM acute lymphoblastic leukemia therapy studies. The treatment plans of study BFM 70/76 (Oct. 1970–Sept. 1976) and study BFM 76/79 (Oct. 1976–March 1979) are outlined in Figs. 1 and 2. All patients received Protocol I (Fig. 3) for remission induction. In study BFM 76/79 a risk index (RI) was established for definition of high risk patients (Table 1). Children with RI ≥3 received a reinforced reinduction protocol (Protocol II, Fig. 4) within the first 6 months after diagnosis. These patients were randomly allocated to either limb B1 or B2.

Diagnosis of ALL was made by morphologic analysis of stained bone marrow smears. Only children with a least 25% blasts in the bone marrow aspirate were diagnosed as having ALL; patients with less than 25% lymphoblasts were considered to be cases of non-Hodgkin's lymphoma and not included in this series. Relapse was diagnosed by the appearance of leukemic cells at any site. Patients who failed to achieve complete remission after 4 weeks of therapy were considered therapeutic failures and counted as relapses as were patients who died during remission induction or in continuous complete remission (CCR).

Methods of statistical analysis were the life table algorithm (Cutler and Ederer 1958) and Cox's regression model (Cox 1972). The date of evaluation for this report was 4 June 1980.

C. Results

Remission rates were comparable in both studies. Two patients with B-cell leukemia, one in study BFM 70/76 and one in study BFM 76/79, did not respond to therapy. Deaths during remission induction (five children in study BFM 70/76 and four children in study

* Supported by the Stiftung Volkswagenwerk

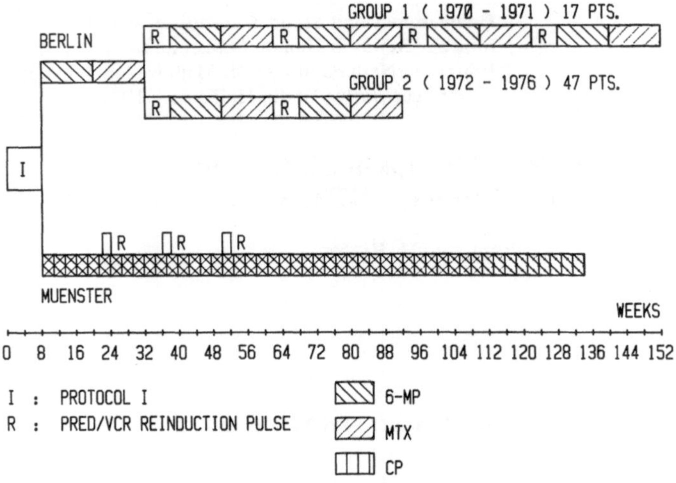

GROUP 1 (1970 - 1971) 17 PTS.

BERLIN

R ///// R ///// R ///// R /////

GROUP 2 (1972 - 1976) 47 PTS.

R ///// R /////

I

[]R []R []R

MUENSTER

WEEKS

0 8 16 24 32 40 48 56 64 72 80 88 96 104 112 120 128 136 144 152

I : PROTOCOL I
R : PRED/VCR REINDUCTION PULSE

6-MP
MTX
CP

Fig. 1. Outline of study BFM 70/76. *PRED*, prednisone; *VCR*, vincristine, *6-MP*, 6-mercaptopurine; *MTX*, methotrexate; *CP*, cyclophosphamide

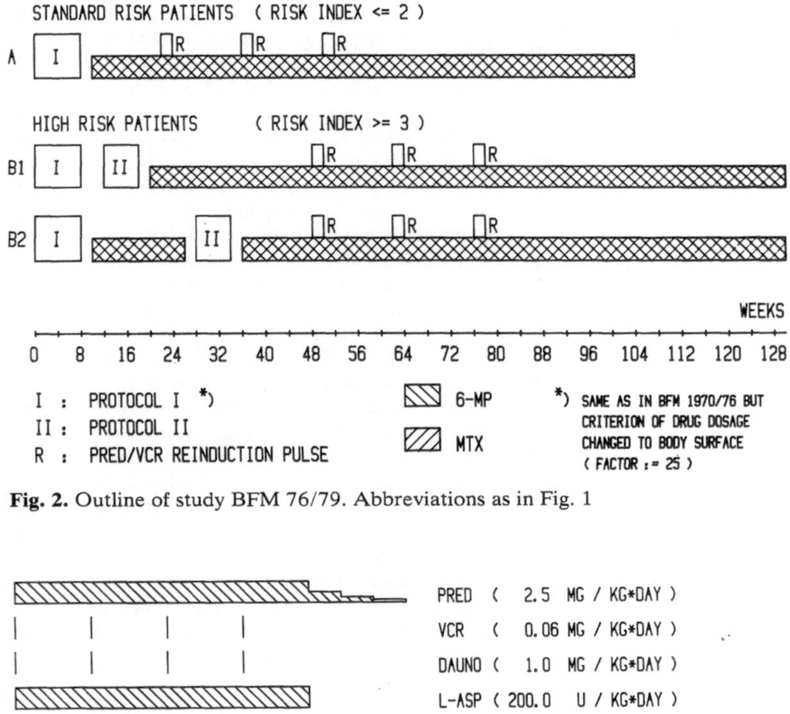

STANDARD RISK PATIENTS (RISK INDEX <= 2)

A I []R []R []R

HIGH RISK PATIENTS (RISK INDEX >= 3)

B1 I II []R []R []R

B2 I II []R []R []R

WEEKS

0 8 16 24 32 40 48 56 64 72 80 88 96 104 112 120 128

I : PROTOCOL I *)
II : PROTOCOL II
R : PRED/VCR REINDUCTION PULSE

6-MP
MTX

*) SAME AS IN BFM 1970/76 BUT CRITERION OF DRUG DOSAGE CHANGED TO BODY SURFACE (FACTOR := 25)

Fig. 2. Outline of study BFM 76/79. Abbreviations as in Fig. 1

PRED (2.5 MG / KG*DAY)
VCR (0.06 MG / KG*DAY)
DAUNO (1.0 MG / KG*DAY)
L-ASP (200.0 U / KG*DAY)

CP (40.0 MG / KG*DAY)
ARA-C (3.0 MG / KG*DAY)
MTX I.T. (0.5 MG / KG*DAY)
6-MP (2.5 MG / KG*DAY)
CNS IRRADIATION

1 8 15 22 29 36 43 50 57
DAYS

Fig. 3. Induction therapy: Protocol I, *PRED*, prednisone; *VCR*, vincristine; *DAUNO*, daunorubicin; *L-ASP*, asparaginase; *CP*, cyclophosphamide; *ARA-C*, cytarabin; *MTX*, methotrexate; *6-MP*, 6.mercaptopurine

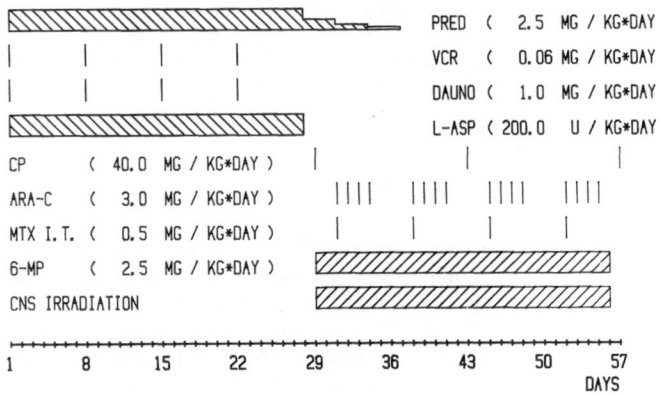

Table 1. Determination of the risk index according to findings at diagnosis

Findings at diagnosis	Score
White blood count≥25E9/L	3
Leukemic cells in the spinal fluid	2
Thymic enlargement	1
Positive acid phosphatase and/or rosette formation test	1
Negative perjodic acid Schiff reaction (PAS reaction) Age<2 years or age≥10 years	1
Significant extranodal mass	1

Risk index: = Score sum

BFM 76/79) were mainly due to infectious complications.

Fourteen patients (eight in study BFM 70/76, six in study BFM 76/79) died during remission. In 11 children death was related to infectious complications. Another three patients died of toxic side effects of therapy (pulmonary fibrosis caused by methotrexate, vincristine induced encephalopathy, and brain stem necrosis of unknown origin).

The probability of continuous complete remission (life table analysis) for patient groups with regard to initial clinical features is summarized in Table 2. Cox regression was used to estimate the influence of commonly

Table 2. Patient characteristics of studies BFM 70/76 and BFM 76/79 with corresponding probability of continuous complete remission (p-CCR) calculated by the life table method after 117 and 44 months, respectively

	BFM 1970/76		BFM 1976/79	
	No. (%)	p-CCR After 117 MTHS	No. (%)	p-CCR After 44 MTHS
Boys	78 (65.5)	0.55 ±/± 0.06	89 (56.3)	0.74 ±/± 0.06
Girls	41 (34.5)	0.57 ±/± 0.08	69 (43.7)	0.78 ±/± 0.06
Age < 2 yrs	10 (8.4)	0.50 ±/± 0.16	15 (9.5)	0.80 ±/± 0.10
Age 2–10 yrs	88 (73.9)	0.57 ±/± 0.06	107 (67.7)	0.85 ±/± 0.04
Age ≥10 yrs	21 (17.6)	0.52 ±/± 0.11	36 (22.8)	0.41 ±/± 0.14
Thymic mass	15 (12.6)	0.47 ±/± 0.13	14 (8.9)	0.74 ±/± 0.14
WBC< 25,000/mm³	79 (66.4)	0.63 ±/± 0.06	107 (67.7)	0.77 ±/± 0.05
WBC≥ 25,000/mm³	40 (33.6)	0.40 ±/± 0.08	51 (32.3)	0.72 ±/± 0.07
Risk index≤2	76 (63.9)	0.65 ±/± 0.06	103 (65.2)	0.77 ±/± 0.05
Risk index≥3	43 (36.1)	0.39 ±/± 0.08	55 (34.8)	0.75 ±/± 0.07
Total	119	0.55 ±/± 0.05	158	0.76 ±/± 0.04

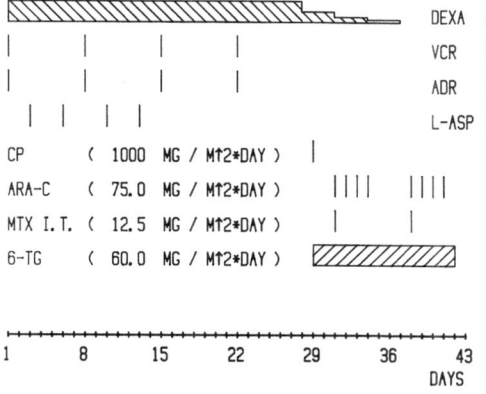

```
                                              DEXA  (  10.0 MG / M↑2*DAY )
  |       |       |       |                    VCR  (   1.5 MG / M↑2*DAY )
  |       |       |       |                    ADR  (  25.0 MG / M↑2*DAY )
    |   |   |   |                            L-ASP  ( 10000    U / M↑2*DAY )
CP       ( 1000  MG / M↑2*DAY )  |
ARA-C    ( 75.0  MG / M↑2*DAY )        ||||   ||||
MTX I.T. ( 12.5  MG / M↑2*DAY )         |      |
6-TG     ( 60.0  MG / M↑2*DAY )    //////////

1       8      15      22      29      36      43
                                              DAYS
```

Fig. 4. Reinforced reinduction therapy: Protocol II. *DEXA,* dexamethasone; *VCR,* vincristine; *ADR,* adriamycin; *L-ASP,* asparaginase; *CP,* cyclophosphamide; *ARA-C,* cytarabin; *MTX,* methotrexate; *6-TG,* 6-thioguanine

Table 3. Influence of initial features on prognosis in study BFM 70/76 obtained by Cox regression analysis

Initial features	P-values for significance
Peripheral blast cell count	<0.001
Spleen enlargement (cm)	<0.001
Liver enlargement (cm)	<0.001
PAS reaction	0.17
Thymic enlargement	0.20
Hemoglobin (g/dl)	0.31
Platelet count	0.31
Age: 0–2, 2–10, ≥10 years	0.44
Acid phosphatase reaction	0.46
Sex	0.65

reported risk factors on prognosis. In study BFM 70/76 one-parametric analysis (Table 3) as well as multiparametric analysis revealed the peripheral blast cell count and enlargement of the liver and spleen to be significant. In study BFM 76/79 only an age over 10 years was found to influence prognosis ($P<0.01$), even when adjustment was made for the remaining features.

Remarkably, prognosis is independent of the presence of T-cell characteristics. In study BFM 76/79 the probability of CCR is exactly the same for T-ALL patients as for non-T-ALL cases (Fig. 5). Of note, however, is that 17/22 patients with T-cell characteristics received therapy B1 or B2 because of their high concomitant WBC.

The main reason for allocating patients to the high risk group (RI≥3) was the initial WBC of ≥25,000/mm³. Combination of initial features other than WBC ≥25,000/mm³ caused a score sum ≥3 in only three patients of study BFM 70/76 and in four patients of study BFM 76/79.

Life table curves correspond well for low risk patients (RI≤2) in both studies after comparable periods of time (Fig. 6). In study BFM 76/79 prognosis could be markedly improved for high risk patients by the addition of Protocol II early in remission (Fig. 7). No significant difference was found between limb B1 and B2. Figure 8 supports the assumption that relapses in high risk patients are really prevented rather than postponed. The probability of any first event was reduced by more than 50% in BFM 76/79 compared to BFM 70/76 in every yearly interval up to 4 years after onset of treatment.

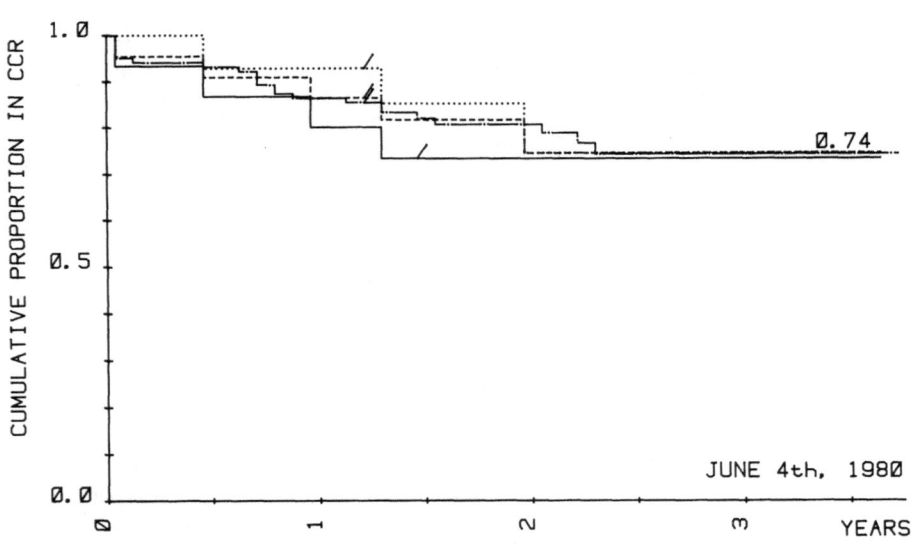

Fig. 5. Study BFM 76/79: Probability of continuous complete remission;/, Last patient of the group; ———, rosette formation test positive (n=15); ....., mediastinal mass (n=14); –––––, mediastinal mass and/or positive E-rosette formation (n=22); and –.–.–, no mediastinal mass and E-rosette formation negative (n=102). Thirty-four patients not investigated

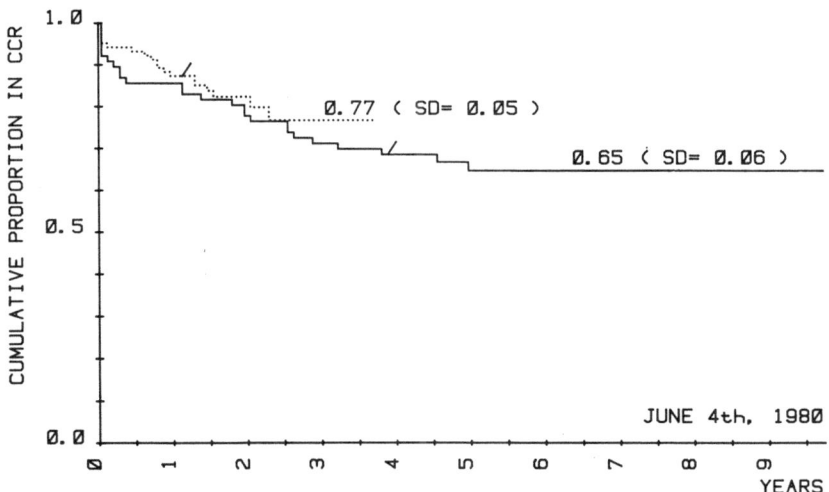

Fig. 6. Comparison of probability of continuous complete remission for low risk patients (RI⩽2). ———, study BFM 70/76 ($n=76$); . . . . ., study BFM 76/79 ($n=103$)

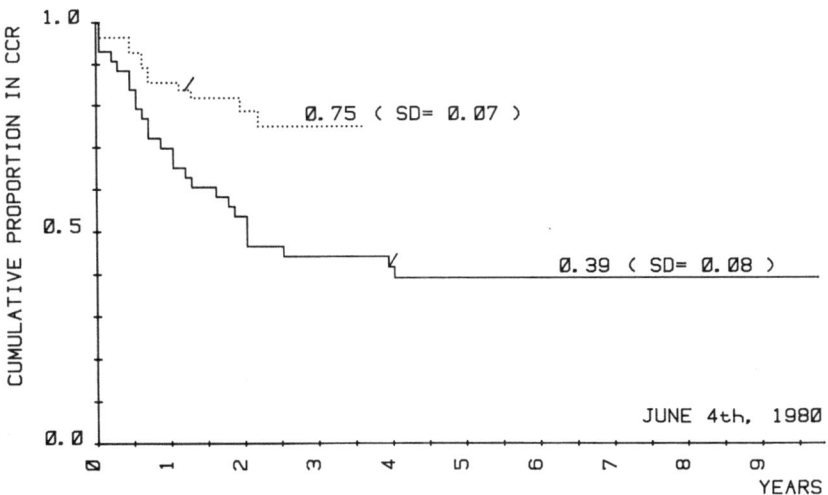

Fig. 7. Comparison of probability of continuous complete remission for high risk patients (RI⩾3). ———, study BFM 70/76 ($n=43$); . . . . . ., study BFM 76/79 ($n=55$)

D. Discussion

Currently used induction therapy for childhood ALL is capable of producing complete remission in about 90%–95% of patients after several weeks. However, complete remission is a very poorly defined condition with respect to prediction of final outcome, since it merely indicates that leukemic cells can no longer be detected. The number of residual leukemic cells that might eventually cause recurrence of the disease is unknown. Combination therapy with vincristine and prednisone, for example, produces remission rates that are similar to but in a large series significantly lower than those obtained with vincristine, prednisone, and asparaginase (Ortega et al. 1977). There is little doubt that multidrug combination che-

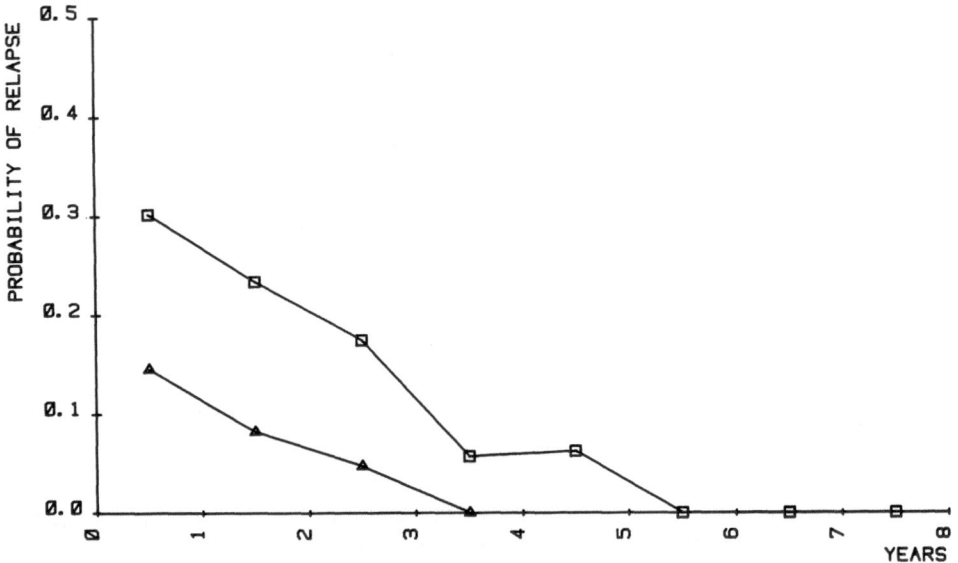

Fig. 8. Probability of any first event during yearly intervals after onset of treatment estimated by life table analysis (induction deaths, deaths in remission, and all sites of relapse included) for high risk patients. □, study BFM 70/76 ($n=43$), Protocol I plus maintenance therapy; △, study BFM 76/79 ($n=55$), Protocol I and Protocol II plus maintenance therapy

motherapy is superior to single or two drug combination therapy, because rapid cytore-duction lessens the chance for persistent leuke-mic cells to develop drug resistance. It is more likely, therefore, that the remission status established after 4 weeks of intensive therapy is "more complete".

Even though results with the original West Berlin protocol were promising, it was evident in 1976 that therapy was insufficient for patients with high initial WBC, a strong indicator of the total leukemic cell burden. About 60% of these patients relapsed, most during the 1st year after onset of treatment. Since conventionally administered reinduction pulses of prednisone and vincristine failed to prevent early relapses, it seemed to be reaso-nable to introduce a second intensive phase of induction therapy at a time when the prolifera-ting residual leukemic cells were not detecta-ble by currently available methods. Hitherto existing results in high risk patients support this concept.

An unexpected finding was the compartati-vely unfavorable result obtained in children over 10 years of age in study BFM 76/79. Despite a shorter observation period and improved therapeutic strategy in this group,

prognosis is worse than in the previous study. One possible explanation might be that the drug dosage was changed from body weight to body surface area. For older patients the calculated surface area dosages are distinctly lower, making up only about 75% of the dosage calculated according to body weight. Since in most therapy protocols drug dosage is based on body surface the question arises whether the significance of age as an adverse prognostic factor might be partially corrected.

Results of study BFM 76/79 indicate that the overall prognosis in childhood ALL is 75% with respect to long-term disease-free survival. We conclude that intensification of chemothe-rapy early in remission is capable of signifi-cantly reducing the relapse rate in high risk patients. Further improvement of prognosis in low risk patients may be achieved by remission induction intensification as was done in the current study BFM 79/81. Future efforts should be aimed at the development of more sensitive methods to determine the individual risk for relapse at diagnosis and to detect residual leukemic cells. This would enable us to design individual and appropriate therapeutic regimens and evaluate the efficacy of therapy early in treatment.

References

Cox DR (1972) Regression models and life-tables. J Stat Soc Bull 34:187–220 – Cutler S, Ederer F (1958) Maximum utilisation of the life table method in analysing survival. J Chronic Dis 4:699–712 – Dow LW, Borella L, Sen L, Aur RJA, George SL, Mauer AM, Simone JV (1977) Initial prognostic factors and lymphoblast-erythrocyte rosette formation in 109 children with acute lymphoblastic leukemia. Blood 50:671–681 – Frei E III, Sallan SE (1978) Acute lymphoblastic leukemia: Treatment. Cancer 42:828–838 – Henze G, Langermann HJ, Lampert F, Neidhardt M, Riehm H (1979) ALL therapy study 1971–1974 of the German Working Group for Leukemia Research and Therapy in childhood: Prognostic significance of initial features and different therapeutic modalities. Klin Paediat 191:114–126 – Mathe G, Pouillart P, Sterescu M, Amiel JL, Schwarzenberg L, Schneider M, Hayat M, de Vassal F, Jasmin C, Lafleur M (1971) Subdivision of classical varieties of acute leukemia. Correlation with prognosis and cure expectancy. Eur J Clin Res 16:1554–560 – Ortega JA, Nesbit ME, Donaldson MH, Weiner J, Hittle R, Karon M (1977) L-asparaginase, vincristine, and prednisone for induction of first remission in acute lymphocytic leukemia. Cancer Res 37:535–540 – Riehm H, Gadner H, Henze G, Langermann HJ, Odenwald E (1980) The Berlin childhood acute lymphoblastic leukemia study, 1970–1976. Am J Pediatr Hematol Oncol 2:299–306 – Robison LL, Sather HN, Coccia PF, Nesbit ME, Hammond GD (1980) Assessment of the interrelationship of prognostic factors in childhood acute lymphoblastic leukemia. Am J Pediatr Hematol Oncol 2:5–13 – Sallan SE, Camitta BM, Cassady JR, Nathan DG, Frei E III (1978) Intermittent combination chemotherapy with adriamycin for childhood acute lymphoblastic leukemia: Clinical results. Blood 51:425–433 – Simone JV, Verzosa MS, Rudy JA (1975) Initial features and prognosis in 363 children with acute lymphocytic leukemia. Cancer 36:2099–2108 – Wagner VM, Baehner RL (1979) Correlation of the FAB morphologic criteria and prognosis in acute lymphocytic leukemia of childhood. Am J Pediatr Hematol Oncol 1:103–106 – Working Party on Leukemia in Childhood (1978) Effects of varying radiation schedule, cyclophosphamide treatment, and duration of treatment in acute lymphoblastic leukemia. Br Med J II: 787–791

Haematology and Blood Transfusion Vol. 26
Modern Trends in Human Leukemia IV
Edited by Neth, Gallo, Graf, Mannweiler, Winkler
© Springer-Verlag Berlin Heidelberg 1981

Recurrent Childhood Lymphocytic Leukemia:
Outcome of Marrow Relapses After Cessation of Therapy*

G. Rivera

A. Introduction

Leukemia therapists have long agreed that relapse – particularly in the bone marrow – signals the end of opportunities to obtain long-lasting remissions. This thinking can be traced to the emergence of drug-resistant lymphoblasts, the hallmark of leukemia in relapse, and to the lack of sufficient numbers of uniformly treated patients for analysis and comparison. It is becoming clear, however, that in patients with recurrent acute lymphocytic leukemia (ALL), treatment responses differ widely. Second hematologic remissions, for instance, are significantly longer in children who relapse after therapy is electively stopped than in those who relapse during therapy (Chessells and Cornbleet 1979; Ekert et al. 1979; Kearney et al. 1979; Rivera et al. 1976, 1978). Furthermore, in some patients, treatment can be stopped altogether for a second time with the possibility of continued disease-free survival (Rivera et al. 1979). The purpose of this article is to review the clinical course of 56 patients who were retreated for marrow relapses that developed after cessation of intensive initial treatment.

B. Patients Studies

From 1966 to 1978, 288 of 645 (0.44) children with ALL who were entered in Total-Therapy Studies I–VIII at St. Jude Children's Research Hospital (SJCRH) had all therapy stopped.

The details of each study group have been presented in earlier publications (Aur et al. 1978; Simone et al. 1972). Treatment was discontinued after 2–3 years of complete remission; thereafter, the patients had marrow and cerebrospinal fluid examinations at intervals ranging from every 2 months during the 1st year to annually after the 5th year off therapy. Of these 288 patients, 72 (0.25) have relapsed. Fifty-six children developed marrow relapses during unmaintained remissions; in 43 only the marrow was involved, whereas in the remaining 13 the testes and central nervous system (CNS) were involved as well. Sixteen additional patients had isolated extramedullary relapses: 11 testicular and 5 CNS (Table 1). This review includes only the 56 patients who developed hematologic relapses with or without other sites of leukemic involvement.

Table 1. Results of stopping therapy in childhood ALL: SJCRH Studies I–VIII[a]

No. of patients entered	645
No. electively removed from treatment	288
No. still in remission (2–14 Yr)	216
No. relapsing	72

Sites of relapse in 72 patients

1. Bone marrow		2. Extramedullary	
BM alone	43	CNS	5
BM + CNS	5	Testicular	11
BM + T	6		
BM + T + CNS	2		
	56		16

[a] As of 1 June 1980. BM, bone marrow; CNS, central nervous system; T, testicular

* Supported by Cancer Center Support (CORE) Grant CA-21765, by Leukemia Program Project Grant CA-20180, and by ALSAC

C. Retreatment Without CNS Prophylaxis

From 1970 to 1973, when no uniform second treatment plan was available, 13 patients who relapsed off therapy were treated again with essentially the same therapy as used originally. CNS prophylaxis at the time of relapse was not used. Only 2 of these 13 patients are living free of disease; both are off therapy for a second time for 39+ and 51+ months and survive 11+ and 14+ years from diagnosis. An additional patient refused further treatment and has been lost to follow-up.

From 1973 to 1976, 17 children with leukemia in relapse were enrolled in the institution's first formal relapse protocol (see Table 2). Each received reinduction chemotherapy with prednisone, vincristine, and adriamycin (4 weeks), and all were randomized at the time of remission to receive or not to receive an intensive phase of chemotherapy with asparaginase and cytosine arabinoside (ara-C) (2 weeks). Continuation therapy consisted of mercaptopurine and methotrexate (MTX) (30 months). CNS prophylaxis was not used. Sixteen patients attained second remissions and were followed for 5–6 years; the median duration of marrow remission was 10 months (range 3–78+). Each child relapsed again: eight in the marrow, six in the CNS, one in the testes, and one in both marrow and CNS. Remission durations were not discernibly different between children who did or did not receive the intensive phase of chemotherapy. In four of the seven patients with new isolated extramedullary relapses, remissions were reinduced and, after 30–44 months of continuous second marrow remission, all therapy was stopped again. In three of these four patients, new marrow relapses developed within 1–7 months; one child remains in remission 48+ months after having treatment stopped for a second time.

The lengths of second remissions in this study varied widely, from 3 to 78+ months, despite uniform application of a standardized treatment. Analysis of the relationships between selected patient variables and the duration of second hematologic remission yielded several significant results. The features analyzed were sex, age, and leukocyte count at diagnosis and at relapse; length of first complete remission; time off therapy to relapse; proportion of blasts disclosed by marrow examination; and number of sites at the time of relapse off therapy. An initial complete remission duration of less than 3 years, a relapse occurring within 6 months of cessation of first therapy, and the presence of marrow plus extramedullary sites of relapse on admission to the study all proved to be unfavorable prognostic indicators.

D. Retreatment Including CNS Prophylaxis

The overall incidence of second marrow and/or extramedullary relapses in the preceding study – 16/16 patients – together with the moderate toxicity encountered during treat-

Table 2. Treatment Programs for recurrent ALL[a]

	First study (No. = 17)	Second study (No. = 23)
Reinduction phase (4 wk)	Pred 40 mg/m^2/day p.o. × 28 VCR 1.5 mg/m^2/wk IV × 4 Adria 40 mg/m^2 IV days 1 and 15	Same as first study
Intensive phase (2 wk)	ASP 10,000 IU/m^2/wk IV × 2 ara-C 300 mg/m^2/wk IV × 2	None
Continuation phase (30 mo)	MP 50 mg/m^2/day p.o. MTX 40 mg/m^2/wk p.o.	ara-C 300 mg/m^2/wk IV MTX 40 mg/m^2/wk p.o.
Late intensive phase (4 wk)	None	Same as reinduction
CNS prophylaxis	None	I.T. MTX 10 mg/m^2 + ara-C 50 mg/m^2 wkly × 4 during induction and every 6 wks during continuation therapy

[a] Pred, prednisone; VCR, vincristine; Adria, adriamycin; ASP, asparaginase; ara-C, cytosine arabinoside; MP, mercaptopurine; MTX, methotrexate; p.o., orally, IV, intravenously; I.T., intrathecally

ment indicated that additional therapy was needed. The proportion of patients having the meninges as a first site of relapse was unusually high, equalling the figure for patients with marrow relapses. This indicated that systemic relapses had nullified the effects of earlier successful CNS prophylaxis. We reasoned that under this circumstance a new prophylactic CNS treatment would be especially beneficial. This hypothesis was tested in a second study in which two major questions were asked. Will the periodic administration of intrathecal chemotherapy, given at the time of relapse and throughout second remission, significantly reduce the incidence of CNS leukemia? Will the administration of a *late* intensive phase of chemotherapy at the end of 30 months of continuation therapy prevent subsequent marrow relapses off therapy?

Briefly, treatment consisted of (1) the same reinduction therapy as in the first study but with the addition of four weekly injections of MTX plus ara-C, (2) 30 months of continuation therapy with ara-C and MTX and intrathecal injections of both agents every 6 weeks, and (3) a late intensive phase of therapy with the same three agents – prednisone, vincristine, adriamycin – successfully used for reinduction of remission (4 weeks) (see Table 2). Then, treatments were stopped a second time.

In these patients intrathecal chemotherapy replaced cranial irradiation because on admission to the study each child had received a course of irradiation to the brain at the time of initial diagnosis. Although the toxicity of a second course of cranial irradiation is not known at present, there is histopathologic evidence that CNS toxicity may be related to high doses of radiation (>2000 rads) (Price and Jamieson 1975). Therefore, rather than administer additional irradiation, we elected to study the effectiveness of intrathecal chemotherapy alone for the prevention of CNS leukemia.

All 23 patients studied in the second protocol attained complete remission and have now been followed for 20 months to 4 years. The median duration of hematologic remission was 14 months (3–50+). Although 14 patients have again relapsed in the marrow, none has developed a CNS relapse. This represents a significant improvement over the high frequency of CNS relapses in the preceding study ($P = 0.02$ by the log rank test). Nine patients remain in continuous second complete remis-

sions for 19 to 50+ months. In five patients, treatment was stopped again, and only one child has developed a subsequent relapse after a year of unmaintained remission. Vomiting, often severe, was the major form of toxicity and was attributed to intravenous as well as intrathecal administration of ara-C.

Periodic prophylaxis with intrathecal chemotherapy effectively prevented CNS leukemia but did not appreciably influence the median duration of marrow remission. In fact, children not receiving a second course of CNS prophylaxis had median remission time of 10 months vs. 14 months for patients in the later study. Combinations of ara-C and MTX for continuation treatment of second remissions were not therapeutically superior to combinations of mercaptopurine and MTX but did induce more pronounced gastrointestinal toxicity. The fact that more than one-half (0.60) of the patients in this group have relapsed again indicates a need for more effective methods of therapy aimed mainly at prevention of marrow relapses.

The final two patients to relapse off therapy were recently entered in a new treatment protocol and are now in remission for 6+ months each.

E. Long-Term Disease-Free Survival

Of the 56 patients reported here, 38 have died of leukemia, one was lost to follow-up, and 17, about one-third, survive (Table 3). Nine survivors are still receiving therapy, and eight are off therapy again. Among those being treated,

Table 3. Outcome of marrow relapses after elective cessation of therapy

No. of patients	56
No. dying of leukemia	38
No. lost to follow-up	1
Survivors in remission	17 (0.30)

Survivors	
In second remission	14
On therapy (6–23+ mo)	7
Off therapy (1–51+ mo)	7
In third remission	3
On therapy (7–18+ mo)	2
Off therapy (6+ mo)	1

seven are in second remission for 6 to 23+ months and two have been reinduced into new remissions after a second relapse off therapy. The durations of their third hematologic remissions are 7+ and 18+ months. Of the eight patients who had treatment stopped for a second time, one completed therapy only recently and six are in unmaintained second remissions for 12+ to 51+ months. Another child who also developed a second relapse off therapy attained a third remission and is now off treatment a third time for 6+ months.

Among the 17 survivors, 14 have had long-term leukemia-free remissions. Their median survival since diagnosis is 9 years (range 5–14 years), with a median of 33+ months (range 19+ to 76+ mo) of continuous complete remission since their last relapse.

F. Discussion

These results demonstrate that prolonged second remissions are attainable in about one-third of the patients who develop a marrow relapse after elective cessation of initial cure-oriented therapy. Most importantly, in a certain proportion of children therapy may be stopped altogether for a second time. Although it is still not possible to predict the likelihood of relapse in individual patients after cessation ot treatment (Simone et al. 1978), statistical analysis of patient variables at the time of relapse can provide a reliable estimate of prognosis. Patients whose first complete remission lasts longer than 3 years, whose first relapse occurs more than 6 months after cessation of therapy, and whose site of relapse is exclusively hematologic have a significantly better chance to attain a extended second remission.

Other large series of patients are not available for comparison. Instances of extended second remissions have been reported, but only in patients who relapsed after unmaintained remissions following short-term initial therapy, i.e., 3–13 months (Leventhal et al. 1975).

When first diagnosed with ALL, none of the children in these studies had clinical or biologic features that are today regarded as carrying a "high risk" for early treatment failure. The most plausible explanation for their variable therapeutic responsiveness is that subpopulations of leukemic cells not eradicated by initial treatment have different growth potentials, which would account for the wide range in duration of second remissions (3 to 78+ months). For the few patients who remain free of leukemia after completing a second course of therapy, one could speculate that there relapses stemmed from the emergence of a new (and hence more drug-sensitive) clone of leukemic cells. Evidence for the emergence of different clones of leukemic cells in previously treated patients is supported by several recent reports (Fisher et al. 1977; Merteksmann et al. 1978; Spector et al. 1979).

The treatment results presented here were obtained by administering a second program of thera y :omparable to that originally given to these children. The only notable exception was that CNS prophylaxis was not repeated in about one-half of the subjects, because at the onset of the study the need for such additional treatment was unknown. Repeating a treatment that has become ineffective would not be recommended today. It should be stressed, however, that even in this circumstance about onethird of our patients responded well to therapy, an outcome that compares favorably to results for initially treated childhood ALL. Ultimately, the prospects for obtaining larger proportions of long-term remissions following relapse will depend on the development of more effective chemotherapy, preferably with agents not used earlier, to suppress the emergence of drug-resistant disease. A new protocol study to test the value of cyclic combination chemotherapy for maintenance of second remissions is underway at this center.

We conclude that children with ALL who develop marrow relapses during unmaintained remissions should be retreated just as aggressively as *newly diagnosed* patients.

Acknowledgments

I thank J.R. Gilbert for criticisms and editorial suggestions throughout preparation of this paper.

References

Aur RJA, Simone JV, Verzosa MS, Hustu HO, Barker LS, Pinkel DP, Rivera G, Dahl GV, Wood A, Stagner S, Mason C (1978) Childhood acute lymphocytic leukemia. Study VIII. Cancer

42:2123–2134 – Chessells JM, Cornbleet M (1979) Combination chemotherapy for bone marrow relapse in childhood lymphoblastic leukemia (ALL). Med Pediatr Oncol 6:359–365 – Ekert H, Ellis WM, Waters KD, Matthews RN (1979) Poor outlook for childhood acute lymphoblastic leukemia with relapse. Med J Aust 2:224–226 – Fisher EL, Lyons RM, Sears DA (1977) Development of chronic myelocytic leukemia during the course of acute lymphatic leukemia in an adult. Am J Hematol 2:291–297 – Kearney PJ, Baumer JH, Howlett BC (1979) Marrow relapse on maintenance chemotherapy in childhood acute lymphoblastic leukemia. Br J Cancer 40:890–897 – Leventhal BG, Levine AS, Graw RG, Simon R, Freireich EJ, Henderson ES (1975) Long-term second remissions in acute lymphocytic leukemia. Cancer 35:1136–1140 – Merteksmann R, Koziner B, Ralph P, Fillipa D, McKenzie S, Arlin ZA, Gee TS, Moore MAS, Clarkson BD (1978) Evidence for distinct lymphocytic and monocytic populations in a patient with terminal transferase-positive acute leukemia. Blood 51:1051 – Price R, Jamieson P (1975) The central nervous system in childhood leukemia. II. Leukoencephalopathy. Cancer 35:306–318 – Rivera G, Pratt CB, Aur RJA, Verzosa M, Hustu HO (1976) Recurrent childhood lymphocytic leukemia following cessation of therapy. Treatment and response. Cancer 37:1679–1686 – Rivera G, Murphy SB, Aur RJA, Verzosa MF, Dahl GV, Mauer AM (1978) Recurrent childhood lymphocytic leukemia. Clinical and cytokinetic studies of cytosine arabinoside and methotrexate for maintenance of second hematologic remission. Cancer 42:2521–2528 – Rivera G, Aur RJA, Dahl GV, Pratt CB, Hustu HO, George SL, Mauer AM (1979) Second cessation of therapy in childhood lymphocytic leukemia. Blood 53:1114–1120 – Simone J, Aur RJA, Hustu HO, Pinkel D (1972) "Total-Therapy" studies of acute lymphocytic leukemia in children. Current results and prospects for cure. Cancer 30:1488–1494 – Simone JV, Aur RJA, Hustu HO, Verzosa M, Pinkel D (1978) Three to ten years after cessation of therapy in children with leukemia. Cancer 42:839–842 – Spector G, Youness E, Culbert SJ (1979) Acute lymphoblastic leukemia followed by acute agranulocytic leukemia in a pediatric patient. Am J Clin Pathol 72:242–245

Haematology and Blood Transfusion Vol. 26
Modern Trends in Human Leukemia IV
Edited by Neth, Gallo, Graf, Mannweiler, Winkler
© Springer-Verlag Berlin Heidelberg 1981

The Treatment of Primary Childhood Acute Lymphocytic Leukemia with Intermediate Dose Methotrexate*

L. F. Sinks, J. J. Wang, and A. I. Freeman

A. Summary

Fifty-four consecutive children with acute lymphocytic leukemia (ALL) were treated from August 1974 until December of 1976 at Rosewell Park Memorial Institute (RPMI) according to a protocol which substituted cranial irradiation with systemic intermediate dose methotrexate (IDM) 500 mg/m² each 3 weeks for a total of 3 courses immediately following induction. Of 54 patients, 52 went into remission (96%). There were 35 standard risk and 17 increased risk patients according to age and presenting white blood count (WBC). As of September 1979 9 of the 35 standard risk patients had relapsed: (five central nervous system (CNS), three systemic, and one testicular. The overall disease control is comparable to other published methods of therapy involving cranial irradiation but has the added advantage of not exposing these children to the long range side effects currently being observed in children who had previously been treated with prophylactic cranial irradiation.

B. Introduction

The last decade and a half has seen dramatic improvement in the survival and actual "cure" of children with ALL. This improvement has been due principally to (1) the use of CNS "prophylaxis" and (2) effective systemic chemotherapy (Aur et al. 1971, 1972, 1973; Holland 1976; Hustu et al. 1973; Pinkel et al. 1977; Simone et al. 1975).

In the first half of the 1960s as improved systemic chemotherapy resulted in longer duration of complete remission, it became apparent that approximately 50% of these children would develop CNS leukemia (Evans et al. 1970). Once they developed CNS leukemia, very few were cured. In the mid-1960s effective methods of CNS prophylaxis were first employed to prevent overt CNS leukemia and eventual systemic relapse and death. In 1968 Cancer and Leukemia Group B (CALGB) in Protocol 6801 utilized prophylactic intrathecal methotrexate (IT MTX) and found that instead of 50% developing overt CNS leukemia, only 23% of the children developed this complication (Holland 1976), which has yet to be improved upon in subsequent CALGB studies. At approximately the same time investigators at St. Jude Cancer Research Center introduced the technique of cranial RT and IT MTX as CNS prophylaxis. This method reduced the incidence of CNS disease to approximately 10% (Aur et al. 1971, 1972, 1973; Hustu et al. 1973; Pinkel et al. 1977), which has not been confirmed in larger cooperative group studies.

However, cranial RT clearly cannot eradicate leukemic cells in sanctuaries other than the cranial cavity, e.g., the gonads, liver, and spleen. Furthermore, there has evolved a growing concern with immediate and long-term toxicity from prophylactic cranial RT. Therefore in 1974 we began a study with the following objectives: (1) to prevent the development of CNS leukemia without employing cranial RT and (2) to intensify systemic therapy and thus eradicate leukemic cells in other sanctuaries, which has been more recently emphasized by late testicular relapses in two cooperative group studies (Land et al. 1979;

* Supported in part by Grant CA 07918 and the Association for Research of Childhood Cancer (AROCC)

Baum et al. 1979). This study was based on clinical pharmacologic data demonstrating that intravenous IDM at a dose of 500 mg/m² given over 24 h was capable of diffusing across the CNS barrier in amounts adequate to eradicate most, if not all, leukemia cells in the CNS (Wang et al. 1976) and, hopefully, simultaneously penetrate other sanctuaries to a like degree. This report describes the clinical results of this study.

C. Materials and Methods

Fifty-four patients with newly diagnosed ALL were treated according to the protocol depicted in Fig. 1, which was instituted in the Department of Pediatrics at RPMI in August 1974. This was conducted as a pilot study and no randomization was planned.

Following induction with steroids, vincristine, and L-asparaginase, three courses of IDM were administered at three weekly intervals. IDM was administered at 500 mg/m², one-third by intravenous (IV) push and two-thirds by IV infusion over 24 h. IT MTX at 12 mg/m² was initially given on day 15, 22, 29 and then administered from ½ to 2 h after the initiation of IV MTX. Twenty-four h following completion of IV MTX, a single dose of citrovorum factor (leucovorin) was given at 12 mg/m². With moderately severe mucosal ulceration, the subsequent course of IDM was delayed until there was complete healing. The next IDM course was then administered at full dosage, but an additional dose of leucovorin at 12 mg/m² was injected 72 h from the start of IDM (48 h after completion of IDM). Following intermediate dose MTX, the patient received maintenance therapy consisting of daily oral 6-mercaptopurine and weekly oral MTX and pulse doses of steroid and vincristine (Fig. 1). Dexamethasone was used interchangeable with prednisone and 15 patients received the former.

All children with ALL or acute undifferentiated leukemia who could not be identified as acute myelocytic leukemia or acute myelomonocytic leukemia were entered on the study. Cell surface markers were not routinely done when this study was initiated.

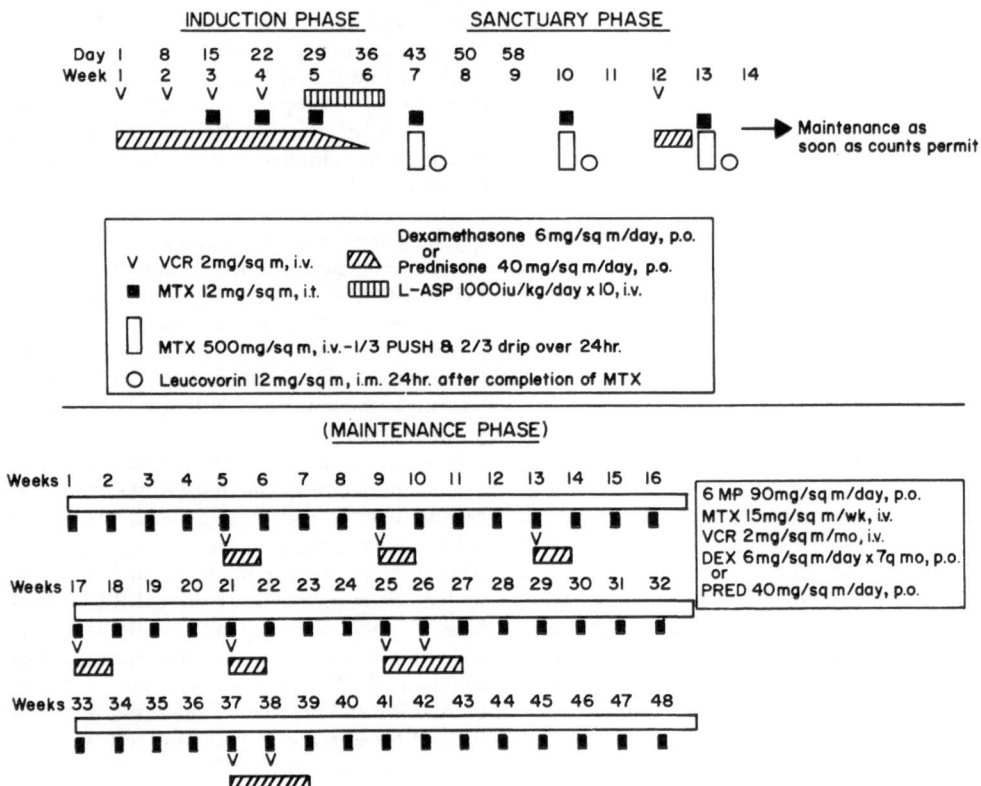

Fig. 1. Schema of treatment in ALL employing IDM

From August 1974 until December 1976, when the study was closed to patient accrual, 54 patients were entered ranging in age from 6 months to 17 years.

Patients were classified as standard risk or increased risk in terms of age or WBC at presentation, i.e., those patients less than 2 years or greater than 10 years of age and those patients who had a WBC greater than 30000/mm³ were defined as being increased risk. There were 19 children classified as increased risk, 17 of which went into remission and 35 children who were standard risk, all of whom went into remission. Two children (increased risk) probably had CNS leukemia at diagnosis – one presented with papilledema, and one had a right facial palsy of central type, but when spinal taps were performed on these two children two weeks later, no blasts were detected in the cerebrospinal fluid (CSF).

Patients with hyperuricemia or elevated blood urea nitrogen levels received appropriate short-term therapy for these conditions prior to beginning antileukemic therapy. Red cell and platelet transfusions were used as needed. Peripheral blood counts and appropriate blood chemical determinations were performed at frequent periodic intervals.

Spinal taps were performed routinely until week 13 of therapy and then at the first symptom or signs indicative of a CNS problem. All children in remission had spinal taps performed from February 1979 through July 1979.

Bone marrow aspirates were examined prior to the onset and again at completion of induction therapy and every 2–3 months thereafter, or at any time the peripheral blood was suspicious of a relapse. The criteria for determining complete remission have been published previously (Ellison et al. 1968). A remission bone marrow has normal granulopoiesis, thrombopoiesis, and erythropoiesis with fewer than 5% lymphblasts and less than 40% lymphocytes plus lymphoblasts. The patient's activity, physical findings, and peripheral blood must have reverted to normal. Induction failure was defined as those patients not achieving a remission bone marrow (less than 5% blasts) by day 42.

Leukoencephalopathy was defined clinically by the persistant unexplained presence of confusion, somnolence, ataxia, spasticity, focal neurologic changes, and seizures (Rubinstein et al. 1975; Kay et al. 1972; Price et al. 1975).

For purposes of analysis, complete remission status was terminated by: (1) bone marrow relapse (greater than 25% blast cells), (2) development of meningeal leukemia (two blasts cells on cytologic preparations of the CNS or ten cells/μl not attributable to chemical meningitis, (3) biopsy-proven leukemic cell infiltration in extramedullary organs, and (4) death while in remission. Patients were taken off chemotherapy after 4 years of continuous sustained remission. There are now 14 standard risk patients and three increased risk off all therapy.

All plots of remission duration were determined by actuarial life table analysis. The duration of remission was calculated through August of 1979.

D. Results

Of 54 patients, 52 (96%) achieved complete remission. The two inductio ailures were both in the increased risk group.

As of 1 September 1979 all patients in continuous remission have been followed for 36 to 72 months. A total of 20 patients (38%) have relapsed. These included: ten CNS relapses, nine systemic relapses, and one testicular relapse. Eleven of 17 increased risk patients (64%) and 9/35 standard risk patients (25%) have relapsed (Table 1).

Table 1. Current analyses

Site of relapse	CNS	10
	Systemic	9
	Testes	1
Risk factor and	Increased risk	11/17
relapse[a]	Standard risk	9/35
Time on study	44–80 months	
Median time on study	52 months	

[a] Number of relapses/number of patients achieving complete remission, June 1980

Of the nine standard risk patients who relapsed, there were five CNS relapses, three systemic relapses and one testicular relapse. Three of the nine havé died (Figs. 2–4).

Of the 11 increased risk patients who relapsed, five were in the CNS and six were systemic. Nine of the eleven patients have died. No CNS relapse was detected in those patients who had cerebrospinal fluid analysis performed routinely from February 1979 through July 1979.

One of the increased risk children who developed CNS leukemia was a 22-month-old male who presented with a central right facial palsy at diagnosis which subsequently disappeared with induction therapy and was thought to be due to CNS leukemia, but a spinal tap was not performed until 2 weeks later and there was no lymphoblasts in the CSF at this time. His CNS relapse occurred 23 months after diagnosis. Eight of the 52 children who entered complete remission have died.

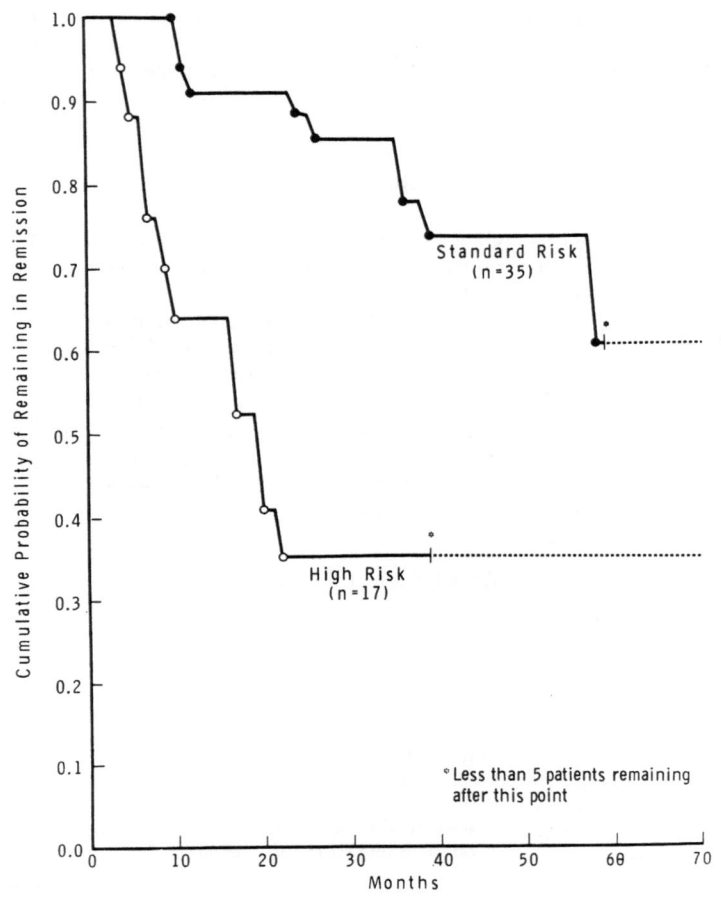

Fig. 2. Duration of *complete* remission employing IDM. Standard risk and high risk (see text)

E. Toxicity

The toxicity (Table 2) from the IDM included:
1. Vomiting occurring in 20/52 patients and was most pronounced during the first 2–4 h after the institution of IDM but occasionally persisted for 24–48 h;

2. Oral ulceration occuring in 20/52 patients with oral mucositis in 14 and pharyngitis in six patients. This was mild in 17/20, i.e., there were small ulcers which did not substantially interfere with orlke;
3. Hematologic toxicity occurring in 12 patients which, however, was minimal in its

Table 2. Toxicity results as of June 1980

Vomiting (with administration)	20/52	
Hematological		
WBC	2 (<3000/mm³)	0 (<1500/mm³)
Hgb	10 (<10 gm%)	0 (<8 gm%)
Platelets	0 (<100,000/mm³)	
Mucositis	14/52 (3 moderate and 11 mild)	
Pharnygitis	6/52	
Hepatic	11/52 (mild)	
Skin	3/52	
Renal	0/52	

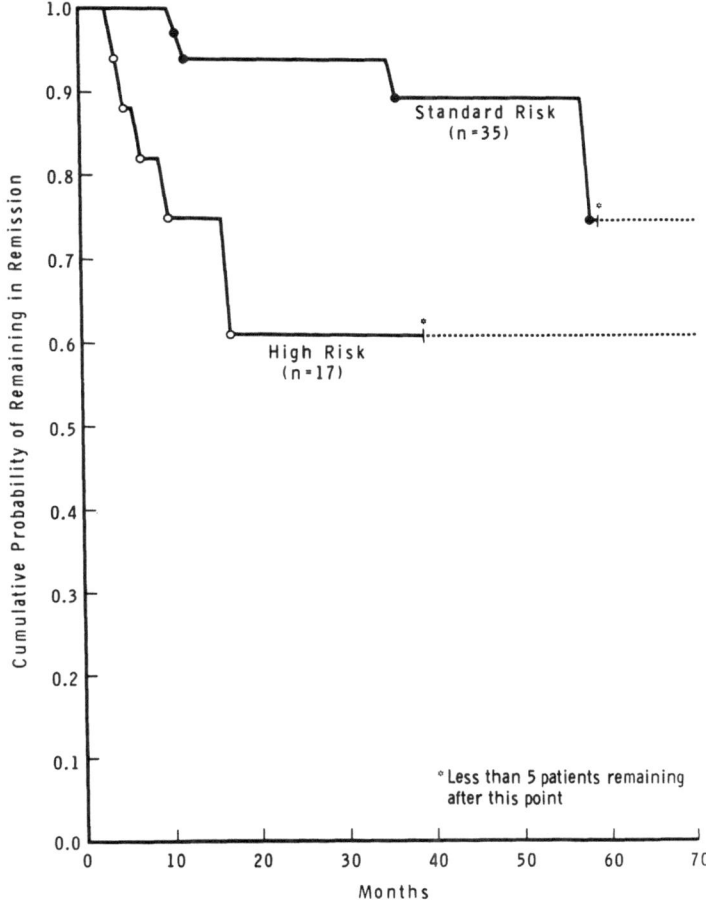

Fig. 3. Disease-free interval systemic[+] remission includes bone marrow and testicular relapse only

° Less than 5 patients remaining after this point

Standard Risk (n=35)

High Risk (n=17)

severity; there were no related clinical manifestations;

4. Hepatic toxicity occurring in 11 patients as evidenced by increased liver enzymes, particularly the SGOT. However, the peak SGOT was less than twice the normal level and returned to normal in all cases; and

5. Transient maculopapular rashes occurring in three cases and lasting for several days.

No case of renal toxicity was noted.

The overall regimen has been very well tolerated. There has been no life-threatening toxicity and no deaths secondary to IDM. Furthermore, there have been no cases of leukoencephalopathy and no interstitial pneumonia associated with IDM. One adolescent experienced anaphylaxis with the first dose of L-asparaginase. There have been neither infectious deaths nor toxic deaths for any patient while in remission on this study.

F. Discussion

The clinical data upon which this study was based was that of the early work of Djerassi who demonstrated the effectiveness of high doses of MTX in ALL (Djerassi et al. 1967). CALGB Protocol 6601 demonstrated that the greatest proportion of children remaining in complete sustained remission were those who received the intensive cycles of IV MTX (18 mg/m^2) daily for 5 days every 2 weeks (i.e., they received 90 mg/m^2 as a total dose every 2 weeks) and reinduction pulses of vincristine and prednisone for a period of 9 months (Holland 1976). In addition, CALGB Protocol 6801 demonstrated that "prophylactic" IT MTX during induction was important in decreasing the overt CNS leukemia. Furthermore, Habhbin et al. (1975) reported data suggesting that intensive systemic chemotherapy

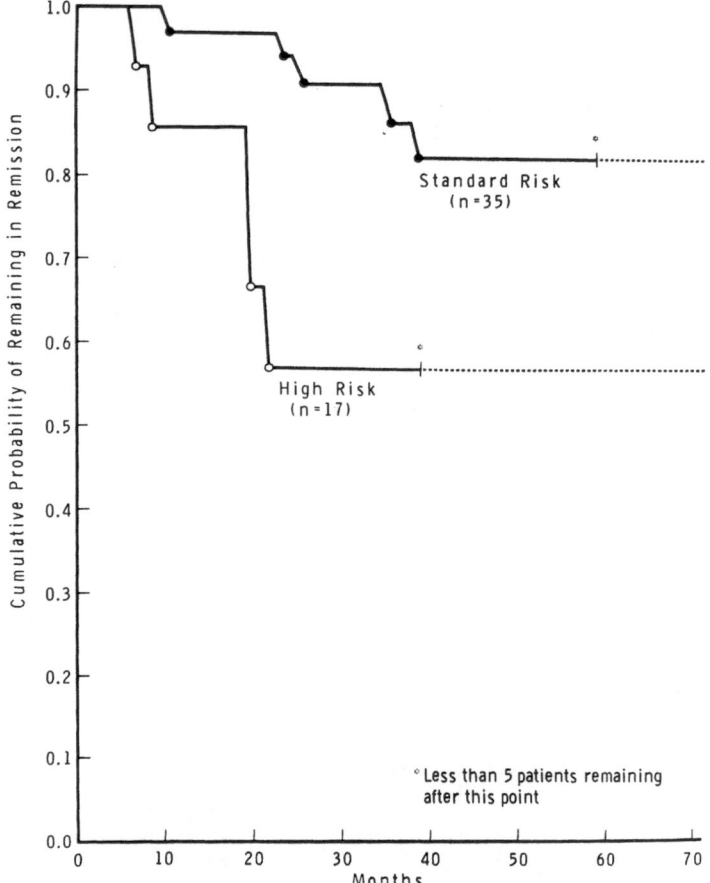

Fig. 4. Disease-free interval
CNS relapse only

may decrease the incidence of CNS leukemia.

The pharmacologic basis of this study includes the following: (1) reports showing that intravenous IDM resulted in MTX levels of 10^{-7} M reaching the CNS axis and diffusing into the CSF (Wang et al. 1976), and (2) the studies of Oldendorf and Danson (1967) using C^{14} sucrose in rabbits and Bourke et al. (1973) using C^{14}-5-flurouracil in monkeys demonstrating that the concomitant use of intrathecal with intravenous injection led to higher levels of drug in the CSF and more even distribution throughout the CNS than with either method alone and the findings that when MTX is given only via lumbar puncture the distribution of MTX throughout the CSF ist very variable (Shapiro et al. 1975). Studies in man corroborate these animal observations, i.e., higher levels of CSF MTX are obtained with conco-

mitant administration of IT and IV MTX than with either technique alone (Shapiro et al. 1975). Thus the technique employed in the present study of simultaneous IDM plus IT MTX enables one to more effectively bathe the CNS axis. The serum MTX levels following 500 mg/m^2 remain at 10^{-5} M for the 24-h infusion period (Wang et al. 1976; Freeman et al. 1977); therefore, it is anticipated that this will afford greater protection to other sanctuary sites such as gonads, liver, and spleen.

The clinical objectives of this study have been attained to a certain degree in the standard risk patient. The first objective to prevent CNS leukemia has been partially achieved as evidenced by the fact that only 5/35 standard risk patients developed CNS leukemia and 10/52 of the entire population experienced this complication (Fig. 4). This incidence is similar to that seen in a comparable cooperative study (CALGB Protocol 7111) (Jones et al. 1977). Furthermore, our objective to dispense with the need for cranial RT now appears even more important that when the study was designed in 1974. A recent study of children treated with prophylactic cranial RT and IT MTX or IT cytosine arabinoside showed that 53% developed abnormal findings as detected by computerized tomography (CT) (Peylan-Ramu et al. 1978). These findings included dilated ventricles, intracerebral calcifications, demyelination, and dilation of subarachnoid space. Signs of endocrinologic long-range effects have been reported as evidenced by a reduction in growth hormone secretion in children treated with prophylactic cranial RT (Shalet et al. 1976). A comparable CT scan study has been undertaken in our 43 patients (Ochs et al. 1978). Only 19% showed abnormal changes, and furthermore, these findings were much less marked than those reported by Peylan-Ramu et al. No calcifications and no patients with decreased attenuation coefficient were seen in any of the 43 cases. In a similar study from Norway, the investigators found only 1 child out of 19 with an abnormal CT scan. These patients had been treated with IDM similar to the schedule described in this report (Kolmannskog et al. 1979). The possible effect of prophylactic cranial RT on psychological, neurologic, and intellectual development is the subject of studies now in progress.

The overall relapse rate in this study is 20/52 and the CNS relapse rate as the initial site of failure is 10/52. Thus, 10/20 relapses occurred first in the CNS.

In a recent comparison by Green et al. it was demonstrated that patients treated at RPMI (standard risk) with IDM (Fig. 2) were maintained in *complete* remission significantly longer than two other groups of patients. One group consisted of those treated with prophylactic IT MTX (Children's Cancer Study Group CCG-101) and the other of those who received IT MTX and prophylactic RT (Sidney Farber Cancer Institute SFCI-73-01). This was in spite of the fact that CNS relapse rate was higher in the IDM-treated group (Fig. 4) compared to the irradiated group (Green et al., to be published). In this same comparison the increased risk group of patients did better in terms of CNS relapse and complete remission when treated with IT MTX and cranial irradiation.

Another large study (CALGB Protocoll 7111) recently reported by Jones et al. (1977) has demonstrated a protective value of cranial RT and IT MTX alone in preventing CNS leukemia but not benefit in the overall complete remission rate. This was the result of an increased incidence of hematological relapse in the patients who received cranial RT. The British Medical Research Council also has observed a higher rate of hematologic relapse in these patients receiving prophylactic craniospinal radiation than in those without CNS prophylaxis (Medical Research Council 1973). In the British study the radiated group, either cranial or craniospinal, had a greater lymphopenia, which may reflect a pertubation of the immune surveillance system and thus lead to a greater systemic relapse (Medical Research Council 1975, 1978).

Moe and Seip (1978) patterned their study in Norway closely after the one reported here; their results are preliminary, but to date there have been only 5 of 69 patients relapsing. Seventy-eight percent of the children have been followed for 18 months or more and are in complete remission.

It appears reasonable on the basis of present information to advance the conclusion that the treatment of children with ALL who fall into the standard risk category (age and WBC) can effectively be treated by IDM plus IT MTX in terms of better overall control of disease. Furthermore, the long-term risks and complications of cranial irradiation (Peylan-Ramu et al. 1978; Medical Research Council 1975; Fishman et al. 1976; Freeman et al. 1973; McIntosh et al. 1977) can be avoided with this type of therapy.

Children who are at increased risk appear to be protected by the use of cranial irradiation, but the way is clear to improve upon the present schedule of IDM in terms of dose escalation and pulse dose administration through the 1st year of remission. Such studies are currently under way in a number of centers.

The second objective, i.e., to intensify systemic treatment (Fig. 3) and thus to prevent other sanctuary site infiltration, has also been reasonably achieved. Only one male child (26 males) developed testicular relapse. We attribute this to effective serum levels of MTX which presumably can eradicate disease in sanctuary sites such as the liver, spleen, and gonads.

In conclusion, we can state that the use of a systemic form of therapy, as opposed to a local form (RT to cranium), appears to confer greater protection to standard risk children with ALL than the use of cranial RT. In addition, we can avoid the long-range complications of cranial RT. In the high risk patients, cranial RT and IT MTX appears superior to the systemic form (IDM); however, manipulation of this form of therapy (increasing dose and pulse therapy) may overcome this disadvantage.

Acknowledgment

Thanks to E. S. Henderson for his comments and help in preparing this manuscript.

We gratefully acknowledge the statistical assistance provided by J. Coombs, Ph. D., Assistant Professor, Division of Biostatistics and Epidemiology, Vincent T. Lombardi Cancer Research Center, Georgetown University Hospital.

References

Aur RJA, Simone JV, Hustu HO, Walters T, Borella L, Pratt L, Pinkel D (1971) Central nervous system therapy and combination chemotherapy of childhood lymphocytic leukemia. Blood 37:272–281 – Aur RJA, Simone JV, Hustu HO, Verzosa MS (1972) A comparative study of central nervous system irradiation and intensive chemotherapy early in remission of childhood acute lymphocytic leukemia. Cancer 29:381–391 – Aur RJA, Hustu HO, Verzosa MS, Wood A, Simone JS (1973) Comparison of two methods of preventing central nervous system leukemia. Blood 42/3:349–357 – Baum E, Sather H, Nachman J, Seinfeld J, Drivit W, Leikin S, Miller D, Joo P, Hammond D (1979) Relapse rates following cessation of chemotherapy during complete remission of acute lymphocytic leukemia. Med Pediatr Oncol 7:25–34 – Bourke RS, West CR, Chheda G, Tower DB (1973) Kinetics of entry and distribution of 5-fluoruracil in cerebrospinal fluid and brain following intravenous injection in a primate. Cancer Res 33:1735–1747 – Djerassi I, Farber S, Abir E, Neikirk W (1967) Continous infusion of methotrexate in children with acute leukemia. Cancer 20:233–242 – Ellison RR, Holland JF, Weil M, Jacquillat C, Boiron M, Bernard J et al. (1968) Arabinosyl cytosine: A useful agent in the treatment of acute leukemia in adults. Blood 32:507–523 – Evans AE, Gilbert ES, Zandstra A (1970) The increasing incidence of central nervous system leukemia in children (Children's cancer study group A). Cancer 26:404–409 – Fishman ML, Bear SC, Cogan DG (1976) Opticatrophy following prophylactic chemotherapy and cranial radiation for acute lymphocytic leukemia. Am J Opthalmol 82/4:571–576 – Freeman JE, Johnson PGB, Volre JM (1973) Somnolence after prophylactic cranial irradiation in children with acute lymphocytic leukemia. Br Med J 4:523–525 – Freeman AI, Wang JJ, Sinks LF (1977) High-dose methotrexate in acute lymphocytic leukemia. Cancer Treat Rep 61/4:727–731 – Green DM, Sather HN, Sallan SE, Nesbit ME Jr, Freeman AI, Cassady JR, Sinks LF, Hammond D, Frei E (1980) A comparison of four methods of central nervous system prophylaxis in childhood acute lymphoblastic leukemia. Lancet 1398–1402 – Haghbin M, Tan CTC, Clarkson BD et al. (1975) Treatment of acute lymphocytic leukemia in children with prophylactic intrathecal methotrexate and intensive systemic chemotherapy. Cancer Res 35:807–811 – Holland JF (1976) Oncologists reply. N Engl J Med 294:440 – Hustu HO, Aur RJA, Verzosa MS, Simone JV, Pinkel D (1973) Prevention of central nervous system leukemia by irradiation. Cancer 32:585–597 – Jones B, Holland JF, Glidewell O, Jacquillat C, Weil M, Pochedly C, Sinks LF, Chevalier L, et al. (1977) Optimal use of L-Asparaginase (NSC-109229) in acute lymphocytic leukemia. Med Pediatr Oncol 3:387–400 – Kay HEM, Knapton PJ, O'Sullivan JP, Wells DG, Harris RF, Innes EM, Surart J, Schwartz FCM, Thompson EN (1972) Encephalopathy in acute leukemia associated with methotrexate therapy. Arch Dis Child 47:344–354 – Kolmannskog S, Moe PJ, Anke IM (1979) Computed tomographic findings of the brain in children with acute lymphocytic leukemia after central nervous system prophylaxis without cranial irradiation. Acta Paediatr Scand 68:254–256 – Land VJ, Berry DH, Herson J, Miale T, Reid H, Silva-Sosa M, Starling K (1979) Long-term survival in childhood acute leukemia: "Late" relapses. Med Pediatr Oncol 7:19–24 – McIntosh S, Fisher D, Rothman SG, Rosenfeld N, Lebel JF, O'Brien RT (1977) Intracranial calcifications in childhood leukemia. J Pediatr 91:909–913 – Medical Research Council: Working party on leukemia in childhood: Treatment of acute lymphocytic leukemia: Effect of "prophylactic" therapy against central nervous leukemia. Br Med J 2:381–384 – Medical Research Council: Working party on leukemia in childhood: Analysis of treatment in childhood leukemia I. Prolonged predisposition to drug induced neutropenia following craniospinal irradiation. Br Med J 244:563–566 – Medical Research Council: Working party on leukemia in childhood: Analysis of treatment in childhood leukemia IV. The critical association between dose fractionation and immunosuppression induced by cranial irradiaton. Cancer 41:108–111 – Moe PJ, Seip M (1978) High dose methotrexate in acute lymphocytic leukemia in childhood. Acta Paediatr Scan 67:265–268 – Ochs JJ, Berger PE, Brecher ML, Sinks LF, Freeman AI (1978) Computed tomography (CT) scans in children with acute lymphocytic leukemia (ALL) following CNS prophylaxis without radiotherapy. Proc. ASCO 19:391 – Oldendorf WH, Danson J (1967) Brain extracellular space and the sink action of cerebrospinal fluid. Arch Neurol 17:196–205 – Peylan-Ramu N, Poplack DG, Pizzo PA, Adornato BT, Dichero, G (1978) Abnormal CT scans in asymptomatic children after prophylactic cranial irradiation and intrathecal chemotherapy. N Engl J Med 298:815–819 – Pinkel D, Hustu HO, Aur RJA, Smith K, Borella LD, Simone JV (1977) Radiotherapy in leukemia and lymphoma in children. Cancer 39/2:817–824 – Price RA, Jamieson PA (1975) The central nervous system in childhood leukemia – II. Subacute leukoencephalopathy. Cancer 35:306–318 – Rubinstein LJ, Herman MM, Wilbur JR (1975) Disseminated leukoencephalopathy: A complication of treated central nervous system leukemia and lymphoma. Cancer 35:291–305 – Shalet SM, Beardswell CG, Jones PH, Pearson D (1976) Growth hormone deficiency after treatment of acute lymphocytic leukemia. Arch Dis Child 51/7:489–493 – Shapiro WR, Young DF, Metha BM (1975) Methotrexate: Distribution in cerebrospinal fluid after intravenous, ventricular and lumbar injections. N Engl J Med 293:161–166 – Simone JV, Aur RJA, Hustu HO, Verzosa M, Pinkel D (1975) Combined modality therapy of acute lymphocytic leukemia. Cancer 35/1:25–35 – Wang JJ, Freeman AI, Sinks LF (1976) Treatment of acute lymphocytic leukemia by high dose intravenous methotrexate. Cancer Res 36:1441–1444

Haematology and Blood Transfusion Vol. 26
Modern Trends in Human Leukemia IV
Edited by Neth, Gallo, Graf, Mannweiler, Winkler
© Springer-Verlag Berlin Heidelberg 1981

Present Problems in Management of Childhood Lymphoblastic Leukaemia: Experience from the Hospital for Sick Children, London

J. M. Chessells, J. Ninane, and K. Tiedemann

The majority of children with acute lymphoblastic leukaemia (ALL) at the Hospital for Sick Children, Great Ormond Street (GOS), are treated in collaborative protocols designed by the United Kingdom Medical Research Council Working Party on Childhood Leukaemia (UKALL trials). Data is presented from patients treated in these trials and in other protocols piloted at GOS for the Working Party.

In the late 1960s children with ALL were treated at GOS with a variety of sequential regimes or short intensive protocols such as the CONCORD (Medical Research Council 1971). Continuing chemotherapy (remission maintenance) with multiple agents as in UKALL I (Medical Research Council 1973) was introduced in 1970 and from 1972 onwards all patients received prophylaxis against development of leukaemic infiltration of the central nervous system (CNS) with cranial irradiation (2400 rads) and a course of intrathecal methotrexate injections and/or spinal irradiation. Long-term follow up of these patients has, as expected, confirmed that CNS prophylaxis increases the proportion of patients achieving long-term *disease-free* survival but has, as yet, failed to show any influence of

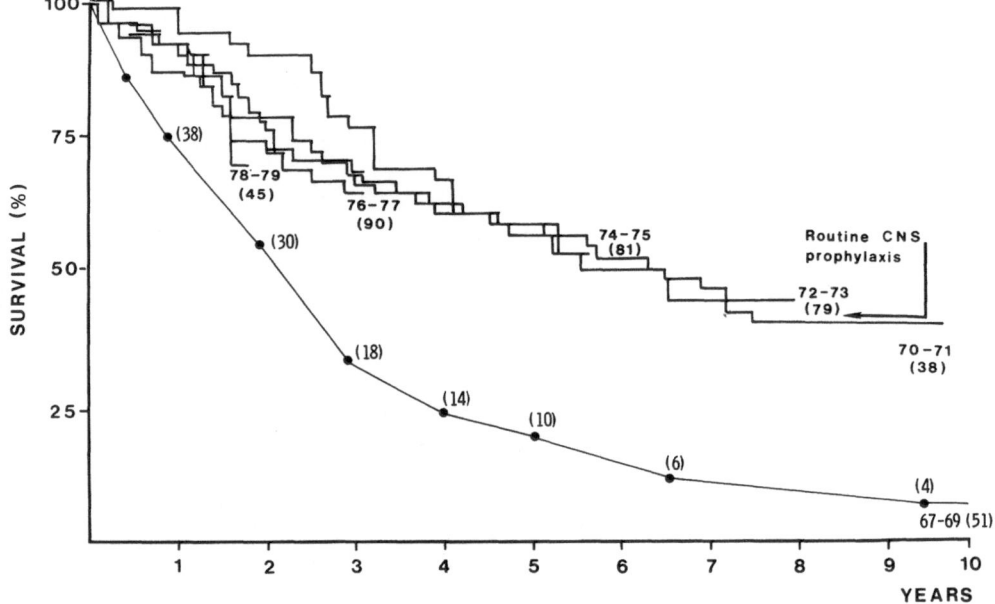

Fig. 1. Survival in all patients with ALL treated in consecutive periods at GOS. *Numbers in parentheses* refer to total numbers of patients in the period

CNS prophylaxis on overall survival or on duration of haematological remission (Figs. 1, 2). The major problem in management, therefore, remains that of haematological relapse, although the proportion of deaths in remission also gives cause for continuing concern.

A. Death in remission

Analysis of data from the first and second UKALL trials showed that death in remission was primarily seen in patients with "standard" prognostic features (aged less than 14 at diagnosis with a pre-treatment leucocyte count of less than $20 \times 10^9/1$) (Medical Research Council 1976). A survey of remission deaths in children at GOS between 1973 and 1977 (Table 1) who all received standard CNS prophylaxis with cranial irradiation and intrathecal methotrexate showed that the most common cause was measles pneumonia, usually occurring in children without overt clinical measles. Two of the four deaths from septicaemia occurred in young infants and one in a splenectomized child receiving prophylactic penicillin. The high incidence of measles pneumonia can be ascribed to the regrettably low uptake of measles vaccine in Britain.

Table 1. Causes of death in remission in 168 children with ALL

Cause	No. patients
Measles	6
Septicaemia	4
Cytomegalovirus	2
Herpes simplex	1
Varicella-zoster	1
Total	14 (8% of cases)

Concern about these complications of treatment led us to explore the relative efficacy and immunosuppression of 6-mercaptopurine and methotrexate given in equivalent dose either continously or intermittently in a 5-day course every three weeks (Fig. 3). The continuous (C) and intermittent (I) arms of this protocol for "standard risk" patients were introduced at GOS in 1974 and the protocol was subsequently adopted as the UKALL V schedule, with introduction of an intermediate (G) schedule. The results of the immunological studies in the three groups of patients have recently been published (Rapson et al. 1980) and show that in patients receiving continuous chemotherapy the blood lymphocyte counts,

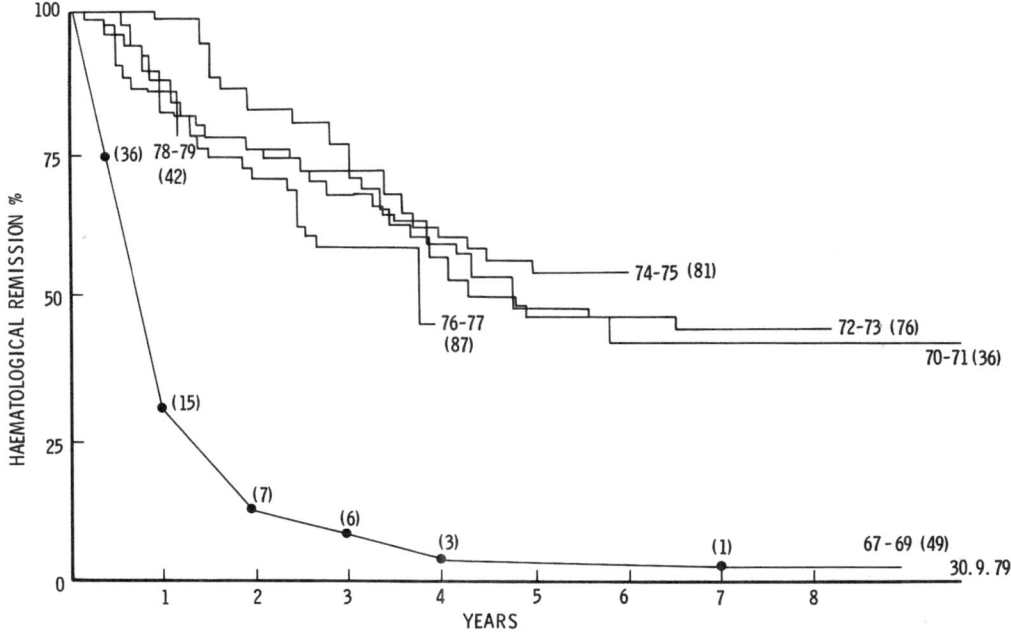

Fig. 2. Duration of first haematological remission in the same group of patients. The improvement between 1969 and 1970 is due to introduction of combination chemotherapy for remission maintenance

109

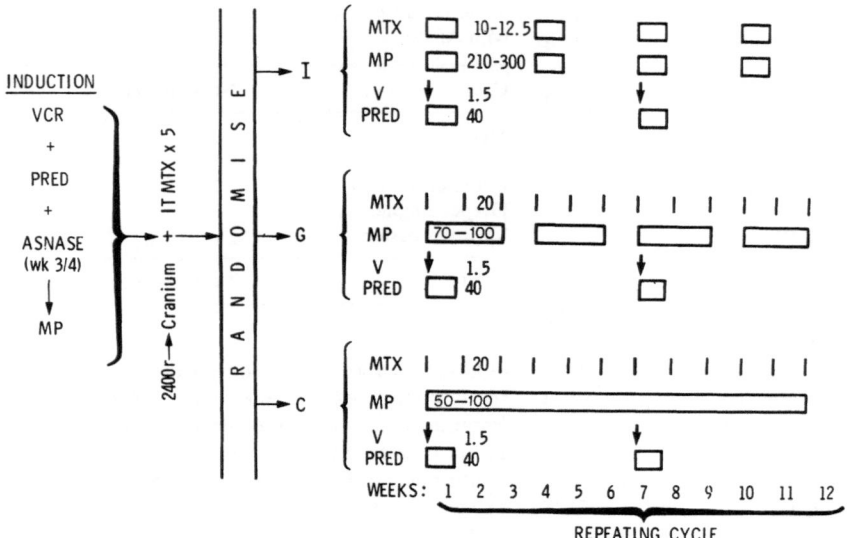

Fig. 3. Design of MRC UKALL V started at GOS in 1974. Doses of drugs are in mg/m² surface area. *Pred*, prednisolone; *V, VCR*, vincristine; *MTX*, methotrexate; and *MP*, 6-mercaptopurine

mitotic response to phytohaemagglutinin and plasma immunoglobulin levels were significantly lower than in patients receiving intermittent therapy. Results in the intermediate G group fell between the other two groups. We have subsequently reviewed the incidence of infection in 115 patients (Table 2) as of January 1980. Patients receiving continuous chemotherapy had a higher incidence of remission deaths, with measles again as the most common agent. The death from measles in the G group occurred in a patient in the first treatment cycle after radiotherapy. The two children in the study who survived measles were both receiving intermittent chemotherapy and in both the illness pursued a normal clinical course. Pneumocystis infection was

confined to the C group but all cases responded to treatment with high dose co-trimoxazole.

Preliminary analysis of remission duration in the three groups of patients shows no significant differences between the three regimes, although schedule I appears marginally inferior (Fig. 4). However, schedule I has also been associated with nausea and mouth ulceration. Because of this, it has proved difficult to achieve the maximum drug dosage in all patients; the intermediate (G) schedule has been adopted for continuing chemotherapy in a subsequent protocol, and we are now starting a program of routine administration of immunoglobulin to all children at risk of measles.

B. Prevention of Marrow Relapse

While these attempts to reduce remission deaths were in progress, the UKALL IV protocol for high risk patients compared the value of early intensive induction with cyclophosphamide, cytosine arabinoside, prednisolone and vincristine to a regime of prednisolone and vincristine (Fig. 5) and compared simple continuing chemotherapy as given in UKALL II (Medical Research Council 1976) with a rotating intermittent multiple drug schedule (Fig. 6). Preliminary analysis of the

Table 2. Infections in UKALL V pilot study

Protocol	C	I	G	Total patients
No. patients	55	37	23	115
Admitted with infection	29	1	9	39
Pneumocystis	7	0	0	7
Deaths in remission (measles)	6(4)	0	2(1)	8

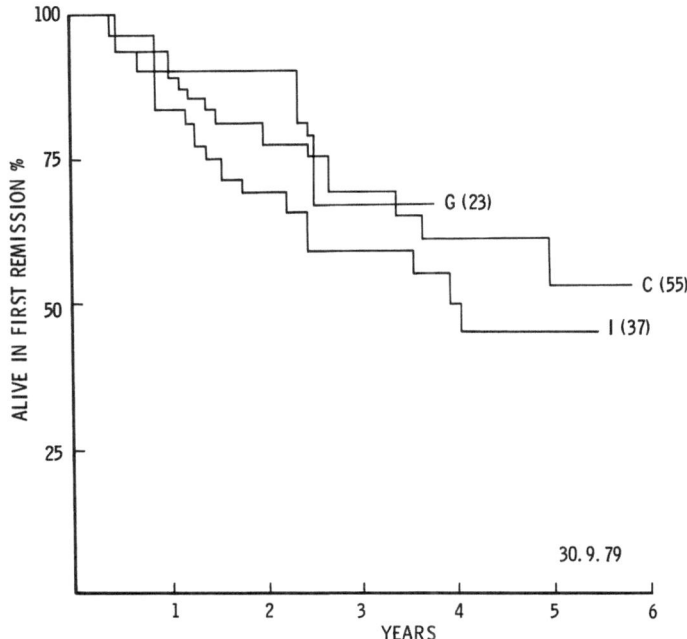

Fig. 4. Duration of first remission in patients on UKALL V schedule. *Numbers in parentheses* refer to total numbers of patients in each group

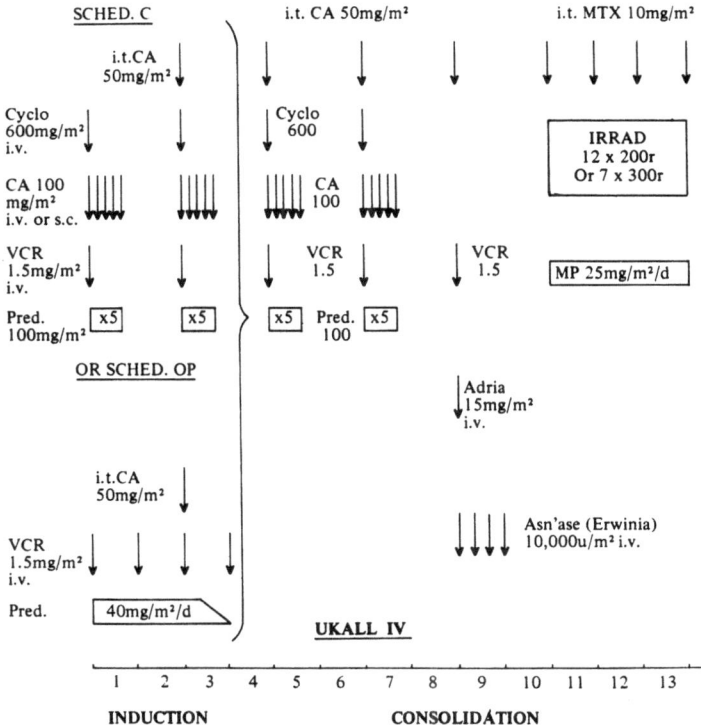

Fig. 5. MRC UKALL IV poor risk patients). Induction regimen with randomization to prednisolone and vincristine or COAP combination chemotherapy. *Cyclo,* cyclophosphamide; *CA,* cytosine arabinoside, *VCR,* vincristine; *Pred,* prednisolone; *Adria,* adriamycin; *MTX,* methotrexate; *MP,* 6-mercaptopurine

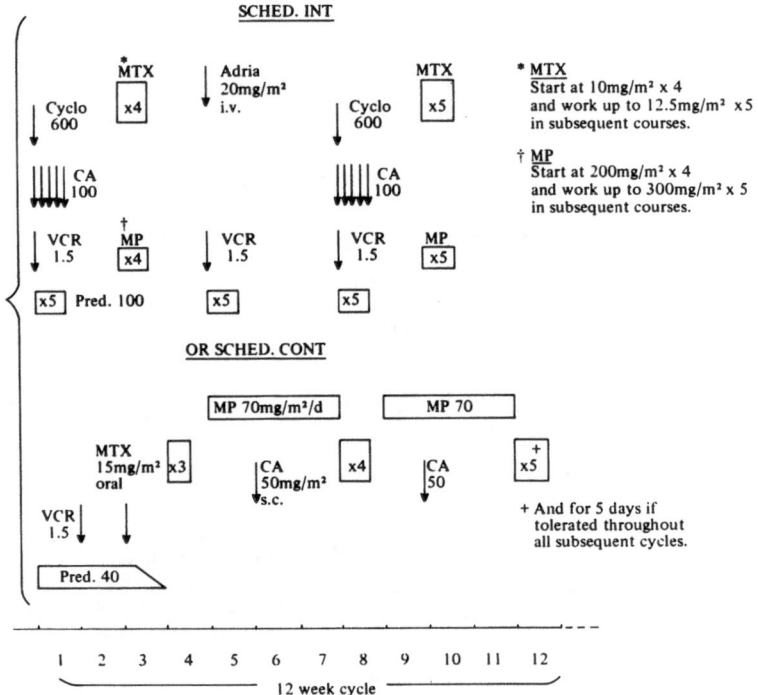

Fig. 6. UKALL IV continuing (maintenance) therapy. Abbreviations as in Figure 5

results is disappointing and shows no advantage for intensive induction or for multiple agent maintenance over the simpler schedules.

These drugs, of course, may not be the optimal ones to use in early induction. We have found that prolonged L-asparaginase in combination with daunorubicin, prednisolone and vincristine is extremely effective in relapsed and resistant ALL (Chessells and Cornbleet 1979) and are at present evaluating this combination of drugs in induction of first remission, with the aim of improving duration of subsequent haematological remission.

C. Sex and Prognosis

Long-term follow up of the MRC UKALL II trial showed that boys fared significantly worse than girls and that this trend was not just due to testicular relapse (Medical Research Council 1978). Similar results have since been reported by others (George et al. 1979). This worse prognosis in boys has been consistently observed in our clinic population (Fig. 7) and is not confined to "poor risk" patients among whom there might be a predominance of T-cell ALL (Chessells 1979). The difference is accounted for partly but not entirely by testicular relapse; boys also have a higher incidence of marrow relapse after stopping treatment than girls (Fig. 8).

The influence of sex on prognosis, unlike that of leucocyte count or the immunological sub-type of the leukaemia (Chessells et al. 1977), becomes apparent well after the first year of treatment at about the time of stopping therapy.

We have two approaches to this problem at present. First, by early intensification of chemotherapy, as previously described, we are attempting to reduce the incidence of marrow relapse. Secondly, we are attempting to detect testicular disease early by routine bilateral wedge biopsy of the testicles in all boys at the time of stopping treatment. So far routine biopsy has been performed in 60 boys with no clinical sign of infiltration; infiltration was histologically detected in six (10%). Three of 54 boys with a negative biopsy have subse-

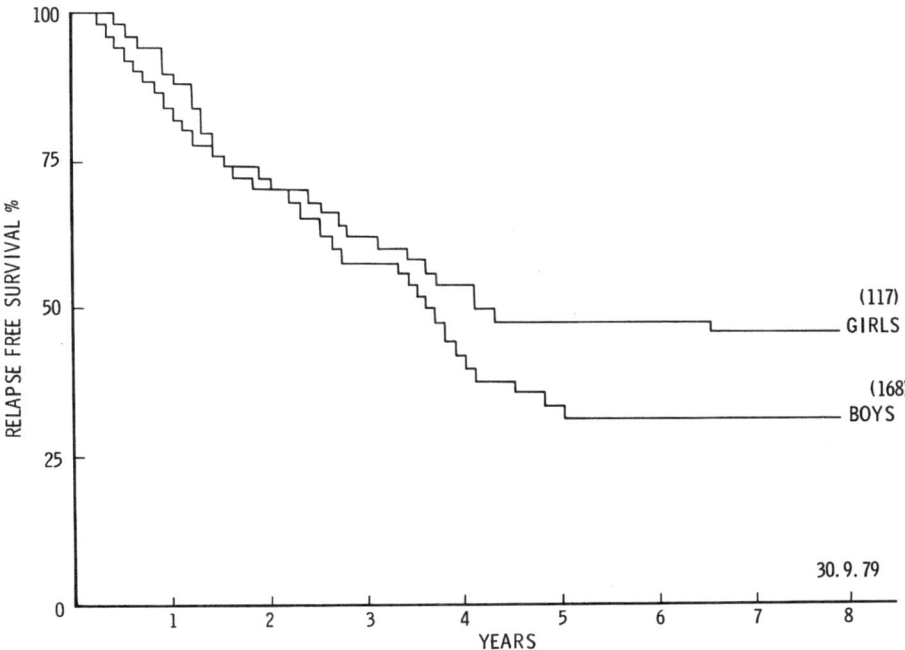

Fig. 7. Relapse-free survival compared in the sexes. GOS 1972–78. Note divergence at 3–5 years

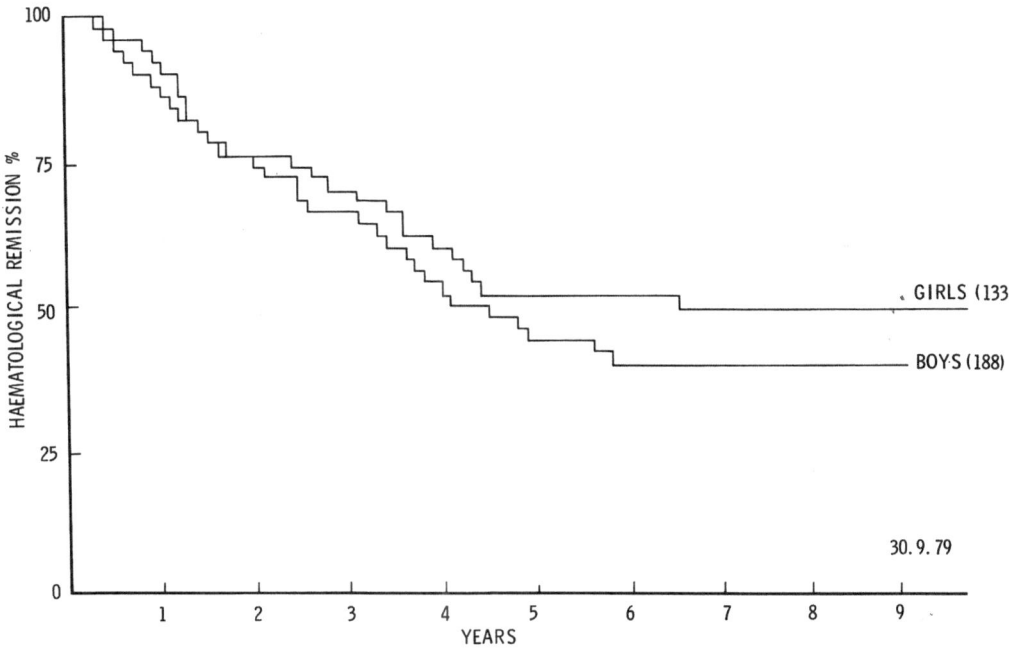

Fig. 8. Haematological remission duration in both sexes, 1970–78. Note similar but less marked divergence

113

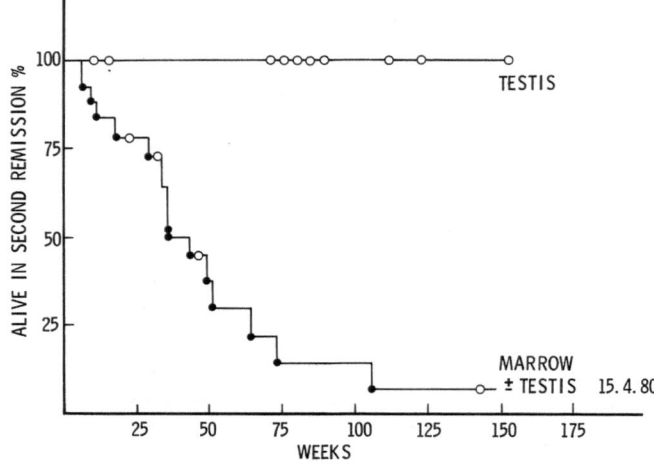

Fig. 9. Comparison of duration of second remission in boys with isolated testicular infiltration at or after stopping chemotherapy and boys with marrow relapse with or without testicular involvement. *Open circles* denote patients still in remission

quently developed testicular leukaemia. Boys with overt or occult infiltration are treated with radiotherapy to both testicles (2400 rads) a course of intrathecal methotrexate injections and 2 years of continuous chemotherapy. Preliminary results in ten boys thus treated are encouraging and show that at least in the short term isolated testicular relapse has a better prognosis than bone marrow relapse (Fig. 9).

D. Conclusions

The two major areas of concern are deaths during continuing (maintenance) treatment and bone marrow relapse. The duration of haematological remission in the series of UKALL trials has not been improved by a variety of manipulations of continuing treatment. It is to be hoped that early intensification of treatment will increase the proportion of patients achieving long-term haematological remission and improve the poor prognosis for boys hitherto observed in the UKALL trials.

References

Chessells JM (1979) Presentation and prognosis in childhood leukaemia. In: Morris Jones PH (ed) Topics in paediatrics I. Haematology and oncology, Pitman Medical, Tunbridge Wells, pp 27–35 – Chessells JM, Cornbleet M (1979) Combination chemotherapy for bone marrow relapse in childhood lymphoblastic leukaemia (ALL). Med Pediatr Oncol 6:359–365 – Chessells JM, Hardisty RM, Rapson NT Greaves MF (1977) Acute lymphoblastic leukaemia in childhood: classification and prognosis. Lancet ii:1307–1309 – George SL, Aur RJA, Mauer AM, Simone JV (1979) A reappraisal of the results of stopping therapy in childhood leukemia. N Engl J Med 300:269–273 – Medical Research Council (1971) Treatment of acute lymphoblastic leukaemia. Comparison of immunotherapy (B.C.G.) intermittent methotrexate, and no therapy after a five-month intensive cytotoxic regimen (Concord Trial). Br Med J 4:189–194 – Medical Research Council (1973) Treatment of acute lymphoblastic leukaemia: central nervous system leukemia. Br Med J 2:381–384 – Medical Research Council (1976) Analysis of treatment in childhood leukaemia. II. Timing and the toxicity of combined 6-mercaptopurine and methotrexate maintenance therapy. Br J Haematol 33:179–188 – Medical Research Council (1978) Effects of varying radiation schedule, cyclophosphamide treatment and duration of treatment in acute lymphoblastic leukaemia. Br Med J 2:787–791 – Rapson NT, Cornbleet MA, Chessells JM, Bennett AJ, Hardisty RM (1980) Immunosuppression and serious infections in children with acute lymphoblastic leukaemia: a comparison of three chemotherapy regimes. Br J Haematol 45:41–52

Haematology and Blood Transfusion Vol. 26
Modern Trends in Human Leukemia IV
Edited by Neth, Gallo, Graf, Mannweiler, Winkler
© Springer-Verlag Berlin Heidelberg 1981

Different Therapy Protocols for High Risk and Standard Risk ALL in Childhood

F. Zintl, W. Plenert, and J. Hermann

Children with acute lymphocytic leukemia can be apparently cured today. The subclassification of ALL in childhood as "high risk" and "standard risk" ALL by means of a determination of immunologic and clinical parameters is of increasing importance. This classification could become the basis for a risk-oriented individual therapy. We present here the current results attained in the treatment of childhood ALL by our Pediatric Hematology and Oncology working group involving 13 treatment centers of the German Democratic Republic.

A. Patients and Methods

I. Study IV

From January 1976 to December 1977 111 previously untreated patients were entered in this study. The outline of therapy is shown in Fig. 1. There were two different treatment groups based upon the presence or absence of high risk factors at the time of diagnosis. The criteria for high risk factors were defined as:

1. Leukocyte count above 20,000 cells/mm³,
2. Age under 2 years and over 10 years,
3. Mediastinal mass,
4. Generalized enlargement of lymph nodes or enlargement of one or more lymph nodes by 3 cm or more,
5. Tumor of other organs,
6. Enlargement of liver or spleen by 5 cm or more, and
7. CNS leukemia at diagnosis.

In the presence of one or more high risk criteria the patients received a consolidation therapy with Ara-C and L-asparaginase.

Of the 111 patients 67 were classified as high risk and 44 as standard risk patients.

As CNS prevention therapy – regardless of their prognostic factors – all children received combined intrathecal injections of methotrexate and prednisolone during induction therapy, early in remission, and periodically throughout the continuation treatment. In addition, 41 patients received preventive cranial irradiation (2400 rad telecobalt) and 68 received intrathecal application of macrocolloidal radiogold (198 Au, 2,5 mCi) (Metz et al. 1977).

II. Study V and LSA₂L₂ Protocol

As of January 1978 treatment was given by two other protocols: study V (Fig. 2) for standard risk patients and LSA₂L₂ protocol for high risk patients (Fig. 3). This latter group also included children with non-Hodgkin lymphomas who had 25% or more tumor cells in the bone marrow. In this study high risk criteria differed from the previous study and was limited to:

1. Leukocyte counts 50,000 per cu mm and more,
2. Mediastinal mass,
3. T-ALL (blast cells form spontaneous rosettes with sheep erythrocytes and/or give a positive reaction with antithymocyte serum),
4. Positive acid phosphatase reaction of the blast cells, and
5. CNS leukemia at diagnosis.

III. Statistical Analysis

The results of each of the three studies were analysed as of 31 December 1979 and the statistical analysis was performed according to the life table method of Cutler and Ederer (1958).

B. Results

I. Study IV

Table 1 depicts the clinical course of the 111 patients entered on study IV. As shown in Fig. 4, no statistical difference could be detected in

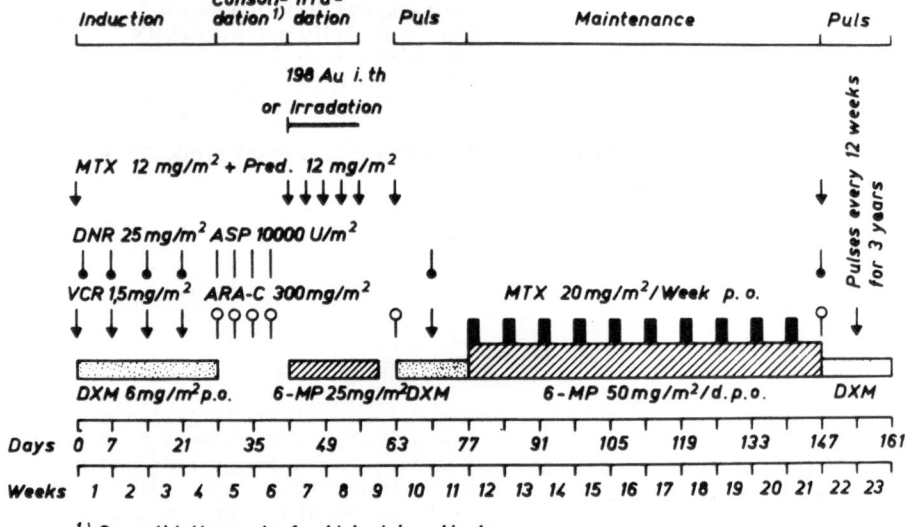

Fig. 1. Outline of therapy for study IV (1976–77)

the outcome of standard and high risk patients entered on study IV. At 3 years the cumulative complete remission rate was 0.56 ± 0.11 for the standard risk group and 0.44 ± 0.07 for the high risk group. Thirty nine patients are still receiving chemotherapy and in 15 treatment has recently been stopped (median time off therapy was 3 months).

II. Study V and LSA₂L₂ Protocol

New treatment programs were introduced in 1978 with the objective of improving these results. The LSA_2L_2 protocol developed by Wollner et al. (1976) for patients with non-Hodgkin lymphoma was used for a newly defined group of high risk patients as described

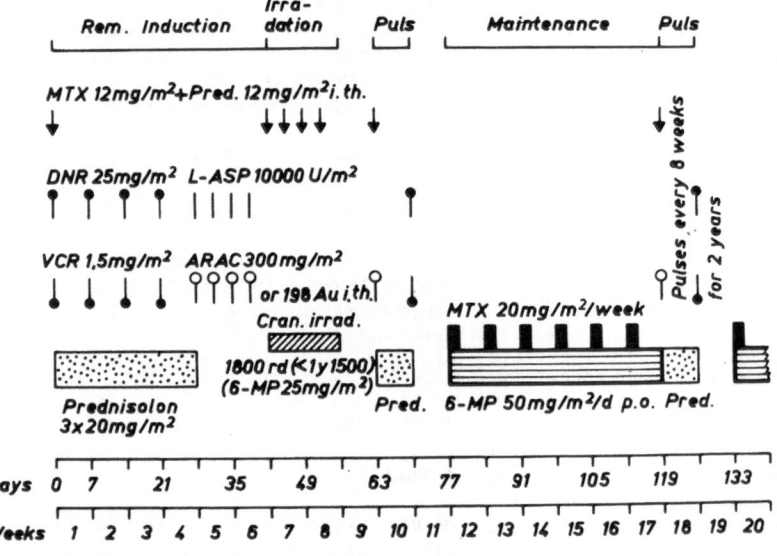

Fig. 2. Outline of therapy for study V (1978–79)

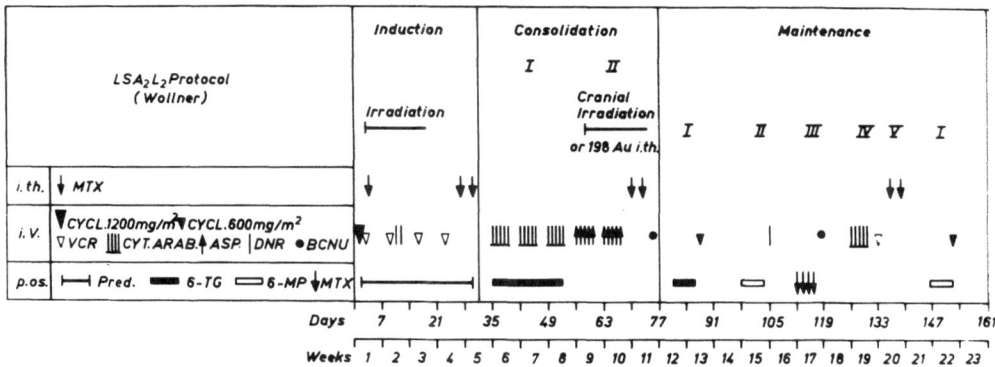

Fig. 3. Outline of therapy for study LSA$_2$L$_2$ (Wollner et al.)

above. At this time only preliminary results are available for these studies. The cumulative complete remission rate at 2 years is 0.79 for 111 standard risk patients and 0.50 for 58 children with high risk leukemia. Thus far the outcome has been significantly worse for patients with leukocyte counts exceeding 100,000 cells/mm^3 (Fig. 6), with mediastinal masses (Fig. 7), and in children under the age of 2 and above the age of 10 years (Fig. 8). The significance of T-cell lymphoblasts and of initial CNS leukemia could not be calculated.

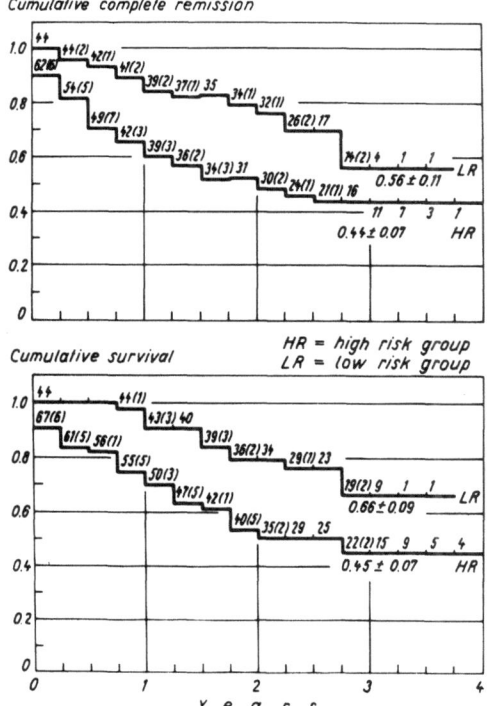

Fig. 4. Survival and relapse-free survival in childhood acute lymphocytic leukemia, study IV

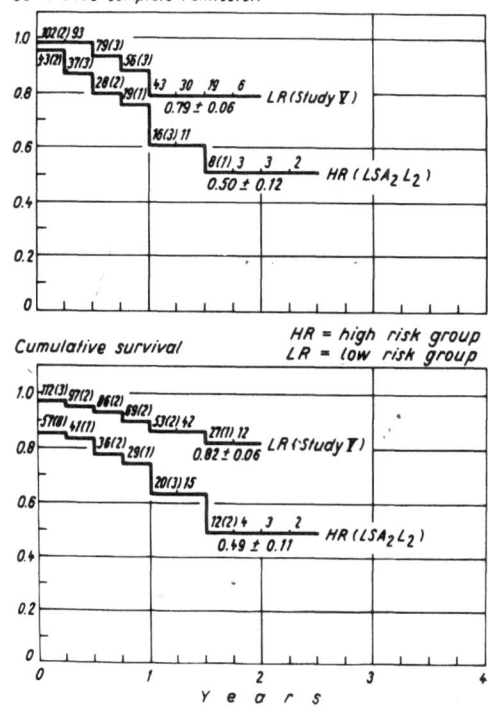

Fig. 5. Survival and relapse-free survival in childhood acute lymphocytic leukemia, studies V and LSA$_2$L$_2$

	High risk	Standard risk	Total	
Number of patients	67	44	111	
Early deaths	5	0	5	
Complete remission	62	44	106	
Number of relapses	34	14	48	
Marrow	28	9	37	
Marrow + CNS	0	3	3	
CNS	4	2	6	
Testes	2	0	2	
Remission deaths	2	2	4	
Cumulative complete remission	0.44 ± 0.07	0.56 ± 0.11	0.50 ± 0.06	

Table 1. Clinical course in study IV (1976–1977)

C. Discussion

The therapeutic value of intensive early therapy for ALL remains controversial. Pinkel has reported that this treatment phase does not reduce the incidence of relapses (Pinkel 1979), while Riehm et al. have concluded that intensified induction treatment definitively improves the final outcome (Riehm et al. 1977). Because of the recognized poor prognosis in patients with high risk leukemia we decided to use more intensive initial therapy in these patients. However the 2 week consolidation therapy with cytosine arabinoside and L-asparaginase

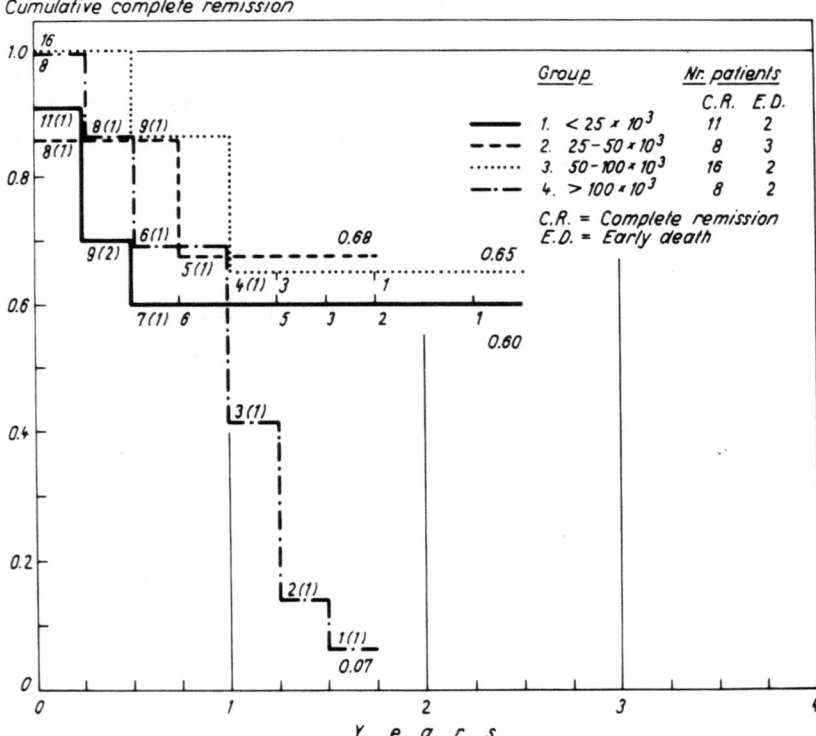

Fig. 6. Relationship of initial WBC to relapse-free survival in childhood acute lymphocytic leukemia, study LSA$_2$L$_2$

	Study V (Standard risk patients)	LSA$_2$L$_2$ (Wollner) (High risk patients)	
Number of patients	111	58	
Early deaths	4	9	
Complete remission	102	44	
Number of relapses	12	12	
Marrow	7	7	
Marrow + CNS	0	0	
CNS	4	4	
Testes	1	1	
Remission deaths	2	2	
Cumulative complete remission	0.79 ± 0.06	0.50 ± 0.12	

Table 2. Clinical course in study V and LSA$_2$L$_2$ (1978–1979)

used in study IV did not prove to be more effective when important features such as leukocyte count over 100,000 cells/mm^3, mediastinal mass, or age under 2 or over 10 years were present. Since different criteria were used to define high risk patients in studies IV and LSA$_2$L$_2$, results cannot be readily compared among both treatment groups. Current information, however, favors the results attained in the LSA$_2$L$_2$ study when single factors are comparatively analyzed, i.e., mediastinal mass, leukocyte count up to 100,000 cells/mm^3, and acid phosphatase reaction by lymphoblasts. For patients with leukocyte counts over

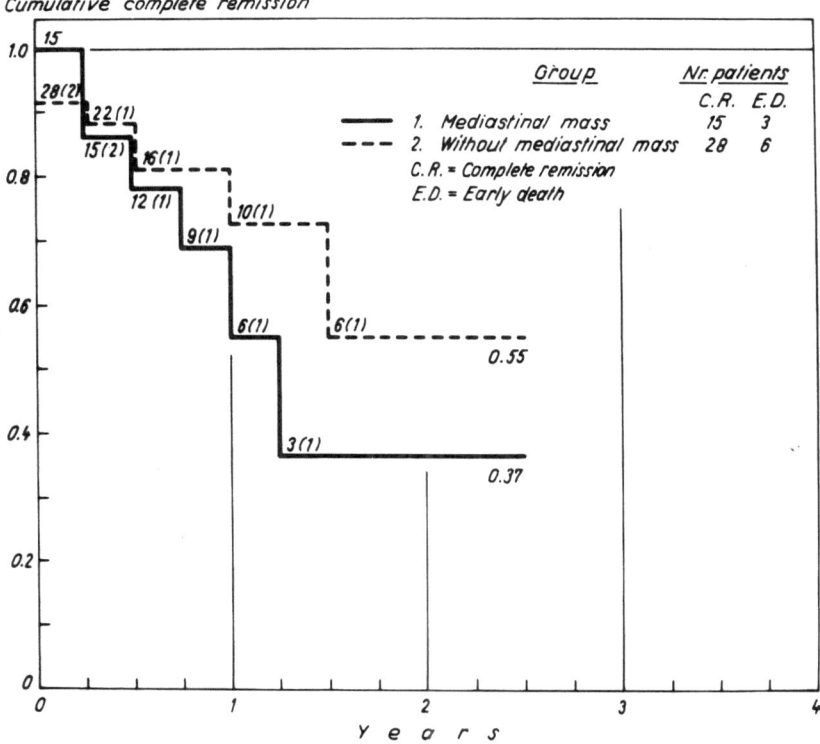

Fig. 7. Relationship of mediastinal mass to relapse-free survival in childhood acute lymphocytic leukemia, study LSA$_2$L$_2$

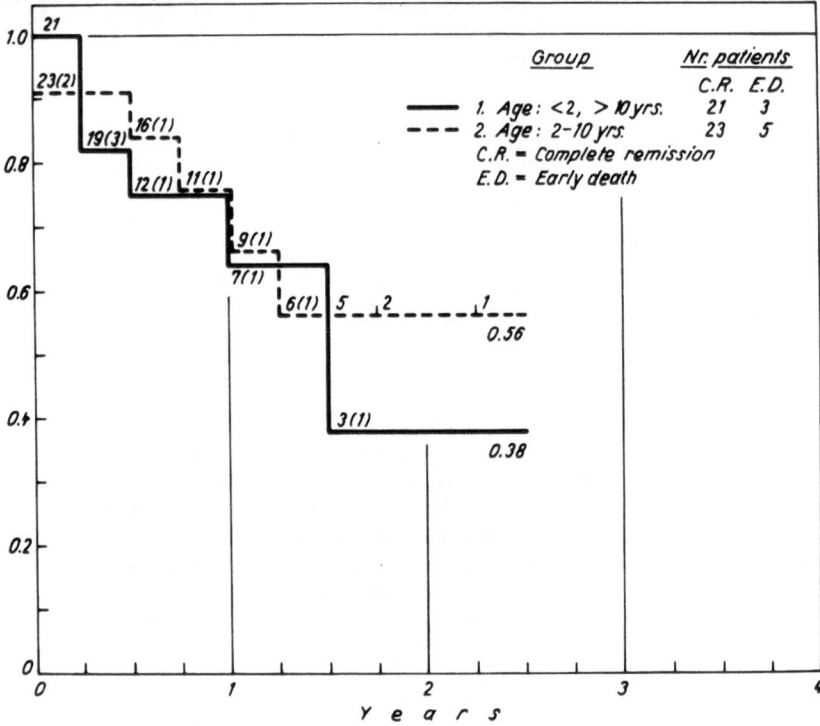

Fig. 8. Relationship of age to relapse-free survival in childhood acute lymphocytic leukemia, study LSA₂L₂

100,000 cells/mm³ the results have not been influenced by this latter therapy.

The division into high and standard risk patients is based on empirical clinical observations. Little is known about the biologic behaviour of the different ALL forms that are responsible of the sensitivity of resistance to cytostatic drugs (Pinkel 1979).

References

Cutler SJ, Ederer F (1958) Maximum utilization of the life table method in analysing survival. J Chronic Dis 8:699–712 – Metz O, Unverricht A, Walter W, Stoll W (1977) Zur Methodik der Meningosis-"Prophylaxe" bei Leukämien und Non-Hodgkin-Lymphomen im Kindesalter mit 198-Goldkolloid. Dtsch Gesundheitswes 32:67–70 – Pinkel D (1979) The ninth annual David Karnofsky lecture. Treatment of acute lymphocytic leukemia. Cancer 43:1128–1137 – Riehm H, Gadner H, Wette K (1977) Die West-Berliner-Studie zur Behandlung der akuten lymphatischen Leukämie des Kindes – Erfahrungsbericht nach 6 Jahren. Klin Päediatr 189:89–102 – Wollner N, Burchenal JH, Lieberman PH, Exelby P, D'Angio G, Murphy ML (1976) Non-Hodgkin's lymphoma in children. Cancer 37:123–134

Haematology and Blood Transfusion Vol. 26
Modern Trends in Human Leukemia IV
Edited by Neth, Gallo, Graf, Mannweiler, Winkler
© Springer-Verlag Berlin Heidelberg 1981

T-Cell Acute Lymphoblastic Leukemia in Children

S. E. Sallan

Newer chemotherapeutic and support programs have resulted in survival of approximately 40%–50% of children with acute lymphoblastic leukemia (ALL) (Sallan et al. 1980; George et al. 1979; Haghbin 1977). It is likely that children who fail conventional therapy programs represent subsets of patients whose disease is biologically distinct, and, as such, require different therapeutic strategies. Approximately 15%–20% of children with ALL have lymphoblasts with surface receptors for sheep erythrocytes or T-cell antigens. In a treatment program at our institution patients with T-cell disease had a median disease-free survival of 12 months compared to 47 months for those with non-T-cell disease ($P=0.0004$) (Fig. 1) (Sallan et al. 1980). The majority of relapses in the T-cell population occurred at extramedullary sites, whereas nearly all of the non-T-cell patients relapsed in the bone marrow. When it became apparent that patients with T-cell disease enjoyed a less than 20% disease-free survival, a new treatment strategy was designed.

A. The Rationale for T-cell ALL Therapy

The treatment program reported herein entails three major differences from conventional ALL regimens: (1) the inclusion of chemotherapeutic agents that are more selective for T-cells; (2) special attention to extramedullary sites; and (3) thymectomy.

Frei and his co-workers (1974) have demonstrated that the most commonly used antileukemic agents, methotrexate and 6-mercaptopurine, are less cytotoxic in experimental murine T-cell leukemias, such as AKR leukemia, than are drugs such as cyclophosphamide

and cytosine arabinoside (Ara-C). Extrapolations from these experimental systems suggested that the treatment of human T-cell leukemia might be facilitated by the incorporation of drugs active in the AKR system. Therefore, we chose to treat with cyclophosphamide, Ara-C, and adriamycin as well as vincristine and prednisone (see schema, Fig. 2).

Because the majority of relapses in patients with T-cell ALL occurred in extramedullary sites (Sallan 1980), our T-cell ALL treatment program attempted to intensify therapy to the testes and central nervous system (CNS). Other investigators have demonstrated that prophylactic testicular irradiation can prevent the occurrence of testicular relapse (Nesbit et al. 1980). Thus, we irradiate both testes of all male T-cell ALL patients to 2400 rad. Although cranial irradiation and intrathecal methotrexate provide relatively good CNS "prophylaxis" (Green et al. 1980), at our institution the majority of failures of this mode of therapy have been T-cell patients. To strengthen CNS therapy we added intermittent high-dose, systemic Ara-C given in a 120 h continuous infusions. Pharmacokinetic studies of continuous infusion of Ara-C suggest that cytotoxic levels of drug can be attained in the cerebrospinal fluid shortly after the institution of the infusion and remain at therapeutic doses throughout the duration of the infusion (Weinstein et al. 1978).

The rationale for thymectomy is based primarily on experimental evidence from AKR systems. It has been shown that the addition of thymectomy to cytotoxic therapy with cyclophosphamide prolonged survival in AKR mice when compared to treatment with cyclophosphamide alone (Athanasiou et al. 1978). In addition, we hypothesized that

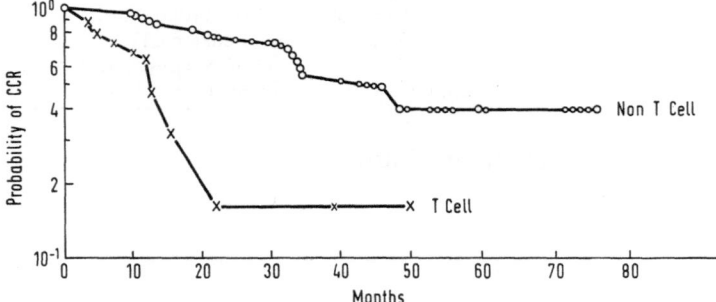

Fig. 1. T-cell and Non-T-cell leukemia disease free survival

lymphocytes may be continuously transformed in the thymus by hormonal factors secreted by thymic epithelial cells. Although high dose radiation therapy could ablate the thymic epithelial cells, it would do so at the cost of added toxicity to both the esophagus and heart when it was used concurrently with adriamycin. Therefore, we chose to ablate the thymus by total thymectomy.

B. Preliminary Results

Since March 1977 17 patients with immunologically proven T-cell ALL have been entered onto the T-cell protocol, 12 from our institution and 5 from Yale-New Haven Medical Center. Two patients died during induction of sepsis and pneumonitis. Of the 15 patients who entered complete remission, 3 have relapsed.

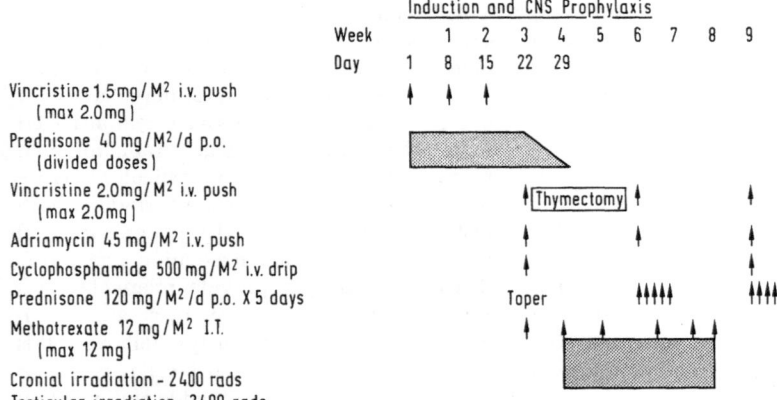

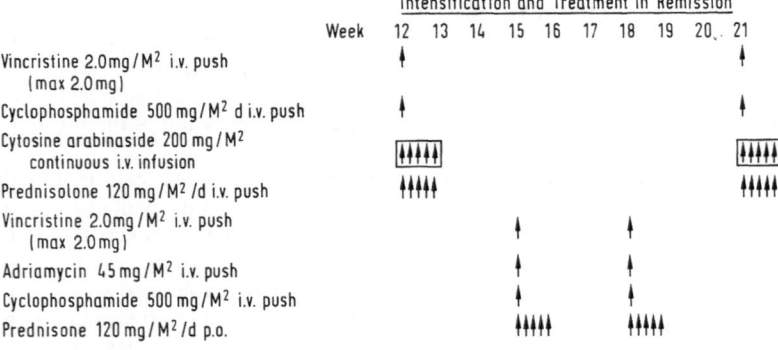

Fig. 2. Schema for treatment of T-cell leukemia

122

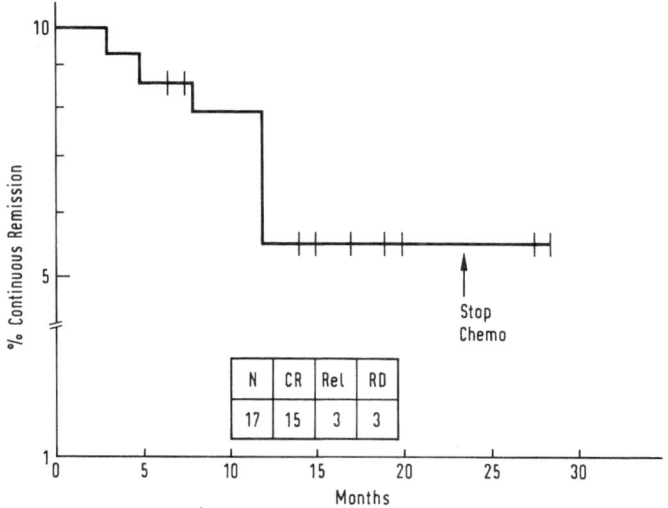

N	CR	Rel	RD
17	15	3	3

Fig. 3. Childhood T-cell ALL

The relapses occurred at 5, 12, and 12 months and were in the bone marrow in the first two patients and the CNS in the third patient. There have also been three remission deaths at 3, 8, and 12 months. The first two deaths were from sepsis (one episode in the only patient who did not have a thymectomy) and the third death resulted from adriamycin-induced cardiomyopathy. Eleven patients remain in continuous remission from 7 + to 28 + months. The median follow-up for the program has been 15 months. Two patients have electively discontinued therapy and remain disease-free for 28 months. The disease-free survival curve for this group is shown in Fig. 3.

C. Summary

Children with T-cell ALL have a biologically distinct subset of disease and require special treatment. This T-cell protocol suggests that the selection of chemotherapeutic agents, the emphasis on extramedullary prophylaxis, and thymectomy may be one rational approach to the treatment of these patients. The therapy program is highly immunosuppressive and requires expertise in pediatric supportive care. Future considerations must recognize the importance of T-cell subsets (Reinherz et al. 1979) as well as the use of antileukemic monoclonal antibodies and other innovative approaches to therapy.

Acknowledgments

The author thanks Dr. Sue McIntosh and Dr. Diane Komp for entering the Yale patients and supplying appropriate follow-up information.

References

Athanasiou A, (1978) The role of thymus in the relapse of leukemia in AKR mice. Proc Am Assoc Cancer Res Am Soc Clin Oncol 19:348 – Frei E III, (1974) Comparative chemotherapy of AKR lymphoma and human hematological neoplasia. Cancer Res 34:184 – George SL, (1979) A reappraisal of the results of stopping therapy in childhood leukemia. N Engl J Med 300:1401 – Green D, (1980) A comparison of four methods of central nervous system prophylaxis in childhood acute lymphoblastic leukemia. Lancet 2:1398–1401 – Haghbin M, (1977) Treatment of acute non-lymphoblastic leukemia in children with multiple-drug protocol. Cancer 40:1417 – Nesbit ME, (1980) Testicular relapse in childhood acute lymphoblastic leukemia: Association with pretreatment patient characteristics and treatment. Cancer 45:2009 – Reinherz EL, (1979) Subset derivation of T-cell acute lymphoblastic leukemia in man. J Clin Invest 64:392 – Sallan SE, (1980) Cell surface antigens: Prognostic implications in childhood acute lymphoblastic leukemia. Blood 55:395 – Weinstein H, (1978) Pharmacology of cytosine arabinoside. Proc Am Assoc Cancer Res Am Soc Clin Oncol 19:157

Haematology and Blood Transfusion Vol. 26
Modern Trends in Human Leukemia IV
Edited by Neth, Gallo, Graf, Mannweiler, Winkler
© Springer-Verlag Berlin Heidelberg 1981

The Concept of GvHD-Suppression by In Vitro Treatment with Antisera*

H. Rodt, S. Thierfelder, H. J. Kolb, B. Netzel, R. J. Haas, K. Wilms, and C. Bender-Götze**

Progress in chemotherapy during the past decade resulted in considerable improvement in treatment of acute leukemias. Once the first relapse occurs, however, prognosis for prolonged survival is poor. The patient finally reaches an end stage of the disease which no longer responds to chemotherapy. In these cases the application of bone marrow transplantation opens up a second chance for a long lasting remission. Leukemic cells were eradicated by a short intensive course of chemotherapy and total body irradiation followed by a marrow infusion from a suitable donor to rescue the patient from the otherwise lethal marrow cell damage. One major obstacle to the successful application of allogeneic bone marrow transplantation is the occurence of immunologic complications when donor and recipient are not monozygous twins and express differences in their histocompatibility properties. The bidirectional immunologic barrier may cause a rejection of the marrow graft or a graft-versus-host reaction induced by immunocompetent T-lymphocytes in the donor marrow. Whereas graft rejection is supressed with increasing success by the intensive conditioning treatment of the leukemic patients, graft-versus-host disease (GvHD) is still a frequent problem of clinical bone marrow transplantation (Thomas et al. 1977). The disease is presumably attributable to a cytopathogenic reaction of immunocompetent donor T lymphocytes of the graft on host target tissues (Slavin and Santos 1973). Even after transplantation of HLA-identical and MLC-negative marrow grafts the occurence of GvHD cannot be excluded due to genetic differences not detected by present histocompatibility typing techniques.

In the past several experimental approaches have been designed to eliminate the GvH-reactive cell populations in the donor marrow by incubating the graft in vitro with specific antibody preparations whose stem cell toxicity had been absorbed by various tissues, in particular non-T lymphocytes (Rodt et al. 1972; Trentin and Judd 1973; Müller-Ruchholtz et al. 1975). Pretreatment of donor spleen marrow with absorbed anti-T cell antisera which reacted with T lymphocytes but spared hemopoietic stem cells suppressed GvHD in over 90% of H-2 incompatible semiallogeneic mice preirradiated with 900 R (Rodt et al. 1972). This observation encouraged us to analyse the effect of absorbed anti-T-cell globulin (ATCG) more systematically in mice and dogs before applying it to the clinical situation.

The present report summarizes data on the prevention of a GvHD by ATCG which have been published elsewhere (Rodt et al. 1972, 1974, 1975, 1977, 1979, 1980; Thierfelder and Rodt 1978; Netzel et al. 1978a; Kolb et al. 1979a, 1980; Rodt 1979). Investigations will be reported in addition on the in vivo elimination mechanism of T cells which had been pretreated with ATCG in vitro. The survey also includes approaches to suppress GvHD by monoclonal antibodies as well as investigations on the chimerism, immunocompetence, and tolerance in the transplanted animals. Complete recovery of immune functions after transfer of ATCG-treated marrow will be

---

* Supported in part by SFB 37/E3, GSF-EURA-TOM BIOD-089-721 and Dieter Schlag-Stiftung, Hannover
** In Cooperation with the Munich Cooperative Group of BMT

shown in chimeras in which hemopoietic stem cells and host thymus differed by both H-2 haplotypes, including Ia specificities (Rodt et al. 1980). Finally the first results of an application of bone marrow incubation in the clinical situation will be described in which the marrow of 14 leukemic patients was preincubated with ATCG to prevent GvHD.

A. Animal Experiments

I. Studies in Mice

1. Effect of ATCG, Its Fragments, or Monoclonal ATh1.1 on GvHD

The principle and main test systems for the study of suppression of GvHD with ATCG in mice are shown in Fig. 1. The following figure (Fig. 2) measures the survival time of lethally irradiated F1-mice injected with parental spleen cells which had been pretreated with anti-T cell globulin. The latter was produced from rabbit ATG or anti-brain serum by absorption with mouse liver or kidney homogenate and B lymphoid cells from a B cell myeloma. The not incubated control group died early with GvHD. Survival of the irradiated mice signals T cell inhibition and preservation of donor-type stem cells.

The use of monoclonal antibodies in another promising modification of the described principle. Monoclonal anti-Theta (Th-1.1) was harvested in ascites form from the hybridoma cells, MRC 0 × 7 (a gift from S. V. Hunt and A. Williams) (Mason and Williams 1980). The hybridoma was made by fusing NS1 myeloma with spleen cells from Balb/c mice immunized with purified rat Th-1. Spleen marrow of AKR/J (H-2k) incubated with monoclonal anti-Theta (Th-1.1) antibody suppressed mortality from GvHD in the majority of (C57BL/6 × CBA)F1 (H-2b/H-2k) hybrids (Fig. 3).

Only incubation of the donor's spleen marrow with complete ATCG molecules prevented GvHD as is shown in Fig. 2. The Fab or F(ab)$_2$ fragments of ATCG did not increase the survival from GvHD. The importance of an intact Fc fragment in ATCG, even in the absence of complement, during incubation is also reflected by data on the fate of ^{51}chromium-labeled lymphnode cells pretreated with ATCG or its fragments and transferred to syngeneic, irradiated mice (Table 1). Opsonization of the labeled lymphocytes in the liver resulted in a high liver/spleen ratio. It occurred only if the T lymphocytes were covered with complete ATCG molecules. Fab or F(ab)$_2$ of ATCG did not cause opsonization of antibody-labeled lymphocytes. In this respect these fragments did not differ from normal rabbit globulin (NRG) (Table 1, exp. I). It is interesting that xenogeneic (rabbit) ATCG showed more pronounced opsonizing capacity than a monoclonal ATh1.1 antibody (L/S Ration ATCG 10.0, ATh1.1 6.7) as shown in Table 1, exp. II.

2. Immunocompetence, Chimerism, and Tolerance in the Recipients

The immune response of parent-to-F1 chimeras was tested using the following indicator system: C57BL/6 marrow cells were incubated with ATCG and transplanted to lethally irradiated (C57BL/6 × CBA)F1 hybrid reci-

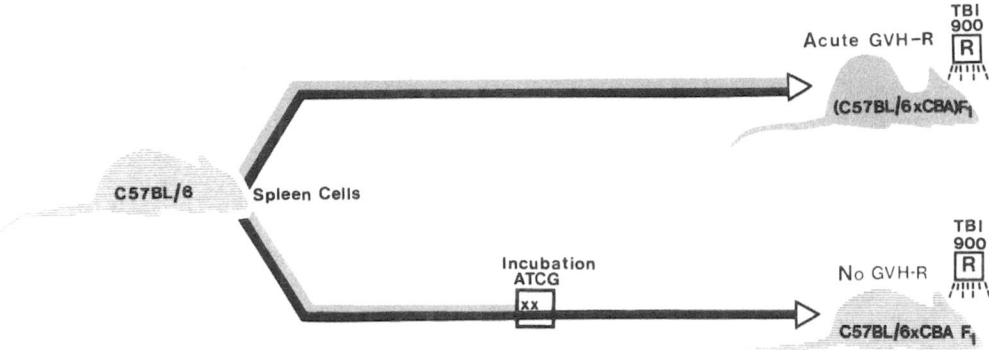

Fig. 1. Suppression of GvHD by incubation of the donor marrow with ATCG

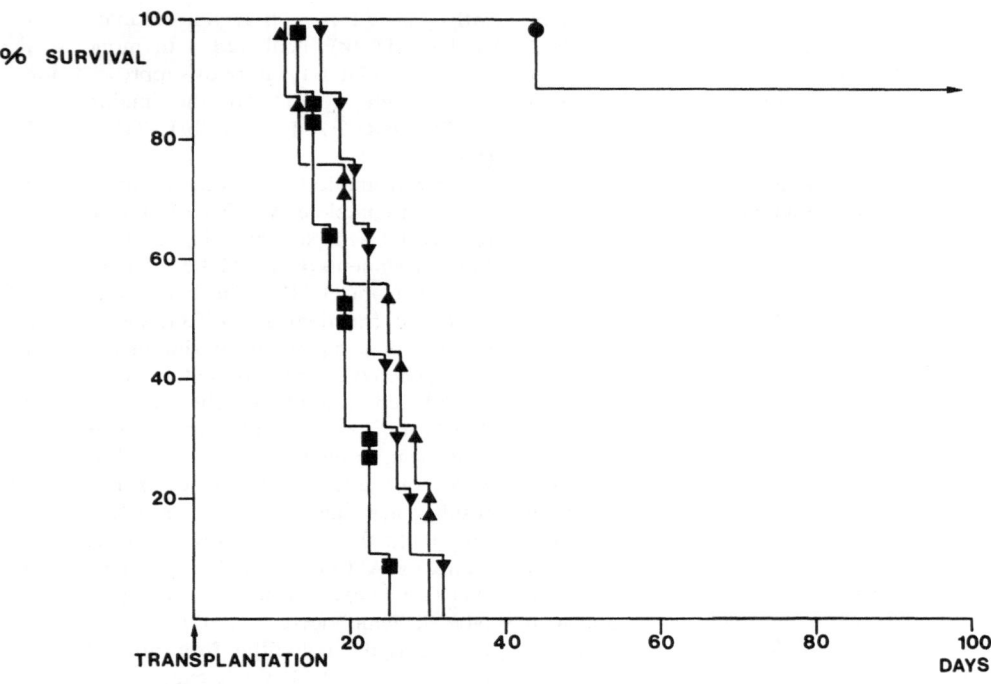

Fig. 2. Survival of lethally irradiated (C57BL/6 × CBA)F1 recipients of C57BL/6 spleen cells pretreated with ATCG (●) or its Fab (▼) or F(ab)₂fragments (▲). ■, no ATCG

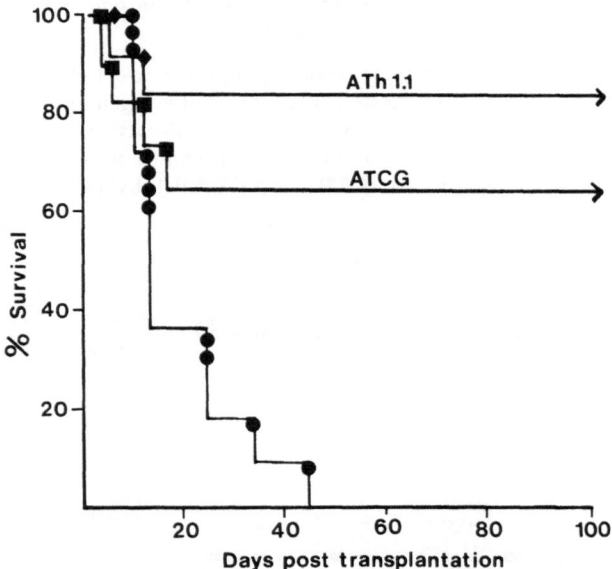

Fig. 3. Survival of lethally irradiated (C57BL/6 × CBA)F1 recipients of C57BL/6 spleen cells pretreated with ATCG (■) or monoclonal ATh1.1 (◆), ●, no ATCG

Table 1. Lymphocyte opsonization in lethally irradiated $(C57Bl/6 \times CBA)F_1$ recipients of Cr^{51}-labeled lymphnode cells. Exp. I: $(C57Bl/6 \times CBA)F_1$ donor cells incubated with ATCG or its $F(ab)_2$ or Fab fragments or normal rabbit globulin (NRG). Exp. II: AKR donor cells incubated with ATCG, monoclonal A-Th1.1, or NRG

Exp. I	ATCG	ATCG F(ab)$_2$	ATCG Fab	NRG
Liver-spleen ratio[a]	8.6 ± 1.2[b]	1.5 ± 0.3	1.3 ± 0.1	1.3 ± 0.1

Exp. II	ATCG	ATh1.1(mono)	NRG
Liver-spleen ratio[a]	10.0 ± 1.7	6.7 ± 0.4	1.7 ± 0.1

[a] calculated as follows: $L/S = cpm(liver)-cpm(backgr.) / cpm(spleen)-cpm(backgr.)$

[b] mean ± standard deviation

pients. The recipients were transplanted at 10 weeks of age (10-W) or at 70 weeks of age (70-W). The latter investigation was performed in order to determine whether the function of old involuted thymuses can be reactivated by bone marrow transplantation. Thymectomized and syngeneically transplanted recipients were used as controls. Sixty days after transplantation the survival of BALB/c skin grafts and the response against sheep red blood cells (SRBC) was analyzed. A recovered immune response against BALB/c skin and SRBC was found in the 10-W, 70-W, and syngeneic chimeras. In contrast thymectomized chimaeras rejected third party skin grafts in a delayed fashion or not at all. Not only cellular but also humoral primary or secondary immune response were low in this group.

The same restauration of immunity as in 10-W chimeras was observed in "old" (70-W) chimaeras whose thymus had already been involuted before transplantation. This suggests that involuted thymuses regain their original function in differentiating T lymphocytes no matter whether the latter derive from syngeneic or semiallogeneic precursor cells.

The recipients are almost complete donor cell chimeras. Cytogenetic studies in the bone marrow and cytotoxic testing of lymphnode and thymus cells revealed more than 90% donor-type cells in the respective tissues (Table 3). The donor cell population remains immunologically tolerant against the tissues of the recipient. When spleen cells of a C57BL/6 → (C57BL/6 × CBA)F1 chimera are used for an adaptive transfer into the footpath of a second F1 host, no enlargement of the popliteal lymph node could be detected when compared with a syngeneic control. Normal C57BL/6 cells on the other hand produced a significant increase of lymphnode of this strain by a GvHR (Fig. 4).

An interesting question was whether stem cells can develop immunocompetence through a fully H-2 and Ia incompatible thymus. This was investigated with the following experi-

Table 2. Immune response of lethally irradiated (C57Bl/6 × CBA)F1 recipients grafted with ATCG-incubated parental bone marrow against SRBC and BALB/c skin grafts

Donors	Recipients[a]	Rejection of BALB/c skin grafts (days)[b]	Response against SRBC[c]		
			Primary, direct	Secondary, direct	Secondary, indirect
CBL	CBL/CBA, 10 weeks of age	13	45 ± 33[d]	62 ± 67	236 ± 114
CBL	CBL/CBA, 70 weeks of age	13	75 ± 74	56 ± 21	241 ± 97
CBL	CBL/CBA, thymectomized	>40	4 ± 3	3 ± 3	4 ± 4
CBL/CBA	CBL/CBA	11	221 ± 56	42 ± 37	389 ± 210

[a] Lethally irradiated with 1000 rad, reconstituted with ATCG-incubated 20×10^{10} donor cells

[b] Mean rejection time of BALB/c(H-2^d) skin grafts, H-2 different to thymus and bone marrow cells

[c] Number of plaque-forming cells (PFC)/2×10^6 spleen cells

[d] PFC ± S.D.

a) Percentage of donor cell mitoses (DCM) in the bone marrow

Table 3. Hemopoietic chimerism of lethally irradiated (C57Bl/6×CBA)F1 recipients of C57BL/6 marrow cells incubated with ATCG

Recipients	%DCM[a]
Recipients transplanted at 10 weeks of age	97
Recipients transplanted at 70 weeks of age	95
Thymectomized recipients	94

b) Percentage of donor type lymphocytes (DL) in the lymphnodes (LyN) and thymus (Thy) determined with anti H-2 sera

Recipients	%DL in LyN[b]	%DL in Thy[b]
Recipients transplanted at 10 weeks of age	>90	100
Recipients transplanted at 70 weeks of age	>90	100
Thymectomized recipients	>90	–

[a] Average of 3 mice
[b] Average of 127 mice

mental design: (C57BL/6×CBA)F1 recipients were thymectomized and transplanted with CBA-thymus tissue under the kidney capsule. After lethal irradiation these animals were reconstituted with T-cell-deprived C57BL/6 marrow cells (group 1). Thymectomized recipients without thymus transplantation (group 2) and (C57BL/6×CBA)F1 recipients with syngeneity between transplanted thymus and transferred bone marrow cells (group 3 and 4) served as controls. All different groups are indicated in Table 4. It was shown that the presence of a CBA thymus under the kidney capsule of irradiated (C57BL/6×CBA)F1 mice induced C57BL/6 precursor cells to immune reactivity which

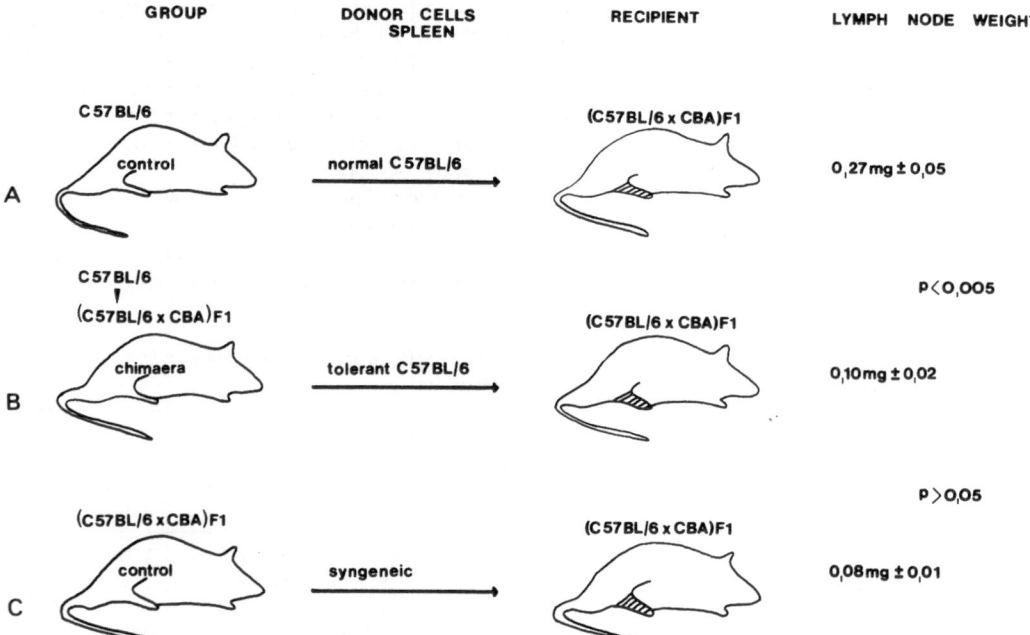

Fig. 4. Investigation of the tolerance of donor cells in the chimeras against the host C57BL/6 spleen cells of parent → F1 chimeras adaptively transferred to the footpath of a second F1 host. The enlargement of the popliteal lymphnode was determined in comparison with the transfer of normal C57BL/6 cells and syngeneic F1 cells

Table 4. Influence of a complete H-2 difference between transplanted thymus tissue and T-cell deprived bone marrow cells on the immune response of (C57BL/6 × CBA)F1 recipient mice against BALB/c skin grafts and SRBC

Group	Transplanted		Rejection of BALB/c skin grafts[b] (days)	Response against SRBC[c]		
	Thymus[a] (H-2)	Bone marrow[b] (H-2)		Primary, direct	Secondary, direct	Secondary indirect
1	CBA (k)	CBL (b)	17	131 ± 90[d]	711 ± 284	1110 ± 306
2	– No –	CBL (b)	>49	9 ± 5	20 ± 18	29 ± 20
3	CBL (b)	CBL (b)	17	56 ± 24	601 ± 304	893 ± 403
4	CBA (k)	CBA (k)	16	413 ± 201	389 ± 189	1178 ± 498

[a] Recipients = (C57BL/6 × CBA)F1 hybrids
[b] Mean rejection time of BALB/c(H-2^d) skin grafts, H-2 different to thymus and bone marrow cells
[c] Number of plaque-forming cells (PFC)/2 × 10^6 spleen cells
[d] PFC ± S.D.

rejected BALB/c skin grafts and responded to sheep red blood cells in the same way as the syngeneic control groups.

II. Studies in Dogs

These studies were performed in order to establish the anti-GvHD effect of an incubation treatment in the dog, which is regarded a model of particular relevance for clinical bone marrow transplantation.

Removal of stem cell toxicity of crude anti-dog-thymocyte globulin was attempted by absorption with spleen cells from new-born puppies. Test systems for T cells in dogs are less well developed than those in mice and man. Also the lack of B lymphocyte cell lines complicated the production of dog ATCG. T cell specificity of dog ATCG was shown by selective immunohistologic staining of thymus-dependent T cell areas in lymphnodes. After absorption the ATCG did not reduce colonies in the CFUc test after incubation and cultivation of dog bone marrow. In vivo leucocyte and platelet recovery were followed after autologous transplantation of bone marrow preincubated or not with ATCG.

ATCG was then applied in canine allogeneic marrow transplantation. The results are shown in Table 5. In a randomly bred species such as the dog the combination of DLA homozygous donors and DLA heterozygous recipients is comparable to the murine parent-to-F1 situation with regard to the known MHC antigen. In this incompatible combination all 1000 rad irradiated recipients died within 27 days of GvHD when receiving untreated bone marrow

grafts. Following in vitro treatment of the donor marrow with ATCG, two dogs died without sustained hemopoietic engraftment, in eight dogs the course of GvHD was remarkably delayed, and eight dogs had hemopoietic recovery without any sign of GvHD. These dogs showed complete chimerism, as indicated by the DLA type of lymphatic cells and by a change of the karyotype in the sex-different combinations.

B. Clinical Aspects

I. Characteristics of Anti-Human T Cell Globulin

The results of the animal experiments suggested an in vitro application for suppression of GvHD in humans, provided that a suitable ATCG for the clinical situation could be produced. Such antisera were raised in rabbits with human thymocytes. Cross reactions of this crude preparation were removed by absorption with liver-kidney homogenate, B lymphocytes from a pool of several CLL patients, and red cells. Table 6 gives complement fixation titers which are the highest against thymocytes. The lower titer against bone marrow cells is due to the low concentration of T cells in human bone marrow. No cross reactions with B lymphocytes, granulocytes, red cells, glomerulo-basal membrane and plasma proteins were found. Comparable results were obtained using the microcytotoxicity test. However, quantitative complement fixation has the advantage over microcytotoxicity that its titers

Table 5. Results of bone marrow transplantation in DLA-incompatible litter mate dogs with and without in vitro treatment of bone marrow with ATCG

No. of dogs	Donor-recipient differences	Marrow cells per kg body weight ($\times 10^8$)	ATCG-treatment of the marrow (charge No./concentration[a]	Death without sustained engraftment (No.)	Death on GvHD (No./mean survival)	Surviving without GvHD[b] (No.)
5	DLA-homozygous marrow into DLA hetero-zygous litter mates	4.1(1.9–6.2)	no	–	5/21 days	–
5	DLA-homozygous marrow into DLA-heterozygous litter mates	4.72.6–7.7)	No. 618/1:100	2	2/65 days	1
5	DLA-homozygous marrow into DLA-heterozygous litter mates	3.3(2.2–4.9)	No. 618/1:200	–	2/48 days	3
3	DLA-homozygous marrow into DLA-heterozygous litter mates	5.0(1.0–8.3)	No. 819/1:100	1	1/44 days	1
3	DLA-homozygous marrow into DLA-heterozygous litter mates	6.7(5.3–7.7	No. 819/1:200	–	–	3
3	DLA-homozygous marrow into DLA-heterozygous litter mates	5.7(4.8–7.0)	No. 819/ 1:400–800	–	3/32 days	–

[a] Final concentration in the incubation volume.
[b] Observation time of the surviving animals 3 months until>2 years.

are not influenced by the variable lysability of the different cell types under investigation. An important question was whether ATCG inhibited stem cell proliferation. Incubation of bone marrow with ATCG did not reduce the number of cells growing in diffusion chambers of forming colonies in agar when compared to the normal rabbit globulin control. Purification of ATCG over DEAE cellulose ion exchange chromatography and ultracentrifugation lead to a preparation lacking contaminants and immune complexes.

II. Application of ATCG to Clinical Bone Marrow Transplantation

Fourteen patients with acute leukemia were transplanted between February 1978 and May 1980 with bone marrow of HLA-compatible siblings. Ten patients were transplanted by members of The Munich Cooperative Group of BMT. These patients received a conditioning regimen including combined chemotherapy and 1000 rad of total body irradiation (TBI) applied by two opposite ^{60}Co sources. Four patients were transplanted in the Medizinische Universitätsklinik, Tübingen, where they received a conditioning treatment with cyclophosphamide and 1000 rad of TBI applied by a linear accelerator. In these cases the lungs were shielded to a total dose of 800 rad. The fractionation and concentration of bone marrow cells using a cell separator were performed as described by Netzel et al. (1978b). The technical approach of marrow incubation in vitro has already been published (Rodt et al. 1979). Six of the patients were transplanted after the second relapse, three patients after the first, and one patient after the third relapse. Four patients were transplanted in remission.

1. Reactivity on blood cell populations (Complement fixation)	
Cells	Titer
Thymocytes	1:1064
Peripheral blood lymphocytes	1: 512
Bone Marrow cells	1: 32
B-lymphocytes (CLL)	neg.
Granulocytes	neg.

2. Reactivity on hemopoietic progenitors		
Cells	Culture system	Effect[a]
AHTCG-incubated bone marrow cells	CFU-C diffusion chamber	No reduction of CFU No reduction of cell numbers and normal differentiation

3. Cross reactions	
Antigen	Reaction
Erythrocytes	No
Glomerulo-basalmembrane	No
Plasmaproteins	No

4. Sterility, absence of pyrogenic substances, and no general toxicity

[a] Compared with normal globulin incubated controls.

Table 6. Properties of anti-human-T-cell globulin used for clinical bone marrow transplantation. For details see: Rodt et al., Experimental Hematology Today, Springer 1979

Five patients had the common type of acute lymphoblastic leukemia (cALL) and six had acute myelogeneous leukemia. Three other patients suffered from ALL of the T-cell type, an erythroleukemia, and an acute undifferentiated leukemia (AUL), respectively (Table 7).

Treatment of bone marrow with ATCG was preceeded by a concentration of the collected bone marrow to about 300 ml (Fig. 5). The recovery of CFUc was more than 80%. The use of a cell separator permitted the recovery of red cells for retransfusion into the bone marrow donor, a particular advantage when the donor is a child. Separation of red cells from the bone marrow is also advantageous in ABO-incompatible patients where hemolysis of donor red cells by preformed antibodies of the patient must be avoided. The final dilution of ATCG of 1:200 of a preparation of 10 mg/ml was derived from our studies in dogs. Injection of the ATCG-pretreated bone marrow over a period of about 20 min caused no immediate symptoms. Transient fever and chills were occasionally observed after bone marrow transfusion with or without ATCG.

In general, engraftment and recovery of bone marrow functions after incubation treatment did not differ from that of earlier transplantations without ATCG. Engraftment was documented by bone marrow cellularity and the rise of peripheral blood cell counts. Of 14 patients, 12 showed an engraftment between day 13 and day 26 after transplantation, which was indicated by a rise in the peripheral granulocyte counts to values between 500–1000/mm^3. This range does not markedly differ from other groups performing BMT without any marrow incubation treatment. Thomas et al. (1977) reported bone marrow engraftment after an average time of 16 days after transplantation in 91 cases with acute leukemia. Seven of the twelve patients were sex mismatched, three showed ABO blood group incompatibility, and in one patient sex and blood group and in another HLA-D and blood group were different. Two patients did not show substantial engraftment. One of these patients was one-way HLA-D different and died very early on day 21 with septicemia. In the other case the HLA-D compatibility could not be clearly documented. This patient in addition showed persisting leukemia at

Table 7. Clinical results in 14 patients with acute leukemias undergoing bone marrow transplantation. For prevention of GvHD the marrow was preincubated with ATCG

Patient	Donor-recipient-diff.			Conditioning[a]	Leukemia, Relapse	Marrow treatment			Clinic[d]				Hospital[f]
	HLA	Sex	ABO			Separat.	ATCG incub[b]	No. of cells[c]	Take	GvHD	Survival time	Outcome	
B.V.	no	+	no	BAC TBI-1000rad	cALL 3. Relapse	+	+	3,3	+	no	>872	Alive in remission	U-K-KI
K.G.	no	+	no	BAC TBI-1000rad	T-ALL 2. Relapse	no	+	4,0	+	no	38	Died on interstitial pneumonitis	M-KI-TU
B.S.	HLA-D?	no	A/B diff.	Ad AC TBI-1000rad	AML 2. Relapse	+	+	8,0	no	no	34	Died on sepsis after 2. BMT without incubation	K-P-KI
S.A.	no	+	A/O diff.	BAC TBI-1000rad	cALL 2. Relapse	+	+	6,0	+	no	190	Died on leukemic relapse	U-K-KI
A.G.	no	no	no	BAC TBI-1000rad	cALL 2. Relapse	+	+	6,0	+	skin (I–II)	215	Died on leukemic relapse	U-K-KI
B.K.	no	+	no	Ad AC TBI-1000rad	AML 1. Relapse	+	+	9,5	+	no	>424	Alive in remission	K-P-KI
T.G.	HLA-D?	+	no	Ad AC TBI-1000rad	Ery-L 2. Relapse	+	+	6,2	no	no	19	Died on pneumonitis	K-P-KI
A.E.	no	no	no	Cy TBI-1000rad[e]	AML 2. Remission	+	+	11,1	+	no	>220	Alive in remission	M-KI-UT
H.G.	no	+	no	BAC TBI-1000rad	AML 1. Relapse	+	+	4,3	+	no	49	Died on interstitial pneumonitis	M-KI-GH
D.S.	no	+	no	Cy TBI-1000rad[e]	AUL 1. Remission	+	+	3,4	+	no	64	Died on interstitial pneumonitis	M-KI-UT
Mu.H.	no	no	AB/O diff.	BAC TBI-1000rad	cALL 2. Relapse	+	+	9,1	+	no	98	Died on leukemic relapse	U-K-KI
Kr.G.	HLA-D HLA-DR ident.	no	O/B diff.	Cy TBI-1000rad[e]	AML 1. Remission	+	+	3,4	+	skin (II)	> 95	Alive in remission	M-KI-UT
H.J.	no	+	no	BAC TBI-1000rad	ALL 1. Relapse	+	+	7,7	+	no	> 53	Alive in remission	U-K-KI
M.I.	no	no	no	Cy TBI-1000rad[e]	AML 1. Remission	+	+	1,8	+	skin (II)	> 52	Alive in remission	M-KI-UT

a BAC=BCNU, Ara C, Cy / Ad AC=Adriablastin, Ara C, Cy
b Final concentration 1:200, incubation at 4° C for 30'
c cells ×10⁸ per kg body weight
d Methotrexate prophylaxis post BMT in all patients

f U-K-KI=Universitätskinderklinik München;
K-P-KI=Kinderpoliklinik der Universität München;
M-KI-TU=I. Medizinische Klinik der TU München;
M-KI-GH=III. Medizinische Klinik, Klinikum Großhadern;
M-KI-UT=Med. Klinik, Universität Tübingen

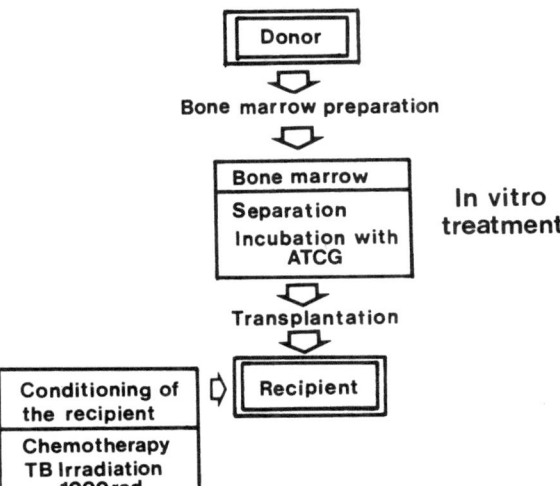

Fig. 5. Follow up of incubation treatment with ATCG in clinical marrow transplantation

autopsy, factors which may have prevented sustained engraftment. None of the patients died of severe GvHD. Three showed a transient skin rash lasting about 2 weeks consistent with a skin GvHD of grade I to II or II. The other patients showed no manifestations of acute GvHD on the skin nor on other tissues. No chronic reactions have been be detected so far, but observation time is too short for final estimations.

Table 7 summarizes the survival and final outcome of the transplanted patients. Of 14 patients ranging between day 872 and day 52 after transplantation, six are in complete remission. The three patients who showed leukemic relapse survived between 98 and 215 days. Two patients died without sustained engraftment on day 21 and day 34 after transplantation of lethal infections. Three patients had a leukemic relapse detected on days 67, 123, and 181 and died due to this complication on days 98, 197, and 215, respectively. All three patients were cases with cALL. The other three patients died of infections and interstitial pneumonitis (I.P.). In one case the I.P. was caused by infection with Pneumocytis carinii. None of the patients with I.P. showed any sign of GvHD.

C. Conclusions

Our data from mice indicate that only complete ATCG antibodies with their Fc fragments suppressed GvHD by opsonization of the donor's T lymphocytes in marrow recipients (Rodt 1979). The consequence of this T cell deprivation is not an immunologically crippled chimera. It has been shown that the marrow recipient's thymus, inspite of H-2 incompatiblity or even involution, induced the transplanted donor-type stem cells to differentiate T cells which were tolerant towards the recipient who was immunocompetent towards third party antigens. It was possible to transfer chimeric spleen cells without incubation to the footpath of secundary (C57BL/6×CBA)F1 recipients without causing local GvHD (Thierfelder et al. 1974). Immunohistologic studies (Rodt et al. 1980) showed that repopulation of T cell areas in lymphoid tissue depended likewise on the presence of the semiallogenic thymus in the host. It is of interest that recovery of immune response occurred eben in chimaeras where stem cells and thymus epithelium differed by both H-2 and Ia haplotypes. The restriction in the context of MHC of thymus and maturing T lymphocytes postulated for certain T cell functions by Zinkernagel et al. (1978) was not found to be a precondition for the recovery of immune response in our chimaeras, not even for virus-specific T cell cytotoxicity (Wagner et al. 1980). Monoclonal antibodies against T cell antigens were also effective in suppression of GvHD. Incubation with ATCG in the canine model was also found to prevent GvHD in a substantial number of DLA-D-A-B one haplotype incompatible dogs (Kolb et al. 1980). It is encouraging that no other immunosuppressive agent had to be added and that in the surviving dogs no symptoms of GvHD were observed. There were, however, dogs which still died from GvHD inspite of an ATCG application. Whether this failure was due to the relatively high dilution of ATCG (1:100–200) remains to be shown, although the production of a good ATCG for dogs is more difficult than for mice and man as pointed out. Our studies on ATCG concerned mainly the suppression of GvHD due to major histocompatibility antigens. In mice ATCG also suppressed GvHD resulting from minor histocompatibility antigens, for instance after transfer of AKR spleen cells to irradiated CBA mice. GvHD in DLA-compatible dogs is absent or relatively weak. A considerable number of dogs would be necessary to document the effect of ATCG on GvHD in DLA identical MLC nonreactive dogs.

So far our human studies concerned only HLA identical MLC nonreactive leukemic siblings, a situation with a still relatively high probability for GvHD. In sex different patients (in 7 out of 14 patients reported here) bone marrow has been reported to cause GvHD more frequently (Storb et al. 1977). Sex difference appears to influence GvHD also in dogs (Kolb et al. 1979b; Vriesendorp et al. 1978). The formal proof that ATCG prevents GvHD in MHC-identical patients requires, of course, a greater number of patients than have been listed in this study. So far our data only prove that ATCG did not interfere with hemopoietic engraftment at dilutions known to be toxic for T cells. The successful animal experiments, however, raise the hope that ATCG may also reduce the incidence of GvHD in clinical marrow transplantation.

References

Kolb HJ, Rieder I, Rodt H, Netzel B, Grosse-Wilde H, Scholz S, Schäfer E, Kolb H, Thierfelder S (1979a) Antilymphocytic antibodies and marrow transplantation. IV. Graft-versus-host tolerance in DLA-incompatible dogs after in-vitro treatment of bone marrow with absorbed antithymocyte globulin. Transplantation 27:242 – Kolb HJ, Rieder I, Grosse-Wilde H, Bodenberger U, Scholz S, Kolb H, Schäffer E, Thierfelder S (1979b) Graft-versus-host desease (GvHD) following marrow graft from DLA-matched canine littermates. Transplant Proc 11:507 – Kolb HJ, Bodenberger U, Rodt HV, Rieder I, Netzel B, Grosse-Wilde H, Scholz S, Thierfelder S (1980) Bone marrow transplantation in DLA-haploidentical canine littermates – Fractionated total body irradiation (FTBI) and in vitro treatment of the marrow graft with anti-T-cell globulin (ATCG) In: Thierfelder S, Rodt H, Kolb H-J (eds) Immunobiology of bone marrow transplantation. Springer, Berlin Heidelberg New York, p 61 – Mason DW, Williams AF (1980) The kinetics of antibody binding to membrane antigens in solution and at the cell surface. Biochem J 187:1 – Müller-Ruchholtz W, Wottge H-U, Müller-Hermelink HK (1975) Selective grafting of hemopoietic cells. Transplant Proc 7:859 – Netzel B, Rodt H, Hoffmann-Fezer G, Thiel E, Thierfelder S (1978a) The effect of crude and differently absorbed anti-human T-cell globulin on granulocytic and erythropoietic colony formation. Exp Hematol 6:410 – Netzel B, Haas RJ, Janka GE, Thierfelder S (1978b) Viability of stem cells (CFU-c) after long term cryopreservation of bone marrow cells from normal adults and children with acute lymphoblastic leukemia in remission. In: Barberg H, Mishler JM, Schäfer U (eds) Cell separation and cryobiology. Schattauer, Stuttgart New YorK – Rodt H (1979) Herstellung und Spezifität heterologer Anti-T-Lymphozytenseren und ihre Anwendung im Rahmen der Knochenmarktransplantation und der Leukämiediagnostik. GSF Bericht H 604 München – Rodt H, Thierfelder S, Eulitz M (1972) Suppression of acute secondary disese by heterologous anti-brain serum. Blut 25:385 – Rodt H, Thierfelder S, Eulitz M (1974) Anti-lymphocytic antibodies and marrow transplantation. III. Effect of heterologous anti-brain antibodies on acute secondary disease in mice. Eur J Immunol 4:25 – Rodt H, Thierfelder S, Thiel E, Götze D, Netzel B, Huhn D, Eulitz M (1975) Identification and quantitation of human T-cell antigen by antisera purified from antibodies cross-reacting with hemopoietic progenitors and other blood cells. Immunogenetics 2:411 – Rodt H, Thierfelder S, Netzel B, Kolb HJ, Thiel E, Niethammer D, Haas RJ (1977) Specific absorbed anti-thymocyte globulin for incubation treatment in human marrow transplantation. Transplant Proc 9:187 – Rodt H, Kolb HJ, Netzel B, Rieder I, Janka G, Belohradsky B, Haas RJ, Thierfelder S (1979) GvHD suppression by incubation of bone marrow grafts with anti-T-cell globulin: effect in the canine model and application to clinical marrow transplantation. Transplant Proc 11:962 – Rodt H, Thierfelder S, Hoffmann-Fezer G (1980) Influence of the recipient thymus on the maturation of T-lymphocytes in H-2 different radiation chimeras In: Thierfelder S, Rodt H, Kolb HJ (eds) Recent trends in the immunbiology of bone marrow transplantation. Springer, Berlin Heidelberg New York, pp 179–191 – Slavin RE, Santos GW (1973) The graft versus host reaction in man after bone marrow transplantation: Pathology, pathogenesis, clinical features and implication. Clin Immunol Immunopathol 1:472 – Storb R, Weiden PL, Prentice R, Buchner CD,

Clift RA, Einstein AB, Fefer A, Johnson FL, Lerner KG, Neimann PE, Sanders JE, Thomas ED (1977) Aplastic anemia (AA) treated by allogeneic marrow transplantation: The Seattle Experience. Transplant Proc 9:181 – Thierfelder S, Rodt H (1977) Antilymphocytic antibodies and marrow transplantation. V. suppression of secondary disease by host-versus-graft reaction. Transplantation 23:87 – Thierfelder S, Rodt H, Netzel B, Thiel E, v. Rössler R (1974) Studies on chimeric tolerance induced with anti-T cell globulin. Exp Hematol 2:299 – Thomas ED, Buckner CD, Banaji M, Clift RA, Fefer A, Flournoy N, Goodell BW, Hickmann RO, Lerner KG, Neiman PE, Sale GE, Sanders JE, Singer J, Stevens M, Storb R, Weiden P (1977) One hundred patients with acute leukemia treated by chemotherapy, total body irradiation and allogeneic marrow transplantation. Blood 49:511 – Trentin IJ, Judd KP (1973) Prevention of acute graft-versus-host (gvh) mortality with spleen-absorbed antithymocyte globulin (ATG). Transplant Proc 5:865 – Vriesendorp HM, Bijnen AB, van Kessel ACM, Obertop H, Westbrock DL (1978) Minor histocompatibility systems in dogs. In: Baum SJ, Ledney GD (eds) Experimental hematology today. Springer, Heidelberg Berlin New York, p. 109 – Wagner H, Röllinghoff M, Rodt H, Thierfelder S (1980) T cell mediated cytotoxic immune reactivity of bone marrow reconstituted chimeric mice. In: Thierfelder S, Rodt H, Kolb HJ (eds) Immunobiology of bone marrow transplantation. Springer, Berlin Heidelberg New York, p. 101 – Zinkernagel RM, Callahan GN, Althage A, Cooper J, Klein PA, Klein J (1978) On the thymus in the differentiation of "H-2 self-recongnition" by T-cells: Evidence for dual recognition. J Exp Med 147:882

Haematology and Blood Transfusion Vol. 26
Modern Trends in Human Leukemia IV
Edited by Neth, Gallo, Graf, Mannweiler, Winkler
© Springer-Verlag Berlin Heidelberg 1981

Bone Marrow Transplantation for the Treatment of Leukemia*

R. Storb

Marrow transplantation from a syngeneic (monozygous twin) or allogeneic [homologous leucocytic antibody (HLA)-identical sibling] donor allows the administration of aggressive antileukemic therapy without regard to marrow toxicity. Until 1975 marrow transplantation was carried out only in patients with advanced relapse after failure of all other therapy. Six of sixteen patients given syngeneic marrow grafts and 13 of 100 patients with allogeneic marrow grafts are still in remission after 5½–10 years (Thomas et al. 1977a,b). An actuarial survival curve according to the method of Kaplan and Meier of the first 100 patients grafted in Seattle after treatment with cyclophosphamide (60 mg/kg/day×2) and total body irradiation (1000 rad at 5–8 rad/min) showed three periods of interest: (1) during the first 4 months the slope was steep because many patients died due to advanced illness, graft-versus-host disease, infections (in particular interstitial pneumonias), and recurrent leukemia; (2) from 4 months to 2 ys the curve showed a much slower rate of decline, primarily due to death from recurrent leukemia; and (3) from 2 to 10 years the curve was almost horizontal with a negligible loss of patients and no recurrent leukemia. This flat portion of the curve corresponded to 13% of the patients, and it is likely that the majority of these survivors are cured of their disease (Thomas et al. 1977b).

A number of transplant groups, including our own, made attempts at reducing the

incidence of leukemic relapse after transplantation by added chemotherapy. This approach proved to be toxic, lengthened the period of maximum pancytopenia, and failed to reduce the rate of recurrent leukemia. Survival after these various approaches proved to be similar to that seen after the cyclophosphamide/total body irradiation regimen used in Seattle.

Current approaches at reducing leukemic relapse and improving long-term survival in patients transplanted with acute leukemia in relapse have involved the use of higher doses of total body irradiation by means of fractionation. Perhaps these efforts are futile, since in an exponential killing process it is difficult to kill the last leukemic cell. Some of the apparent cures may have occurred because of destruction of leukemic cells by immune reactions of the grafted cells against non-HLA antigens and/or leukemia-associated antigens of the host. Such a possibility is suggested by the observation of a graft-vs-leukemia effect in man (Weiden et al. 1979).

The demonstration that a treatment regimen is effective in the otherwise refractory end stage patient with acute leukemia constitutes a rational basis for its application earlier in the course of the disease. Accordingly, the Seattle group initiated a study in early 1976 of treating patients with acute nonlymphoblastic leukemia by marrow grafting in first or subsequent remission and those with acute lymphoblastic leukemia in second or subsequent remission using the basic conditioning regimen of cyclophosphamide and total body irradiation used since 1971. We assumed that patients with leukemia in remission would be more readily cured, since the number of leukemic cells in the body could be expected to be small and cells

---

* This investigation was supported by Grant Numbers CA 18029, CA 15704, and CA 18221, awarded by the National Cancer Institute. U.S.-Dept. of Health, Education and Welfare

should not have become resistant to therapy. Moreover, previous experience had shown that patients in good clinical condition and with good blood cell values at the time of transplantation had a much better chance of surviving the transplantation procedure.

A. Acute Nonlymphoblastic Leukemia in First or Subsequent Remission

Patients with acute nonlymphoblastic leukemia have a poor prognosis with chemotherapy. The median duration of the first remission is approximately one year and onyl 15%–20% of the patients are alive at 3 years. A Kaplan-Meier plot of survival with a logarithmic ordinate for the fraction of patients surviving usually shows no evidence of a plateau (Powles et al. 1980b). Our past observation that marrow transplantation could lead to an operational cure of 13% of end stage refractory patients made it ethically acceptable to consider marrow grafting for acute nonlymphoblastic leukemia in first remission. The first 19 patients were transplanted between March 1976 and March 1978 at a median of 4 months following initial treatment or 2½ months following the achievement of the first complete remission (Thomas et al. 1979b). Of the 19 patients, 12 are alive in continued unmaintained remission with a functioning marrow graft between 27 and 48 months after transplantation. Nine of the twelve are entirely well, while three have mild chronic graft-vs-host disease with Karnofsky performance scores of 80%–90%. A Kaplan-Meier plot of the probability of survival shows a plateau at 65% with the long-term survivors far out on the plateau and presumably cured of their disease. Six of the nineteen patients died from graft-vs-host disease and/or interstitial pneumonia.

Of particular interest is the fact that only 1 of the 19 patients has had a recurrence of leukemia. Forty-eight patients have now been transplanted in first remission, and again recurrence has been limited to that single patient. Evidently the chemo-radiotherapy regimen used is capable of eradicating the leukemic cell population in most of these patients. In contrast, patients grafted in second remission have a leukemic recurrence rate of 35%.

More recently, the Seattle results in acute nonlymphoblastic leukemia in first remission have been confirmed by reports from the marrow transplant teams at the City of Hope in Duarte, California (Blume et al. 1980) and at the Royal Marsden Hospital in Sutton, Surrey, England (Powles et al. 1980a).

B. Acute Lymphoblastic Leukemia in Second or Subsequent Remission

Approximately 50% of the patients with acute lymphoblastic leukemia, particularly children, can be cured by combination chemotherapy. However, once marrow relapse has occurred, only 5% of the patients treated with conventional chemotherapy are alive at 2 years after relapse (Chessels and Cornbleet 1979). Transplantation of patients with this disease in second or subsequent remission would entail the risk of losing some of them early after grafting due to grafts-vs-host disease and/or infections. However, this risk seemed acceptable if other patients could be "cured" of their disease.

The first 22 patients were grafted between April 1976 and December 1977 (Thomas et al. 1979a). Three patients died of interstitial pneumonia within three months of transplantation. Eleven patients died of recurrent leukemia within 27 months of grafting. The latest relapse was in the central nervous system of a patient who had active central nervous system leukemia at the time of grafting. The median survival of this group of transplanted patients was 1 year compared to the 6–8 months usually observed after combination chemotherapy. Eight patients are surviving between 32–41 months after transplantation in unmaintained remission. Seven of the eight are without problems and one has moderately severe chronic graft-vs-host disease with a Karnofsky performance score of 70%. It is clear that recurrent leukemia was the major problem in patients with acute lymphoblastic leukemia transplanted in second or subsequent remission. These recurrences were in cells of host type indicating that the conditioning regimen was ineffective in eradicating residual leukemic cells in approximately 50% of the patients. Further improvement in survival in patients with acute lymphoblastic leukemia hinges on the development of new preparative regimens.

C. Chronic Myelogenous Leukemia

The Seattle team has carried out six marrow grafts from monozygous twins for chronic myelogenous leukemic in blast crisis and one of these patients continues to be in unmaintained remission with disappearance of the Philadelphia chromosome 53 months after transplantation. Four of 22 patients with chronic myelogenous leukemia in blast crisis treated by marrow grafts from HLA identical siblings are alive in unmaintained remission 8, 15, 27, and 31 months after grafting, while the remainder died either of transplantation associated complications of recurrent blast crisis.

In an attempt to improve the results in patients with chronic myelogenous leukemia, a study was initiated during the chronic phase of the disease for those patients who had a healthy monozygous twin (Fefer et al. 1977). The objective was to eradicate the Philadelphia chromosome positive clone by chemotherapy and total body irradiation and, thus, to prevent the transformation into blast crisis and cure the disease. An initial group of four patients was treated with a combination of dimethylbusulfan, cyclophosphamide, and total body irradiation followed by marrow infusion. Complete hematologic and cytogenetic remissions were induced in all four. One patient has relapsed 30 months after transplantation and is now back in the original state of chronic myelogenous leukemia. The other three are clinically, hematologically, and cytogenetically normal 36, 39, and 44 months after transplantation. It is possible that the Philadelphia chromosome positive clone has been eradicated. Obviously a longer follow-up of these three patients and of seven similar patients grafted since the initial report is in order.

References

Blume KG, Beutler E, Bross KJ, Chillar RK, Ellington OB, Fahey JL, Farbstein MJ, Forman SJ, Schmidt GM, Scott EP, Spruce WE, Turner MA, Wolf JL (1980) Bone marrow ablation and allogeneic marrow transplantation in acute leukemia. N Engl J Med 302:1041–1046 – Chessels JM, Cornbleet M (1979) Combination chemotherapy for bone marrow relapse in childhood lymphoblastic leukemia (ALL). Med Pediatr Oncol 6:359–365 – Fefer A, Buckner CD, Thomas ED, Cheever MA, Clift RA, Glucksberg H, Neiman PE, Storb R (1977) Cure of hematologic neoplasia with transplantation of marrow from identical twins. N Engl J Med 297:146–148 – Fefer A, Cheever MA, Thomas ED, Boyd C, Ramberg R, Glucksberg H, Buckner CD, Storb R (1979) Disappearance of Ph[1]-positive cells in four patients with chronic granulocytic leukemia after chemotherapy, irradiation and marrow transplantation from an identical twin. N Engl J Med 300:333–337 – Powles RL, Morgenstern G, Clink HM, Hedley D, Bandini G, Lumley H, Watson JG, Lawson D, Spence D, Barrett A, Jameson B, Lawler S, Kay HEM, McElwain TJ (1980a) The place of bone-marrow transplantation in acute myelogenous leukemia. Lancet I:1047–1050 – Powles RL, Palu G, Raghavan D (1980b) The curability of acute leukemia. In: Roath S (ed) Topical review of haematology. Wright, London, pp 186–219 – Thomas ED, Buckner CD, Banaji M, Clift RA, Fefer A, Flournoy N, Goodell BW, Hickman RO, Lerner KG, Neiman PE, Sale GE, Sanders JE, Singer J, Stevens M, Storb R, Weiden PL (1977a) One hundred patients with acute leukemia treated by chemotherapy, total body irradiation, and allogeneic marrow transplantation. Blood 49:511–533 – Thomas ED, Flournoy N, Buckner CD, Clift RA, Fefer A, Neiman PE, Storb R (1977b) Cure of leukemia by marrow transplantation. Leuk Res 1:67–70 – Thomas ED, Sanders JE, Flournoy N, Johnson FL, Buckner CD, Clift RA, Fefer A, Goodell BW, Storb R, Weiden PL (1979a) Marrow transplantation for patients with acute lymphoblastic leukemia in remission. Blood 54:468–476 – Thomas ED, Buckner CD, Clift RA, Fefer A, Johnson FL, Neiman PE, Sale GE, Sanders JE, Singer JW, Shulman H, Storb R, Weiden PL (1979b) Marrow transplantation for acute nonlymphoblastic leukemia in first remission. N Engl J Med 301:597–599 – Weiden PL, Flournoy N, Thomas ED, Prentice R, Fefer A, Buckner CD, Storb R (1979) Antileukemic effect of graft-versus-host disease in human recipients of allogeneic marrow grafts. N Engl J Med 300:1068–1073

Haematology and Blood Transfusion Vol. 26
Modern Trends in Human Leukemia IV
Edited by Neth, Gallo, Graf, Mannweiler, Winkler
© Springer-Verlag Berlin Heidelberg 1981

Allogeneic Bone Marrow Transplantation for Acute Myeloid Leukemia in First Remission

G. R. Morgenstern and R. L. Powles

Evidence that conventional treatment (chemotherapy and/or immunotherapy) produces a substantial number of cures in acute myeloid leukaemia (AML) is lacking (Powles et al. 1980a). Thomas et al. (1977) showed that there was a proportion of long-term survivors of a group of AML patients treated with high-dose cyclophosphamide, total body irradiation (TBI) and allogeneic bone marrow transplantation (BMT).

The purpose of the study reported here is to define the place for BMT in the treatment of AML and involves a comparison of two groups of first remission patients treated either with BMT or chemoimmunotherapy. This study is an extension of the results published earlier this year (Powles et al. 1980c).

A. Patients and Methods

Since August 1977, 33 1st remission AML patients have received a BMT – 27 from HLA-identical and MLC-compatible sibling donors, two from identical twin donors and four from related mis-matched donors (three sibling and one paternal, incompatible

in MLC). The outcome of the matched allografted patients has been compared with the simultaneous group of 33 patients with AML in first remission, who lacking a suitable donor did not receive a transplant and were maintained on chemotherapy and immunotherapy.

Patients details are shown in Table 1. Remission was induced by various regimes using cytosine arabinoside, thioguanine and anthracycline-daunorubicin alone or with adriamycin, or rubidazone. Consolidation with the same three agents or with thioguanine and cytosine arabinoside followed. Twenty of the transplanted patients had their remission induction given elsewhere and were referred to our unit when in remission. Those patients who did not receive a transplant were given maintenance chemotherapy consisting of courses of cytosine arabinoside (10 mg/kg as 24 h intravenous infusion) followed by daunorubicin (1.5 mg/kg intravenously), given at intervals of 2, 4, 6, 8, 10 and 12 weeks after consolidation for a total period of 42 weeks (Powles et al. 1979), or 3 day courses of cytosine arabinoside (1.5 mg/kg sub-cutaneously, 12 hourly) and 6-thioguanine (80 mg orally, 12 hourly) given every 3 weeks for 27 weeks. In addition they received continuous weekly immunotherapy consisting of subcutaneous injections of irradiated myeloblasts and intradermal BCG.

	Allografted (27)	Non-transplanted (33)
M:F	14:13	14:19
Age-mean (range)	24.8 (8–46)	29.4 (3–47)
Diagnosis: M1	3	2
M2	4	14
M3	1	1
M4	14	14
M5	1	2
M6	4	0
Time to CR-median (range)	10.6 weeks (2–53)	7.7 weeks (3–17)

Table 1. Details of patients studied

Patients with a suitable donor received a transplant as soon as practicable after achieving remission. They were conditioned according to the Seattle schedule with high-dose cyclophosphamide (60 mg/kg intravenously for two doses) followed by total body irradiation (1,000 rad mean midline dose given from a cobalt source at 2.5 rad/min). No anti-leukaemic chemotherapy was given after transplantation except low-dose methotrexate (Mtx) for six patients to prevent graft versus host disease. Subsequently, Cyclosporin A (CSA) was used instead of Mtx for 21 patients (Powles et al. 1980b). Patients were nursed in cubicles with filtered positive pressure ventilation, received sterile food and non-absorbable anti-microbials as gut decontamination. Systemic antibiotics and platelet transfusions were given as indicated. No patient required granulocyte transfusions. They were discharged from hospital after marrow reconstitution, 3 to 4 weeks after transplantation.

B. Results

Actuarial analysis of complete remission duration is shown in Figure 1. Of the 33 patients treated with chemo-immunotherapy 20 have relapsed with a median remission duration of 12 months compared with four of the matched allografted patients. This difference is highly significant ($P<0.001$) using the log-rank test.

Twelve of the 33 chemo-immunotherapy patients have died (11 of relapse and one of infection while in remission) with a median survival of 21 months from date of complete remission. There have been five deaths in the 27 matched allografted patients, one of relapse, four of GVHD with or without pneumonitis, (two of these patients received methotrexate prophylaxis and one only a short course of CSA). Actuarial analysis of survival from complete remission of these two groups (Fig. 2) shows that while there is not at present a statistically significant difference between them, at no time do the transplanted patients fare worse and they have a 75% 3 year actuarial survival compared with 45% for the chemoimmunotherapy patients.

Survival from graft date is shown in Figure 3. Nineteen (70%) matched allografted patients remain alive in continuous remission compared with 12 (33%) of chemoimmunotherapy patients ($P=<0.01$).

The syngeneic and mis-matched allografts received the same conditioning regimen and supportive care. The mis-matched allografts all received prolonged CSA as prophylaxis against GVHD. Their outcome is shown in Table 2.

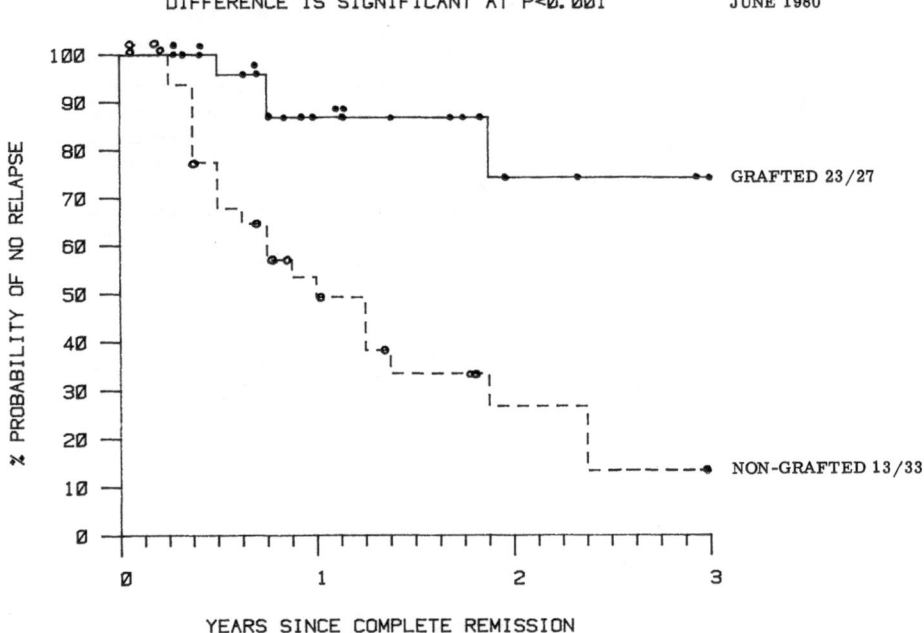

Fig. 1. Actuarial life table analysis of complete remission duration

140

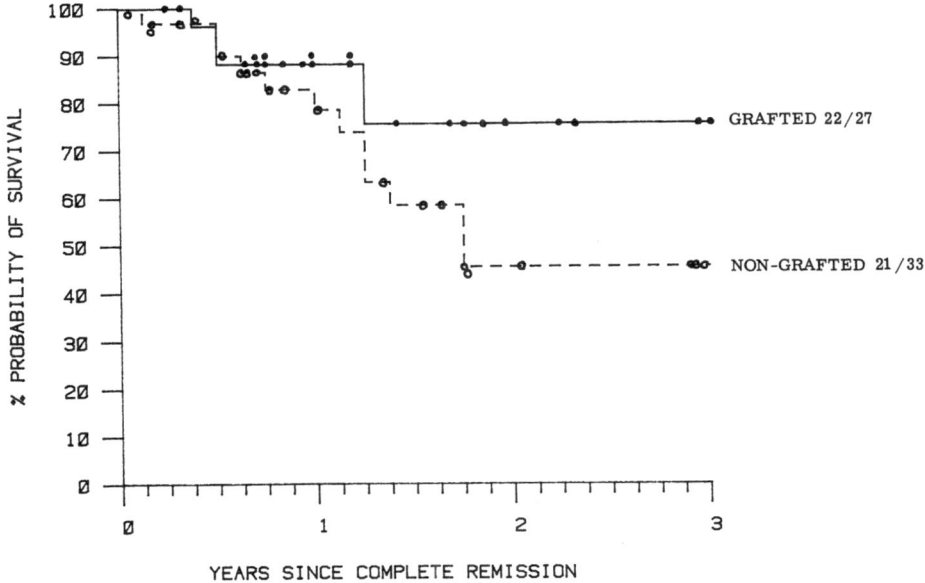

Fig. 2. Actuarial life table analysis of survival from complete remission date

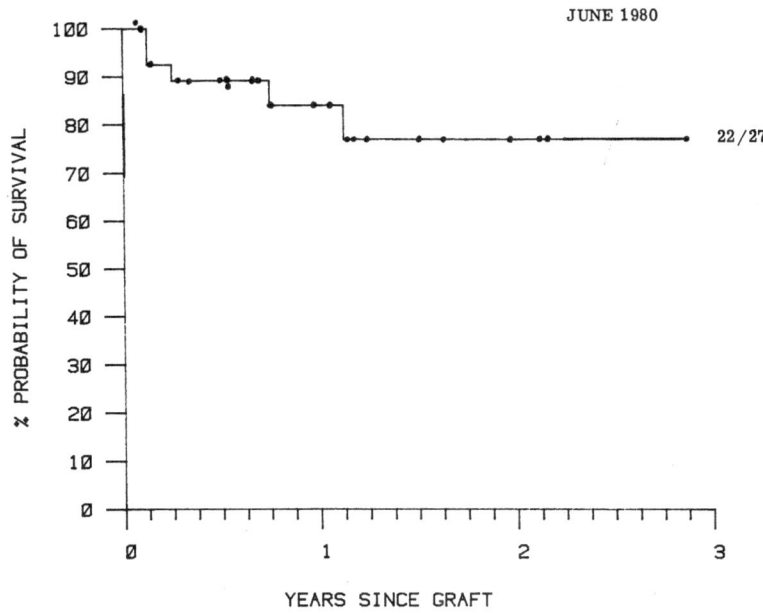

Fig. 3. Actuarial life table analysis of survival from transplant date

	No.	Recurrent Leukaemia		Other deaths
		Total	Died	
Matched allograft:				
CSA prophylaxis	21	3 (14%)	1	2 GVHD
Mtx prophylaxis	6	1 (17%)	0	2 GVHD
Mis-matched allograft	4	1	1	1 pulmonary oedema
Syngeneic graft	2	1	1	0

Table 2. Outcome of patients transplanted for AML in first remission

C. Discussion and Conclusions

The results show clearly that allogeneic BMT significantly reduces the risk of relapse in AML in first remission compared with conventional chemoimmunotherapy, although it is too early to state what the long-term (greater than 2 years) remission rate may be.

The transplanted patients at no time fare worse than the non-transplanted controls, despite four deaths from GVHD. With the greatly reduced mortality from GVHD in patients on long-term CSA (Powles et al. 1980b) this may be a much less severe problem in future. Of the 21 patients with AML in first remission who received CSA after matched allografts 20 received the drug for a period of at least 4 months (Powles et al. 1980b) and 18 are alive and 16 (80%) free from leukaemia.

Cyclosporin A does not seem to influence the relapse rate after transplantation when compared with methotrexate; so far only 3 of the 21 matched patients on CSA have had recurrent leukaemia (Table 2).

We feel that patients under the age of 45 with AML in a first remission who have a suitable donor should be offered as an alternative to chemoimmunotherapy a bone marrow transplant, but at present this should only be done in a suitably experienced centre.

References

Powles RL, Selby PJ, Palu G, (1979) The nature of remission in acute myeloblastic leukaemia. Lancet II:674–76 – Powles RL, Palu G, Raghavan D (1980a) The curability of acute leukaemia. In: Roath S (ed) Topical reviews in haematology. Wright, London, pp 186–219 – Powles RL, Clink HM, Spence D (1980b) Cyclosporin A to prevent graft-versus-host disease in man after allogeneic bone marrow transplantation. Lancet I:327–29 – Powles RL, Morgenstern G, Clink HM (1980c) The place of bone marrow transplantation in acute myelogenous leukaemia. Lancet I:1047–50 – Thomas ED, Buckner CD, Banaji M (1977) One hundred patients with acute leukaemia treated by chemotherapy, total body irradiation and allogeneic marrow transplantation. Blood 49:511–33

Haematology and Blood Transfusion Vol. 26
Modern Trends in Human Leukemia IV
Edited by Neth, Gallo, Graf, Mannweiler, Winkler
© Springer-Verlag Berlin Heidelberg 1981

Use of Erythrocyte Ghosts for Therapy

M. Furusawa and T. Iino

When a mixture of erythrocytes (RBCs) and a foreign substance is dialysed against a hypotonic saline, the hemoglobin is replaced with the substance (Furusawa et al. 1976). The resultant ghosts containing foreign substances could be used for various therapeutic purposes.

A. Intracellular Microinjections or "Fusion Injections"

Fusion between cells and RBC ghosts containing foreign substances results in the introduction of the substances into the cells (Furusawa et al. 1974). With this technique any substance smaller than 6×10^7 dalton can be injected into the cytoplasm. An accurate quantitative injection can be performed using a combination of this method together with a cell sorter (Yamaizumi et al. 1978). It is significant that there is no limitation in the number of target cells subjected to microinjection. This fusion injection technique could be used for alleviating or repairing defective cells. That is, drugs, nucleic acids, or enzymes of normal counterparts can be introduced into these cells, then injected back to the patient. Because the cells and RBCs used can be obtained from the individual to be injected, there would be no risk of rejection (Furusawa 1980). In spite of such advantages it has an inevitable weak point in that intranuclear injections are impossible. Recently we developed a new instrument, namely an "injectoscope", by which one can easily perform intranuclear microinjections without employing a conventional micromanipulator (Furusawa et al. 1980; Yamamoto and Furusawa 1978).

B. Drug Administrations

RBC ghosts loaded with drugs may serve as a good tool for the treatment of some diseases, especially hepatic diseases. When mouse RBC ghosts loaded with proteins were injected into a vein, they disappeared from the circulation blood within 30 min and accumulated exclusively in the liver and spleen. The transfused ghosts may be trapped by Kupffer's cells or macrophages where the loaded substance might be liberated. In clinical therapy a specific drug for a given disease can be loaded in the RBCs of the patient. Then, the drug-loaded ghost cells could be injected intravenously to the same patient. Thus a concentrated amount of the drug could be administered to the liver. Accordingly, it can be expected to diminish subsidiary ill effects of the drug. The fate of the drug thus introduced remains to be examined.

C. Immunization

In humans two important requirements for a successful immunization are (1) a high antibody producing efficiency and (2) minimized side effects. Our preliminary study demonstrated that the intraperitoneal injection of RBC ghosts loaded with dinitrophenol-conjugated ovalbumin (DNP-OA) gave rise to a significant increase of anti-DNP antibody production without artificial adjuvant.

The introduction of DNP-OA into the ghosts was carried out as follows: A mixture of 1 volume of packed RBCs from ICR mice and 9 volumes of PBS containing 10 mg/ml of DNP-OA was dialysed to ten fold diluted PBS until hemolysis had been accomplished and followed by dialysis against isotonic PBS. In addition, a sample containing 1 mg/ml of DNP-OA entrapped in 2×10^9 ghosts was prepared. For sensitization were the ghosts loaded with DNP-OA were intraperitoneally injected into additional mice of the same strain. For controls, free DNP-OA, a mixture of vacant ghosts and DNP-OA, vacant ghosts, and an emulsion with Freund's complete adjuvant were injected. The antisera were collected on the 11th day. The second sensitization was performed on the 11th day after the first injection, and the sera obtained after an additional 11 days. A passive hemagglutination (PHA) test was used for the titration of serum antibody (anti-DNP). The result is summarized in Table 1. Compared with free DNP-OA, ghosts loaded with DNP-OA resulted in a significant increase of anti-DNP production, even in the primary response. In the secondary response higher titers were obtained when the ghosts loaded with DNP-OA were used, although the titers were lower than those with the emulsion. The most striking difference is seen between the sensitization with free DNP-OA and the ghosts loaded with DNP-OA of 25 µg in the secon-

dary response: no detectable antibody was obtained in the former while 2^4 to 2^9 in the titer were observed in the latter.

The present experiment clearly shows that sensitization with antigens entrapped in the RBC ghosts produces a significant amount of antibodies without adjuvant when intraperitoneally introduced. An in vitro study suggests that antigen-loaded ghosts are positively engulfed by abdominal macrophages. If so, the leakage of antigens from the ghosts is minimized. This would raise the antibody forming efficiency and diminish subsidiary ill effects involved. As neither adjuvants nor artficial carriers such as liposomes (Poste et al. 1976) are used in the present method, their possible harmful effects can be avoided.

References

Furusawa M (1980) Cellular microinjection by cell fusion: Technique and applications in biology and medicine. Int Rev Cytol 62:29–67 – Furusawa M, Nishimura T, Yamaizumi M, Okada Y (1974) Injection of foreign substances into single cells by

Table 1. Anti-DNP antibody production in mice receiving intraperitoneal injections of RBC ghosts loaded with DNP-OA as compared to the positive and negative controls (Iino & Furusawa, unpublished)[a]

Means of DNP-OA administration	Dose of DNP-OA in a single injection (µg)	PHA titer ($\log_2$)					
		Primary response			Secondary response		
		Average	(Range)	No. of animals	Average	(Range)	No. of animals
Dissolved in PBS	0	0.4	(0– 2)	8			
	25	0.0		4	0.0		4
	100	1.6	(1– 2)	7	3.8	(2– 5)	4
	400	2.1	(1– 4)	7	5.8	(5– 7)	4
Entrapped in ghosts	0	1.0	(0– 4)	7	1.0	(0– 3)	6
	25	3.5	(0– 7)	8	6.5	(4– 9)	8
	100	5.7	(2– 8)	11	6.5	(5– 8)	6
	400	6.0	(5– 7)	7	8.8	(8–12)	6
DNP-OA/ ghost mixture	25	0.3	(0– 1)	4	0.8	(0– 3)	5
	100	3.3	(1– 5)	4	3.5	(3– 4)	4
	400	4.7	(4– 5)	3	6.7	(6– 7)	3
Emulsion with adjuvant	25	6.3	(5– 7)	4	8.8	(7–10)	4
	100	8.3	(5–12)	8	10.8	(8–12)	8
	400	7.5	(5– 9)	8	12.5	(11–15)	6

[a] DNP = dinitrophenol; DNP-OA = dinitrophenol-conjugated ovalbumin

cell fusion. Nature 249:449–450 – Furusawa M, Yamaizumi M, Nishimura T, Uchida T, Okada Y (1976) Use of erythrocyte ghosts for injection of substances into animal cells by cell fusion. Methods Cell Biol 14:73–80 – Furusawa M, Yamamoto F, Hashiguchi M, Swetly P, Zlatanova J (1980) Studies on Friend cell differentiation using a new microinjection technique. In: Rossi GB (ed) In vivo and in vitro erythropoiesis: The Friend system. Amsterdam, Elsevier/North-Holland Biomedical Press, pp 193–198 – Poste G, Papahadjopoulos D, Vail W (1976) Lipid vesicles as carrier for introducing biologically active materials into cells. Methods Cell Biol 14:33–71 – Yamaizumi M, Mekada E, Uchida T, Okada Y (1978) One molecule of diphtheria toxin fragment A introduced into a cell can kill the cell. Cell 15:245–250 – Yamamoto F, Furusawa M (1978) A simple microinjection technique not employing a micromanipulator. Exp Cell Res 117:441–445

Haematology and Blood Transfusion Vol. 26
Modern Trends in Human Leukemia IV
Edited by Neth, Gallo, Graf, Mannweiler, Winkler
© Springer-Verlag Berlin Heidelberg 1981

A Possible Biochemical Basis for the Use of Hyperthermia in the Treatment of Cancer and Virus Infection

B. Hardesty, A. B. Henderson and G. Kramer

There are numerous reports of tumors that have regressed or disapeared after artificial hyperthermia or a concurrent disease that caused high fever. Generally, local or whole body hyperthermia in the range of 41°–45°C has been involved. Overgaard (1978) has reviewed this literature. Current aspects of hyperthermia in the treatment of cancer has been the subject of several recent conferences (Converence on Hyperthermia in Cancer Treatment 1979; Thermal Characteristics of Tumors: Applications in Detection and Treatment 1980). A number of hypotheses have been advanced to account for these phenomena. Most of these have emphasized elevated blood glucose levels, hyperacidification, and breakdown of capillary circulation (Ardenne and Krüger 1979) or cytoplasmic damage resulting from changes in certain environmental factors such as hypoxia, increased acidity, and insufficient nutrition (Overgaard 1978).

Protein synthesis in intact cells and cell-free systems also is sensitive to inhibition by temperature in the range of 41°C to 45°C. The inhibition is reversible in intact cells and results in breakdown of polysomes without degradation of mRNA (Schochetman and Perry 1972; Goldstein and Penman 1973). The kinetics of protein synthesis inhibition caused by heating reticulocyte lysates to temperatures in the range of 41°C to 45°C are very similar to the novel inhibition curves observed with heme deficiency or double-stranded RNA (dsRNA) (Bonanou-Tzedaki et al. 1978a). Inhibition of protein synthesis is associated with a reduction in binding of Met-tRNA$_f$ to 40S ribosomal subunits (Bonanou-Tzedaki et al. 1978b). This binding reaction is mediated by peptide initiation factor 2 (eIF-2). We found that two components with inhibitory activity are activa-

ted by high pressure (Henderson and Hardesty 1978) or heat (Henderson et al. 1979). Both factors cause inhibition of protein synthesis when they are added to reticulocyte lysates. One is an acidic, heat-stable protein (HS) with an apparent molecular weight of about 30,000 daltons as estimated by gel filtration chromatography. HS has been purified more than 5,000-fold from reticulocyte lysates but has not been obtained in homogeneous form. An inhibition curve for a typical preparation of HS is shown in Fig. 1. We estimate that there is less than 30 µg of recoverable HS per 100 g of

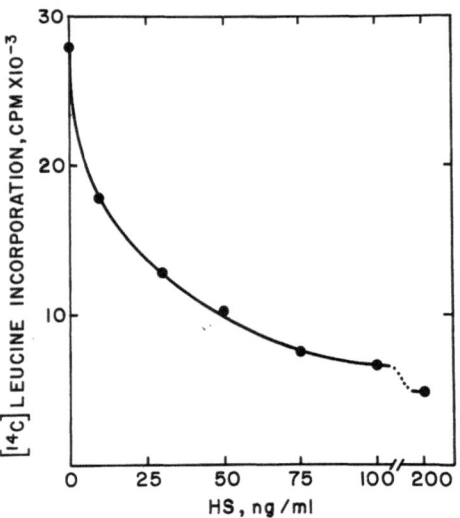

Fig. 1 Heat stable (HS) inhibition of protein synthesis. HS$_i$, purified as described by Henderson et al. (1979), was activated by heating at 100° for 3 min. Aliquots were added to the reticulocyte lysate to give the indicated final concentration. Incorporation of [^{14}C]leucine (40 ci/mol) into protein was measured

protein in the postribosomal supernatant of rabbit reticulocytes. This corresponds to less than a few thousand molecules of HS per reticulocyte.

HS can be converted from an inactive form (HS_i) to an active species by heat or pressure. Activation of highly purified HS during a 5-min incubation at different temperatures is depicted in Fig. 2. Under these conditions appreciable activation is seen at 37°C. It is likely that HS is stabilized by other components in intact cells. HS has the unusual property of reverting to an inactive form if it is held at 0°C for 24–48 h. Table 1 shows the results of an experiment in which HS was cycled between the inactive and active form by repeated heating at 100°C for 3 min, followed by 24 h on ice. There is little or no loss of HS activity during this procedure. HS has little or no detectable inhibitory activity in the absence of the second factor, HL, which is a heat-labile protein of about 43,000 daltons. It appears that HS functions to inhibit protein synthesis by a catalytic, irreversible conversion of an inactive form of HL, HL_i, to an active species. The reaction is ATP-dependent but phosphorylation does not appear to be involved (Henderson et al., 1979).

The mechanism by which HS and HL inhibit protein synthesis appears to involve phospho-

Table 1. Interconversion of HS_i and HS by heating to 100°C followed by cold. A solution of purified HS similar to that used for the experiment of Fig. 1 was heated at 100°C for 3 min, then allowed to stand on ice for 24 h. The cycle of heating and standing in the cold was repeated as indicated. Aliquots containing 0.1 µg of HS protein were assayed in the reticulocyte lysate as described for Fig. 1

Cycle number	Leucine incorporation into protein, cpm $\times 10^{-3}$	
	Unheated	Heated
1	28	8.9
2	29	9.3
3	28	9.1
4	27	8.6
5	28	10.1

rylation of the smallest subunit of eIF-2, eIF-2α, by the specific protein kinase that is also activated in the absence of heme. This eIF-2α kinase appears to contain a peptide of about 100,000 daltons that is phosphorylated during activation by either HS-HL or by heme deficiency (Kramer et al. 1980). Antibodies against the eIF-2α kinase of the HCR system block inhibition by HS or HL. However, it should be emphasized that activation of this protein kinase by HS and HL occurs in the presence of heme. Thus HS and HL appear to form the distal elements of a cascade-type sequence of reactions that lead to inhibition of protein synthesis by phosphorylation of eIF-2α. The relationship of the known components of the HS-HL and HCR systems that are involved in phosphorylation and dephosphorylation of eIF-2 is shown in Fig. 3.

Also shown in Fig. 3 is the relation of the components of the interferon-dsRNA system that appear to lead to phosphorylation of the same three sites of eIF-2α that are phosphorylated by the 100,000 dalton protein kinase of the HS-HL and HCR system (Samuel 1979). The protein kinase of the interferon-dsRNA system involves a 67,000 dalton peptide that also is phosphorylated during activation of the kinase. This occurs in the presence of dsRNA.

It is not established that the HS-HL system is activated during whole body or tissue hyperthermia. However, the biochemical studies indicated above considered with the effects of elevated temperature on protein synthesis apparatus of cells in culture make this seem likely. In turn, it appears that hyperthermia

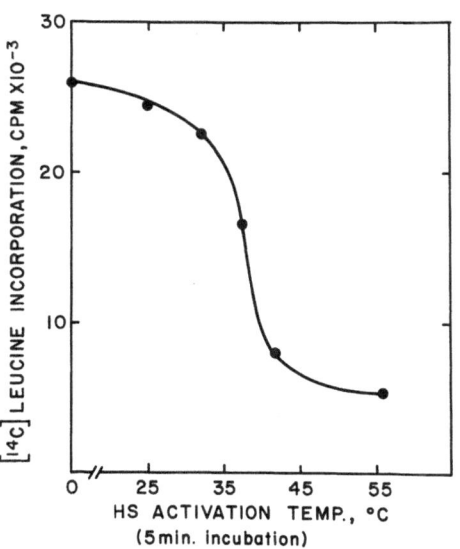

Fig. 2. Heat activation of HS. HS_i was heated at the indicated temperature for 5 min, then inhibitory activity (100 µg HS protein/ml) was measured in the reticulocyte lysate system as described for Fig. 1

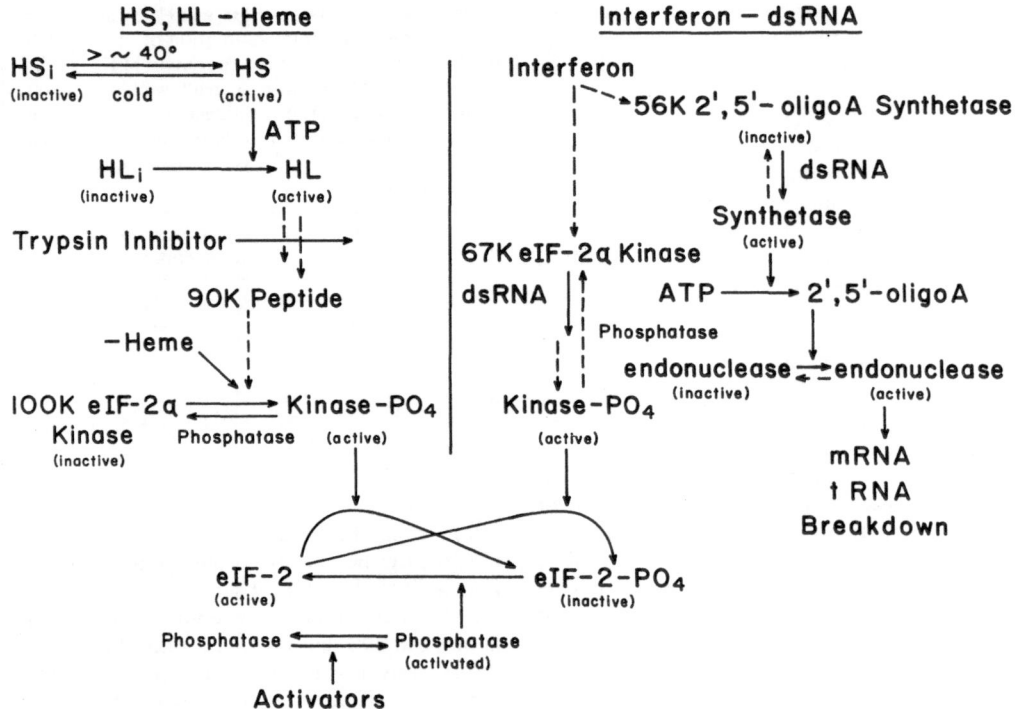

Fig. 3. Comparison of protein synthesis inhibition by HS-HL and by interferon-dsRNA. *Dashed lines* indicated unknown or uncertain relationship

and interferon may function by equivalent biochemical mechanisms to reduce the rate of peptide initiation. A change in this rate may not only slow the rate of cell growth but may also alter the relative proportion of proteins formed from different competing mRNA species (Kramer et al. 1980), thus altering the basic composition and physiology of the cell. Such a change brought on by activation of HS during high fever may constitute a basic defense mechanism for limiting translation of viral mRNA during viral infections and might be exploited for the treatment of cancer by hyperthermia.

References

Ardenne M von, Krüger W (1980) Ann NY Acad Sci 335:356–361 – Bonanou-Tzedaki SA, Smith KE, Sheeran BA, Arnstein HRV (1978a) Eur J Biochem 84:591–600 – Bonanou-Tzedaki SA, Smith KE, Sheeran BA, Arnstein HRV (1978b) Eur J Biochem 84:601–610 – Conference on Hyperthermia in Cancer Treatment (1979) Cancer Res 39:2231–2340 – Goldstein ES, Penman S (1973) J Mol Biol 80:243–254 – Henderson AB, Hardesty B (1978) Biochem Biophys Res Commun 83:715–723 – Henderson AB, Miller AH, Hardesty B (1979) Proc Natl Acad Sci USA 76:2605–2609 – Kramer G, Henderson AB, Grankowski N, Hardesty B (1980). In: Chamblis G, Craven G, Davies J, Davis K, Kahan L, Nomura M (eds) RIBOSOMES: Structure, function and genetics; University Park Press, Baltimore, pp 825–845 – Overgaard J (1978) Cancer 39:2637–2646 – Samuel CE (1979) Proc Natl Acad Sci USA 76:600–604 – Schochetman G, Perry RP (1972) J Mol Biol 63:577–590 – Thermal Characteristics of Tumors: Applications in Detection and Treatment (1980) Jain RK, Gullino PM (eds) Ann NY Acad Sci 335:542

Cytogenetic Aspects of Lymphomas

Haematology and Blood Transfusion Vol. 26
Modern Trends in Human Leukemia IV
Edited by Neth, Gallo, Graf, Mannweiler, Winkler
© Springer-Verlag Berlin Heidelberg 1981

The Implications of Nonrandom Chromosome Changes for Malignant Transformation*

J. D. Rowley

The role of chromosome abnormalities in malignant transformation has been debated for more than 60 years (Boveri 1914). The evidence that chromosome changes play a fundamental role and that they perhaps may even be the ultimate transformation event in some malignancies is becoming ever more compelling. This view is contrary to that held by most investigators even a few years ago. The change in attitude is the result of new technologic advances which allow cytogeneticists to identify precisely each human chromosome and parts of chromosomes as well. Application of the same chromosome banding techniques to the cytogenetic study of animal cancers has provided data that confirm observations of specific nonrandom chromosome abnormalities in virtually every human tumor that has been adequately studied (Mitelman and Levan 1978; Rowley 1978; Sandberg 1980). The evidence obtained from the study of human leukemias is summarized in chapter four.

These nonrandom chromosome changes consist of gains or losses of part or all of certain specific chromosomes and of structural abnormalities, which are most frequently relatively consistent translocations and are presumed to be reciprocal. The nonrandom translocations that we observe in malignant cells would represent those that provide a particular cell

type with a selective advantage vis-a-vis the cells with a normal karyotype. There is very strong evidence that many malignancies, for example, chronic myelogenous leukemia and Burkitt lymphoma, are of clonal origin. This means that a particular translocation in a single cell gives rise to the tumor or to the leukemia that ultimately overwhelms the host. Other rearrangements may be neutral, and the cells therefore will survive but will not proliferate differentially; still others may be lethal and thus would be eliminated. In such a model, the chromosome change is fundamental to malignant transformation.

Two questions are raised by these observations. First, how do such chromosome changes occur, and second, why do they occur? There is very little experimental evidence that is helpful in answering either of these fundamental questions. They clearly provide a focus for future research.

A. Production of Consistent Translocations

The mechanism for the production of specific, consistent reciprocal translocations is unknown. Chromosome breaks and rearrangements may occur continuously at random and with a low frequency, and only those with a selective advantage will be observed (Nowell 1976; Rowley 1977). Alternatively, certain chromosome regions may be especially vulnerable to breaks and, therefore, to rearrangements. In the rat, Sugiyama (1971) showed that a particular region on No. 2 was broken when bone marrow cells from animals given DMBA were examined. In man, however, trisomy for lq is not necessarily related to

* This work was supported in part by grants CA-16910 and CA-23954 from the National Cancer Institute, U.S. Dept. of Health, Education, and Welfare, and by the University of Chicago Cancer Research Foundation. The Franklin McLean Memorial Research Institute was operated by The University of Chicago for the U.S. Department of Energy under Contract EY-76-C-02-0069

fragile sites (Rowley 1977). Thus, a comparison of the break points seen in hematologic disorders that involve balanced reciprocal translocations with those leading to trisomy lq revealed a clear difference in preferential break points, depending on whether the rearrangement resulted in a balanced or an unbalanced aberration.

Other possible explanations depend on either (1) chromosomal proximity, since translocations may occur more frequently when two chromosomes are close together, or (2) regions of homologous DNA that might pair preferentially and then be involved in rearrangements. Many of the affected human chromosomes, e.g., Nos. 1, 9, 14, 15, 21, and 22, are involved in nucleolar organization which would lead to a close physical association. All partial trisomies which result from a break in the centromere of No. 1 involve translocations of lq to the nucleolar organizing region of other chromosomes, specifically Nos. 9, 13, 15, and 22 (Rowley 1977). In the mouse, chromosome No. 15 also contains ribosomal cistrons (rRNA) (Henderson et al. 1974). Sugiyama et al. (1978) noted that in rat malignancies aneuploidies frequently involve chromosomes with late-replicating DNA or those which have rDNA and late-replicating DNA. They have suggested that nucleolus-associated late-replicating DNA rather than rDNA is involved in the origin of nonrandom chromosome abnormalities.

On the other hand, if chromosome proximity or homologous DNA sequences were the mechanism, this should lead to an increased frequency of rearrangements such as t(9q+;22q−) or t(8q−;14q+) in patients with constitutional abnormalities, but this has not been observed. It is possible that either or both of these mechanisms are subject to selection; a translocation might occur because the chromosomes are close together, but only certain specific rearrangements might have a proliferative advantage which results in malignancy and thus allows them to be detected.

One other possible mechanism which should be considered concerns transposable genetic elements that can cause large-scale rearrangements of adjacent DNA sequences (Rowley 1977). Not only do these elements exert control over adjacent sequences, but the type of control, that is, an increase or a decrease in gene product, is related to their position and orientation in the gene locus. Whereas they can cause nonrandom chromosomal deletions adjacent to themselves, these controlling elements can also move to another chromosomal location, and they may transpose some of the adjacent chromosomal material with them. The evidence for the presence of transposable elements in mammalian cells is tenuous, but a more precisely defined gene map is required for the detection of such nonhomologous recombinations.

B. Function of Nonrandom Changes

Our ignorance of how nonrandom changes occur is matched by our ignorance as to why they occur. The question to be examined now relates to the kinds of gene loci that can provide a proliferative advantage.

I. Host Genome

First, two points should be emphasized; one concerns the genetic heterogeneity of the human population, and the second, the variety of cells involved in malignancy. There is convincing evidence from animal experiments that the genetic constitution of an inbred strain of rats or mice plays a critical role in the frequency and type of malignancies that develop. Some of the factors controlling the differential susceptibility of mice to leukemia not only have been identified but also have been mapped to particular chromosomes, and their behavior as typical Mendelian genes has been demonstrated (Ihle et al. 1979; Lilly and Pincus 1973; Rowe 1973; Rowe and Kozak 1979). These genes have been shown to be viral sequences that are integrated into particular sites on chromosomes; these sites vary for different inbred mouse strains and for different murine leukemia viruses.

Certain genetic traits in man predispose to cancer, such as Bloom syndrome, Fanconi anemia, and ataxia-telangiectasia (German 1972). We recognize the existence of cancer-prone families, of inherited genetic susceptibility to specific types of malignancy, such as retinoblastoma and breast cancer, and of the inheritance of lesions which have a high propensity for becoming malignant, such as familial colonic polyps (Mulvihill et al. 1977). How many gene loci are there in man which in some way control resistance or susceptibility to a particular malignancy? We have no way of knowing at present. These genes may influence the types of chromosome changes that are present in malignant cells.

The second factor affecting the karyotypic pattern relates to the different cells that are at risk of becoming malignant and the varying states of maturation of these cells. The catalog of the nonrandom changes in various tumors maintained by Mitelman and Levan (1978) provides clear evidence that the same chromosomes, for example, Nos. 1 and 8, may be affected in a variety of tumors. On the other hand, some chromosomes seem to be involved in neoplasia affecting a particular tissue; the involvement of No. 14 in lymphoid malignancies and the loss of No. 7 in myeloid abnormalities might be suitable examples. All of the consistent translocations are relatively restricted to a particular cell lineage. Given the great genetic diversity, the number of different cell types that might become malignant, and the variety of carcinogens to which these cells are exposed, it is surprising that nonrandom karyotypic changes can be detected at all.

II. Chromosome Changes Related to Gene Dosage

Gains or losses of chromosomes directly affect the number of functioning structural gene copies and therefore alter the amount of gene product in the cell. Although this is only speculative at present, the action of translocations may be to modify the regulation of gene function and therefore to alter the amount of gene product in the cell. There is ample evidence that as cells evolve to a more malignant state many of them gain one or more extra copies of particular chromosomes which must carry genes that provide a proliferative advantage. In some instances, particularly in secondary leukemias, chromosome material is lost; this may allow putative recessive transforming genes to alter the cell (Comings 1973). Alternatively, the loss may shift the balance between genes for the expression and those for the suppression of malignancy (Sachs 1978).

1. Homogeneously Staining Regions and Double Minute Chromosomes

One of the most rapidly moving areas of current investigation involves chromosomes of unusual morphology such as homogeneously staining regions (HSR), reiteration of apparently identical sequences of dark-light bands,

double minutes (DM), and selective gene amplification. Homogeneously staining regions (HSR) were first described by Biedler and Spengler (1976) in drug-resistant Chinese hamster cell lines and in human neuroblastoma cell lines. Within the HSR, replication was synchronous and rapid and was completed before the midpoint of the DNA synthesis period. Similar HSR regions have been described in other human neuroblastoma cell lines by Balaban-Malenbaum and Gilbert (1977). Some animal tumor cells also have HSR (Levan et al. 1977).

Double minutes are small, paired DNA-containing structures that are palestaining with various banding techniques. They appear to lack a centromere and are apparently carried through cell division by attaching themselves to remnants of nucleolar material or by "hitchhiking" on the ends of chromosomes (Levan and Levan 1978). Variable numbers up to 100 DM per cell are found in malignant cells from a number of human tumors as well as those induced in experimental animals.

Neither HSR nor DM are commonly described in hematologic malignancies, for reasons that are not clear. I have seen DM in only five patients with various types of acute leukemia in more than 150 cases studied, and I have never seen them in any form of CML. The apparent absence of HSR may be explained by their altered appearance in hematologic malignancies. One patient in the leukemic phase of histiocytic lymphoma had several unusual marker chromosomes that contained multiple repeats of alternating dark and light bands (Brynes et al. 1978). Biedler and Spengler (1977) have recently reported what may be an analogous phenomenon in drug-resistant Chinese hamster cell lines. Evidence relating HSR and DM has recently been obtained from a human neuroblastoma. (Balaban-Malenbaum and Gilbert 1977) in which about one-half of the cells contained a long HSR in 5q, whereas the other one-half of the cells contained two normal No. 5s and DM. The HSR and DM were never seen in the same cell, although there was clear cytogenetic evidence that both subpopulations had a common precursor.

2. Evidence for Gene Amplification

The function of HSR and DM within the cells is largely unknown. Structure and function have been correlated in an elegant fashion in the drug-resistant Chinese hamster cell lines described by Biedler et al. (1976). When cells from these lines were exposed to methotrexate or methasquin, they developed extraordinarily high levels of dihydrofolate reductase (EC1.5.1.3-DHFR) in association with their drug resistance. Of the 13 independently derived drug-resistant cell lines, only those with greater than 100-fold increases in enzyme activity contained HSR-bearing chromosomes. In some cell lines, HSR represented as much as 6% of the chromosome complement.

In studies of various methotrexate-resistant mouse cell lines, Alt et al. (1978) have shown that the relative number of DHFR gene copies is proportional to the cellular level of DHFR and DHFR mRNA sequences. Giemsa banding studies of a methotrexate-resistant murine lymphoblastoid cell line (Dolnick et al. 1979) showed a large HSR on chromosome No. 2. Molecular hybridization studies in situ indicate that the DHFR genes are localized in this HSR. Similar observations have been made in a methotrexate-resistant Chinese hamster ovary cell line (Nunberg et al. 1978). Evidence from other tumors suggests that amplification of genes coding for 18S and 28S ribosomal RNA may occur (Miller et al. 1979).

All of these data taken together indicate that HSR and DM provide the chromosomal evidence of gene amplification which, in the case of these particular drug-resistant lines, represents amplification for the DHFR gene. The nature of the genes that are amplified in human neuroblastomas, in other human tumors, and in animal tumors is unknown. Recent technical advances provide the tools with which these significant questions can be answered.

C. Conclusion

The relatively consistent chromosome changes, especially specific translocations, that are closely associated with particular neoplasms provide convincing evidence for the fundamental role of these changes in the transformation of a normal cell to a malignant cell. In some tumors these changes may be too small to be detected, and the cells would appear with present techniques to have a normal karyotype.

When one considers the number of nonrandom changes that are seen in a malignancy such as ANLL, it is clear that not just one gene but rather a class of genes is involved. Our knowledge of the human gene map has developed concurrently with our understanding of the consistent chromosome changes in malignancy (McKusick and Ruddle 1977). It is now possible to try to correlate the chromosomes that are affected with the genes that they carry. Clearly, these efforts are preliminary, since relatively few genes have been mapped, and since some of the chromosomes that are most frequently abnormal have few genetic markers. In such a preliminary attempt in 1977 (Rowley 1977), I observed that chromosomes carrying genes related to nucleic acid biosynthesis and also the specific chromosome region associated with these genes were frequently involved in rearrangements associated with hematologic malignancies. More recently, Owerbach et al. (1978) reported that a gene for the large external transformation-sensitive (LETS) protein is located on chromosome No. 8. They noted that because LETS protein has been implicated in tumorigenicity and cellular transformation, its localization to a human chromosome associated with malignancies may prove to be a significant observation.

In the future we will be able to determine the break points in translocations very precisely, to measure the function of genes at these break points, and to compare the activity of these genes in cells with translocations with their activity in normal cells. In other types of abnormalities such as HSR or DM we will be able to identify the genes involved in this process of gene amplification. Such information will be the basis for understanding how chromosome changes provide selected cells in certain individuals with a growth advantage that results in malignancy.

References

Alt FW, Kellems RE, Bertino JR, Schimke RT (1978) Selective multiplication of dihydrofolate reductase genes in methotrexateresistant variants of cultured murine cells. J Biol Chem 253:1357–1370 – Balaban-Malenbaum G, Gilbert F (1977) Double minute chromosomes and the homogeneously staining regions in chromosomes of a human neuroblastoma cell line. Science 198:739–741 – Biedler JL, Spengler BA (1976) Metaphase chromosome anomaly: Association with drug resistance and cellspecific products. Science 191:185–187 – Biedler JL, Spengler BA (1977) Abnormally banded metaphase chromosome regions in cells with low levels of resistance to antifolates. In Vitro 13:200 – Boveri T (1914) Zur Frage der Entstehung maligner Tumoren. Fischer, Jena – Brynes RK, Golomb HM, Gelder F, Desser RK, Rowley JD (1978) The leukemic phase of histiocytic lymphoma. Am J Clin Pathol 89:550–558 – Comings DE (1973) A general theory of carcinogenesis. Proc Natl Acad Sci USA 70:3324–3328 – Dolnick BJ, Berenson RJ, Bertino JR, Kaufman RJ, Nunberg HH, Schimke RT (1979) Correlation of dihydrofolate reductase elevation with gene amplification in a homogeneously staining chromosomal region. J Cell Biol 83:394–402 – German J (1972) Genes which increase chromosomal instability in somatic cells and predispose to cancer. Prog Med Genet 8:61–101 – Henderson AS, Eicher EM, Yu MT, Atwood KC (1974) The chromosomal location of ribosomal DNA in the mouse. Chromosoma 49:155–160 – Ihle JN, Joseph DR, Domofor JJ Jr (1979) Genetic linkage of C3H/HeJ and BALB/c endogenous extropic C-type viruses to phosphoglucomutase-1 on chromosome 5. Science 204:71–73 – Levan A, Levan G (1978) Have double minutes functioning centromeres? Hereditas 88:81–92 – Levan G, Mandahl N, Bengtsson BO, Levan A (1977) Experimental elimination and recovery of double minute chromosomes in malignant cell populations. Hereditas 86:75–90 – Lilly F, Pincus T (1973) Genetic control of murine viral leukemogenesis. Adv Cancer Res 17:231–277 – McKusick VA, Ruddle FH (1977) The status of the gene map of the human chromosomes. Science 196:390–405 – Miller OJ, Tantravahi R, Miller DA, Yu L-C, Szabo P, Prensky W (1979) Marked increase in ribosomal RNA gene multiplicity in a rat hepatoma cell line. Chromosoma 71:183–195 – Mitelman F, Levan G (1978) Clustering of aberrations to specific chromosomes in human neoplasms. III. Incidence and geographic distribution of chromosome aberrations in 856 cases. Hereditas 89:207–232 – Mulvihill JJ, Miller RW, Fraumeni JF Jr (eds) (1977) Progress in cancer research and therapy. Genetics of human cancer, vol 3. Raven, National Cancer Institute, National Institute of Health, Bethesda, MD – Nowell PC (1976) The clonal evolution of tumor cell poulations. Science 194:23–28 – Nunberg JH, Kaufman RJ, Schimke RT, Urlaub G, Chasin LA (1978) Amplified dihydrofolate reductase genes are localized to a homogeneously staining region fo a single chromosome in a methotrexate resistant chinese hamster ovary cell line. Proc Natl Acad Sci USA 75:5553–5556 – Owerbach D, Doyle D, Shows TB (1978) Genetics of the large, external, transformation sensitive (LETS) protein: Assignment of a gene coding for expression of LETS to human chromosome 8. Proc Natl Acad Sci USA 75:5640–5644 – Rowe WP (1973) Genetic factors in the natural history of murine leukemia virus infection. GHA Clowes Memorial Lecture. Cancer Res 33:3061–3068 – Rowe WP, Kozak CA (1979) Genetic mapping of the ecotropic murine leukemia virus-inducing lccus of BALB/c mouse to chromosome 5. Science 204:69–71 – Rowley JD (1977) Mapping of human chromosomal regions related to neoplasia: Evidence from chromosomes 1 and 17. Proc Natl Acad Sci USA 74:5729–5733 – Rowley JD A possible role for nonrandom chromosomal changes in human hematologic malignancies. In: De la Chapelle A, Sorsa M (eds) (1977) Chromosomes Today 6. Elsevier/North-Holland, Amsterdam, pp 345–359 – Rowley JD (1978) Chromosomes in leukemia and lymphoma. Semin Hematol 15:301–319 – Sachs L (1978) Control of normal cell differentiation and the phenotypic reversion of malignancy in myeloid leukemia. Nature 274:535–539 – Sandberg AA (1980) Chromosomes in human cancer and leukemia. Elsevier/North-Holland, New York – Sugiyama T (1971) Specific vulnerability of the largest telocentric chromosome of rat bone marrow cells to 7, 12-dimethylbenz(α)anthracene J Natl Cancer Inst 47:1267–1276 – Sugiyama T, Uenaka H, Ueda N, Fukuhara S, Maeda S (1978) Reproducible chromosome changes of polycyclic hydrocarbon-induced rat leukemia: Incidence and chromosome banding pattern. J Natl Cancer Inst 60:153–160

Haematology and Blood Transfusion Vol. 26
Modern Trends in Human Leukemia IV
Edited by Neth, Gallo, Graf, Mannweiler, Winkler
© Springer-Verlag Berlin Heidelberg 1981

Regional Gene Mapping of Human Chromosomes Purified by Flow Sorting

A. V. Carrano, R. V. Lebo, L. C. Yu, and Y. W. Kan

A. Introduction

Analysis and sorting of chromosomes using fluorescence-based high speed flow systems was reported in 1975 (Gray et al. 1975a). In the ensuing 5 years these principles have been applied to karyotype analysis (Gray et al. 1975b; Stubblefield et al. 1975; Carrano et al. 1976, 1978, 1979a,b; Otto and Oldiges 1978; Gray et al., 1979) and to chromosome biochemistry and cytochemistry (Sawin et al. 1979; Lebo et al. 1979; Langlois et al. 1980). The results of these investigations indicate that the use of these systems for chromosome analysis and sorting is an important adjunct to existing cytogenetic techniques and a primary resource for molecular cytogenetic studies of individual chromosomes. This brief report describes one application of this approach, namely, regional gene mapping of human chromosomes.

B. Methodology for Flow Systems Analysis and Sorting of Chromosomes

For human studies metaphase chromosomes are routinely isolated from diploid fibroblast cultures. Cells are grown in roller bottles, metaphase cells accumulated by the addition of Colcemid, and the cultures rotated to dislodge the mitotic cells. These cells are then collected by centrifugation, distributed into aliquots of 8×10^6 cells, and resuspended in hypotonic KCl (0.075 M) at 4° C for 30 min. After centrifugation each cell aliquot is resuspended in 0.5 ml chromosome isolation buffer (25 mM Tris-HCl, pH 7.5/0.75 M hexylene glycol/0.5 mM CaCl$_2$/1.0 mM MgCl$_2$) and sheared with a Virtis homogenizer. The isolated chromosomes are then stained with an appropriate fluorochrome. For high resolution human chromosome analysis 33258 Hoechst (2 µg/ml, final concentration) has been excellent. The final suspension containing approximately $2-4 \times 10^8$ stained chromosomes in about 1 ml buffer is used directly for analysis and sorting.

The principles and operational aspects of flow cytometry and sorting have been previously described (Van Dilla et al. 1974; Horan and Wheeless 1977). Basically, the stained chromosomes flow in a narrow stream past a laser beam of high intensity UV light (360 nm at 0.7 – 1.0 W). The size of the chromosome stream and width of the laser beam are such that the emitted fluorescence can be measured from single chromosomes at rates of several thousand per second. Separation of chromosomes with a preselected fluorescence intensity is accomplished by electronically charging and deflecting liquid droplets containing the chromosome of interest. Two preselected "windows" of fluorescence intensity are sorted simultaneously. Sort rates for human chromosomes generally range from 100 to 200 chromosomes per second. Thus to collect 5×10^6 human chromosomes (about 1 µg DNA for an average size human metaphase chromosome) requires about 7–14 h. The sorted chromosomes can be fixed onto microscope slides for cytologic analysis or collected in tubes for subsequent DNA extraction.

C. Application to Regional Gene Mapping

There are three requirements for regional gene mapping: (1) the ability to resolve the chromosome of interest in the flow distribution; (2)

a DNA probe specific for the gene to be mapped; and (3) cell strains possessing rearrangements of the chromosome to be mapped. The regional mapping of the human β-, γ-, and δ-globin genes illustrates the principles involved.

The 33258 Hoechst distribution of a normal human diploid fibroblast strain is shown in Fig. 1. The ordinate represents the relative number of chromosomes measured and the abscissa, the relative fluorescence intensity. Fifteen peaks are distinguishable and each can be characterized by a mode and area determined by computer fit. The peak mode is a measure of the relative Hoechst fluorescence and the area a measure of the relative number of chromosomes in the peak. These values are given in the figure and the chromosomes associated with each peak (identified by quinacrine banding analysis of the sorted chromosomes) are shown on the top of the distribution. There is reasonably good agreement between the relative Hoechst fluorescence and DNA stain content of the chromosomes, although there are exceptions, e.g., chromosomes 18 and 19. The variations between the observed and expected number of chromosomes for some peaks are attributed primarily to inaccuracies in the fit code. The purity of the chromosomes obtained by sorting is also shown. This ranges from 63% to 98%. Since only four chromosome types (No. 5, 6, 13, and 18) are compeletely resolved, identifying a gene on any other chromosome requires segregation of at least one homolog of the chromosome from the peak – hence the utility of chromosomal rearrangements.

In order to map the β-, γ-, and δ-globin genes we purified chromosomes from several peaks in the distribution. The DNA from each was extracted, digested with EcoRl, and applied to a single well on an agarose gel. After electrophoresis the DNA was transferred to nitrocellulose filters and the filters hybridized with ^{32}P-labeled cDNA prepared by reverse transcription of human globin mRNA. The filters were then washed, dried, and exposed for autoradiography. Positive hybridization occurred between the cDNA for the β-, γ-, and δ-globin genes and DNA extracted from the peak containing chromosomes 9 through 12.

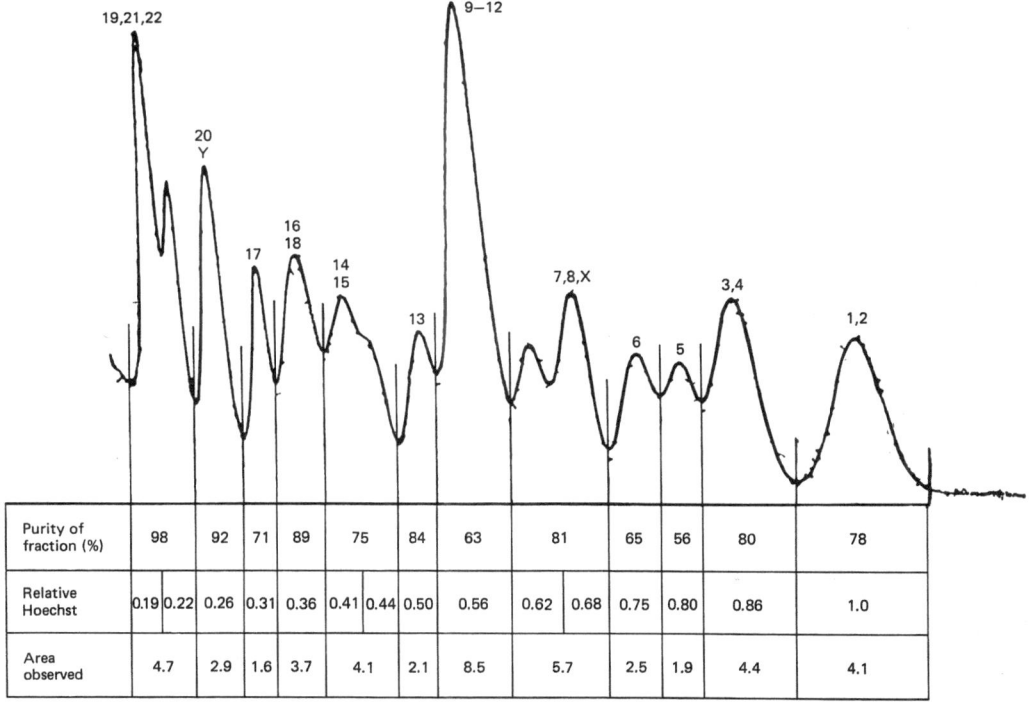

Purity of fraction (%)	98	92	71	89	75	84	63	81	65	56	80	78
Relative Hoechst	0.19 0.22	0.26	0.31	0.36	0.41 0.44	0.50	0.56	0.62	0.68	0.75 0.80	0.86	1.0
Area observed	4.7	2.9	1.6	3.7	4.1	2.1	8.5	5.7	2.5	1.9	4.4	4.1

Fig. 1. Flow distribution of metaphase chromosomes isolated from diploid human fibroblasts and stained with 33258 Hoechst. The *ordinate* represents the number of chromosomes analyzed and the *abscissa*, the fluorescence intensity

157

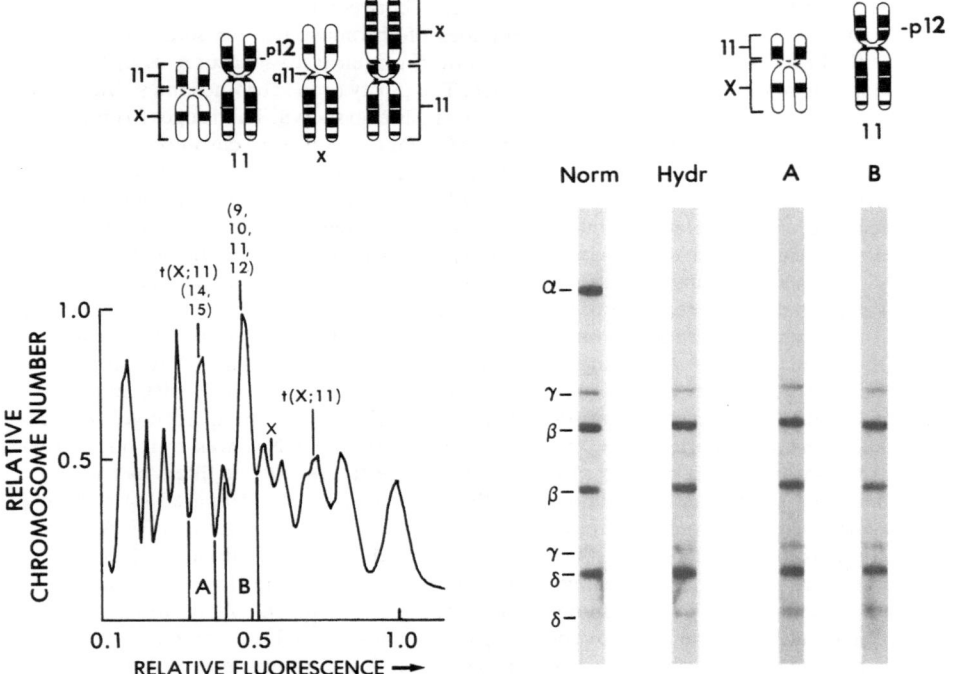

Fig. 2. *Left:* The 33258 Hoechst flow distribution of a human fibroblast strain carrying a translocation, t(X;11) (q11;p12). The normal and derivative chromosomes are shown above the distribution. *Right:* Autoradiographs of ^{32}P-labeled cDNA from human globin RNA hybridized to restricted total cell DNA from a normal *Norm* and hydrops *(Hydr)* individual or to restricted DNA from chromosomes sorted from peaks A and B. The location of the α-, β-, γ-, and δ-globin EcoRl restriction fragments are indicated

Since these genes had been provisionally mapped to chromosome 11 by somatic cell hybridization (Deisseroth et al. 1978), we used three translocations of chromosome 11 to further localize the genes. The 33258 Hoechst flow distribution, the nature of the third translocation, and the autoradiographs from the restricted DNA are shown in Fig. 2. As illustrated by the chromosome diagram above the flow distribution, peak B contained one normal chromosome 11, while peak A contained chromosomes 14, 15, and the derivative chromosome consisting essentially of the short arm of the X and the short arm of chromosome 11 (bands pl2 → pter). The other derivative chromosome containing the remainder of chromosomes 11 and X shifted to a higher fluorescence intensity. The restriction enzyme patterns of total cell DNA from a normal individual are shown in the gel at the left. A single band is present for α-globin, while two bands each are present for β-, γ-, and δ-globin.

The total hydrops DNA lacking the α-globin is shown in the next gel. Gels A and B were prepared from DNA extracted from chromosome peaks A and B in the flow distribution. Positive hybridization in both gels identified the location of the β-, γ-, and δ-globin genes to chromosome 11, bands p12 → pter. This is supported by independent somatic cell hybridization studies (Gusella et al. 1979).

D. Conclusions

In addition to gene mapping studies, chromosomes purified by flow sorting have potential application to gene transfer and to the molecular biology of chromosome structure and function. It should now be possible to examine DNA or protein unique to a single chromosome and, for example, to examine the DNA associated with specific chromosomal alterations in hematological disorders such as the translocation between chromosomes 9 and 22 in chronic myelogenous leukemia (Rowley 1973; Mayall et al. 1977). The full potential of this flow systems approach to chromosome analysis has not yet been realized.

Acknowledgment

This work was conducted under the auspices of the U.S. Department of Energy by the Lawrence Livermore Laboratory under contract number W-7405-ENG-48 and also supported by Grants AM 16666 and HL 20985 from the National Institutes of Health and a grant from the March of Dimes.

Notice

This report was prepared as an account of work sponsored by the United States Government. Neither the United States nor the United States Department of Energy, nor any of their employees, nor any of their contractors, subcontractors, or their employees, makes any warranty, express or implied, or assumes any legal liability or responsibility for the accuracy, completeness or usefulness of any information, apparatus, product or process disclosed, or represents that its use would not infringe privately-owned rights.

References

Carrano AV, Gray JW, Moore II, DH, Minkler JL, Mayall BH, van Dilla MA, Mendelsohn ML (1976) Purification of the chromosomes of the Indian muntjac by flow sorting. J Histochem Cytochem 24:348–354 – Carrano AV, Gray JW, van Dilla MA (1978) Flow cytogenetics: Progress towards chromosomal aberration detection. In: Evans HJ, Lloyd DC (eds) Mutagen-induced chromosome damage in man. Edinburgh University Press, Edinburgh pp 326–338 – Carrano AV, Gray JW, Langlois RG, Burkhart-Schultz KJ, van Dilla MA (1979a) Measurement and purification of human chromosomes by flow cytometry and sorting. Proc Natl Acad Sci USA 76:1382–1384 – Carrano AV, van Dilla MA, Gray JW (1979b) Flow cytogenetics: A new approach to chromosome analysis. In: Melamed MR, Mullaney PF, Mendelsohn ML (eds) Flow cytometry and sorting. Wiley New York, pp 421–451 – Deisseroth A, Nienhuis A, Lawrence J, Giles R, Turner P, Ruddle FH (1978) Chromosomal location of human β-globin gene on human chromosome 11 in somatic cell hybrids. Proc Natl Acad Sci USA 75:1456–1460 – Gray JW, Carrano AV, Steinmetz LL, van Dilla MA, Moore II DH, Mayall BH, Mendelsohn ML (1975a) Chromosome measurement and sorting by flow systems. Proc Natl Acad Sci USA 72:1231–1234 – Gray JW, Carrano AV, Moore II DH, Steinmetz LL, Minkler JL, Mayall BH, Mendelsohn ML, van Dilla MA (1975b) High-speed quantitative karyotyping by flow microfluorometry. Clin Chem 21:1258–1262 – Gray JW, Langlois RA, Carrano AV, Burkhart-Schultz K, van Dilla MA (1979) High resolution chromosome analysis: One and two parameter flow cytometry. Chromosoma 73:9–27 – Gusella J, Varsanyi-Breiner A, Kao FT, Jones C, Puck TT, Keys C, Orkin S, Housman D (1979) Precise localization of human β-globin gene complex on chromosome 11. Proc Natl Acad Sci USA 76:5239–5243 – Horan PK, Wheeless LL Jr (1977) Quantitative single cell analysis and sorting. Science 198:149–157 – Langlois RG, Carrano AV, Gray JW, van Dilla MA (1980) Cytochemical studies of metaphase chromosomes by flow cytometry. Chromosoma 77:229–251 – Lebo RV, Carrano AV, Burkhart-Schultz K, Dozy AM, Yu LC, Kan YW (1979) Assignment of human β-, γ-, and δ-globin genes to the short arm of chromosome 11 by chromosome sorting and DNA restriction enzyme analysis. Proc Natl Acad Sci USA 76:5804–5808 – Mayall BH, Carrano AV, Moore DH II, Rowley JD (1977) Quantification by DNA-based cytophotometry of the 9q+/22q− chromosomal translocation associated with chronic myelogenous leukemia. Cancer Res 37:3590–3593 – Otto F, Oldiges H (1978) Requirements and procedures for chromosomal measurements for rapid karyotype analysis in mammalian cells. In: Lutz D (ed) Cytophotometry, vol III. European Press, Ghent, pp 393–400 – Rowley JD (1973) A new consistent chromosomal abnormality in chronic myelogenous leukemia identified by quinacrine fluorescence and giemsa staining. Nature 243:290–293 – Sawin VL, Rowley JD, Carrano AV (1979) Transcription and hybridization of ^{125}I-cRNA from flow sorted chromosomes. Chromosoma 70:293–304 – Stubblefield E, Deaven L, Cram LS (1975) Flow microfluorometric analysis of isolated Chinese hamster chromosomes. Exp Cell Res 94:464–468 – Van Dilla MA, Steinmetz LL, Davis DT, Calvert RN, Gray JW (1974) High speed cell analysis and sorting with flow systems: biological applications and new approaches. IEEE Trans Nucl Sci 21:714–720

Haematology and Blood Transfusion Vol. 26
Modern Trends in Human Leukemia IV
Edited by Neth, Gallo, Graf, Mannweiler, Winkler
© Springer-Verlag Berlin Heidelberg 1981

The Different Origin of Primary and Secondary Chromosome Aberrations in Cancer

G. Levan and F. Mitelman

A. Abstract

We have proposed a hypothetical model to explain the role of chromosomal aberrations in malignant development. In this model we postulate two kinds of chromosomal changes: (1) *primary, active changes* caused by direct interaction between the oncogenic agent and the hereditary material of the host cell. These changes are mainly somatic mutations, but may also be associated with directed structural changes visible in the microscope; and (2) *secondary, passive changes* arising randomly by nondisjunction and structural rearrangements. They are followed by selection of cells with changes that amplify the primary change and thus appear as nonrandom chromosome patterns.

This hypothesis is discussed in the light of 1827 cases of human malignancy in which we have recently surveyed and systematized chromosomal aberrations. Special support for the idea of somatic mutations as the initiator of malignant development comes from work of Knudson and collaborators in human retinoblastoma. The Ph[1] chromosome, predominant during the chronic phase of chronic myeloid leukemia (CML), is proposed as an instance of a primary change, whereas the chromosome changes during the blastic crisis of CML will illustrate the secondary changes. The most common of these secondary changes is actually the doubling of the Ph[1] and thus an amplification of the primary change. The increase in number of copies of a specific chromosome reported by Green and collaborators demonstrates that this kind of amplification can result in direct response to the need for a specific gene located in that chromosome.

B. Introduction

Towards the end of the nineteenth century it became known from the work of pathologists that malignant cells were often liable to chromosome aberrations. Boveri in 1914 hypothesized that these aberrations actually were the cause of the malignant growth. At that time, technical difficulties in the study of mammalian chromosomes effectively put a stop to any thorough investigation of chromosome aberrations in tumors. Improvements in methodology in the early 1950s made detailed studies feasible, but only after the introduction of chromosome banding in the early 1970s could chromosomal and subchromosomal changes in tumor materials be analyzed with great precision. The results from both experimental and human tumors were significant: clear nonrandom patterns of aberrations became discernible. There were, however, considerable difficulties in interpreting the findings. Firstly, there were usually many different types of changes even within a clinically well defined group of tumors. Secondly, there was a variable degree of "background noise", i.e., chromosome changes that did not fall into the nonrandom pattern. Thirdly, there were cases of malignant tumors in which even refined chromosome banding did not reveal any aberrations.

C. Chromosome Aberrations in Human Malignancies

We have attempted to collect data as completely as possible from all human tumors that have been studied carefully by chromosome banding techniques. The bulk of the material

Myelo-proliferative disorders	Chronic myeloid leukemia (CML)	
	t(9;22) and other aberrations	361
	Aberrant translocations	94
	Acute myeloid leukemia (AML)	496
	Polycythemia vera (PV)	86
	Myelodyscrasia (MD)	278
Lympho-proliferative disorders	Malignant lymphomas (ML)	105
	Burkitt's lymphoma (BL)	24
	Acute lymphocytic leukemia (ALL)	156
	Chronic lymphocytic leukemia (CLL)	30
	Monoclonal gammopathies (MG)	23
Solid tumors	Benign mesenchymal tumors (BMT)	56
	Benign epithelial tumors (BET)	9
	Carcinomas (CA)	87
	Malignant melanomas (MM)	8
	Neurogenic tumors (NT)	7
	Sarcomas (SA)	7

Table 1. Subdivision of 1827 cases of human neoplasms with chromosome aberrations identified by banding techniques

comes from the published cases in the literature. In addition, there are unpublished cases from our own laboratory and from other laboratories, the latter kindly made available by the original investigators. All in all we have collected and systematized 1827 cases of human malignancies exhibiting chromosome aberrations. This figure does not include about 2000 cases of chronic myeloid leukemia that have the Ph^1-translocation as the only aberration. According to the diagnoses the material has been subdivided into 15 classes (Table 1).

The aberrations of each patient with a parti-cular disease may be scored and surveyed in histograms such as the one in Fig. 1. This diagram represents 496 cases of acute myeloid leukemia. We think it must be obvious to all that the various chromosome types are affected by aberrations in a nonrandom fashion. Clearly chromosomes Nos. 7, 8, 17, and 21 are selectively involved in aberrations. It should be noted, however, that the nonrandom elevation of the aberrations in these chromosomes is blurred by the random aberrations occasional-ly affecting all chromosomes and causing the rather high background level of aberrations.

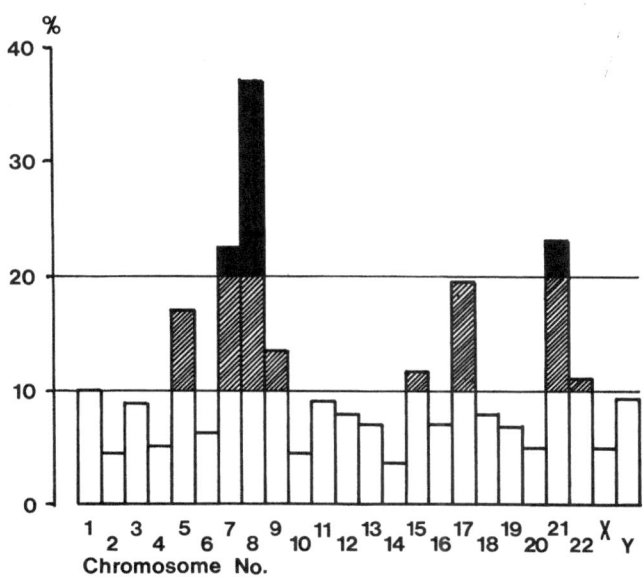

Fig. 1. Histogram of per cent aberrations affecting the 24 human chromosome types in 496 patients with acute myeloid leukemia

161

Table 2. Selective involvement of chromosome types in 15 classes of human neoplasms

Tumor type[a]	Chromosome No.																							
	1	2	3	4	5	6	7	8	9	10	11	12	13	14	15	16	17	18	19	20	21	22	X	Y
CML								8	9								17					22		
AML					5		7	8									17				21			
PV	1							8	9											20				
MD					5		7	8												20	21			
ML	1	3							9					14										
BL							7	8						14										
ALL	1													14							21	22		
CLL	1													14			17							
MG	1	3												14										
BMT								8														22		
BET								8						14										
CA	1	3			5		7	8																
MM	1								9															
NT	1																					22		
SA													13	14										
No. of times involved	8	–	3	–	3	–	4	8	4	–	–	–	1	7	–	–	3	–	–	2	3	4	–	–

[a] Key to abbreviations of the tumor types, see Table 1

D. Clustering of Aberrations to Specific Chromosomes

Similar histograms have been prepared for all the different tumor classes listed in Table 1. When the chromosomes affected most commonly in each class are selected, the picture of Table 2 emerges. It is clear from this table that not only are aberrations nonrandom within each tumor class, but there is also a tendency for the aberrations to cluster to specific chromosomes when different classes are compared. Thus, chromosomes 1, 3, 5, 7, 8, 9, 14, 17, 21, and 22 exhibit nonrandom involvement in three or more types of malignancy, whereas 12 chromosome types never show any indication of a selective involvement.

These data from the human tumors are corroborated and strengthened when similar data from experimental tumors are taken into account as well. Thus, sarcomas of the rat, the mouse, and the Chinese hamster all show involvement of specific chromosomes. The same is true of rat leukemias and is especially consistent in mouse leukemias. Virtually 100% of mouse T-cell leukemias exhibit triso-

my No. 15 (Wiener et al. 1978a,b; Chan et al. 1979).

E. The Significance of Chromosome aberrations in Malignancy – A Hypothesis

Thus, banding studies have conclusively demonstrated that chromosome aberrations in tumors are nonrandom. Unfortunately, this knowledge does not immediately throw light on the question what significance this nonrandom involvement has to tumor initiation and development. Levan and Mitelman (1977) proposed a model of interpretation, which may still be useful as a working hypothesis (Fig. 2). According to this model there are two kinds of chromosome changes with different modes of generation: (1) primary or active changes, which arise through direct interaction between the oncogenic agent and the genetic material of the cell, and (2) secondary or passive changes, which arise at random in the proliferating cell population and are subject to subsequent selection. The effect of the primary

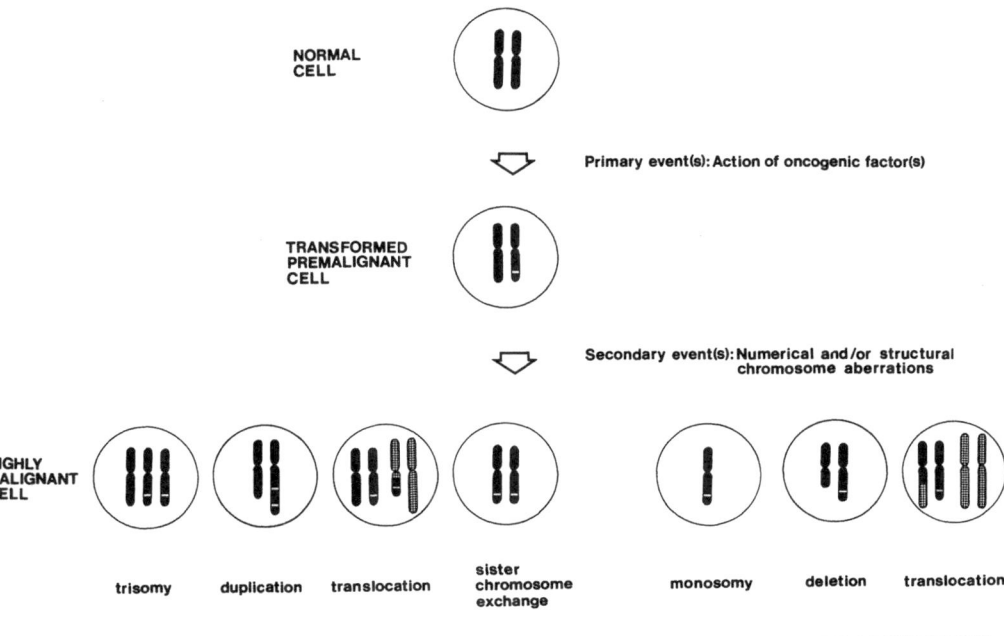

Fig. 2. Hypothetical scheme of chromosomal events in the origin and development of cancer

changes is to transform the cell into an autonomous parasite and the effect of the secondary changes is to stepwise render the parasitic cell population more and more malignant. In the model it is assumed that the primary changes usually are submicroscopic somatic mutations. Secondary changes cause chromosome imbalance to amplify the primary changes and arise from structural rearrangements and nondisjunction.

F. Somatic Mutation in the Initiation of Malignancy

There are still considerable differences in opinion about the role of somatic mutation in cancer. Even though no direct evidence exists that somatic mutation constitutes the initial step in oncogenesis, many facts are compatible with this assumption. Strong support comes from the fact that most carcinogens have proven to be potent mutagens.

The work of Knudson in human hereditary cancers also tends to support the somatic mutation theory (Knudson et al. 1975). In retinoblastoma, both sporadic and hereditary cases exist. According to Knudson's hypothesis two specific somatic mutations in homologous loci are required for a tumor to develop. This highly unlikely event must be very rare and is the cause of the low incidence of sporadic retinoblastoma. In hereditary retinoblastoma, on the other hand, the first mutation is inherited and thus present in advance in all somatic cells. Due to the great number of cells involved in the development of the retina, the probability is now high that the second mutation will take place in at least one cell, making this cell fully malignant. This hypothetical scheme is supported by the fact that sporadic cases virtually always are unifocal, whereas the majority of the hereditary cases are multifocal.

Recently, some hereditary cases have been studied where one of the mutations apparently is substituted for by small chromosomal deletions (Nove et al. 1979). These deletions all affect chromosome 13 and when different cases are compared the common segment lost is band 13q14. It is well known from genetic studies that expression of a recessive mutant phenotype may be achieved either by a second mutation in the homologous locus or by a deletion affecting the same locus.

The conclusion from the discussion so far is that one or more somatic mutation is the initiating step in at least some tumors. The somatic mutation may be substituted for by a deletion and possibly also by other specific chromosomal aberrations. It is characteristic of the primary chromosome changes that they are quite specific and directed towards one or more genes probably concerned with growth regulation and differentiation in the affected tissue.

G. The Ph^1 Chromosome – an Example of a Primary Chromosome Aberration

The chromosomes of an ample number of cases of Ph^1-positive human chronic myeloid leukemia (CML) have been studied with modern banding techniques. The total number of cases is not known, since many of them have not been published, but they must amount to several thousands. The great majority of them show one very specific aberration: a translocation between chromosome Nos. 9 and 22. Usually, patients with this aberration alone are clinically in the chronic phase of the disease – when the blastic crisis sets in, secondary chromosome aberrations ordinarily develop.

Thus CML quite nicely follows the scheme: a primary specific change followed by secondary less specific changes, a process which is parallelled by the development of the disease from a less malignant to a highly malignant state. It is, of course, possible to hypothesize that the Ph^1-positive cells arise not through the action of some specific mechanism but through selection from a large number of equally frequent translocations. There is, however, overwhelming evidence against this interpretation. A number of Ph^1-positive leukemias have been detected in which the translocation is not the typical t(9;22) but some other change (Table 3). In all cases one of the translocation partners is the deleted No. 22, but the other is not No. 9 but either another chromosome or the translocation is complex involving more than two chromosomes. There are also three cases where Ph^1 appears to represent a true deletion. All these chromosomal variants are associated with a disease indistinguishable from typical t(9;22) CML. The first conclusion from these data is that the significant change in CML is the deletion of No. 22. The second is that selection from a random population of translocations is excluded. Obviously, the t(9;22) is immensely overrepresented and other translocations leading to del(22) underrepresented. The conclusion must be that t(9;22) in CML is a chromo-

Table 3. Aberrant translocation patterns in 94 cases of Ph^1-positive CML

Translocation	No. of cases	Translocation	No. of cases	Translocation	No. of cases
t(X;22)	1	t(X;9;22)	1	t(X;9;17;22)	1
t(2;22)	2	t(1;9;22)	4	t(1;4;20;22)	1
t(3;22)	1	t(2;9;22)	4	t(3;4;9;22)	1
t(4;22)	1	t(3;9;22)	7	t(4;9;17;22)	1
t(5;22)	1	t(4;9;22)	2	t(7;9;11;22)	1
t(6;22)	2	t(5;9;22)	2	t(9;13;15;22)	1
t(7;22)	2	t(6;9;22)	3	t(9;16;17;22)	1
t(9;22)ab	1	t(7;9;22)	4	t(9;10;15;19;22)	1
t(10;22)	2	t(8;9;22)	1		
t(11;22)	2	t(9;10;22)	2	del (22)	3
t(12;22)	4	t(9;11;22)	3		
t(13;22)	1	t(9;13;22)	2		
t(14;22)	3	t(9;14;22)	3		
t(15;22)	2	t(9;15;22)	1		
t(16;22)	3	t(9;17;22)	2		
t(17;22)	6	t(17;17;22)	1		
t(19;22)	4	t(21;22;22)	1		
t(21;22)	1				
t(22;22)	1				

some change of the primary type, induced by a highly specific mechanism which is slightly error prone and occasionally produces an aberrant translocation.

H. Secondary Chromosome Aberrations Are Due to Random Changes and Subsequent Selection

The cell that has been transformed by a primary change into a premalignant or malignant state begins to divide without being restricted by the homeostasis. Secondary chromosome changes will occur in a random fashion due to the mechanisms frequent in transformed cells, i.e. nondisjunction and chromosome breakage and reunion. Most abnormal cells thus originated will be at selective disadvantage and never attain any importance in the population. If, however, a secondary change occurs which amplifies the effect of the primary chance, the cell thus changed will be at selective advantage and divide faster than the surrounding cells. Since cell division is a prerequisite for secondary changes to become manifest, further changes will have an increased change of arising. In this way increased division rate will generate cells with even more increased division rate in the mode of a vicious circle.

It is this process, we feel, that leads to the nonrandom distribution of secondary chromosome changes mentioned in the beginning of the paper. Conversely, it is possible to deduce from the distribution of aberrations which chromosomes were originally affected by a primary change. Thus, it is significant that the most common secondary change in CML is the duplication by nondisjunction of the Ph^1-chromosome.

It has been long recognized that malignant cell populations give the impression of existing in a condition of perpetual change and selection. Direct evidence that this may involve genetic responses leading to the amplification of specific genes is scarce. Proof that such a mechanism can be at work has been obtained in certain experiments of Green et al. (1971). Growth of human-mouse cell hybrids, selected in the HAT medium, is dependent on the human TK+ gene situated on the No. 17 chromosome. Normally, such a hybrid will carry only one No. 17 chromosome. Green and collaborators drastically decreased the thymi-dine concentration in the HAT medium and then selected clones with the best growth potential. These clones proved to contain both two and three copies of the TK+ chromosome. The obvious conclusion of this experiment was that this system selected for randomly occurring nondisjunction products in the cell population and may thus serve as a model for the appearance of secondary changes in malignant development.

I. Is it Reasonable to Postulate That Both Significant and Insignificant Chromosome Aberrations may be Found in Neoplastic Cells?

A fact, which has seemed very difficult to reconcile with the thought of specific and significant chromosome involvement in the origin and early development of tumors, is the presence of a background level of random aberrations in many materials. It does not appear biologically reasonable that both significant and insignificant aberrations should be manifest in tumor cell populations. Recent work by Wiener and collaborators has thrown light on this question. In a series of elegant experiments these workers have shown that mouse T-cell leukemias very specifically exhibit No. 15 trisomy (Wiener et al. 1978a,b). Furthermore, by using four strains of Robertsonian translocation mice (2n=38) with rob(1;15), rob(4;15), rob(5;15) and rob (6;15), respectively, they were able to show that T-cell leukemias in these animals display trisomy for the entire translocation chromosome (Spira et al. 1979). Clearly, these neoplasms require trisomy 15 for their development and are not bothered by carrying trisomy for an insignificant chromosome as well, as long as the required No. 15 trisomy is present. We feel that this is a general feature of tumor cell populations that may explain the high level of background aberrations in some tumors.

Acknowledgements

Financial support of this work by grants from the Swedish Cancer Society, the John and Augusta Persson Foundation of Medical Research, and CANCIRCO is gratefully acknowledged.

165

References

Chan FHP, Ball JK, Sergovich FR (1979) Trisomy 15 in murine thymomas induced by chemical carcinogens, X-irradiation, and an endogenous murine leukemia virus. J Natl Cancer Inst 62:605–610 – Green H, Wang R, Kehinde O, Meuth M (1971) Multiple human TK chromosomes in human-mouse somatic cell hybrids. Nature (London) New Biol 234:138–140 – Knudson AG, Heathcote HW, Brown BW (1975) Mutation and childhood cancer: A probabilistic model for the incidence of retinoblastoma. Proc Natl Acad Sci 72:5116–5120 – Levan G, Mitelman F (1977) Chromosomes and the etiology of cancer. In: Chapelle A de la, Sorsa M (eds) Chromosomes today, vol 6. Elsevier/North-Holland, Amsterdam, pp 363–371 – Nove J, Little JB, Weichselbaum RR, Nichols WW, Hoffman E (1979) Retinoblastoma, chromosome 13, and in vitro cellular radiosensitivity. Cytogenet Cell Genet 24:176–184 – Spira J, Wiener F, Ohno S, Klein G (1979) Is trisomy cause or consequence of murine T-cell leukemia development? Studies on Robertsonian translocation mice. Proc Natl Acad Sci 76:6619–6621 – Wiener F, Ohno S, Spira J, Haran-Ghera N, Klein G (1978a) Chromosome changes (trisomies #15 and 17) associated with tumor progression in leukemias induced by radiation leukemia virus. J Natl Cancer Inst 61:227–237 – Wiener F, Spira J, Ohno S, Haran-Ghera N, Klein G (1978b) Chromosome changes (trisomy 15) in murine T-cell leukemia induced by 7,12-dimethyl-benz(α)anthracene (DMBA). Int J Cancer 22:447–453

Haematology and Blood Transfusion Vol. 26
Modern Trends in Human Leukemia IV
Edited by Neth, Gallo, Graf, Mannweiler, Winkler
© Springer-Verlag Berlin Heidelberg 1981

Insertion of New Genes into Bone Marrow Cells of Mice

M. J. Cline, H. D. Stang, K. Mercola, and W. Salser

A. Summary

Drug resistance genes such as those coding for
a methotrexate-resistant dihydrofolate reductase (DHFR) or the thymidine kinase from
herpes simplex virus can be used to confer
a proliferative advantage on bone marrow cells
of mice. As a result of this proliferative
advantage, transformed cells become the predominant population in the bone marrow.
Efficient gene expression was obtained for
both the thymidine kinase and DHFR genes
inserted into mouse bone marrow. Such
gene insertion techniques may ultimately
lead to the cure of life-threatening globinopa-
thies such as sickle cell disease or the beta
thalassemias. They may also be useful in
reducing the hematopoietic toxicity of anticancer drugs.

B. Introduction

We have developed techniques for the insertion of new genes into bone marrow stem cells
of living mice. By selective procedures we can
favor the proliferation of transformed stem
cells carrying the inserted genes (Cline et al.
1980; Mercola et al. 1980). We have shown
that such cells transformed with the genes
coding for DHFR or herpes simplex virus
thymidine kinase (HSV-tk) produce high levels of the active enzymes specified by these
genes (Salser et al., to be published).

In these experiments we focused on procedures which might eventually have clinical
relevance for the treatment of genetic diseases
of the hematopoietic system such as sickle cell
disease. This constrained out approach to
procedures which could potentially be used to
insert functioning globin genes into the great
majority of bone marrow stem cells.

We utilized the technique of cell transformation by calcium precipitates of DNA as developed by Bachetti and Graham (1977) and
modified by Wigler et al. (1978). This procedure allows the insertion of quite large DNA
sequences; the mouse DHFR gene which we
have inserted is at least 42 kilobases (kb) in
size (Nunberg et al. 1980).

C. Use of Selection Techniques

An essential component of our strategy has
been to develop selective procedures favoring
the proliferation of transformed cells in living
animals. In this way even a small number of
cells with the desired gene insertions could
gain a proliferative advantage so that they
would ultimately predominate in the bone marrow population. We selected a strategy based
on selective pressure by the chemotherapeutic
agent, methotrexate (MTX). MTX binds to the
enzyme DHFR and inhibits the synthesis of
thymidine monophosphate (TMP) and DNA
synthesis. Our first strategy involved the insertion of altered DHFR genes coding for an
enzyme resistant to MTX. Our second strategy
involved the insertion of HSV-tk genes which
code for the enzyme that catalyzes the conversion of thymidine to TMP and enables the cells
to grow in the presence of MTX by utilizing the
salvage pathway of DNA synthesis more efficiently. The HSV-tk enzyme has a greater
affinity for its substrate than does the normal
mammalian enzyme. We reasoned that this
might confer an additional advantage to cells
incorporating and expressing the viral gene.
The K_m for the virus enzyme is estimated to be

0.4 μM thymidine (Klemperer and Haynes 1967) whereas that for the normal mouse enzyme is estimated as $9\mu M$ thymidine (Chang and Prusoff 1974).

D. 3T6-Rl Cells Have a MTX-resistant DHFR

We isolated DNA from mouse 3T6 cells containing reiterated DHFR structural genes (Kellums et al. 1979). These cells, designated 3T6-Rl, contain about 30 copies of the DHFR structural gene and produce correspondingly elevated levels of the enzyme (Kellums et al. 1979). We found that the 3T6-Rl DHFR activity is strikingly resistant to MTX (Salser et al., to be published).

The 3T6-Rl cells appear to contain two DHFR activities; one, comprising about 25% of the total activity, is sensitive to MTX; the other, which represents about 75% of the total activity, is highly resistant to MTX.

E. Transformation of Mouse Bone Marrow Cells with DHFR Genes

We established an escalating schedule of MTX treatment which would select for drug-resistant hematopoietic cells without killing animals (Cline et al. 1980). We used a syngeneic pair of mouse strains (CBA/Ca and CBA/T6T6), one of which carries a distinctive T6T6 chromosomal marker. This enabled us to follow the two cell types independently and determine whether the transformation procedure was successful. In a successful transformation the cell type receiving the methotrexate-resistant (MTX^R) genes should show a marked growth advantage and come to predominate in recipient animals treated with MTX. This cell type could be identified by its distinctive karyotype.

The experiment shown in Table 1 illustrates the type of results obtained. The T6T6 marked cells transformed with MTX^R DHFR genes showed 75%–96% predominance in the bone marrow of recipient animals after treatment with MTX for 33 to 65 days. Control experiments show that these results are not due to any inherent advantage of the T6T6 cells over Ca cells.

Treatment of the recipient animals with MTX is essential if the cell type transformed with MTX^R DNA is to become dominant. When MTX treatment is omitted the MTX^R DNA-transformed cell karyotypes are typically found at levels of only 33%–40% (Cline et al. 1980).

Success of these experiments was judged by appropriate karyotype predominance. It was not feasible to establish insertion of a new DHFR gene by Southern hybridization analysis because of the origin of the mutant DHFR gene from murine sources. In independent experiments it was possible to demonstrate insertion of the human beta globin gene by cotransformation with MTX^R DHFR (Salser et al., to be published).

Table 1. Karyotype analysis of marrow cells of CBA/Ca mice receiving a 1:1 mixture of control Ca and T6 marrow cells transformed with MTX-resistant DNA (Ref. 1)

Recipient	Period with Mtx (days)	Period without MTX (days)	Karyotype (% T6)
Primary 1	0–33	–	79
Primary 2	0–40	–	75
Primary 3	0–47	–	75
Primary 3	0–47	48–68	83
Secondary 3	47–61	–	88, 88, 100[a]
Primary 4	0–54	–	75
Secondary 4	54–72	–	83
Primary 5	0–65	–	96
Primary 5	0–65	66–113	63

[a] Three secondary recipients

Spleens were removed from primary and secondary recipients of transformed marrow from four independent experiments and assayed for DHFR. MTX treatment was terminated 5–7 days before collection of tissue from these mice for the DHFR assays. Spleens were collected from 12 control animals chosen to match those of the experimental group. A radiometric assay for DHFR was performed on sonicated cell-free extracts of spleen (Hillcoat et al. 1967; Hayman et al. 1968). DHFR-specific activity was two- to fourfold greater in the spleen extracts of animals receiving transformed bone marrow than in controls (Cline et al. 1980).

F. Transformation of Mouse Bone Marrow with HSV-tk Genes

The strategy of the experiments was similar to that employed for selection of expression of the DHFR gene. Mouse bone marrow cells with the T6T6 chromosomal marker were treated in vitro with a calcium microprecipitate of the HSV-tk gene. The treated marrow was mixed in a ratio of 1:1.5 with "mock" transformed CBA/Ca marrow cells lacking the chromosomal marker. Karyotype analysis was used to determine whether there was a predominance of T6T6 marked cells indicating successful gene therapy. As shown in Table 2, high levels of the T6T6 karyotype were frequently observed in the treated animals and occasionally in

Table 2. Karyotype analysis of bone marrow cells of irradiated CBA/Ca mice receiving A 1:1.5 mixture of CBA/T6 marrow transformed with HSVtk gene and "mock" transformed CBA/Ca (Ref. 2)

Recipient	Period with Mtx (days)	Karyotype (% T6)
Primary 1	0–32	74
Primary 2	0–47	84
Primary 3	None	35
Controls (20)	0–90	38 ± 10

untreated animals, but never in controls which received mixtures of Ca and T6T6 marked cells in which *both* cell types had been mocked transformed. In selected cases where T6T6 predominance was observed, DNA was extracted and then digested with appropriate restriction enzymes and subjected to Southern blot analysis in order to test for the presence of HSV-tk gene sequences. HSV-tk gene sequences were shown to be present, confirming the success of the transformation procedure (Mercola et al. 1980).

Pyrimidine kinase assays showed that the spleen extracts from transformed animals contain the expected unique enzyme activity which can convert ^{125}I dC to ^{125}I dCMP, and activity not seen in extracts similarly prepared from normal mice (Salser et al., to be published).

We concluded that the HSV-tk gene confers a proliferative advantage on mouse bone marrow cells in the presence and sometimes in the absence of selective drug therapy with MTX. This may indicate that the salvage pathway for DNA synthesis is somewhat limiting to the growth of normal bone marrow cells and that cells with an enhanced salvage pathway capacity have an advantage during repopulation of the irradiated bone marrow.

G. Discussion

We have shown the insertion of genes into the bone marrow of living mice is feasible. Because cells which have been altered in a desired way may have a proliferative advantage, they may eventually constitute the majority of the cells in the bone marrow. We have also shown that these procedures can be used to introduce a gene such as that coding for human beta globin, which by itself would confer no selective advantage on the recipient cells (Salser et al., to be published).

It is our hope that such gene insertion techniques may eventually be used to treat a variety of human diseases more effectively. The hemoglobinopathies and some hematopoietic malignancies are natural targets for such an approach.

References

Bachetti S, Graham F (1977) Transfer of the gene for thymidine kinase to thymidine kinase-deficient human cells by purified herpes simplex viral DNA. Proc Natl Acad Sci USA 74:1590–1594 – Chang Y-C, Prusoff WH (1974) Mouse ascites sarcoma 280 deoxythymidine kinase. General properties and inhibition studies. Biochemistry 13:1179–1185 – Cline MJ, Stang H, Mercola K, Morse D, Ruprecht R, Browne J, Salser W (1980) Gene transfer in intact animals. Nature 284:422–425 – Hayman R, McCready R, van der Weyden M (1968) A rapid radiometric assay for dihydrofolate reductase. Anal Biochem 87:460–465 – Hillcoat BL, Sweet V, Bertino JR (1967) Increase of dihydrofolate reductase activity in cultured mammalian cells after exposure to methotrexate. Proc Natl Acad Sci USA 58:1632–1637 – Kellums R, Morhenn V, Pfendt E, Alt F, Schimke R (1979) Polyoma virus and cyclic AMP-mediated control of dihydrofolate reductase on RNA abundance in methotrexate-resistant mouse fibroblasts. J Biol Chem 254:309–318 – Klemperer HG, Haynes GR (1967) A virus-specific thymidine kinase in BHNZl cells infected with herpes simplex virus. Virology 31:120–128 – Mercola KE, Stang HD, Browne J, Salser W, Cline MJ (1980) Insertion of a new gene of viral origin into bone marrow cells of mice. Science 208:1033–1035 – Nunberg JH, Kaufman RJ, Chang ACY, Cohen SN, Schimke RT (1980) Structure and genomic organization of the mouse dihydrofolate reductase gene. Cell 19:355–364 – Salser W, Tong BD, Stang HD, Browne JK, Mercola K, Bar-Eli M, Cline MJ (to be published) Gene therapy techniques: Use of drug resistance selections in intact animals to insert human globin genes into bone-marrow cells of living mice. – Wigler M, Pellicer A, Silverstein S, Axel R (1978) Biochemical transfer of single-copy eucaryotic genes using total cellular DNA as donor. Cell 14:725–731

Haematology and Blood Transfusion Vol. 26
Modern Trends in Human Leukemia IV
Edited by Neth, Gallo, Graf, Mannweiler, Winkler
© Springer-Verlag Berlin Heidelberg 1981

Organization of the Methotrexate Resistant Mouse L5178YR Dihydrofolate Reductase Gene and Transformation of Human HCT-8 Cells by This Gene

D. I. Scheer, S. Srimatkandada, B. A. Kamen, S. Dube, and J. R. Bertino

A. Introduction

Gene amplification has been recently shown to play a pivotal role in the development of resistance to the folate analogue, methotrexate (MTX), in several cell culture systems (Schimke et al. 1978). Stepwise increases in the concentration of MTX supplied to the medium in which the murine lymphoblastoid line L5178Y was cultivated resulted in the development of 100,000-fold elevation in resistance (Dolnick et al. 1979). The resistant line, L5178YR, was able to grow in the presence of millimolar concentrations of MTX, and it was shown that these cells had a 300-fold elevation in the activity of the target enzyme, dihydrofolate reductase (DHFR). Moreover, the increase in DHFR activity could be correlated with a proportional increase in DHFR-specific mRNA (300-fold) as well as a 300 fold-increase in DHFR gene copies.

To clarify the mechanism of the amplification event as well as gain insight into the regulation of the DHFR gene an analysis has been made of the DNA sequence organization of the DHFR gene. Further, DNA-mediated gene transfer has been employed to transform a human colon carcinoma line (HCT-8) with DHFR genes from the L5178YR line.

B. Methods and Materials

I. Cell Culture

Mouse L5178Y and L5178YR lines were maintained in Fischer's medium with 10% horse serum. Human colon carcinoma, HCT-8, was maintained in RPMI medium containing 20% fetal calf serum.

II. Isolation of DNAs

Essentially as described by Blin and Stafford (1976)

III. Transformation

Essentially as described by Graham and van der Eb (1973) with minor modifications.

IV. Enzymology

Essentially as described by Hayman et al (1978) for DHFR and by Lomax and Greenberg (1967) for TMP synthetase, with modifications by Dolnick and Cheng (1977) and Kamen et al. (1976) for the cofactor binding studies.

V. Southern Blot Hybridization

Southern blot hybridization was done essentially as described by Southern (1975) with modifications by Wahl et al. (1979). Cloned DHFR cDNA probes were kindly provided by Dr. R. Schimke (See Chang et al. 1978).

C. Results and Discussion

Data obtained from our laboratory as well as that of Schimke (Nunberg et al. 1980) suggests that the murine DHFR gene is interrupted by at least five intervening sequences. Figure 1 depicts a Southern blot of amplified L5178YR DNA which has been cleaved by several enzymes, transferred to DBM paper, and hybridized with the cloned DHFR cDNA probes (pDHFR 21 and 26). Since none of the indicated enzymes cleave within the structural gene, the patterns of fragmentation result from sites provided by the intervening sequences. From limited and complete Pst1 digestion

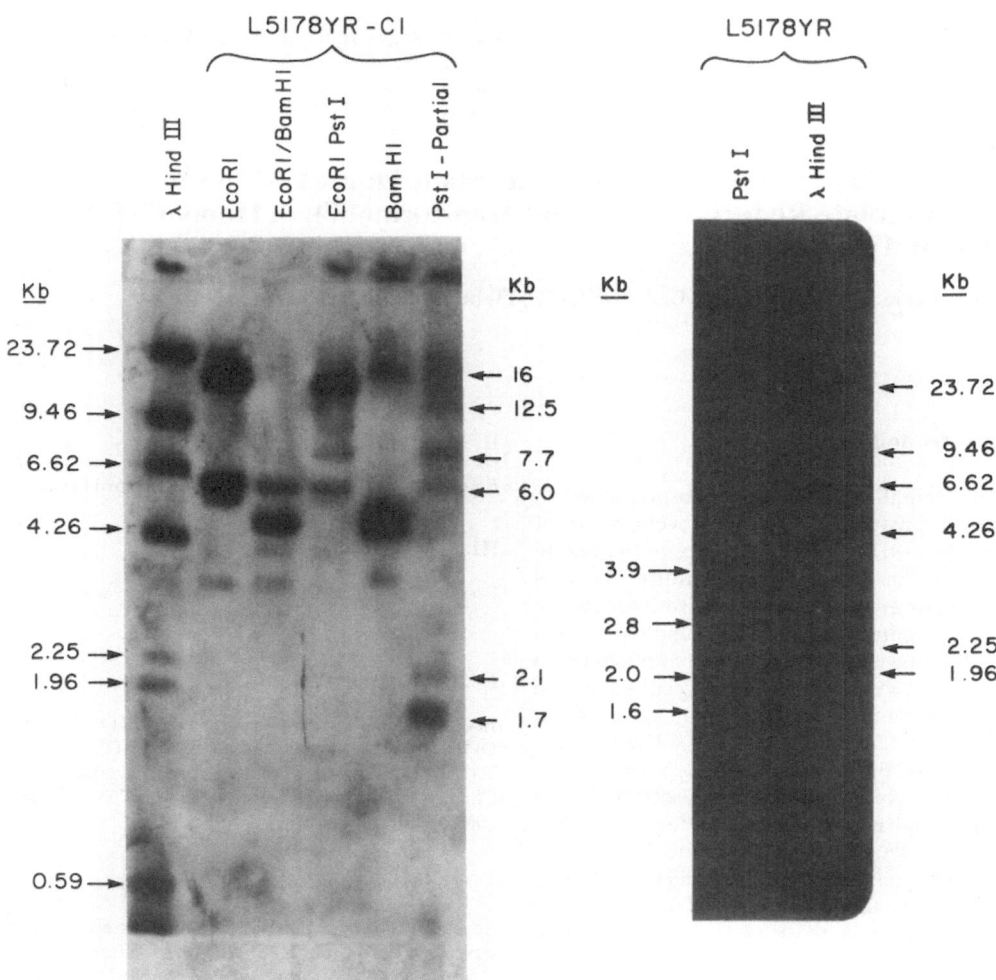

Fig. 1. Southern blot hybridization of L5178YR DNA. *Left* DNA was cleaved with the indicated restriction endonucleases *(Eco R1)* and electrophoresed on 0.8% Agarose, transferred to DBM paper, and hybridized with ^{32}P-labelled pDHFR 21 cDNA probe. *Right* Similar conditions as above except the hybridization was carried with ^{32}P-labelled pDHFR 26 DNA probe. λDNA cleaved with HindIII and labelled with ^{32}P was used as molecular weight marker. *Kb,* kilo base

intervening sequence structure as well as gene size may be deduced. A minimum size estimate for the gene is 45 kilobase pairs. This figure agrees with the estimate of Nunberg et al. (1980) that the DHFR gene is at least 42 Kb in size.

Transformation of the human colon carcinoma (HCT-8) line was obtained with L5178YR DNA as a $CaPO_4$ precipitate. Selection for transformants was carried out at concentrations of MTX ranging from $10^{-7}M$ to $10^{-3}M$.

Two transformant lines remain stably resistant after approximately 12 months, one at $10^{-7}M$ and a second at $10^{-6}M$ (C_1HCT 8-6). C_1HCT 8-6 was analyzed for levels of DHFR enzyme activity and found to contain a ten fold elevation compared to parental HCT-8. Further, in examining other enzymes in the folate pathway it was found that TMP-synthetase was also elevated in this line by five fold.

To determine the species of the elevated enzyme in C_1HCT 8-6 cofactor binding studies

172

were carried out with ^{3}H-MTX in the presence of excess NADPH. Under the conditions of assay C_1HCT 8-6 enzyme exhibits MTX binding that closely approximates the kinetics expected for mouse (L5178YR C3 enzyme), whereas the HCT-8 enzyme binds MTX with a K_D at least 100-fold higher than L5178YR C3 enzyme (data not shown).

Southern blot hybridization analysis of the human DHFR gene and the transformed DHFR gene is depicted in Fig. 2. Results indicate a qualitative as well as a quantitative difference in the sequences corresponding to the DHFR gene from the two sources. That the C_1HCT 8-6 pattern corresponds to mouse is supported by the following observations. The cell line exhibits a stably resistant phenotype in the absence of drug selection for a period of 6 months. Thus, the information has most

likely become associated with the recipient genome. And, assuming an integrative recombination event as depicted in Fig. 3, a truncation from the 3' terminal fragment (EcoR1 16 kb) consisting of approximately 10 kb would result in the observed restriction pattern that is, the 6.1 kb, 5.8 kb, and a ca. 6 kb fragment. The presence of a minor higher molecular weight (14 kb) fragment in the C_1HCT 8-6, which is absent from the human gene, is a further argument for mouse information in the transformed line. Since the line has not been cloned, it is possible that a heterogeneous cell population could account for isolated integrative events that correspond to less sequence loss at the 3' end of the gene. Thus, a 14 kb fragment could result from a 2 kb truncation from the 16 kb fragment. At the 5' end earlier data indicated the presence of a 2.3

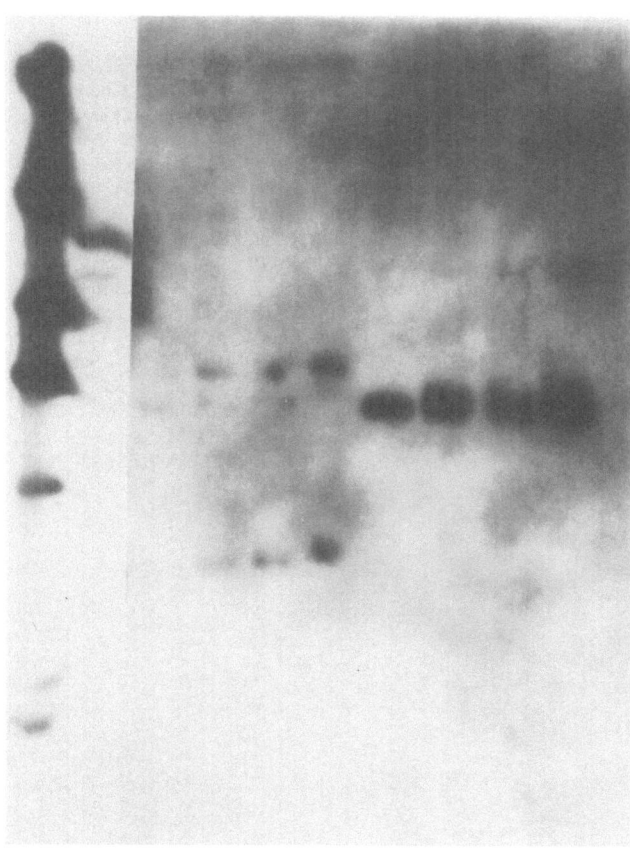

Fig. 2. Southern blot hybridization of human placental DNA (lanes 3 to 6) and C_1HCT8-6 DNA (lanes 7 to 10). Restriction endonuclease *(EcoR1)* was employed for both DNAs. Conditions were otherwise similar to those of Fig. 1. Lanes 3 to 6 and lanes 7 through 10 demonstrate hybridization with increasing concentrations (e.g., 2.5 mcg. to 10 mcg.) for each DNA

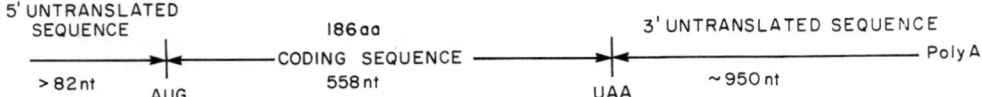

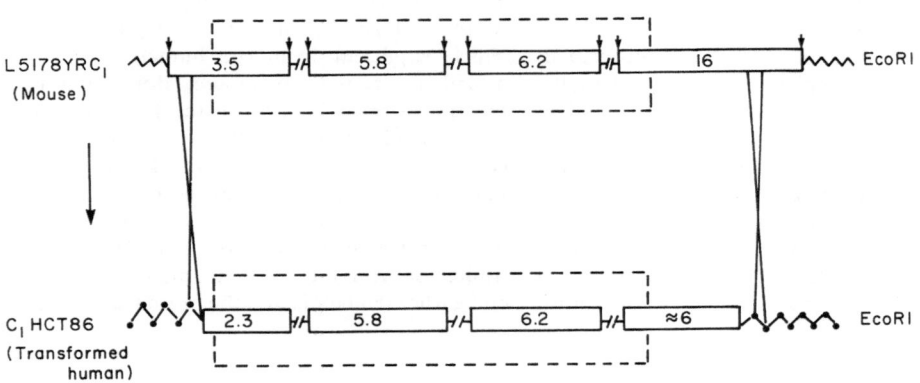

Fig. 3. Proposed model for the integration of the DHFR gene in the recipient human genome. *EcoRI*, restriction endonuclease. Data from upper panel adapted from Nunberg et al. (1980)

kb fragment which might result from a truncation of the 3.5 kb fragment during integration. However, we are trying to resolve whether such is the case in the light of more recent data where the 5′ terminal fragment appears to be 3.5 kb. Definitive structural data on the transformed sequence awaits the characterization of fragments of the gene obtained by molecular cloning.

References

Blin N, Stafford W (1976) Nucleic Acid Research 3:2303–2308 – Chang ACY, Nunberg JH, Kaufman RJ, Ehrlick HA, Schimke RT, Cohen SN (1978) Nature 275:617–624 – Dolnick BJ, Cheng YC (1977) J Biol Chem 252:7697–7703 – Dolnick BJ, Berenson RJ, Bertino JR, Kaufman RJ, Nunberg JH, Schimke RT (1979) J Cell Biol 83:394–402 – Graham FL, van der Eb AJ (1973) Virology 52:456–467 – Hayman R, McGready R, van der Weyden MB (1978) Anal Biochem 87:460–465 – Kamen BA, Takach PL, Vatev R, Caston JD (1976) Anal Biochem 70:54–63 – Lomax MI, Greenberg GR (1967) J Biol Chem 242:109–113 – Nunberg JH, Kaufman RJ, Chang ACY, Cohen SN, Schimke RT (1980) Cell 19:355–364 – Schimke RT, Kaufman RJ, Alt FW, Kellems RF (1978) Science 202:1051–1055 – Southern EM (1975) J Mol Biol 98:503–517 – Wahl GM, Stern M, Stark GR (1979) Proc Natl Acad Sci USA 76:3683–3687

Haematology and Blood Transfusion Vol. 26
Modern Trends in Human Leukemia IV
Edited by Neth, Gallo, Graf, Mannweiler, Winkler
© Springer-Verlag Berlin Heidelberg 1981

Structure of the Lysozyme Gene and Expression in the Oviduct and Macrophages

H. Hauser, T. Graf, H. Beug, I. Greiser-Wilke, W. Lindenmaier, M. Grez, H. Land, K. Giesecke, and G. Schütz

A. Introduction

Lysozyme, a specific differentiation marker for the myeloid lineage of hematopoietic differentiation in mammals (Hansen 1974), is also found in chicken hematopoietic cells (macrophages) (H. Hauser, unpublished work). In the mature hen oviduct lysozyme is produced as one of the major egg white proteins under the control of steroid hormones (Palmiter 1972; Hynes et al. 1979; Schutz et al. 1978).

We show that in chicken macrophages and oviduct cells the same mRNAs are transcribed from a single lysozyme gene. In macrophages, however, the lysozyme gene is expressed at a much lower rate and does not seem to be under the control of steroid hormones.

B. Organization of the Chicken Lysozyme Gene

The lysozyme structural gene is interrupted by three introns on the genomic DNA (Fig. 1). Hybridization data indicate that this gene is probably represented only once per haploid genome (Nguyen-Huu et al. 1979; Lindenmaier et al. 1980). Restriction mapping of sperm, oviduct, and erythrocyte DNA leads to the conclusion that the organization of the coding, intervening, and surrounding sequences of the lysozyme gene are identical or very similar in these tissues. This indicates that gene rearrangement during differentiation does not occur (Sippel et al. 1980).

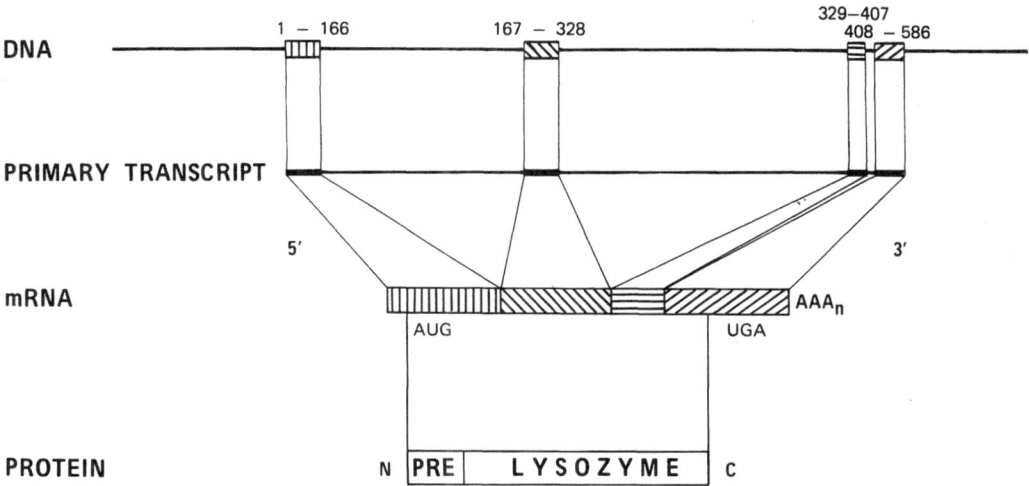

Fig. 1. Schematic representation of the structure and expression of the chicken lysozyme gene

C. Expression of the Chicken Lysozyme Gene in Oviduct

Treatment of young chicks with estrogen leads to the differentiation and proliferation of the oviduct cells and the production of the egg white proteins and their specific mRNAs. Hormone withdrawal leads to deinduction of the egg white protein specific mRNAs. Readministration of estrogen to withdrawn animals reinduces the accumulation of the specific egg white protein mRNAs. This accumulation is due to changes in the rate of transcription of the egg white protein genes and selective stabilization of their mRNAs (Hynes et al. 1979; Schütz et al. 1978; Palmiter and Carey 1974; Swaneck et al. 1979).

To understand the mechanism by which the functional lysozyme mRNA is generated from the split gene, we have analyzed oviduct nuclear RNA containing lysozyme-specific sequences by size analysis (Northern hybridization), S1 nuclease mapping, and electron microscopy. Active mRNA is produced by sequential splicing of the intervening sequences from the primary transcript. This can be seen in the electron micrographs presented in Fig. 2. From these data we could show that the 5' and 3' end of lysozyme pre-mRNA appear to be conserved during mRNA maturation.

D. Expression of the Chicken Lysozyme Gene in Macrophages

Lysozyme is also synthesized in chicken macrophages. The synthesis, however, does not seem to be under the control of steroid hormones (H. Hauser, unpublished work). To compare the lysozyme mRNA from oviduct and macrophages we have hybridized lysozyme cDNA obtained from highly purified oviduct lysozyme mRNA to poly(A) containing RNA from macrophages. Size analysis of the hybrids after S1 digestion indicates that macrophage lysozyme mRNA is homologous to

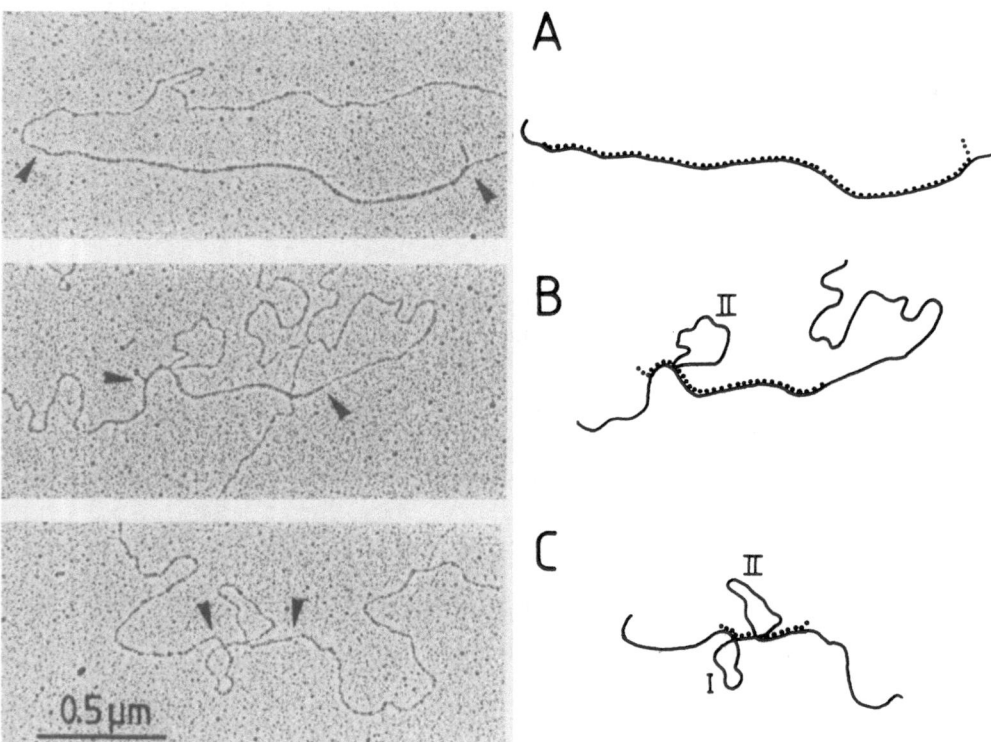

Fig. 2. Analysis of nuclear lysozyme specific-RNA. Nuclear RNA was hybridized to cloned lysozyme DNA in conditions favorable for the formation of hybrids but preventing DNA-DNA duplex formation (Lindenmaier et al. 1980)

the lysozyme cDNA prepared from oviduct mRNA (Fig. 3). Together with the data from chromosomal gene analysis these data indicate that the chicken macrophage lysozyme mRNA

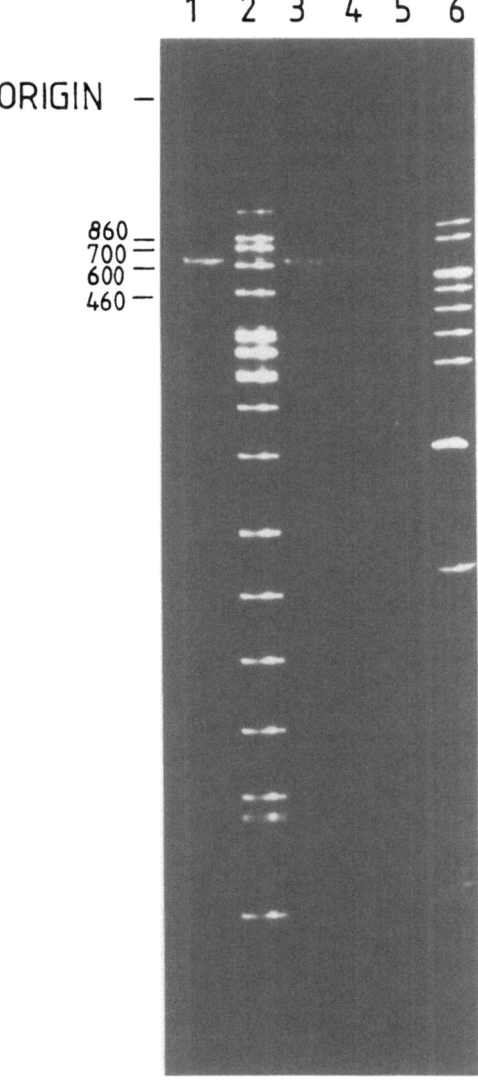

ORIGIN —

860
700
600
460

Fig. 3. The lysozyme mRNA sequence isolated from the oviduct is contained in lysozyme mRNA from macrophages. Total poly(A)-containing RNA from macrophages *(Lane 1)* and oviduct *(Lane 3)* were hybridized to full-length cDNA prepared from lysozyme mRNA purified from the oviduct. The hybrids were treated with S1-nuclease and electrophoresed on a DNA sequencing gel. *Lanes 4 and 5,* cDNA alone before and after S1-nuclease digestion; *Lanes 2 and 6,* DNA size markers

is transcribed from the same gene as in the oviduct.

The avian retroviruses AMV and MC29 transform preferentially cellular precursors of myeloblasts and macrophages, respectively, and appear to block their differentiation (Graf and Beug 1978). Specific markers of myeloid differentiation indicate that the transformed cell lines are promyeloblasts (AMV-transformed) and promacrophages (MC29-transformed) (Beug et al. 1979). Bone marrow cell lines transformed by AMV and MC29 were found to secrete different amounts of lysozyme independently of the addition of hormones (Table 1).

The AMV transformed cell line can be induced by exposure to Na-butyrate so synthesize 20-fold higher levels of lysozyme than untreated cells (Fig. 4). Quantitations of the lysozyme mRNA is in progress to analyze whether the induction of the enzyme is regulated at the level of transcription.

The results described provide a new model to compare the different molecular mechanisms involved in regulation of the chicken lysozyme gene. In oviduct cells the lysozyme gene is expressed under the control of steroid hormones. In mature macrophages, however, it is expressed constitutively. Induction of expression during cell differentiation can be studied in myeloid cell lines.

References

Beug H, von Kirchbach A, Döderlein G, Conscience J-F, Graf T (1979) Chicken hematopoietic cells transformed by seven strains of defective avian leukemia viruses display three distinct phenotypes of differentiation. Cell 18:375–390 – Graf T, Beug H (1978) Avian leukemia viruses – interaction with their target cells in vivo and in vitro. Biochim Biophys Acta 516:269–299 – Hansen NE (1974) Plasma lysozyme – a measure of neutrophil turnover. Ser Haematol 7:1–87 – Hynes NE, Groner B, Sippel AE, Jeep S, Wurtz T, Nguyen-Huu MC, Giesecke K, Schütz G (1979) Control of cellular content of chicken egg-white protein-specific RNA during estrogen administration and withdrawal. Biochemistry 18:616 – Lindenmaier W, Nguyen-Huu MC, Lurz R, Stratmann M, Blin N, Wurtz T, Hauser HJ, Sippel AE, Schütz G (1980) Arragement of coding and intervening sequences of the chicken lysozyme gene. Proc Natl Acad Sci USA 76:6196 – Nguyen-Huu MC, Stratmann M, Groner B, Land H, Lindenmaier W, Wurtz T, Giesecke K, Sippel AE, Schütz G (1979) The chicken lysozyme

Table 1. The lysozyme protein content in the cell supernatant was determined by its enzymatic activity with the lysozyme plaque assay 24 h after medium change. The mRNA concentrations were determined by cDNA excess hybridization with cDNAs from purified lysozyme and ovalbumin mRNA. Lysozyme gene expression in different cells

Cell type	Source	Lysozyme protein	Lysozyme mRNA (molecules/cell)	Ovalbumin mRNA (molecules/cell)
Tubular gland cells	Laying hen oviduct	+++	29,000	80,000
Tubular gland cells	Hormone-withdrawn chicken oviduct	N.D.	5	5
Macrophages primary culture	Chicken	+	100–300	N.D.
MC29 (RAV-2) HBC1	MC29-transformed chicken bone marrow cells (cell line)	+	30–60	N.D.
AMV DU 1765	AMV-transformed chicken bone marrow cells (cell line)	+	5–20	<0.01
AEV6 C-2	AEV-transformed chicken bone marrow cells (cell line)	−	<0.01	<0.01

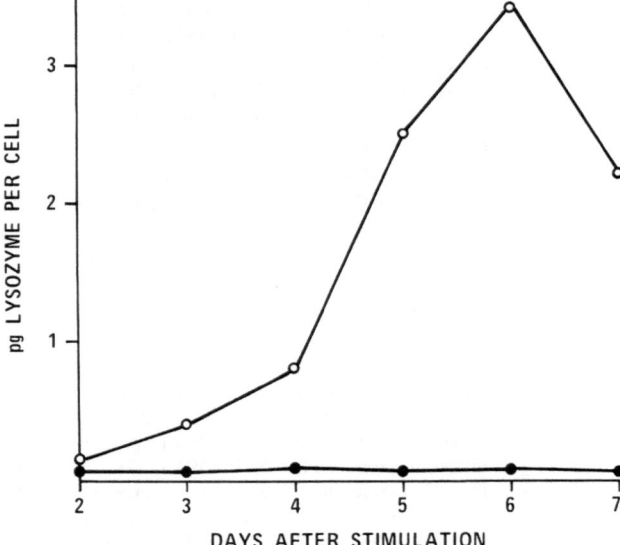

Fig. 4. Stimulation of lysozyme production in AMV-transformed cells by Na-butyrate. AMV DU 1765 cells (see also Table 1) were grown in the presence of 1 mM Na-butyrate (o). The cell density was adjusted every two days to 10^6 cells/ml. 50% of the culture medium was renewed every 2 days. The lysozyme protein content in the cell supernatant was determined by its enzymatic activity with the lysozyme plaque assay

structural gene contains several intervening sequences. Proc Natl Acad Sci USA 76:76 – Palmiter RD (1972) Regulation of protein synthesis in chick oviduct. Independent regulation of ovalbumin, conalbumin, ovomucoid, and lysozyme induction. J Biol Chem 247:6450–6458 – Palmiter RD, Carey NH (1974) Rapid inactivation of ovalbumin messenger RNA after acute withdrawal of estrogen. Proc Natl Acad Sci USA 71:2357–2361 – Schütz G, Nguyen-Huu MC, Giesecke K, Hynes NE, Groner B, Wurtz T, Sippel AE (1978) Hormonal control of egg-white protein mRNA synthesis in the chicken oviduct. Cold Spring Harbor Symp Quant Biol 42:617 – Sippel AE, Nyguyen-Huu MC, Lindenmaier W, Blin N, Lurz R, Hauser H, Giesecke K, Land H, Grez M, Schütz G (1980) Mechanism of induction of egg-white proteins by steroid hormones. In: Beato M(ed) Steroid induced uterine protein. Elsevier, New York, pp 297–314 – Swaneck GE, Nordstrom JL, Kreuzaler F, Tsai MJ, O'Malley BW (1979) Effect of estrogen on gene expression in chicken oviduct: Evidence for transcriptional control of ovalbumin gene. Proc Natl Acad Sci USA 76:1049–1053

Haematology and Blood Transfusion Vol. 26
Modern Trends in Human Leukemia IV
Edited by Neth, Gallo, Graf, Mannweiler, Winkler
© Springer-Verlag Berlin Heidelberg 1981

Some Recent Trends in Studies of Human Lymphoid Cells: B-Cells, Epstein-Barr Virus, and Transformation

J. Zeuthen and G. Klein

A. Introduction

In this brief review we will discuss some recent trends in work on regulatory mechanisms involved in the selective expression of differentiated markers in human B-cell lines as well as the types of controls involved in the expression and function of Epstein-Barr virus (EBV) associated markers in human cells. A problem of special interest in this connection is the relation of the expression of EBV functions to the expression of "transformation".

In man EBV is a lymphotropic herpesvirus (Epstein and Achong 1979). Its main target is the human B-lymphocyte (Jondal and Klein 1973), though EBV may be able to infect other cell types, provided that the membrane barrier is surpassed. EBV is known to be the causative agent of infectious mononucleosis (IM) (Henle and Henle 1979) and is associated with the two completely different human malignancies: African Burkitt's lymphoma (BL), i.e. malignant proliferation of B-cells (Fialkow et al. 1970), and nasopharyngeal carcinoma (NPC), i.e. malignant proliferation of epithelial carcinoma cells (Klein 1979). In both of these cases, the presence of the EBV genome is demonstrated by the presence of EBV DNA as well as by the presence of EBV-specific antigens. The case of NPC in itself indicates that cell types other than B-lymphocytes under the right conditions can be infected by EBV. In addition to in vitro transformed lymphoblastoid cell lines (LCL), a wide variety of B-cell lines of BL origin are available; so far it has not been possible to grow cell lines from NPC tumors.

B. Lymphoid Cell Lines

Infection of B-lymphocytes by EBV regularly leads to transformation ("immortalization") into LCL (Pope 1979). Normally, B-lymphocytes are transitory cells located within a chain of differentiation which proceeds from primitive stem cells toward mature, immunoglobulin-secreting end cells (i.e., plasma cells). EBV cannot infect either stem cells or plasma cells. Infection of B-lymphocytes is sharply restricted to surface immunoglobulin and complement (C3) receptor positive B-cells (Einhorn et al. 1978). The EBV receptor is closely related to, and perhaps identical with, the complement (C3) receptor on B-cells (Jondal et al. 1976). The cell lines of BL origin in contrast to uncloned LCL cells appear to represent clones of proliferating neoplastic cells (Van Furth et al. 1972; Fialkow et al. 1973; Béchet et al. 1974). In contrast to myeloma cell lines which represent the plasma cell type of differentiation and secrete immunoglobulin at a high rate (Matsuoka et al. 1968), BL-derived cell lines correspond to an intermediate step in B-cell differentiation and synthesize immunoglobulins, usually IgM, which are almost exclusively destined for plasma membrane integration (Klein et al. 1970; Eskeland and Klein 1971). LCL cells appear to represent a step which is intermediate between BL and myeloma cells, and immunoglobulin secretion is observed (Nilsson and Pontén 1975). Rosetting B-cells with antigen coated erythrocytes prior to in vitro EBV transformation has permitted the establishment of LCL clones that produce human monoclonal antihapten antibodies (Steinitz et al. 1977, 1978; Kozbor et al. 1979), anti-Rh (D) antibodies (Koskimies 1980), anti-streptococcal antibodies (Steinitz et al. 1979), and Rheumatoid Factor (IgM anti-IgG) (Steinitz et al., to be published).

In addition to immunoglobulin expression, other B-cell markers are useful in characterizing the state of differentiation of lymphoid cell lines. The F_c, complement (C3), and EBV receptors are fully expressed by BL cells, but their expression is decreased in LCL lines and absent on myeloma lines. Ia-like antigens are expressed by both BL and LCL cells, but their expression is decreased on myeloma cells. Insulin receptors are not expressed by typical BL cells but are expressed by LCL cells. These patterns of expression are related to the expression of these markers during the normal B-cell lineage (Nilsson 1978).

C. Chromosome studies on LCL and BL Cell Lines

All newly established LCL lines have been found to be normal diploid or to reflect the karyotype of the patient from which they were established. The lines studied have included LCL lines established spontaneously from blood of patients with acute IM (Jarvis et al. 1974) and leukemia (Hellriegel et al. 1977) as well as lines established from cord and adult peripheral blood by means of exogenous EBV or by cocultivation with X-irradiated EBV-producing cells (Jarvis et al. 1974; Hellriegel et al. 1977; Zech et al. 1976). In lines cultivated for longer times secondary changes towards aneuploidy are very often seen and gains appear to be more frequent than losses of chromosomes. Chromosome gains are not random, since trisomy is often found for chromosomes 3, 7, 8, 9, and 12; the trisomy 7 is particularly interesting, since it is found in both BL and non-BL lymphoma lines (Zech et al. 1976; Steel et al. 1977). Freshly established LCL lines from normal donors usually clone at low frequency (<2%) and are nontumorigenic in nude mice, while some long-term cultivated lines were found to be tumorigenic in nude mice (Nilsson et al. 1977).

Most BL cell lines are aneuploid. The chromosome 14 marker, first detected by Manolov and Manolova (1972) in BL biopsy cells and BL cell lines, has subsequently been identified in all BL cell lines examined with only a few exceptions. The chromosome 14 marker was originally described as an extra

band located at the end of the long arm of one chromosome 14 (14q+). Zech et al. (1976) were able to identify the translocation of a segment from the end of one of the long arms of chromosome 8 to chromosome 14 [t(8;14)(q24;q32).]. Similar chromosome abnormalities have been identified in other malignant lymphomas, but here the donor chromosomes were often variable. The specificity of the 14q+ anomaly in BL has recently been questioned by Van Den Berghe et al. (1979), who found a t(2;8)(p12;q23) in a child with typical European BL, which points to the possibility that chromosome 8 (8q−) may be more specific for the disease than the 14q+. Other chromosomal changes are often found in BL lines, such as trisomy 7 (Zech et al. 1976; Steel et al. 1977). Since this change is also found in long-term cultured LCL cells and a certain preferential retention of chromosome 7 has also been observed in hybrid cells where human chromosomes are lost, it is a possibility that these changes are selected for in tissue culture. In two BL lines (DAUDI and NA-MALWA) a region in the long arm of one chromosome 15 was lost or translocated (Zech et al. 1976; Zeuthen et al. 1977). The deletion of this region (q14-q21) was associated with the complete absence of β_2-microglobulin (DAUDI) or a reduction (NAMALWA) (Zeuthen et al. 1977). The gene for β_2-micro-globulin is located on chromosome 15 (Good-fellow et al. 1975), and the extent of this interstitial deletion agrees well with more recent regional mapping data (Oliver et al. 1978). The karyotype of DAUDI cells is interesting also in the sense that it shows no further changes than the del(15) chromosome and the t(8;14) marker from the normal diploid karyotype in contrast to other commonly used BL cell lines. In various mutant sublines of DAUDI we have found identical karyotypes with so far only one exception (DAUDI-ouab^r-TG^r) which in addition showed trisomy 7 as well as a 3q+ marker. The picture for other commonly used BL sublines (e.g., RAJI and NAMALWA) is much more complicated.

The EBV-negative lymphoma line BJAB, though reported to be derived from an African BL patient (Menezes et al. 1975), clearly lacks the 14q+ marker; in this case the original diagnosis may be doubtful, however. The EBV-negative American BL line RAMOS (Klein et al. 1975) has a 14q+ marker (Klein et al. 1976). The BJAB cell line in contrast to RAMOS is nontumorigenic in nude mice and also clones with low efficiency in agarose. Interestingly, the relatively nontransformed phenotype of BJAB dominates in hybrids with the highly transformed RAJI line, since these are low tumorigenic and clone with low efficiency in agarose (I. Ernberg, B.C. Giovanella, J. Zeuthen, unpublished). The two different EBV-negative lines have been converted to EBV-positive sublines by infection with two different strains of EBV (B95-8 and P3HR-1) (Klein et al. 1976a; Fresen and Zur Hausen 1976; Steinitz and Klein 1975). The converted sublines did not differ from their parents with respect to surface immunoglobulin or F_c receptors, but a significant increase in both EBV and complement (C3) receptors was observed (Klein et al. 1976a). All the EBV converted sublines have shown an increasingly transformed phenotype as evidenced by increased resistance to saturation, decreased serum dependence, decreased capping of surface markers, increased lectin agglutinability, and an increased ability to activate the alternative complement pathway (Steinitz and Klein 1975, 1976, 1977; Yefenof and Klein 1976; McConnell et al. 1978; Yefenof et al. 1977; Montagnier and Gruest 1979). Analyses of the karyotypes of the EBV converted lines as compared to their EBV negative parents do not indicate any consistent chromosomal changes which could explain their changed growth characteristics.

The precise role of chromosome 14 anomalies in the development of lymphomas in unknown, but it has been suggested that the rearrangement of the distal part of the long arm somehow can be advantageous for the lymphoid cells during the suggested stepwise development of an autonomous BL clone (Zech et al. 1976). This suggestion is supported by the finding of rearrangements of chromosome 14 in ataxia telangiectasia (AT), a hereditary disease associated with increased chromosome breakage as well as lymphoid neoplasia (McCaw et al. 1975). Most AT patients have clones marked by a translocation involving chromosome 14. The breaks observed in chromosome 14 have always been in the long arm at the q11-q12 region, and the other chromosomes involved in the translocations observed have been chromosomes 7, 8, 14, and X. Chromosome 14 rearrangements are found in varying proportions (2%–5%) in lymphocytes, and breakage and chromosome 14 rearrangements are highly reduced in EBV-transformed LCL lines (Cohen et al. 1979). LCL lines derived from AT patients clone at slightly increased frequencies compared to lines from normal individuals or AT carriers. By successive cloning of an AT-derived LCL lines, subclones cloning at high efficiency which are also tumorigenic in nude mice were isolated, but we have not been able to correlate this secondary change with specific chromosomal changes (I. Ernberg et al., unpublished work). It is, however, possible that in vivo selected tumorigenic subclones could show specific canges.

The individuality of the different BL lines with respect to chromosome markers have proven of great value for our work on the characterization of different hybrid cell lines obtained by fusion of BL cells. The regular presence of these markers in the parental cells and their hybrids has made it possible to identify hybrid cells by detailed chromosome analysis. An example of the identification of a typical hybrid cell (in this case DAUDI/P3HR-1) (Ber et al. 1978) is indicated in Fig. 1.

D. Studies with Hybrid Cells

In hybrids between the two BL derived cell lines RAJI and NAMALWA (Rosén et al. 1977), which express either small amounts of IgM $\varkappa$ (RAJI) or large amounts of IgMλ(NAMALWA) it was possible to quantitate the amounts of the two different types of light chains produced by the hybrid by means of radioimmunoassay. In spite of some variability between various clones tested, it appears that the hybrids expressed the same level of $\varkappa$ and λ light chains as expressed by the parents individually. We can conclude that the exclusion of one of the light chains (λ or $\varkappa$) in BL cells probably does not operate through soluble repressing factors or activating substances, since the production of $\varkappa$ and λ proceeded simultaneously and at fixed levels in the hybrid clones. The event of allelic exclusion has presumably already taken place by the programming of the genome (i.e., the V-C joining step) and has taken place on only one of the two homologous chromosomes for each immunoglobulin gene family (Bernard et al. 1978). In subsequent studies the analysis of immunoglobulin gene expression was extended to

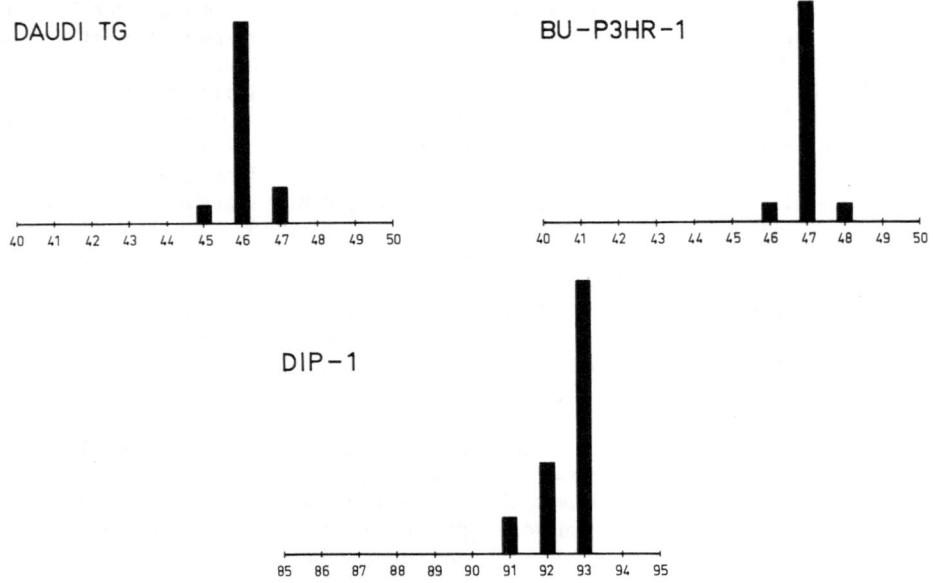

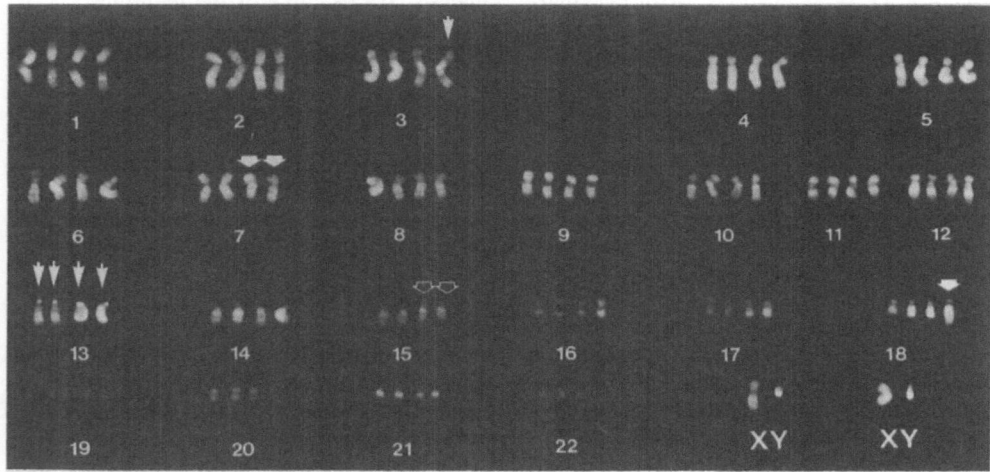

Fig. 1. Distribution of chromosome numbers in metaphases from two BL parental cell variants [*DAUDI-TG (HPRT-)* and *BU-P3HR-1 (TK-)*] and the hybrid *(DIP-1)* derived by fusion and selection of hybrids on selective HAT medium (selecting against growth of the two parents). The DIP-1 hybrid modal chromosome number is the sum of the two parents. Below is shown the karyogram of the DIP-1 hybrid. Marker chromosomes from the DAUDI-TG line are indicated by ↺, marker chromosomes from BU-P3HR-1 by ⬇, and chromosome 3 and 13 markers by ↓. (From Ber et al. 1978), by permission from the International Union Against Cancer)

other hybrid combinations. Two hybrids, RA-JI/DAUDI (8A) and RAJI/BJAB, showed more complex features than observed previously (Klein et al. 1977b), while DAUDI/P3HR-1 (Ber et al. 1978) was similar to the DAUDI parent. The RAJI/DAUDI (8A) hybrid showed a pronounced suppression of surface and intracellular immunoglobulin synthesis with amounts of μ and $\varkappa$ chains similar to the low-level expressing RAJI parent (Klein et al. 1977b). The DAUDI line has an unusual structure of its 8S surface IgM, with an associated extra band of 33,000 daltons present in addition to the 23,500 and 75,000 dalton bands corresponding to light and heavy chains, respectively (Singer and Williamson 1979). The 33K component has been suggested to be an Ia antigen, covalently bound to μ chains (Singer and Williamson 1979). A possibility is that the RAJI parent interferes with the assembly of this structure and makes it impossible for the DAUDI structure ($\mu + \varkappa + Ia$) to integrate properly into the plasma membrane. A related possibility would be that the RAJI parent, being closer to the pre-B cell stage, "extinguishes" the high degree of differentiation of DAUDI cells. However, our recent results on another RAJI/DAUDI hybrid (DITRUD) of a different derivation gave conflicting results from those obtained with our first RAJI/DAUDI hybrid, since here IgM and $\varkappa$ chains were expressed at almost as high a level as for DAUDI on the cell surface (Zeuthen et al., to be published). An illustration of the expression of surface IgM analyzed by means of flow microfluorimetry is given in Fig. 2. To understand this difference, it must be born in mind that the first (8A) hybrid was isolated as adherent cells on selective HAT medium, since the RAJI parent used was both adherent and HPRT- (Allan and Harrison 1980), and the second (DITRUD) was isolated in suspension after fusion of DAUDI (HPRT-) and RAJI (TK-) cells (Zeuthen et al., to be published). Recent results have indicated that the cell shape is correlated with the expression of the differentiated phenotype (Allan and Harrison 1980), and a likely possibility is, therefore, that the selection of adherent cells in our first fusions has worked against the full expression of the differentiated marker (in this case surface IgM $\varkappa$).

In hybrids of lymphoid cells with cells of other differentiation lineages immunoglobulin synthesis may be totally extinguished (Zeuthen and Nilsson 1976). We, therefore, found it of interest to investigate whether hybrids of BL cells with other hematopoietic cells would show the same type of restriction. A hybrid between the human erythroleukemic cell line K562 [inducible for hemoglobin synthesis by haemin (Rutherford et al. 1979)], and

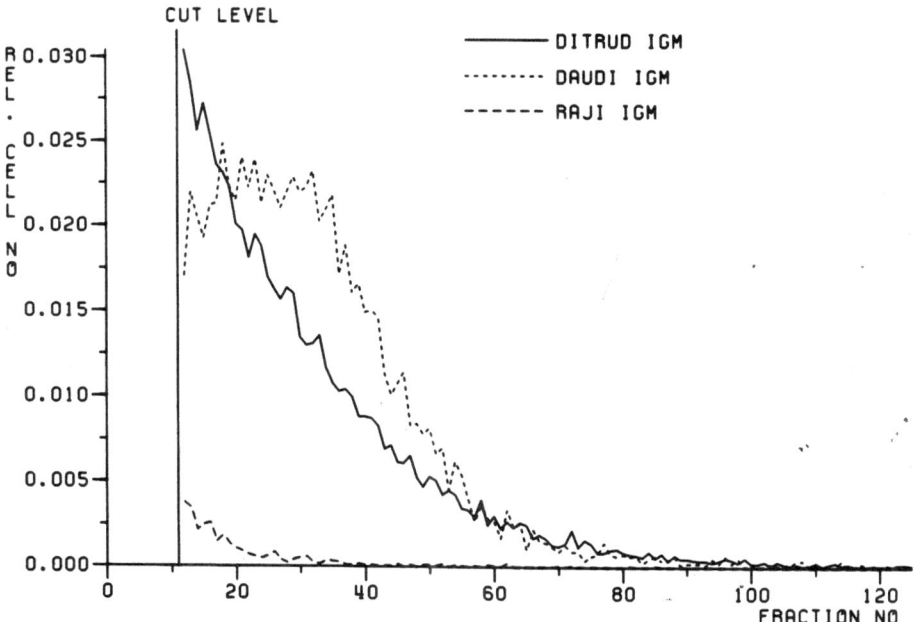

Fig. 2. An example of surface immunoglobulin expression on a RAJI/DAUDI hybrid [*DITRUD*, (Zeuthen et al., to be published)] and its two parental cells characterized by means of flow microfluorimetry after surface immunoglobulin staining for IgM. The analysis was carried out by means of a fluorescence activated cell sorter (FACS) and evaluated by a computer program. Unspecifically stained cells (<cut level) have been left out, and the percentages of cells above this level were: 3.9% (RAJI), 79.5% (DAUDI), and 68.7% (DITRUD). For discussion see text

P3HR-1 (Klein et al. 1980) showed a complete suppression of EBV receptors, and a DAUDI/K562 hybrid showed a complete suppression of surface IgM in addition to other lymphoid markers (Zeuthen et al., to be published). Both of these two hybrid combinations had similarly high levels of heme as the K562 parent and were inducible for hemoglobin synthesis by addition of hemin. An example of the induction of hemoglobin-positive cells stained by benzidine is illustrated in Fig. 3. These results indicate a relative dominance of erythroid differentiation at the expense of lymphoid differentiation in the hybrids of BL cells with the K562 line, which in many respects behaves like a relatively undifferentiated stem cell line. An additional hybrid between the human promyelocytic leukemic cell line HL 60 (Collins et al. 1977) and P3HR-1 (HP-1) was isolated recently (Koeffler, personal communication) and shows retention of B-cell Ia antigens but loss of the myeloid markers that characterize the HL-60 parent. In comparison with K562, HL-60 is more differentiated, and this might explain the fact that a reverse pattern of loss of differentiation is seen in this case.

In contrast to differentiated markers, the cellular "household" functions are usually coexpressed in cell hybrids. This has been the case for isoenzyme markers, which in addition to our chromosomal characterization have been a useful tool in the identification of hybrid cells. One curious deficiency of BL cells is a loss of soluble malic enzyme (ME_S), though this enzyme is expressed by other cell types (Povey et al., to be published). ME_S is re-expressed in hybrids of BL cells with mouse fibroblasts and in the two hybrids with K562.

The HLA specificities of the parental cells are coexpressed in hybrids. A special case here is the hybrids with DAUDI cells (β_2-microglobulin and HLA negative), where we found expression of completely new HLA specificities (A10,B38,B17) (Klein et al. 1977b; Fellous et al. 1977). We have interpreted this observation to indicate genetic complementation of the β_2-microglobulin deficiency of DAUDI to bring out its hidden HLA specificities in the form of new β_2-microglobulin-HLA dimer molecules on the cell membrane. The K562 line shows a similar lack of surface expressed HLA and β_2-microglobulin to DAUDI, though its intracellular content of β_2-microglobulin is normal (Zeuthen et al. 1977). This membrane defect is partially dominant in the P3HR-1/K562 hybrid (Klein et al. 1980), since only one P3HR-1 derived specificity (HLA-A3) could be detected in low amounts on the hybrid. In spite of this, complementation of the two kinds of defects were observed in the DAUDI/K562 hybrid by the expression of low amounts of HLA-B17, one of the "hidden" specificities characteristic of DAUDI cells (Zeuthen et al., to be published). A direct analysis of solubilized membrane proteins from this hybrid by crossed radioimmunoelectrophoresis (Plesner 1978) confirmed the presence of β_2-microglobulin-HLA dimer molecules in low concentration.

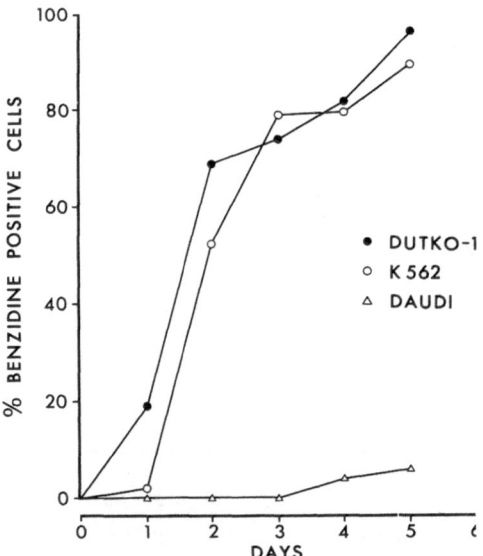

Fig. 3. Induction of benzidine-positive cells by 0.1 mM hemin in cultures of DAUDI, K562, and their hybrid *(DUTKO)* (Zeuthen et al., to be published). For discussion see text

E. Expression of EBV, the EBNA Antigen, and Transformation

Multiple copies of EBV viral genomes are present in EBV-carrying cells of both BL and LCL origin (Adams 1979). These cells invariably contain the EBV-determined nuclear antigen EBNA (Reedman and Klein 1973). While EBNA is always expressed if the EBV genome is present, the early antigens (EA) and viral capsid antigens (VCA) are only expressed during the lytic cycle (Ernberg and Klein

1979). The EBV-carrying cell lines can be classified into three cathegories: nonproducers (EBNA+, EA−, VCA−), abortive producers (EBNA+, EA+, VCA−), and finally producers (EBNA+, EA+, VCA+). The number of cells entering the lytic cycle can be amplified by inducers (IUdR, Na-butyrate, TPA) whose only common denominator is a known effect on differentiation in a variety of cell systems. Abortive producers such as RAJI switch on EA production in a small proportion of cells, but these do not proceed further to viral DNA synthesis and VCA production (Gergely et al. 1971). The block in the abortive producer cell lines could either be due to viral defectiveness or to negative cellular controls. The latter is more likely, since we have recently found that hybridization of RAJI with BJAB lifts the block to viral DNA replication and subsequent VCA production.

Other combinations in cell hybrids have given us further information with respect to the types of controls involved. With certain minor variations, the picture is consistent: When producer BL lines are fused with nonproducers, producer status tends to dominate over nonproducer status and inducibility over noninducibility (Ber et al. 1978; Nyormoi et al. 1973; Klein et al. 1976b, 1977b; Moar et al. 1978). This suggests that the controls appear to be of a positive nature. The results on the RAJI/BJAB hybrid and the observation that inducers used interfere with differentiation, while standard mutagenic or carcinogenic agents are noninducers (Zur Hausen et al. 1979), strongly suggests that the controls are cellular rather than viral.

It is of interest that EBV production and inducibility in many cases parallel the behavior of other B-cell markers in cell hybrids. In the cases where BL cells were hybridized with fibroblasts, virus production and inducibility were switched off in spite of the continued presence of EBV-DNA in multiple genome copies per cell and uninfluenced expression of EBNA (Klein et al. 1974; Glaser et al. 1977). In the P3HR-1/K562 hybrid a similar complete block against EA and VCA inducibility was observed using the three inducers IUdR, Na-butyrate and TPA (Klein et al. 1980). The DAUDI/K562 hybrid (Zeuthen et al., to be published), however, was inducible, probably due to a higher number of EBV copies.

An exception to the rule of extinction of EBV inducibility in hybrids of BL cells with other lineages are hybrids with human carcinoma cells (Glaser and Rapp 1972; Glaser and Nonoyama 1973; Tanaka et al. 1977; Baron and Strominger 1978), were the hybrids were completely permissive. This observation might be of some relevance to NPC, since epithelial carcinoma cells might be more compatible with EBV production than other human cells of non-B-cell origin.

Like the T antigens of the small DNA viruses, EBNA is a DNA binding protein (Lenoir et al. 1976; Luka et al. 1977, 1978, to be published). Purified EBNA antigen has a molecular weight of $\sim$180,000 daltons and consists of two major components of 48,000 and 53,000 daltons (Luka et al., to be published). While the 48K component is probably virus coded, the 53K component is also found in EBV-negative lymphoma lines, but not in T-cell derived cell lines. It is, therefore, possible that the 53K protein is a nuclear protein characteristic of malignant B-cells. A similar 53K component has been found in SV40 T antigen (McCormick and Harlow 1980), suggesting a further analogy between EBV and the much smaller papovaviruses. In recent experiments we have used fusion of EBNA loaded erythrocyte ghosts with quiescent cells to "microinject" (Klein et al. 1980, Zeuthen, unpublished work). In these experiments a stimulation of cellular DNA synthesis was observed to occur after microinjection (Fig. 4). In experiments with the isolated 48K and 53K components, the 53K component appears to have this activity. These observations are similar to the stimulation of DNA synthesis in quiescent cells after microinjection of the SV40 T antigen (Tjian et al. 1978).

A quantitative relation between SV40 T antigen levels and viral late gene expression was recently described (Graessmann et al. 1978): SV40-infected cells with levels of T antigen above a certain treshold value expressed late viral genes. An interpretation of this observation is that an excess of T antigen is required to saturate binding sites on cellular DNA and in addition provide sufficient molecules to initiate DNA replication (and late gene expression). A similar mechanism could perhaps control the induction of viral DNA synthesis and VCA production in BL cells. Measurements by immunofluorimetry of EBNA in induced cultures of RAJI, DAUDI, and P3HR-1 cells show that EBNA immunofluorescence after induction is doubled after induction in the

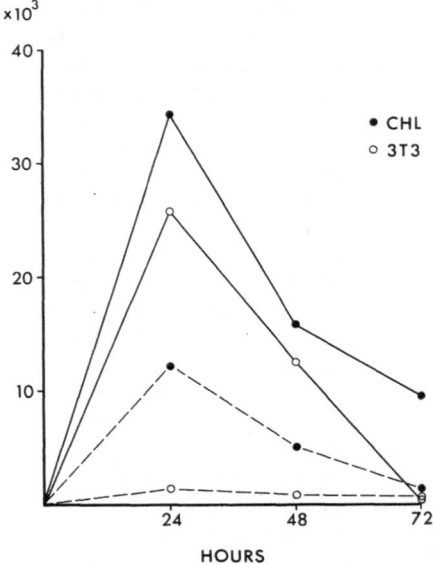

Fig. 4. Stimulation of the rates of DNA synthesis in contact-inhibited monolayers of primary chinese hamster lung *(CHL)* cells and in monolayers of mouse 3T3 cells after erythrocyte ghost mediated microinjection of purified EBNA antigen. Rates of DNA synthesis were followed by pulse labeling of replicate slides with 1 uC$_i$/ml (^{3}H)-thymidine for 2 h for each time point. *Solid lines* indicate cultures microinjected with EBNA, *broken lines* cells microinjected with a mock preparation (HMG proteins from EBV-negative cells). (Zeuthen, unpublished work)

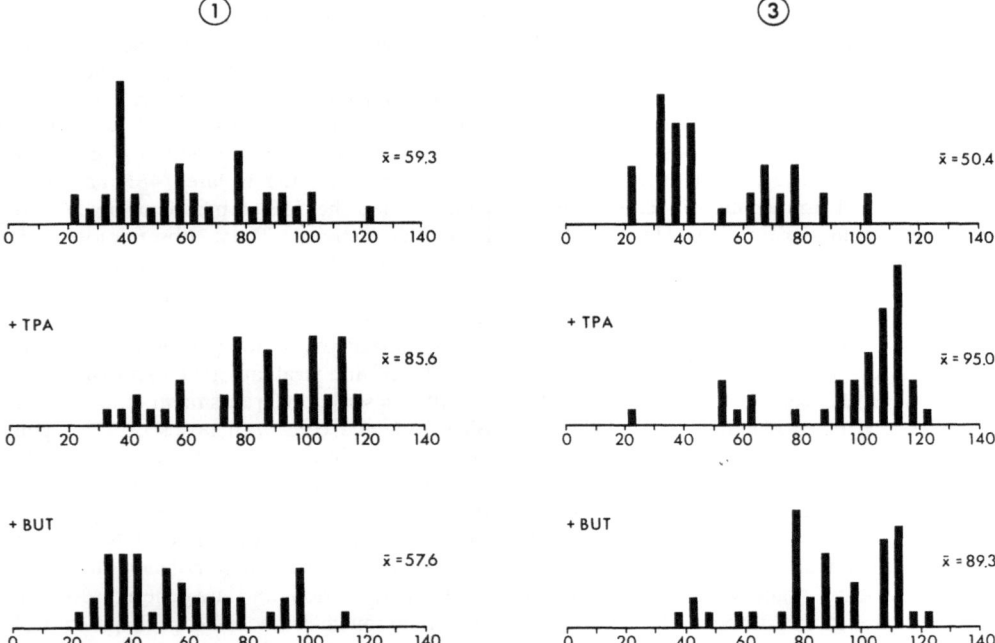

Fig. 5. Quantitative immunofluorimetric measurements of EBNA immunofluorescence stained (Reedman and Klein 1973) slides prepared from control, TPA, and Na-butyrate induced cultures of DAUDI cells, 1 and 3 days after start of the experiment. In the induced cultures the average immunofluorescence values approximately double; this effect was not observed with the abortive producer RAJI line (Zeuthen and Ernberg, unpublished work). For discussion see text

186

producer lines (DAUDI and P3HR-1), but in fact reduced for the abortive producer RAJI line (Zeuthen and Ernberg, unpublished work). These observations could indicate a role of EBNA in the control of viral DNA synthesis and could possibly indicate a defect in RAJI cells responsible for its abortive producer status. An example of these measurements is shown in Fig. 5.

Microinjection by capillaries has been used in attempts to infect cells that lack EBV receptors with EBV-DNA or EBV viral particles. In experiments where fibroblasts were injected with P3HR-1 EBV-DNA, cells were induced to produce EA (Graessmann et al. 1980). Using a similar technique, we injected human amnion epithelial cells with a $100\times$ concentrated supernatant of B95-8 cells and found 50%–100% of the injected cells to become positive for EBNA (Zeuthen J, Rosenbaum S, Sørensen ET, unpublished) (Fig. 6).

Only a few batches of concentrated B95-8 viruses were effective in inducing EBNA, probably due to the limiting concentration of EBV particles. Attempts to select for growth of EBNA positive cells by further cultivation were unsuccesful and the infection achieved by microinjection of EBV in amnion epithelial cells can possibly be abortive.

Acknowledgements

We thank our colleagues for stimulating collaboration, discussions, and exchange of information. It will be evident from this article that without this it would have been impossible to collect the data. The projects have been generously supported by the Danish Cancer Society, the Danish Natural Science Research Council, Contract No. N01 CP 33316 from the Division of Cancer Cause and Prevention, National Cancer Institute, Public Health Service Reserach Grant No. 55R01 CA 14054-05, and the Swedish Cancer Society.

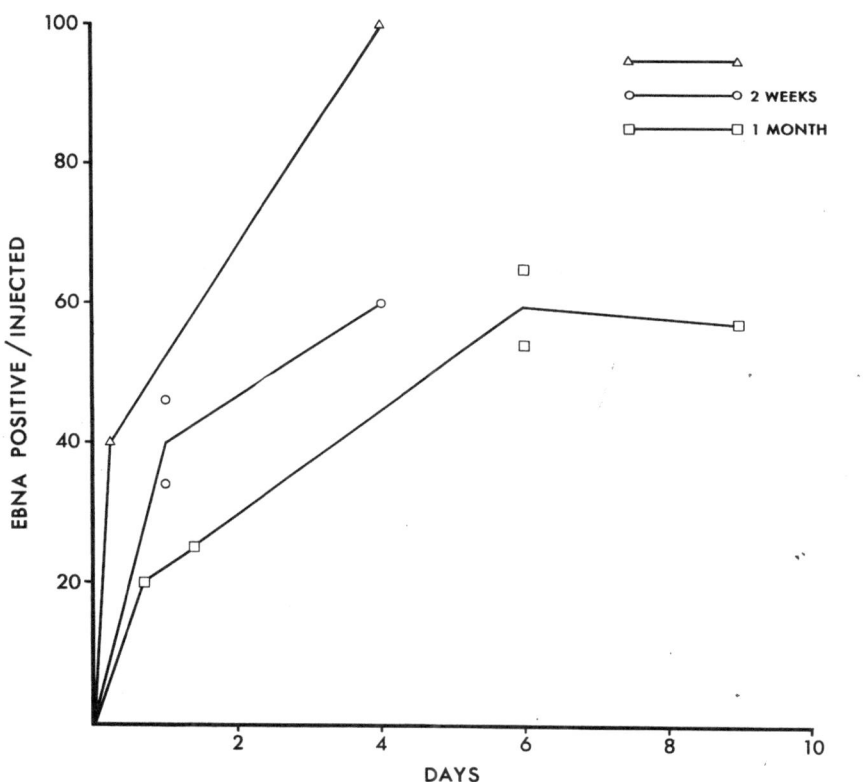

Fig. 6. Appearance of EBNA positive human amnion epithelial cells after microinjection by microcapillaries of a $100\times$ concentrated supernatant of B95-8 cells (inducing 10% EBNA positive RAMOS (EBV-negative) cells at 1:320 dilution) in three successive experiments with the same preparation of B95-8 stored for various times (0, 2 weeks and 1 month) at 4°C. (Zeuthen et al., unpublished)

References

Adams A (1979) The state of the virus genome in transformed cells and its relationship to host cell DNA. In: Epstein MA, Achong BG (eds) The Epstein-Barr virus. Springer, Berlin, p 155 – Allan M, Harrison P (1980) Co-expression of differentiation markers in hybrids between Friend cells and lymphoid cells and the influence of cell shape. Cell 19:437 – Baron D, Strominger JL (1978) Partial purification and properties of the Epstein-Barr virus – associated nuclear antigen. J Biol Chem 253:2875 – Béchet JM, Fialkow RJ, Nilsson K, Klein G (1974) Immunoglobulin synthesis and glucose-6-phosphate dehydrogenase as cell markers in human lymphoblastoid cell lines. Exp Cell Res 89:275 – Ber R, Klein G, Moar M, Povey S, Rosén A, Westman A, Yefenof E, Zeuthen J (1978) Somatic cell hybrids between human lymphoma lines. IV. Establishment and characterization of a P3HR-1/DAUDI hybrid. Int J Cancer 21:707 – Bernard O, Hozumi N, Tonegawa S (1978) Sequences of mouse immunoglobulin light chain genes before and after somatic changes. Cell 15:1133 – Clements GB, Klein G, Povey S (1975) Production by EBV infection of an EBNA-positive subline from an EBNA-negative human lymphoma cell line without detectable EBV DNA. Int J Cancer 16:125 – Cohen MM, Sagi M, Ben-Zur Z, Schaap T, Voss R, Kohn G (1979) Ataxia telangiectasia: Chromosomal stability in continuous lymphoblastoid cell lines. Cytogenet Cell Genet 23:44 – Collins SJ, Gallo RC, Gallagher RE (1977) Continuous growth and differentiation of human myeloid leukaemic cells in suspension culture. Nature 270:347 – Einhorn L, Steinitz M, Yefenof E, Ernberg I, Bakacs T, Klein G (1978) Epstein-Barr virus (EBV) receptors complement receptors, and EBV infectability of different lymphocyte fractions of human peripheral blood. II. Epstein-Barr virus studies. Cell Immunol 35:43 – Epstein MA, Achong BG (1979) Discovery and general biology of the virus. In: Epstein MA, Achong BG (eds) The Epstein-Barr virus. Berlin, Springer, p 1 – Ernberg I, Klein G (1979) EB virus-induced antigens. In: The Epstein MA, Achong BG (eds) The Epstein-Barr virus. Springer, Berlin, p 39 – Eskeland T, Klein E (1971) Isolation of 7S IgM and kappa chains from the surface membrane of tissue culture cells derived from a Burkitt lymphoma. J Immunol 107:1367 – Fellous M, Kamoun M, Wiels J, Dausset J, Clements G, Zeuthen J, Klein G (1977) Induction of HLA expression in Daudi cells after cell fusion. Immunogenetics 5:423 – Fialkow PJ, Klein G, Gartler SM, Clifford P (1970) Clonal origin for individual Burkitt tumors. Lancet I;384 – Fialkow PJ, Klein E, Klein G, Clifford P, Singh S (1973) Immunoglobulin and glucose-6-phosphate dehydrogenase as markers of cellular origin in Burkitt lymphoma. J Exp Med 138:89 – Fresen KO, zur Hausen H (1976) Establishment of EBNA-expressing cell lines by infection of Epstein-Barr virus (EBV)-genome-negative human lymphoma cells with different EBV strains. Int J Cancer 17:161 – Gergely L, Klein G, Ernberg I (1971) The action of DNA antagonists on Epstein-Barr virus (EBV)-associated early antigens (EA) in Burkitt lymphoma lines. Int J Cancer 7:293 – Glaser R, Nonoyama M (1973) Epstein-Barr virus: Detection of the genome in somatic cell hybrids of Burkitt lymphoblastoid cells. Science 179:492 – Glaser R, Rapp F (1972) Rescue of Epstein-Barr virus from somatic cell hybrids of Burkitt lymphoblastoid cells. J Virol 10:288 – Glaser R, Ablashi DV, Nonoyama M, Henle W, Easton J (1977) Enhanced oncogenic behavior of human and mouse cells after cellular hybridization with Burkitt tumor cells. Proc Natl Acad Sci USA 74:2574 – Goodfellow PN, Jones EA, van Heyningen V, Solomon E, Bobrow M, Miggiano V, Bodmer WP (1975) The β_2-microglobulin gene is on chromosome 15 and not in the HLA region. Nature 254:267 – Graessmann A, Graessmann M, Guhl E, Mueller C (1978) Quantitative correlation between simian virus 40 T-antigen synthesis and late viral gene expression in permissive and non-permissive cells. J Cell Biol 77:R1 – Graessmann A, Wolf H, Bornkamm GW (1980) Expression of Epstein-Barr virus genes in different cell types after microinjection of viral DNA. Proc Natl Acad Sci USA 77:433 – Hellriegel KP, Diehl V, Krause PH, Meier S, Blankenstein M, Busche W (1977) The significance of chromosomal findings for the differentiation between lymphoma and lymphoblastoid cell lines. In: Thierfelder S, Rodt H, Thiel E (eds) Hematology and blood transfusion. Immunological diagnosis of leukemias and lymphomas. Springer, Berlin, p. 307 – Henle G, Henle W (1979) The virus as the etiologic agent of infectious mononucleosis. In: Epstein MA, Achong BG (eds) The Epstein-Barr virus. Springer, Berlin, p 297 – Jarvis JE, Ball G, Rickinson AB, Epstein MA (1974) Cytogenetic studies on human lymphoblastoid cell lines from Burkitt's lymphoma and other sources. Int J Cancer 14:716 – Jondal M, Klein G (1973) Surface markers on human B and T lymphocytes. II. Presence of Epstein-Barr virus (EBV) receptors on B lymphocytes. J Exp Med 138:1365 – Jondal M, Klein G, Oldstone M, Bokish V, Yefenof E (1976), Surface markers on human B and T lymphocytes. VIII. Association between complement and Epstein-Barr virus (EBV) receptors on human lymphoid cells. Scand J Immunol 5:401 – Klein G (1979) The relationship of the virus to nasopharyngeal carcinoma. In: Epstein MA, Achong BG (eds) The Epstein-Barr virus. Springer, Berlin, p 339 – Klein E, Eskeland T, Inoue M, Strom R, Johansson B (1970) Surface immunoglobulin moieties on lymphoid cells. Exp Cell Res 62:133 – Klein G, Wiener F, Zech L, zur Hausen H, Reedman B (1974) Segregation of the EBV-determined nuclear antigen (EBNA) in somatic cell hybrids derived from the fusion of a mouse fibroblast and a human Burkitt line. Int J Cancer 14:54 – Klein

G, Giovanella B, Westman A, Stehlin J, Mumford D (1975) An EBV-genome-negative cell line established from an American Burkitt lymphoma: Receptor characteristics, EBV infectability and permanent conversion into EBV-positive sublines by in vitro infection. Intervirology 5:319 – Klein G, Zeuthen J, Terasaki P, Billing R, Honig R, Jondal M, Westman A, Clements G (1976a) Inducibility of the Epstein-Barr virus (EBV) cycle and surface marker properties of EBV-negative lymphoma lines and their in vitro EBV-converted sublines. Int J Cancer 18:639 – Klein G, Clements G, Zeuthen J, Westman A (1976b) Somatic cell hybrid between human lymphoma lines. II. Spontaneous and induced patterns of the Epstein-Barr virus (EBV) cycle. Int J Cancer 17:71515 – Klein G, Terasaki P, Billing R, Honig R, Jondal M, Rosén A, Zeuthen J, Clements G (1977a) Somatic cell hybrids between human lymphoma lines. III. Surface markers. Int J Cancer 19:66 – Klein G, Clements G, Zeuthen J, Westman A (1977b) Spontaneous and induced patterns of the Epstein-Barr virus (EBV) cycle in a new set of somatic cell hybrids. Cancer Lett 3:91 – Klein G, Zeuthen J, Eriksson I, Terasaki P, Bernoco M, Rosén A, Masucci G, Povey S, Ber R (1980) Hybridization of a myeloid leukemia – derived human cell line (K562) with a human Burkitt's lymphoma line (P3HR-1). J Natl Cancer Inst 64:725 – Klein G, Luka J, Zeuthen J (1980) Epstein-Barr virus (EBV)-induced transformation and the role of the nuclear antigen (EBNA). Cold Spring Harbor Symp Quant Biol 44:253 – Koskimies S (1980) A human lymphoblastoid cell line producing specific antibody against Rh-D antigen. Scand J Immunol 11:73 – Kozbor D, Steinitz M, Klein G, Koskimies S, Mäkelä O (1979) Establishment of anti-TNP antibody producing human lymphoid lines by preselection for hapten binding followed by EBV transformation. Scand J Immunol 10:187 – Lenoir G, Berthelon MC, Faure MC, de Thé G (1976) Characterization of Epstein-Barr virus antigens. I. Biochemical analysis of the complement-fixing soluble antigen and relationship with Epstein-Barr virus – associated nuclear antigen. J Virol 17:672 – Luka J, Siegert W, Klein G (1977) Solubilization of the Epstein-Barr virus determined nuclear antigen and its characterization as a DNA-binding protein. J Virol 22:1 – Luka J, Lindahl T, Klein G (1978) Purification of the Epstein-Barr virus determined nuclear antigen from Epstein-Barr virus transformed human lymphoid cell lines. J Virol 27:604 – Luka J, Jörnvall H, Klein G (to be published) Purification and biochemical characterization of the Epstein-Barr virus (EBV) determined nuclear antigen (EBNA) and and an associated protein with a 53K subunit. – Manolov G, Manolova Y (1972) marker band in one chromosome 14 from Burkitt lymphomas. Nature 237:33 – Matsuoka Y, Takahashi M, Yagi Y, Moore GE, Pressman D (1968) Synthesis and secretion of immunoglobulins by established cell lines of human hematopoietic origin.

J Immunol 101:1111 – McCaw KB, Hecht F, Harnden DG, Teplitz RJ (1975) Somatic rearrangement of chromosome 14 in human lymphocytes. Proc Natl Acad Sci USA 72:2071 – McConnell I, Klein G, Lint TF, Lachmann PJ (1978) Activation of the alternative complement pathway by human B cell lymphoma lines is associated with Epstein-Barr virus transformation of the cells. Eur J. Immunol 8:453 – McCormick F, Harlow E (1980) Association of a murine 53,000-dalton phosphoprotein with simian virus 40 large-T antigen in transformed cells. J Virol 34:213 – Menezes J, Leibold W, Klein G, Clements G (1975) Establishment of an Epstein-Barr virus (EBV)-negative lymphoblastoid B cell line (BJA-B) from an exceptional, EBV-genome-negative African Burkitt's lymphoma. Biomedicine 22:276 – Moar MH, Ber R, Klein G, Westman A, Eriksson I (1978) Somatic cell hybrids between human lymphoma lines. V. IUdR inducibility and P3HR-1 superinfectability of Daudi/HeLa (DAD) and Daudi/P3HR-1 (DIP-1) cell lines. Int J Cancer 22:669 – Montagnier L, Gruest J (1979) Cell-density-dependence for growth in agarose of two human lymphoma lines and its decrease after Epstein-Barr virus conversion. Int J Cancer 23:71 – Nilsson K (1978) Established human lymphoid cell lines as models for B-lymphocyte differentiation. In: Serrou B, Rosenfeld C (eds) Human lymphocyte differentiation: Its application to cancer. North-Holland, Amsterdam, p 307 – Nilsson K, Pontén J (1975) Classification and biological nature of established human hematopoietic cell lines. Int J Cancer 15:321 – Nilsson K, Giovanella BC, Stehlin JS, Klein G (1977) Tumorigenicity of human hematopoietic cell lines in athymic nude mice. Int J Cancer 19:337 – Nyormoi O, Klein G, Adams A, Dombos L (1973) Sensitivity to EBV superinfection and IUdR inducibility of hybrid cells formed between a sensitive and a relatively resistant Burkitt lymphoma cell line. Int J Cancer 12:396 – Oliver N, Francke U, Pellegrino MA (1978) Regional assignment of genes for mannose phosphate isomerase, pyruvate kinase 3, and β_2-microglobulin expression on human chromosome 15 by hybridization of cells from a t(15;22) (q14;q13.3) translocation carrier. Cytogenet Cell Genet 22:506 – Plesner T (1978) Lymphocyte associated β_2-microglobulin studied by crossed radioimmunoelectrophoresis. Scand J Immunol 8:363 – Pope JH (1979) Transformation by the virus in vitro. In: Epstein MA, Achong BG (eds) The Epstein-Barr virus. Springer, Berlin p 205 – Povey S, Jeremiah S, Arthur E, Ber R, Fialkow PJ, Gardiner E, Goodfellow PN, Karande A, Quintero M, Steel CM, Zeuthen J (to be published) Deficiency of malic enzyme: A possible marker for malignancy in lymphoid cells Ann Hum Genet – Reedman B, Klein G (1973) Cellular localization of an Epstein-Barr virus (EBV)-associated complement-fixing antigen in producer and non-producer lymphoblastoid cell lines. Int J Cancer 11:499 – Rosén A, Clements G, Klein G, Zeuthen J (1977) Double immunoglobulin production in cloned somatic cell hybrids between two human lymphoid lines. Cell 11:139 – Rutherford TR, Clegg JB, Weatherall DJ (1979) K562 human leukaemic cells synthesize embryonic haemoglobin in response to haemin. Nature 280:164 – Singer PA, Williamson AR (1979) A novel interaction involving a polypeptide chain (P33) in covalent linkage with IgM on the surface of a Burkitt lymphoma cell line (Daudi). Eur J Immunol 9:224 – Steel CM, Woodward MA, Davidson C, Philipson J, Arthur E (1977) Non-random chromosome gains in human lymphoblastoid cell lines. Nature 270:349 – Steinitz M, Klein G (1975) Comparison between growth characteristics of an Epstein-Barr virus (EBV)-genome negative lymphoma line and its EBV-converted subline in vitro. Proc Natl Acad Sci USA 72:3518 – Steinitz M, Klein G (1976) Epstein-Barr virus (EBV)-induced change in saturation density and serum dependence of established, EBV-negative lymphoma lines in vitro. Virology 70:570 – Steinitz M, Klein G (1977) Further studies on the differences in serum dependence in EBV-negative lymphoma lines and their in vitro converted, virus-genome carrying sublines. Eur J Cancer 13:1269 – Steinitz M, Klein G, Koskimies S, Mäkelä O (1977) EB virus-induced B-lymphocyte cell lines producing specific antibody. Nature 269:420 – Steinitz M, Koskimies S, Klein G, Mäkelä O (1978) Establishment of specific antibody producing human cell lines by antigen preselection and EBV transformation. Curr Top Microbiol Immunol 81:156 – Steinitz M, Seppälä I, Klein G, Koskimies S, Mäkelä O (1979) Immunobiology 156:41 – Steinitz M, Izak G, Cohen S, Ehrenfeld M, Flechner J (to be published) Continuous production of rheumatoid factor by in vitro EBV-transformed lymphocytes. Nature – Tanaka A, Nonoyama M, Glaser R (1977) Transcription of latent Epstein-Barr virus genomes in human epithelial/Burkitt hybrid cells. Virology 82:63 – Tjian R, Fey G, Graessmann A (1978) Biological activity of purified simian virus 40 T antigen proteins. Proc Natl Acad Sci USA 75:1279 – Van den Berghe, H, Parloir C, Gosseye S, Englebienne V, Cornu G, Sokal G (1979) Variant translocation in Burkitt lymphoma Cancer Genet Cytogenet 1:9 – Van Furth R, Gorter H, Nadkarni JS, Klein E, Clifford P (1972) Synthesis of immunoglobulins by biopsied tissues and cell lines from Burkitt's lymphoma. Immunology 22:847 – Yefenof E, Klein G (1976) Difference in antibody induced redistribution of membrane IgM in EBV-genome free and EBV-positive human lymphoid cells. Exp Cell Res 99:175 – Yefenof E, Klein G, Ben-Bassat H, Lundin L (1977) Differences in the ConA-induced redistribution and agglutination patterns of EBV genome-free and EBV-carrying human lymphoma lines. Exp Cell Res 108:185 – Zech L, Haglund U, Nilsson K, Klein G (1976) Characteristic chromosomal abnormalities in biopsies and lymphoid cell lines from patients with Burkitt and non-Burkitt lymphomas. Int J Cancer 17:47 – Zeuthen J, Nilsson K (1976) Hybridization of a human myeloma permanent cell line with mouse cells. Cell Differ 4:355 – Zeuthen J, Friedrich U, Rosén A, Klein E (1977) Structural abnormalities in chromosome 15 in cell lines with reduced expression of Beta-2 microglobulin. Immunogenetics 4:567 – Zeuthen J, Klein G, Ber R, Masucci G, Bisballe S, Povey S, Terasaki P, Ralph P (to be published) Human lymphoma/lymphoma and lymphoma/leukemia hybrids. I. Isolation, characterization, cell surface and B-cell marker studies. J Natl Cancer Inst – Zur Hausen H, Bornkamm GW, Schmidt R, Hecker E (1979) Tumor initiators and promotors in the induction of Epstein-Barr virus. Proc Natl Acad Sci USA 76:782

Haematology and Blood Transfusion Vol. 26
Modern Trends in Human Leukemia IV
Edited by Neth, Gallo, Graf, Mannweiler, Winkler
© Springer-Verlag Berlin Heidelberg 1981

Epstein-Barr Virus: Its Site of Persistence and Its Role in the Development of Carcinomas

H. Wolf, E. Wilmes and G. J. Bayliss

A. Introduction

Epstein-Barr virus (EBV) causes in man infectious mononucleosis as a "primary" disease. Burkitt's Lymphoma and Nasopharyngeal Carcinoma may be considered as "secondary" diseases developing only in persons with long preceeding EBV infection.

Following the primary infection with EBV, virus can be isolated from the salivary duct (Morgan et al. 1979) and from throat swabs for months or years (Gerber et al. 1972; Chang and Golden 1971), and B-lymphocytes are lifelong carriers of EBV genomes (Nilsson et al. 1971) and can be used to establish lymphoblastoid cell lines (Pope 1967; Rickinson et al. 1980). For the nasopharyngeal carcinoma, where serology (for review see Henle and Henle 1979) suggested that EBV is regularly associated with the disease, it has been shown by in situ hybridization (Wolf et al. 1973) and other unrelated techniques involving cell separation (Desgranges et al. 1975) or passage through nude mice (Klein et al. 1974) that EBV is indeed regularly present in the epithelioid tumor cells. The ability of EBV to induce tumors in nonhuman primates (Shope et al. 1973; Wolfe and Deinhardt 1978) and the proof of EBV DNA in tumors from these animals (Wolf et al. 1975b) have added further evidence for an etiologic relationship of EBV to the development of neoplasia in man.

B. Results

I. Site of EBV Persistence in the Body

Epstein-Barr virus is associated with B-lymphocytes (Pope 1967). It is, however, not clear whether spontaneous activation of EBV genomes in carrier lymphocytes, which are present in the lymphocyte rich area of the oropharynx, is responsible for lifelong persistence of antibody titers directed against EBV-related antigens and the shedding of virus into the oropharynx or whether EBV resides in addition in specific sites of the body and is produced there, resembling somehow the situation of Marek's disease virus of chicken. That virus is found in T-lymphocytes and produced and spread from the epithelium of feather follicles (Calnek and Hitchner 1969). In situ hybridizations using sections from the parotic gland as well as from tonsils and other tissues of the ear-nose-throat area were performed in an attempt to find cells which harbor EBV genomes. EBV producing cells (P3HR1), EBV carrier Raji cells containing about 50 EBV genomes/cell, and EBV genome negative BJA-B cells were included as controls.

Figure 1 shows that only cells in the sections from the parotic gland contained detectable numbers of grains indicating the presence of EBV DNA. The number of grains per cell seems to be in the range of or higher than that seen in Raji cells which carry 50 viral genomes per cell, though clearly lower than that seen in the virus producing P3HR1 cells. The fact that no producer-type cells were found had to be expected, as the biopsies were taken from healthy adults for reasons not related to EBV infections. The induction of a lytic cycle has to be a rare event, since it leads to cell destruction and would, if it happened on a larger scale, cause necrosis.

Because in situ hybridization, in some cases, may give artifactual results, a confirmation of the results with an independent method would

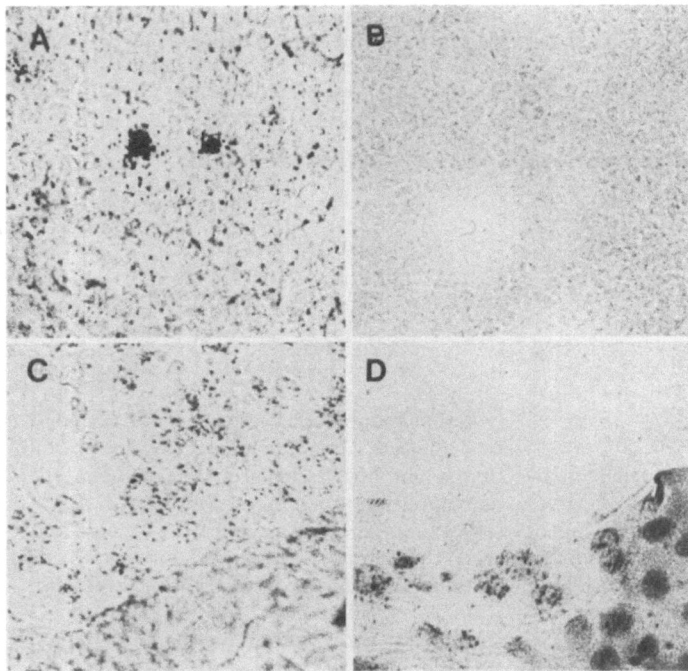

Fig. 1. P3HR1(**A**), frozen sections from tonsils (**B**), and parotid glands (**C, D**) were hybridized with 50,000 cpm H³-labeled, nick-translated EBV DNA and exposed with photoemulsion (Wolf and Wilmes 1981)

add confidence. Reassociation kinetics experiments under stringent conditions gave results in agreement with those from in situ hybridization and substantiate the presence of EBV genomes in parotic gland tissue (Fig. 2).

It is suggested that spontaneous activation of EBV in peripheral lymphocytes is a very rare event and neither the source of virus in the saliva nor the reason for the lifelong persistence of antibodies to EBV-related antigens.

II. Antibodies to EBV Specified Antigens in Carcinomas of the Postnasal Space and Other Locations Within the Waldeyer's Ring

During acute infection with EBV IgM and IgG antibodies directed against EBV-specified antigens are regulary observed, and in the case of IgG antibodies against Virus Capsid Antigen (VCA) and the EBV-specified nuclear antigen (EBNA) persist lifelong after primary exposure to EBV. It was first described by Henle and Henle (1976) that serum-IgA antibodies to VCA and early antigen (EA) were significantly associated with the EBV-linked neoplasias Burkitt's Lymphoma and Nasopharyngeal Carcinoma. We were able to confirm the data

obtained with a Chinese population with 62 cases collected within 2 years in Munich and found that IgA antibodies against VCA are closely associated with NPC and are therefore already of high diagnostic value in a single antibody determination (Wilmes et al. 1979). Successful therapy (radiation) was regularly followed by a decrease in antibody titers (Fig. 3a). In seven cases the VCA-IgA antibody level rose after initial decrease.

In three of these cases careful examination and sample biopsies revealed that new tumors had developed. Thus regular determination of anti-VCA IgA antibodies seem to be of high value as an early marker for relapse. Similar high antibodies levels, including IgA antibodies for EBV antigens, have been found recently in tumors of other locations than the nasopharynx, namely, three lymphoepithelial carcinomas and one undifferentiated carcinoma of the tonsil, two undifferentiated carcinomas at the root of the tongue, and one lymphoepithelial carcinoma of the soft palate. All these locations fall within the Waldeyer's ring. Although these observations are based on serology only and need confirmation by the demonstration of EBV DNA in tumor biopsies, they seem to be of interest because the

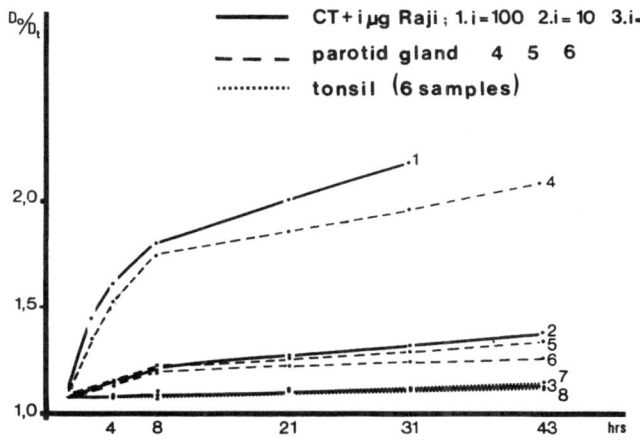

Fig. 2. Each DNA was hybridized in a DNA concentration of 2 mg/ml with 60,000 cmp/ml nick-translated EBV DNA (10^7 cpm/ug). Hydroxylapatite columns were used to separate double stranded from single stranded DNA (for details see Wolf and Wilmes 1981)

Waldeyer's ring is a histologically unique site with respect to the close contact between lymphocytes and epithelial cells (Döhnert 1977).

III. Cell Fusion Ability of EBV-Infected Cells

The EBV genomes containing lymphocytes can be found in the peripheral blood throughout the life of every human following primary infection with EBV. From peripheral blood of persons with prior EBV infection spontaneously growing lymphoblastoid cell lines of the B type, which contain EBV genomes, can be established (Nilsson et al. 1971; Pope 1967; Rickinson et al. 1980). The majority of these permanently growing cell lines do not produce EBV or viral antigens other than EBNA. Superinfection with EBV, however, leads to the synthesis of viral proteins (Bayliss and Wolf, to be published) and, dependent on the multiplicity of infection, to the synthesis of progeny virus. When such viable lymphoblastoid cells are immobilized on anti-lymphocyte globulin (ALG) coated surfaces to yield a dense monolayer (Bayliss and Wolf 1979), they allow the observation of the effects of virus infection in specific cells. As early as 2 h post infection with EBV the formation of polycaryocytes could be observed (Fig. 4a).

This fusion could be blocked by UV irradiation of the virus, by treatment with neutralizing antibodies, or by the addition of sodium azide or cycloheximide to the cultures. Amino acid

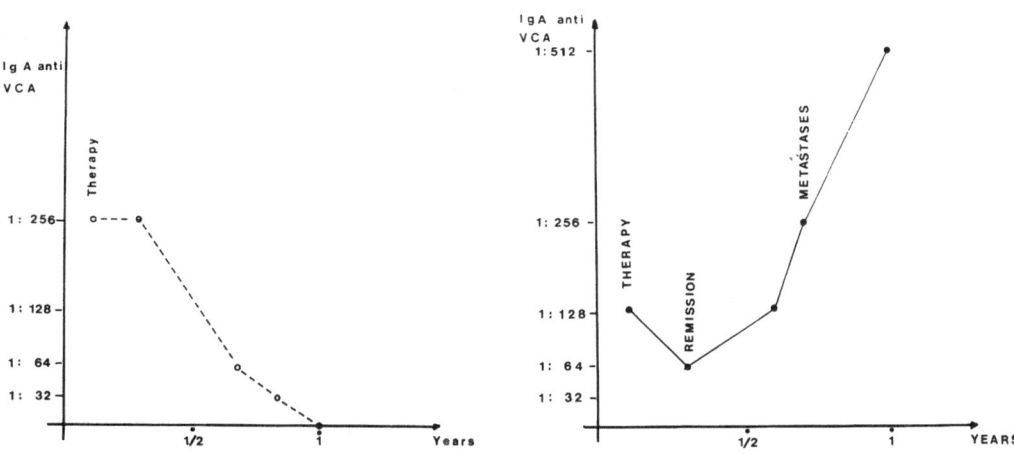

Fig. 3. IgA *anti-VCA* (virus capsid antigen) titers of two patients determined during an observation of 1 year

193

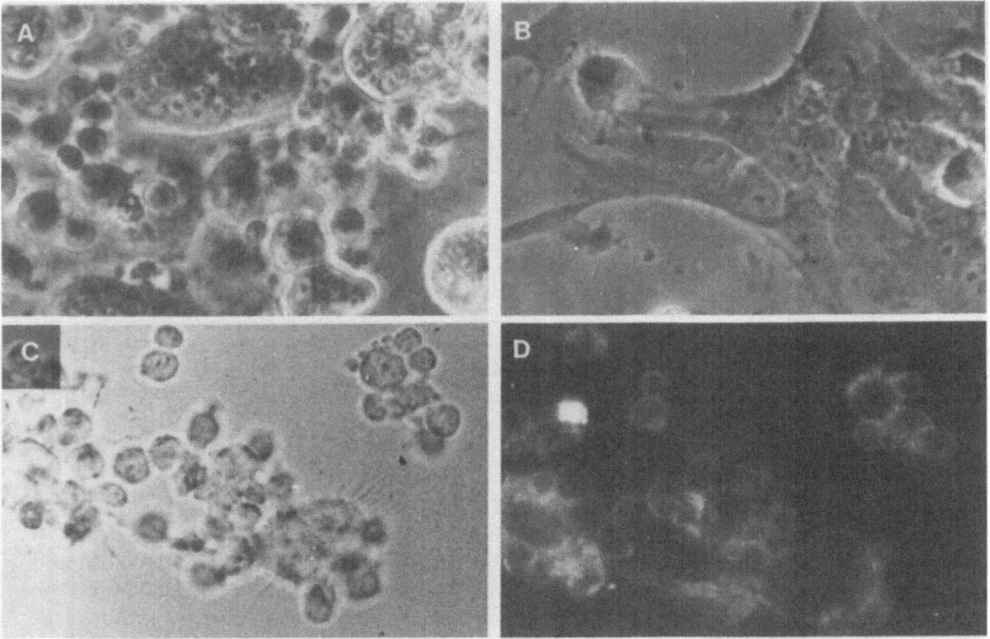

Fig. 4. A Phase contrast picture of a polycaryocyte from Raji cells which were immobilized and superinfected with EBV (8 h. P.I.) **B** Polycaryocyte (seven nuclei) between superinfected Raji cells and a human fibroblast. **C** and **D** polycaryocyte formed in a mixture of 10% superinfected Raji cells and 90% T-cells immooilized on plates. **D** shows areas of clear membrane fluorescence after staining with an anti-T-cell serum (a gift from H Rodt)

analogues (L-canavanine, L-azetidine) or inhibitors of DNA replication (hydroxyurea, phophonoacetic acid) had no such inhibitory effect. The latter drugs have been shown to permit the synthesis of at least a subset of virus-induced proteins in EBV-superinfected Raji cells. The fusion-inducing viral proteins in lymphoblastoid cells can also be produced by the resident EBV genomes of Raji cells, as treatment of these cells with 50 µg/ml of iododesoxyuridine or 20 ng/ml 12-0-tetrade-canylphorbol-13-acetate (TPA) leads to the partial activation of the resident EBV genes (zur Hausen et al. 1979). EA can be detected within these cells and they have the ability to fuse to recipient cells. It is not mandatory for the recipient cells to carry EBV receptors on their surface. When superinfected Raji cells are mixed with human fibroblasts or lymphoblastoid cells of the T type (Jurkat, devoid of EBV genomes or EBV receptors) they form polycaryocytes with these cells (Fig. 4b,c). The participation of these T cells in the polycaryocyte can be clearly demonstrated by membrane fluorescence with specific anti-T-cell

sera (Fig. 4d) (Bayliss and Wolf 1980). When monolayers of Raji cells on ALG-coated surfaces are subconfluent, spontaneous synthesis of EA can be observed in up to 5% of the cells (Bayliss and Wolf 1979). When treated with ALG in suspension, no EA synthesis is observed in Raji cells. Anti-IgM sera on the other hand have been shown (Tovey et al. 1978) to have the potential to induce EA in Raji cells in suspension. The differential effect of ALG in suspension as compared to the effect when ALG is fixed on surfaces upon EA induction in Raji cells may be due to the inhibitory effect the ALG serum had on cell growth. ALG at concentrations of 1.6 to 16 µg/ml even depressed the induction of EA in Raji cells by IUdR. It has been postulated earlier (Hampar et al. 1976) that active cell growth is required for activation of EBV. From these observations one might conclude that the presence of autoantibodies in patients with EBV-carrying lymphocytes could induce the synthesis of EBV-spcified antigens which would, upon cell death, stimulate the production of antibodies.

C. Discussion

During infectious mononucleosis and the following lifelong carrier state EBV seems to be restricted to B-lymphocytes and the carrier-producer cells in the parotic gland. In case of the nasopharyngeal carcinoma, however, it has been shown that EBV genomes reside in the epithelioid tumor cells (Wolf et al. 1973; Desgranges et al. 1975; Klein et al. 1974; Wolf et al. 1975). This finding prompted the question how these EBV genomes came into the tumor cells. Epithelial cells are believed to be devoid of receptors for EBV. All attempts to infect other cells than B-lymphocytes with EBV in vitro failed. The negative results from binding studies using labeled EBV and the failure of induce viral antigens in primary cultures of nasopharyngeal tissue (Wolf, unplublished work) do not support the presence of EBV receptors in these cells. This conflict led to the suggestion that other agents like paramyxoviruses may induce fusion of EBV genome containing lymphocytes and epithelial cells (Gazzolo et al. 1972). Under the condition of close cell to cell contact (Döhnert 1977) we were able to demonstrate in vitro that EBV is able to induce cell fusion. One might speculate that similar events take place in vivo. The exceptional close contact of lymphocytes and epithelial cells found in the Waldeyer's ring of the throat may provide the necessary conditions for cell fusion. The activation of EBV genes in EBV genome carrying lymphocytes may be induced by a variety of influences, including drugs like IUdR or tumor promoters like TPA. If fusion occurs in nature one should be able to observe cells with more than the normal set of chromosomes. This is, however, not necessarily so because induction of the lytic cycle of EBV replication leads to the pulverization of the cellular genome (Seigneurin et al. 1977). Thus only fusion soon after induction of a lymphocyte would lead to the transfer of both viral and cellular DNA, whereas fusion late after induction may not lead to the transfer of cellular chromosomes but only to the transfer of possibly protected circular EB viral DNA.

Finerty et al. (1978) studied the karyotypes of cells from nasopharyngeal carcinomas and found that indeed three out of five had near triploid and two near diploid karyotypes. The postulated interaction of several factors may explain the location of the tumor in the body as well as the increased risk for the development of this tumor in certain areas of the world, especially in Cantonese China. The geographic distribution might be due to the spread of certain substances activating EBV with high efficiency in carrier lymphocytes. Alternatively, endemic virus strains may vary in their fusion inducing ability. Some observations may point in that direction but need further confirmation. The age of first exposure may play an important additional role as early transfer of EBV genomes to epithelial cells could be esential for the evolution of proliferating malignant cells.

Acknowledgments

This work was supported by DFG Wo 227/2, SFB 51 (A 21) and SFB 37 (C 14).

References

Bayliss GJ, Wolf H (1979) Immobilization of viable lymphoblastoid cells on solid supports. In: John D, Lapin B, Blakeslee J (eds) Advances in comparative leukemia research. Elsevier, New York, 381–382 – Bayliss GJ, Wolf H (to be published) The regulated expression of Epstein-Barr Virus: III. Proteins specified by EBV during the lytic cycle. J Gen Virol – Bayliss GJ, Wolf H (1980) Epstein-Barr virus induced cell fusion. Nature 287:164–165 – Calnek BW, Hitchner SB (1969) Localization of viral antigen in chickens infected with Marek's disease herpes virus. J Natl Cancer Inst 43:935–949 – Chang S, Golden D (1971) Transformation of human leukocytes by throat washing from infectious mononucleosis patients. Nature 243:359–360 – Desgranges C, Wolf H, de Thé G, Shanmugaratnam K, Cammoun N, Ellouz R, Klein G, Lennert K, Munoz N, zurHausen H (1975) Nasopharyngeal carcinoma: X. Presence of Epstein-Barr genomes in separated epithelial cells of tumors in patients from Singapore, Tunisia end Kenya. Int J Cancer 16:7–15 – Döhnert G (1977) Über lymphoepitheliale Geschwülste. Erkenntnisse anhand der Gewebekultur und vergleichender klinischer, morphologischer und virologischer Untersuchungen. In: Sitzungsbericht der Heidelberger Akademie der Wissenschaften, 3. Abhandlung. Springer, Berlin Heidelberg New York – Finerty S, Jarvis JE, Epstein MA, Trumper PA, Ball G, Giovanella BC (1978) Cytogenetics of malignant epithelial cells and lymphoblastoid cell lines from nasopharyngeal carcinoma. Br J Cancer 37:231–239 – Gazzolo L, de Thé G, Vuillaume M, H HC (1972) Nasopharyngeal carcinoma: II. Ultrastructure of normal mucosa, tumor biopsies and subsequent epithelial growth in vitro. J Natl Cancer

Inst 48:73–86 – Gerber P, Lucas S, Nonoyama M, Perlin E, Goldstein LJ (1972) Oral excretion of Epstein-Barr virus by healthy subjects and patients with infectious mononucleosis. Lancet 11:988–989 – Hampar B, Lenoir G, Nonoyama M, Derge JG, Chang S-Y (1976) Cell cycle dependence for activation of Epstein-Barr virus by inhibitors of protein synthesis or medium deficient in arginine. Virology 69:660–668 – Henle G, Henle W (1976) Epstein-Barr virus specific IgA serum antibodies as an outstanding feature of nasopharyngeal carcinoma. Int J Cancer 17:1 – Henle W, Henle G (1979) Seroepidemiology of the virus. In: Epstein MA, Achong BG (eds) The Epstein-Barr virus. Springer, Berlin Heidelberg ew York, pp 61–78 – Klein G, Giovanella B, Lindahl T, Fialkow P, Singh S, Stehlin J (1974) Direct evidence for the presence of EBV DNA cells from patients with poorly differentiated carcinoma of the nasopharynx. Proc Natl Acad Sci USA 71:4737–4741 – Morgan DG, Miller G, Niederman JC, Smith HW, Dowaliby JM (1979) Site of Epstein-Barr virus replication in the oropharynx. Lancet I:1154–1155 – Nilsson K, Klein G, Henle W, Henle G (1971) The establishment of lymphoblastoid lines from adult and fetal human lymphoid tissue and its dependence on EBV. Int J Cancer 8:443–450 – Pope JH (1967) Establishment of cell lines from peripheral leucocytes in infectious mononucleosis. Nature 216:810–811 – Rickinson AB, Moos DJ, Pope JH, Ahlberg N (1980) Long-term T-cell-mediated immunity to Epstein-Barr virus in man: IV. Development of T-cell memory in convalescent infectious mononucleosis patients. Int J Cancer 25:59–65 – Seigneurin J-M, Vuillaume M, Lenoir G, de Thé G (1977) Replication of Epstein-Barr virus: Ultrastructural and immunofluorescent studies of P3HR1-superinfected Raji cells. J Virol 24:836–845 – Shope T, Dechairo D, Miller G (1973) Malignant lymphoma in cotton-top marmosets following inoculation of Epstein-Barr virus. Proc Natl Acad Sci USA 70:2487–2491 – Tovey MG, Lenoir G, Begon-Lours J (1978) Activation of latent EBV by antibody to human IgM. Nature 276:270–272 – Wilmes E, Wolf H (1981) Der Nachweis von Epstein-Barr-Virus-Genomen in der Ohrspeicheldrüse. Laryngol Rhinol Otol (Stuttg) 60:7–10 – Wilmes E, Wolf H, Deinhardt F, Naumann HH (1979) Die Bedeutung von Epstein-Barr-Virus-Antikörpern für Diagnose und Verlauf des Nasopharynxkarzinoms. Laryngol Rhinol Otol (Stuttg.) 58:911–915 – Wolf H, zurHausen H, Becker V (1973) EB viral genomes in epithelial nasopharyngeal cells. Nature (London) New Biol 244:245–247 – Wolf H, Werner J, zur Hausen H (1975b) EBV DNA in nonlymphoid cells of nasopharyngeal carcinomas and in a malignant lymphoma obtained after inoculation of EBV into cotton-top marmosets. Cold Spring Harbor Symp Quant Biol 39:791–796 – Wolf H, zur Hausen H, Klein G, Becker V, Henle G, Henle W (1975b) Attempts to detect virus-specific DNA sequences in human tumors: III. Epstein-Barr viral DNA in non-lymphoid nasopharyngeal carcinoma cells. Med Microbiol Immunol 161:15–21 – Wolfe LG, Deinhard F (1978) Overview of viral oncology studies in saguinus and callithrix species. In: Primates Med 10:96–118 – zur Hausen H, Bornkamm GW, Schmidt R, Hecker E: Tumor initiators and promoters in the induction of Epstein-Barr virus. Proc Natl Acad Sci USA 76:782–785 (1979)

Haematology and Blood Transfusion Vol. 26
Modern Trends in Human Leukemia IV
Edited by Neth, Gallo, Graf, Mannweiler, Winkler
© Springer-Verlag Berlin Heidelberg 1981

Episomal and Nonepisomal Herpesvirus DNA in Lymphoid Tumor Cell Lines

C. Kaschka-Dierich, I. Bauer, B. Fleckenstein, and R. C. Desrosiers

A. Introduction

Herpesviruses are able to persist for years or for life in certain cells of the host organism, for example, in neural tissue and cells of the lymphatic series. Little is known at the molecular level about the mode of herpesvirus persistence and the factors determining reactivation to secondary diseases, oncogenic transformation of appropriate target cells, elimination of virus-transformed cells by the immune system, and eventual outgrowth as a malignant tumor. The DNA of Epstein-Barr virus (EBV) is able to form circular molecules and to persist in human tumor tissues and lymphoblastoid tumor cell lines in the form of episomal viral genomes (Kaschka-Dierich et al. 1976; Lindahl et al. 1976). Some viral DNA, however, was found consistently to band with host cell DNA upon consecutive density centrifugations in CsCl gradients (Adams et al. 1973; Adams 1979). This has led to the conclusion that some EBV DNA is integrated into chromosomal DNA in transformed cells. There are, however, at least two problems with this interpretation. First, it is difficult to rule out all artifactual explanations, and secondly, methylation of viral DNA could cause a density shift toward the density of cellular DNA.

In an attempt to learn more about mechanisms of herpesvirus persistence and oncogenic transformation, we have concentrated our efforts on the highly oncogenic herpesviruses of New World primates, *Herpesvirus saimiri* (*H. saimiri*) and *Herpesvirus ateles* (*H. ateles*). A lytic system for growth and the peculiar genome structure of these viruses offer advantages in the biochemical analyses of persisting viral DNA.

B. Structure of Episomal DNA

The complete genomes (M-genomes) of *H. saimiri* particles are linear duplex DNA molecules of slightly variable length, mostly with molecular weights between 96 and 110×10^6, which corresponds to about 136 to 166 kilo base pairs (KB). The M-genome contains a long, internal, unique segment of L-DNA [71.6 megadaltons (md)] with 36% guanine plus cytosine (G and C) and two terminal segments of repetitive H-DNA (71% G and C) which are variable in length. The repeat units of H-DNA have a 830,000 mol.wt.; they are strictly arranged in tandem, and the H-DNA sequences from both ends of the molecule are oriented in the same direction (Bornkamm et al. 1976; Fleckenstein 1979). *H. ateles* shares the characteristic features of this genome structure; L-DNA sequences in M-genomes of *H. ateles* contain 38% G and C; and the repetitive H-DNA termini have 75% G and C (Fleckenstein et al. 1978).

Autopsy materials from tumors induced by these viruses and lymphoid tumor cell lines contain substantial amounts of viral L- and H-DNA (Fleckenstein et al. 1977). Noninte-grated circular superhelical viral DNA could be isolated from *H. saimiri* and *H. ateles*-transformed cells by isopycnic and velocity centrifugation (Werner et al. 1977). Surprisingly, the size of viral episomal DNA in at least two of the cell lines exceeds that of virion DNA. The lymphoid tumor cell line No. 1670, derived from the infiltrated spleen of a cotton top marmoset *(Saguinus oedipus)*, carries circular viral DNA molecules of 131.5 md. Partial denaturation mapping in the electron microscope, computer alignment of the denaturation maps, and blot hybridizations with purified radioactive virion DNA have been used to determine the structure of the viral episomes in tumor cell line No. 1670. Figure 1 summarizes our current understanding of the arrangement of L-DNA and H-DNA sequences in 1670 episomal DNA. The circular molecules contain two L-DNA regions and two H-regions. Both L-DNA segments are in the same orientation, and the shorter L-segment is a subset of the longer one. The longer L-DNA region appears to represent most of the L-region of virion M-DNA; however an internal piece of 12.5 md which encompasses the EcoRI D and H fragments of virion DNA is missing in the episome. The short L-region corresponds to about one half of virion L-DNA only. Thus, *H. saimiri* episomes of this cell line are a form of defective molecules.

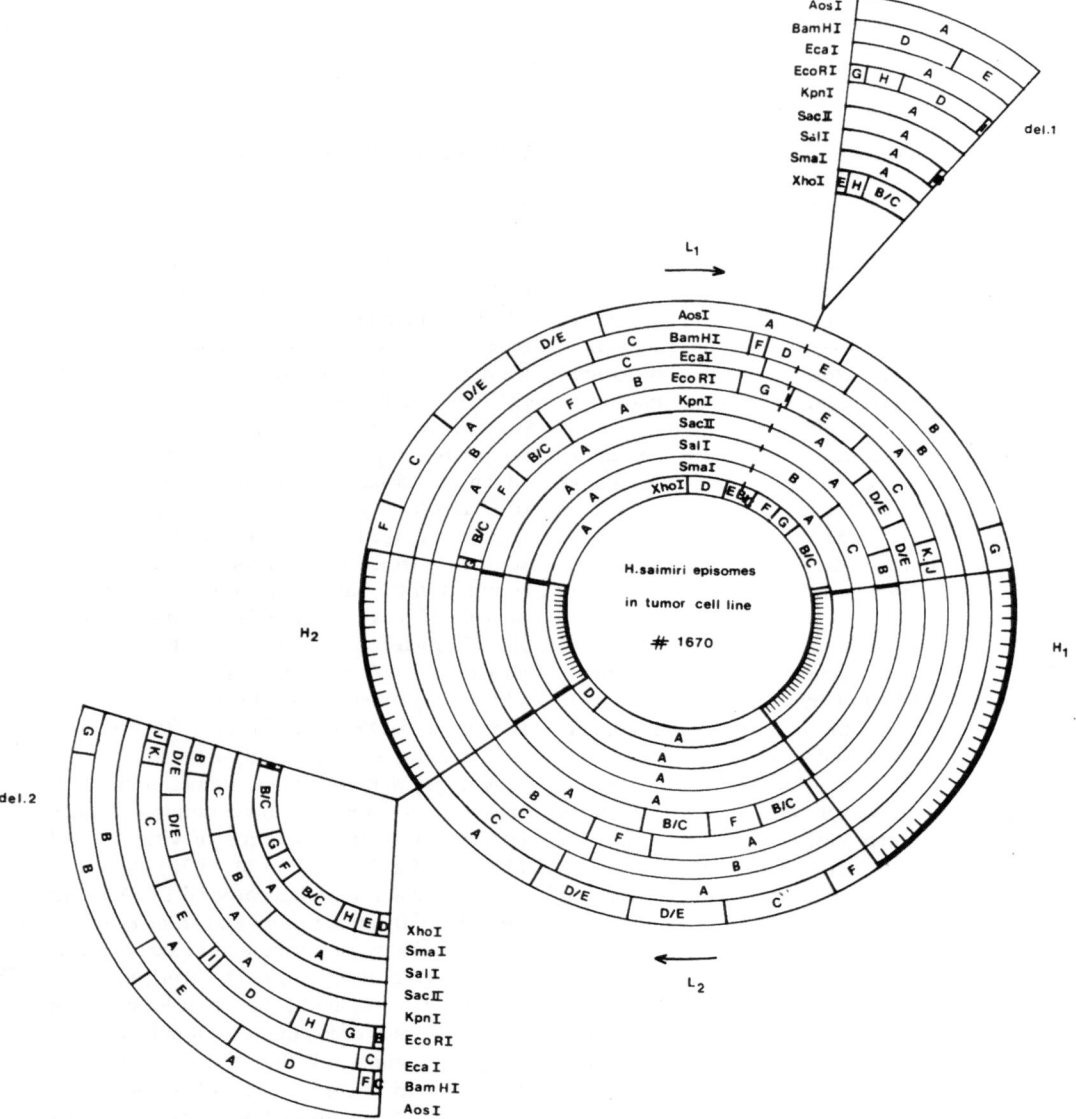

Fig. 1. Schematic representation of the arrangement of *H. saimiri* L- and H-DNA sequences in episomes from lymphoid tumor cell line No. 1670. Missing L-DNA segments are delineated as sectors outside the episome. The correlation between the cleavage maps of virion DNA and episomes was obtained by partial denaturation mapping in the electron microscope and by blot hybridizations

C. Nonepisomal Viral DNA

We have used DNA purified by ethidium bromide – cesium chloride gradients to separately analyze episomal and nonepisomal (linear) viral DNA by Southern transfer and hybridization to ^{32}P virion DNA. The EcoRI fragment D (9.8 md) and the EcoRI fragment H (4.0 md) cannot be detected as discrete bands in

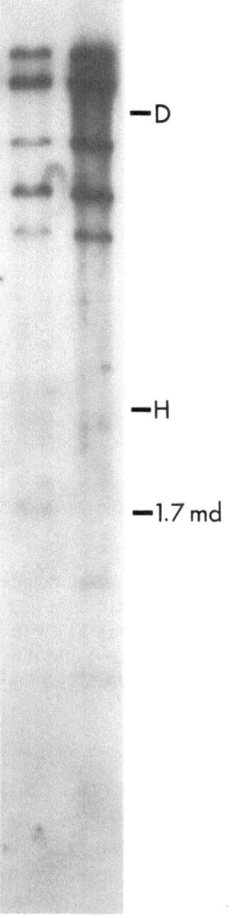

Fig. 2. Hybridization of DNA fragments from lymphoid tumor cell line 1670 to ^{32}P-labeled *H. saimiri* DNA. Nonepisomal DNA (the linear DNA fraction containing the bulk of cellular DNA) and episomal DNA was isolated from 1670 cells by centrifugation in ethidium bromide-cesium chloride gradients. The DNAs were cleaved with *endo* R. *Eco* RI and *Xma* I, transferred to nitrocellulose and hybridized to ^{32}P virion DNA. *Left lane,* nonepisomal DNA; *right lane,* episomal DNA

these blot hybridizations with 1670 DNA (Fig. 2). However, when EcoRI fragment D was isolated and used as a radioactive probe in solution hybridizations with total DNA from 1670 cells, the reassociation rate was accelerated in comparison to self hybridization in the presence of salmon sperm DNA (Fig. 3). This indicates that sequences of the EcoRI D fragment are indeed present in the 1670 cell DNA. These experiments must be extended using cloned DNA fragments and blot hybridization to determine the nature of the hybridizing sequences. It is possible that EcoRI D and H are absent as discrete fragments because they have been excised in an integration event, but further work is necessary to show this.

With some restriction endonucleases the linear DNA fraction described above yields discrete fragments not found in isolated episomal DNA. For example, digestion of isolated linear DNA of 1670 cells with endo R EcoRI and XmaI yields a 1.7 md fragment not observed with isolated episomal DNA (Fig. 2). Further work is needed to determine the nature of this viral nonepisomal DNA.

D. Methylation of Viral DNA

In the course of structural analyses of viral DNA in transformed cells by blot hybridizations we observed a striking resistance of intracellular viral DNA against the action of several restriction endonucleases. This has led us to conclude that viral H-DNA is extensively methylated in nonproducer cell lines (Desrosiers et al. 1979). Methylation of mammalian DNA has previously been found almost exclusively within the dinucleotide CG, forming 5-methylcytosine. Enzymes like endo R. Hpa II, Sac II, Sma I, which possess CG in their recognition site and are inhibited by methylation were found to cleave incompletely in the viral H-DNA from *H. saimiri*-transformed nonproducer cell lines No. 1670 and 70 N2, irrespective of DNA extraction procedure and excess of restriction enzyme. Enzymes without CG in their recognition site like endo R. Pst I, Pvu II, and Sac I cleave virion H-DNA and viral H-DNA from transformed cells identically. Msp I is an isoschizomer of Hpa II but unlike Hpa II cleaves whether or not the C of the CG dinucleotide is methylated. Viral H-DNA of 1670 cells, although resistant to cleavage by Hpa II, was cleaved to the same

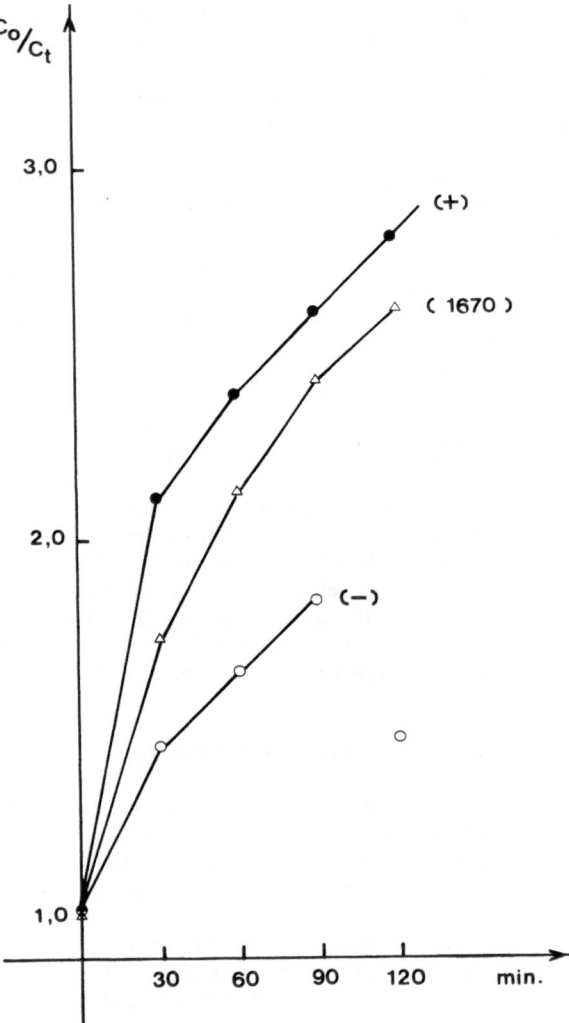

Fig. 3. Reassociation of ³H-labeled *EcoRI* D fragment (3.7×10^4 cpm/μg) of *H. saimiri* L-DNA (strain 11) with DNA from 1670 cells (–△–) and 4.8 μg/ml purified virion M-DNA (–●–); self hybridization (–○–)

extent as virion DNA by Msp I. Using these restriction endonuclease criteria, we were not able to detect methylation of viral H-DNA in three transformed lymphoid cell lines producing virus. In addition, viral H-DNA in 1670 cells appeared somewhat more methylated than in 70 N2 cells.

A different approach for the detection of methylation in viral DNA was developed by measuring the buoyant density of viral DNA in transformed cells. The density of DNA in cesium chloride gradients is lowered by 5-methylation of cytosine (Kirk et al. 1967). As shown in Fig. 4A), the viral DNA of 1670 cells is found at lower density than cellular DNA, in

spite of a significantly higher G and C content in viral DNA. Consistent with blot hybridizations, DNA from 70 N2 cells shows only a slighter density shift (Fig. 4B), apparently due to a lower degree of methylation. Inhibitors of methylation may suppress the density shift of viral episomes in cesium chloride. After treating 1670 cells with 5′deoxy-5′-isobutyl adenosine (SIBA) or S-adenosyl homocystein (SAH) over 6 days, most viral DNA is found at about 1.710 g/ml which is the density to be expected from the average G and C content.

It remains to be seen if methylation of viral DNA plays a role in the lack of complete gene expression of *H. saimiri* in nonproducer lym-

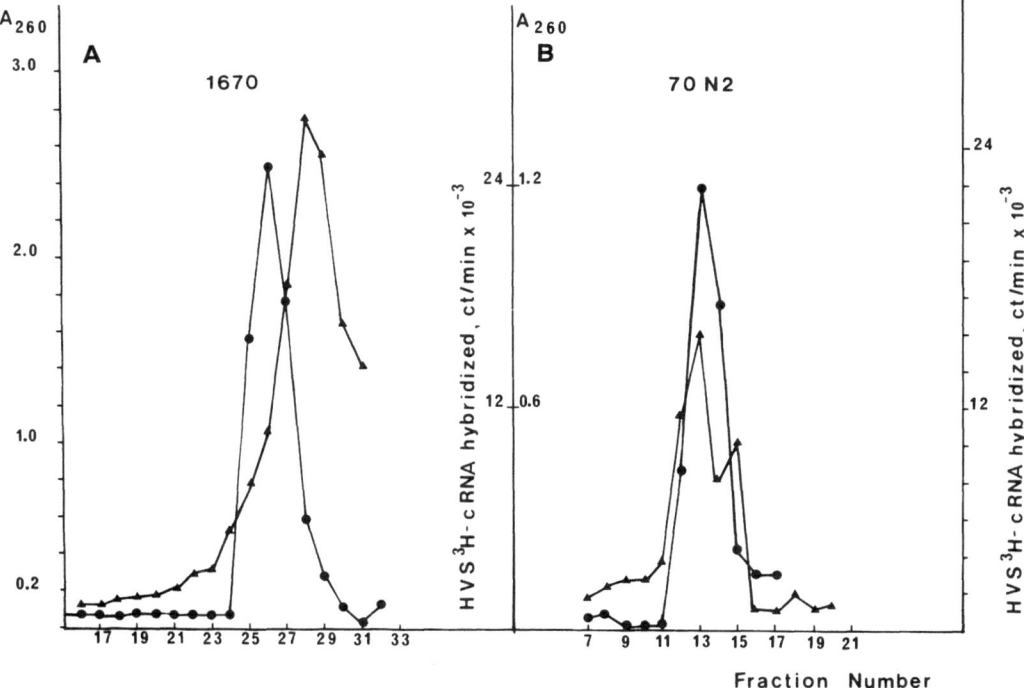

Fig. 4. Density centrifugation of DNA from cell lines No. 1670 (**A**) and 70 N2 (**B**) in cesium chloride. Cellular DNA (−●−); viral DNA monitored by ^{3}HcRNA hybridization on filters (−▲−)

phoid cell lines. The expression or lack of expression of hemoglobin and ovalbumin genes have also been linked to the state of their DNA methylation (McGhee and Ginder 1979; Mendel and Chambon 1979). Similar correlations were described for gene expression of adenovirus and mouse mammary tumor virus in transformed cells (Cohen 1980, Sutter and Doerfler 1980). If DNA methylation is indeed involved in gene expression, a multitude of virus-host interactions could be affected. DNA methylation could conceivably play a role in the control of gene expression in herpesvirus latency and oncogenic transformation.

E. Tumor Promotors and Methylation of Viral DNA in Transformed Cells

Since tumor promotors of the phorbol ester group like 12–0 tetradecanoyl-phorbol 13-acetate (TPA) are potent inducers of herpesvirus gene expression in tumor cell lines (zur Hausen et al. 1978), we recently asked whether these drugs may influence the state of methylation in *H. saimiri*-transformed lymphoid tumor cell lines. Preliminary experiments have shown that treatment of 1670 cells with TPA results in a significant increase of buoyant density for a substantial part of viral DNA (Fig. 5). Again, we do not know yet what the functional role of suppression of methylation may be in cells treated with a tumor promoting phorbol ester.

F. Summary

Tumor cell lines derived from *Herpesvirus saimiri (H. saimiri)*- and *Herpesvirus ateles (H. ateles)*-induced lymphomas of New World primates and rabbits contain multiple copies of viral genomes. Partial denaturation mapping and blot hybridizations of episomal DNA from lymphoid tumor cell line No. 1670 showed that a 12.5md-fragment is missing which represents the EcoRI D- and H-fragments of virion L-DNA. However, the missing piece can be demonstrated in total cellular DNA by reasso-

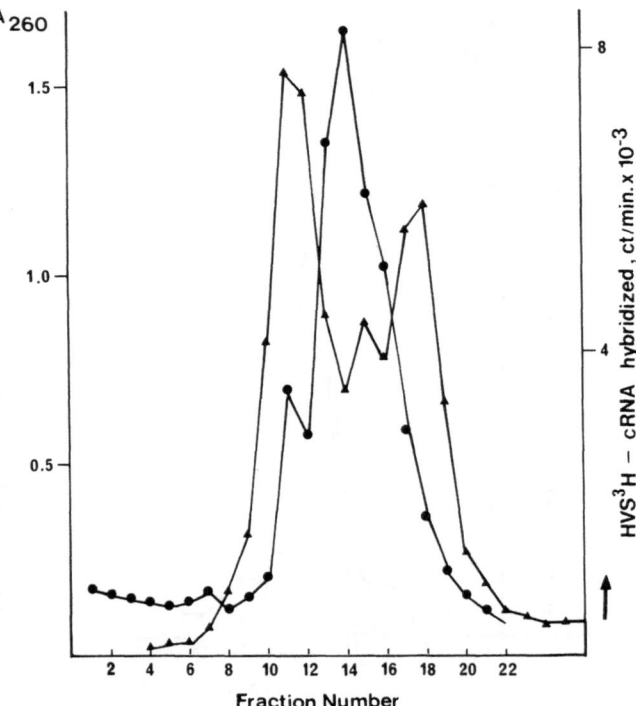

Fig. 5. Density centrifugation of DNA from cell line No. 1670, treated with 40 ng/ml TPA for 3 days. –●– cellular DNA –▲– viral DNA

ciation kinetics, possibly because it persists in integrated form. Both episomal and nonepisomal H-DNA are heavily methylated in a number of the lymphoid cell lines, and methylation may be reduced by conventional methylation inhibitors (S-adenosyl homocystein, SIBA) as well as by the tumor promoting phorbol ester TPA.

Acknowledgments

The work was supported by Stiftung Volkswagenwerk, Wilhelm-Sander-Stiftung, Deutsche Forschungsgemeinschaft, by contract No. 1 CP 81005 from the Virus Cancer Program of the National Cancer Institute, and by a fellowship from the Medical Foundation of Boston, Inc.

References

Adams A (1979). The state of the virus genome in transformed cells and its relationship to host cell DNA. Epstein MA, Achong BG (eds) In: The Epstein-Barr virus. Springer Verlag, Berlin Heidelberg New York, pp 155–183 – Adams A, Lindahl T, Klein G (1973). Linear association between cellular DNA and Epstein-Barr virus DNA in a human lymphoblastoid cell line. Proc Natl Acad Sci USA 70:2888–2892 – Bornkamm GW, Delius H, Fleckenstein B, Werner F-J, Mulder C (1976) The structure of Herpesvirus saimiri genomes: arrangement of heavy and light sequences within the M genome. J Virol 19:154–161 – Christman J, Price P, Pedrinan L, Acs G (1977) Correlation between hypomethylation of DNA and expression of globin genes in Friend Erythroleukemia cells. Eur J Biochem 81:53–61 – Cohen JC (1980) Methylation of milk-borne and genetically transmitted mouse mammary tumor virus proviral DNA. Cell 19:653–662 – Desrosiers RC, Mulder C, Fleckenstein B (1979) Methylation of Herpesvirus saimiri DNA in lymphoid tumor cell lines. Proc Natl Acad Sci USA 76:3839–3843 – Fleckenstein B (1979) Oncogenic herpesviruses of non-human primates. Biochim Biophys Acta 560:301–342 – Fleckenstein B, Müller I, Werner F-J (1977) The presence of Herpesvirus saimiri genomes in virus-transformed cells. Int J Cancer 19:546–554 – Fleckenstein B, Bornkamm GW, Mulder C, Werner F-J, Daniel MD, Falk LA, Delius H (1978) Herpesvirus ateles DNA and its homology with Herpesvirus saimiri nucleic acid. J Virol 25:361–373 – Kaschka-Dierich C, Adams A, Lindahl T, Bornkamm GW, Bjursell G, Klein G, Giovanella BC, Singh S (1976) Intracellular forms of Epstein Barr virus DNA in human tumour cells in vivo. Nature 260:302–306 – Kirk JTO (1967) Effect of methylation of cytosine residues on the buoyant density of DNA in cesium chloride solution. J Mol Biol 28:171–172 – Lindahl T, Adams A, Bjursell G, Bornkamm GW, Kaschka-Dierich C, Jehn U (1976) Covalently closed circular duplex DNA of Epstein-Barr virus in a human lymphoid cell line. J Mol Biol 102:511–530 – McGhee JD, Ginder GD (1979) Specific DNA methylation sites in the vicinity of the chicken beta-globin genes. Nature 280:419–420 – Mandel JL, Chambon P (1979) DNA Methylation: Organ specific variations in the methylation pattern within and around ovalbumin and other chicken genes. Nucleic Acids Res 7:2081–2103 – Sutter D, Doerfler W (1980) Methylation of integrated adenovirus type 12 DNA sequences in transformed cells is inversely correlated with viral gene expression. Proc Natl Acad Sci (USA) 77:253–256 – Werner F-J. Bornkamm GW, Fleckenstein B (1977) Episomal viral DNA in a Herpesvirus saimiri-transformed lymphoid cell line. J Virol 22:794–803 – Werner F-J, Desrosiers RC, Mulder C, Bornkamm GW, Fleckenstein B (1978) Physical mapping of viral episomes in Herpesvirus saimiri transformed lymphoid cells In: Stevens JG, Todaro GJ, Fox CF (eds) Persistent viruses. Academic Press, New York, pp 189–200 – zur Hausen H, O'Neill FJ, Freese UK Hecker E (1978) Persisting oncogenic herpesvirus induced by tumor promoter TPA. Nature 272:373-375

Haematology and Blood Transfusion Vol. 26
Modern Trends in Human Leukemia IV
Edited by Neth, Gallo, Graf, Mannweiler, Winkler
© Springer-Verlag Berlin Heidelberg 1981

B-Lymphotropic Papovavirus (LPV) – Infections of Man?

L. Brade, L. Gissmann, N. Mueller-Lantzsch, and H. zur Hausen

A. Introduction

A possibly new subgroup of papovaviruses has been isolated which appears to be characterized by its highly restricted host range which does not seem to extend beyond proliferating lymphoblasts. A virus revealing this host range derived from transformed African green monkey (AGM) lymphoblasts in described.

B. Results

I. Origin of Lymphotropic Papovaviruses

Papovavirus-like particles were observed by electron microscopy in supernatants of two Epstein-Barr virus (EBV)-transformed lymphoblastoid lines established from individual AGM. One of these lines originated from an inguinal lymph node synthesized in addition a paramyxovirus-like agent (zur Hausen and Gissmann 1979). The second line was derived from the peripheral blood of a different monkey. Cells of both lines revealed cytopathic changes. The papovavirus obtained from lymphoblasts of the peripheral blood has not yet been further characterized. Papovavirus particles were also demonstrated in a human lymphoblastoid cell line (CCRF-SB) originally derived from a leukemic child (zur Hausen and Gissmann 1979). In the following only the papovavirus found in the lymphoblasts derived from the inguinal lymphnode (LK-line) will be described.

II. Host Range

Only B-lymphoblasts obtained from AGM (Böcker et al 1980) and one EBV-negative human line BJA-B (Klein et al. 1974) were susceptible to this papovavirus. It is of interest that conversion of BJA-B cells to EBV genome carriers significantly reduced the number of cells producing AGM papovavirus. Because of its lymphotropic host range which seems to be unique among identified papovaviruses, it is tentatively designated as lymphotropic papovavirus (LPV).

III. Biochemical Characterization

The molecular weight of LPV was determined by gel electrophoresis of cleaved and uncleaved LPV DNA by using SV 40 DNA as marker. The DNA proved to be slightly smaller than SV 40 (3.2×10^6 as compared to 3.3×10^6 for SV 40 DNA (zur Hausen and Gissmann 1979; Dugaiczyk et al. 1975). The analysis of the cleavage pattern and of cross-hybridization with SV 40 DNA by the blotting technique (Southern 1975) has been reported before (zur Hausen and Gissmann 1979). The cleavage pattern of DNA from LPV differs from cleavage patterns of other characterized polyoma-like viruses. As seen in Fig. 1a LPV (left) and SV 40 (right) show completely different fragment patterns after Hae III cleavage. Figure 1b depicts LPVDNA after more than 1 year of continuous passage of the virus in human BJA-B cells. Heterogeneity seems to be due to accumulation of defective DNA molecules.

IV. Serologic Characterization

Apart from biochemical differences, the virus differs antigenetically from all characterized papovaviruses thus far. Antibodies of capsid or

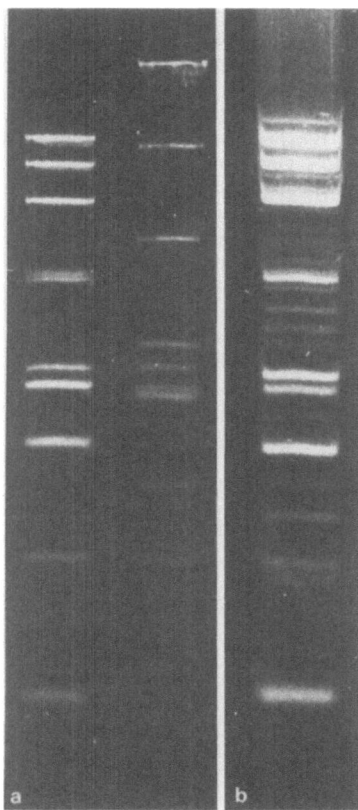

Fig. 1. a Polyacrylamide gelelectrophoresis (4%) of AGM-LPV DNA *(left)* and SV 40 DNA *(right)* after cleavage with Hae III restriction endonuclease. **b** AGM-LPV DNA after more than 1 year of continuous passage of the virus in human BJA-B cells

T antigens of SV 40 or BK virus did not crossreact with LPV in the indirect immunofluorescence test (IFT). Approximately 70% of AGM sera reacted with LPV antigens in IFT. Inoculation of four seronegative animals with LPV resulted in an antibody response within 3 days, suggesting a booster reaction. It appears, therefore, that these animals had low titers of antibodies that were not detected by IFT. The existence of human antibodies to LPV in different age groups was examined. The IFT was used to test 558 sera for antibodies, starting with a serum dilution of 1:10. Only a low number (about 10%) of sera in age groups between 0.5–29 years were found to be positive. In the decade from 30–39 years a sharp rise (to 30%) in the number of positive

sera is noted, resulting in about 30% of positive sera in all age groups above 30 years (40–59, 60–79, ⩾80). The titer range of positive sera varied considerably (up to 1:640) but showed no age dependence.

No disease-specific reactivity has been demonstrated thus far, although patients with symptoms involving the lymphatic system (by excluding EBV and CMV infections) showed a significantly higher percentage of reactive sera (zur Hausen et al. 1980). The percentage of positive sera in 247 patients (23.4%) tested for infectious hepatitis was about twofold higher than that observed in other groups of 221 patients (12.2%). The geometric mean titer was 1:72 in the "hepatitis group" and 1:59 in the other group. The specificity of the IFT was confirmed by immunoprecipitation (IP) studies. ^{35}S-methione-labeled cell extracts from persistently infected BJA-B-LK and from freshly infected BJA-B cells were immunoprecipitated with different sera defined by IFT (this method is described in detail by Mueller-Lantzsch et al. 1980). By this method we could prove that virus-specific antigens and not cellular antigens were involved in immunoprecipitation reactions with positive sera. AGM as well as human sera reacting in immunofluorescence with LPV antigens precipitated polypeptides of about 40 K. Neither IFT-negative sera reacted in IP with infected cells nor did IP-positive sera with uninfected cells.

From IFT-positive sera eight high-titered sera were selected for neutralization studies. They were able to neutralize completely viral infectivity as revealed by IFT.

C. Discussion

A novel member of the papovavirus group has been isolated from EBV-transformed AGM B-lymphoblasts which is characterized by its lymphotropic host range. The virus is widely spread among African green monkeys. Of human sera from adults above the age of 30, 30% reveal antibodies reacting with LP viral antigens. Sera which are highly reactive in IFT are able to neutralize LP viral infectivity. Human sera which react with LPV antigens in IFT also can precipitate viral proteins with a molecular weight of about 40 K. In analogy with SV 40 these proteins might be the major capsid proteins. (Girard et al. 1970, Hirt et al.

1971). The data suggest that an immunologically crossreacting agent also exists in man.

The existence of lymphotropic papovaviruses shows the diversity of host range within this virus group. The presence of papovavirus-like particles in a human lymphoblastoid line (CCRF-SB) may indicate that lymphotropic papovaviruses could represent a distinct subgroup of polyoma-like agents. It should be of interest to elucidate the possible role in the etiology of proliferative diseases, particularly of the lymphopoietic system.

Acknowledgments

The skillful technical assistance of Mrs. Gabriele Menzel is gratefully acknowledged. This work was supported by the Deutsche Forschungsgemeinschaft (SFB 31 – Medizinische Virologie; Tumorentstehung und -Entwicklung).

References

Böcker JF, Tiedemann KH, Bornkamm GW, zur Hausen H (1980) Characterization of an EBV-like virus from African green monkey lymphoblasts. Virology 101:291–295 – Dugaiczyk A, Boyer HW, Goodman HM (1975) Digestion of Eco RI endonuclease – generated DNA fragments into linear and circular structures. J Mol Biol 96:171–184 – Girard M, Marty L, Suarez F (1970) Capsid proteins of simian virus 40. Biochem Biophys Res Commun 40:197–102 – Hirt B Gesteland RF (1971) Characterization of the proteins of SV40 and polyoma virus. Lepetit coll Biol Med 2:98–103 – Klein G, Lindahl T, Jondal M, Leibold W, Menézes J, Nilson K, Sundström C (1974) Continuous lymphoid cell lines with characteristics of B cells (bone-marrow derived) lacking the Epstein-Barr virus genome and derived from three human lymphomas. Proc Natl Acad Sci USA 71:3283–3286 – Mueller-Lantzsch N, Georg B, Yamamoto N, zur Hausen H (1980) Epstein-Barr virus – induced proteins. II. Analysis of surface polypeptides from EBV-producing and -superinfected cells by immunoprecipitation. Virology 102:401–411 – Southern EM (1975) Detection of specific sequences among DNA fragments separated by gel electrophoresis. J Mol Biol 98:503–517 – zur Hausen H, Gissmann L (1979) Lymphotropic papovaviruses isolated from African green monkey and human cells. Med Microbiol Immunol (Berl) 167:137–153 – zur Hausen H, Gissmann L, Mincheva A, Böcker JF (1980) Characterization of a lymphotropic papovavirus. In: Essex M, Todaro G, zur Hausen H (eds) Viruses in naturally occuring cancer. Cold Spring Harbor Laboratory, New York, Vol. A, pp 365–372

Haematology and Blood Transfusion Vol. 26
Modern Trends in Human Leukemia IV
Edited by Neth, Gallo, Graf, Mannweiler, Winkler
© Springer-Verlag Berlin Heidelberg 1981

Immunopathology of the X-Linked Lymphoproliferative Syndrome*

D. T. Purtilo

A. Abstract

The immunopathogenesis of 25 kindreds affecting 100 males with the X-linked lymphoproliferative syndrome (XLP) is being studied comprehensively by our registry and laboratory group. XLP is a combined variable immune deficiency with Epstein-Barr virus (EBV) induced phenotypes of: (1) fatal infectious mononucleosis (IM), (2) chronic IM progressive to malignant lymphoma, (3) acute IM progressive to acquired agammaglobulinemia or (4) malignant lymphoma. Cytogenetic studies of peripheral blood lymphocytes from 15 surviving males and 21 carrier females reveal random karyotype errors in several kindreds. Often polyclonal Ig or selective IgM increases and lymphocytosis with plasmacytoid forms typifies the IM phenotypes. Weakly reactive EBV-specific antibodies are found and anti-EB nuclear antigen is lacking. Antibodies to EBV are paradoxically elevated in female carriers. Initially all lymphoid tissues show immunoblastic proliferation with plasma cell differentiation and focal to extensive necrosis. Thymus gland and other lymphoid organs become depleted in T cell regions and Hassall's corpuscles may become destroyed. Multinucleated giant cells may be seen destroying the corpuscles or calcified corpuscles are found. The lymphoid infiltrates and lesions resemble graft-versus-host response in the fatal IM phenotype. Extensive necrosis in lymph nodes and deficient Ig secretion of B-cells characterize acquired agammaglobulinemia phenotypes. The malignant lymphomas span the spectrum of B cell differentiation with most being immunoblastic sarcomas. One case probably was monoclonal thus far, others are being studied. EBV DNA hybridization of tissues from 7 patients with fatal IM revealed 1 to 20 EBV genome equivalents per cell. The patients lacked appropriate EBV antibody responses. Our studies of XLP support the hypothesis that immune deficiency the EBV permits chronic and fatal lymphoproliferative diseases in XLP following EBV infections. Owing to this knowledge, rational bases for prevention by genetic counseling and by providing high titer gammaglobulin and antiviral therapy is being attempted.

B. Introduction

Our studies of the X-linked lymphoproliferative syndrome demonstrate the interaction between genetic predisposition to oncogenesis triggered by an environmental agent (EBV) in immunodeficient males. Prior to discussing XLP, the immunopathogenesis of Burkitt lymphoma (BL) and IM is reviewed.

The results of studies done by numerous investigators during the past two decades substantiate the view that EBV can be an oncogenic agent in immunodeficient individuals. A brief historical review follows for focusing our discussion of EBV-induced oncogenesis in immune deficient persons. Denis Burkitt, working in tropical Africa, delineated a new malignant lymphoma which often involves the jaws or abdominal organs (Burkitt 1958). Endemic African Burkitt lymphoma (AfBL) is present in areas of hyperendemic malaria. A hematopathology committee of WHO has defined BL pathologically (Berard et al. 1969).

---

* This study was supported in part by a grant from the National Institutes of Health, CA 23561-02

William Dameshek observed that infectious mononucleosis (IM) is a lymphoma-like illness which, though often serious, is rarely fatal (Dameshek and Gunz 1964). Diagnosis of IM requires fulfillment of a triad of clinical, hematologic, and serologic criteria. Werner and Gertrude Henle (1968) demonstrated that EBV was the etiologic agent of IM. Specific antibody responses to EBV form against early antigen and are transient, whereas viral capsid antibodies (VCA) and EB nuclear-associated antigen (EBNA) persist throughout life. Approximately 90% of adults have EBV antibodies to EBV, indicating past infection.

In 1964 Epstein and Barr identified in vitro a unique herpesvirus in a BL-derived cell line (Epstein et al. 1964). EBNA was identified in EBV-transformed B cells by Reedman and Klein in 1973 by immunofluorescence (Reedman and Klein 1973). Many investigators have attempted to determine whether EBV is an oncogenic virus in human beings. Three major EBV-associated diseases occur: IM in adolescents in Western countries, BL in the tropics, and nasopharyngeal carcinoma (NPC) in Southeast Asia. Although EBV has been demonstrated in tumor tissue derived from BL and NPC, absolute proof that EBV is an oncogenic virus is lacking (Klein 1975)

C. Immune Responses to Epstein-Barr Virus

Investigators agree that EBV triggers polyclonal proliferation of B-cells. Major questions remaining are: What stops this proliferation? Can IM be regarded as an aborted malignancy of transformed B cells? Figure 1 summarizes immune responses to EBV in primary infection and in reactivation of virus due to acquired immunodeficiency.

A first line of defense against primary EBV infection and reactivation of infection may be natural killer (NK) cells. The role of interferon as an immunomodulator has been the subject of recent intensive studies. Interferon is a potent modulator of spontaneous NK activity in mouse and man (Stebbing 1979; Klein et al. to be published; Saksela et al. to be published). NK show cytotoxic activity for a variety of tumor cell lines as well as normal cell lines infected with certain viruses (Heberman et al.

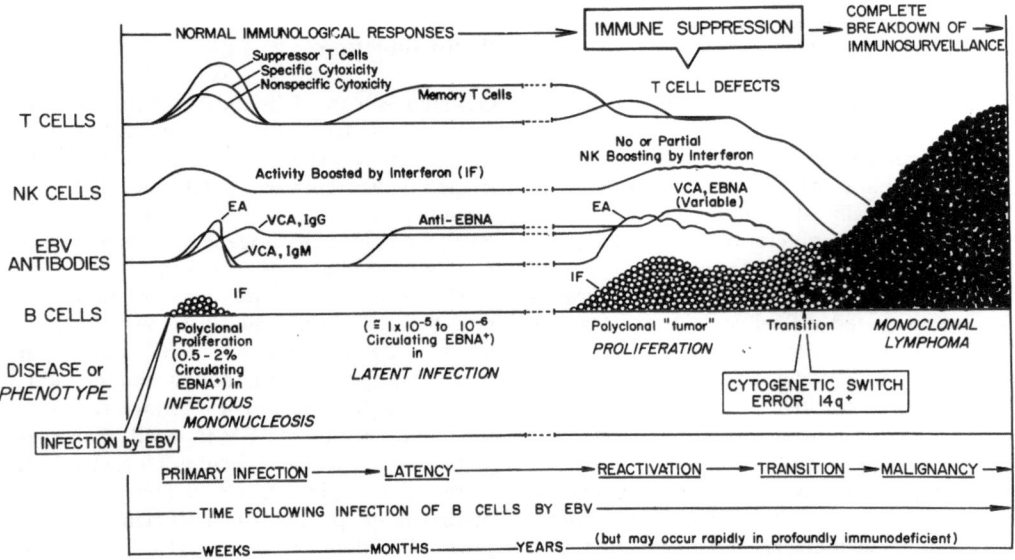

Fig. 1. Hypothesis summarizing humoral and cellular immune responses occurring after primary infection by Epstein-Barr virus (EBV) (*left portion* of diagram). On the *right* acquired immunodeficiency, as in renal transplant recipients, with reactivation of EBV and consequent polyclonal proliferation of B cells is depicted. Males with X-linked lymphoproliferative syndrome who respond or fail to respond to primary EBV infection are displayed on the *right side* of diagram. (Publicated with the permission of Academic Press)

1979). The lymphocyte subpopulation in man responsible for NK activity is currently unknown, although recent evidence favors the T and null lymphocyte subpopulations (Beverly and Knight 1979). Ascertainment of the importance of each of these mechanisms for elimination of EBV-infected or -transformed clones needs further study. Changes in lymphotoxicity of peripheral leukocytes against autologous and allogeneic LCL are demonstrable in IM (Bausher et al. 1973; Junge et al. 1971). The atypical lymphocytes of patients with acute IM reflect an immunologic struggle. EBV infects and causes B-cell proliferation; then T cells respond. The precise magnitude of the B and T cell proliferation is unknown. B cell proliferation is polyclonal, short lived, and precedes the outpouring of T cells (Papermichael et al. 1974; Pattengale et al. 1974). Klein and colleagues have found that approximately 0.5%–2% of circulating B cells contain EBNA during the first week of illness (Klein, et al. 1976). Haynes et al. (1979) have determined that both T and B cells increase in acute mononucleosis and the T cells lack Fc receptors for IgG or IgM.

The subpopulation of B cells infectable by EBV has not been identified; most B cells become transformed by EBV, resulting in a polyclonal proliferation (Pagano and Okasinski 1978). It is noteworthy that bone marrow is not usually involved in IM (Carter and Penman 1969). This finding indicates that a subpopulation of B lymphocytes susceptible to EBV infection traffic to tonsils, lymph nodes, and spleen.

Several laboratories have demonstrated that the atypical T lymphocytes which are characteristic during infectious mononucleosis have cytotoxic activity for EBV-infected lymphoblastoid cell lines (Royston et al. 1976; Hutt et al. 1975; Svedmyr and Jondal 1975). Their data suggest that cytotoxic T lymphocytes may be responsible for the control of EBV-induced B lymphocyte proliferation. Lymphocytes from patients obtained from blood during the initial 2 weeks of overt IM are significantly more cytotoxic than are controls. Cytotoxicity declines proportionately to the number of circulating atypical lymphocytes (Hutt et al. 1975). Results of in vitro studies suggest that in vivo cytotoxicity aborts B cell proliferation. Exactly how B cells are killed by cytotoxic T cell is not known. In addition, suppressor T cells become activated during B cell prolife-

ration (Tosato et al. 1979; Haynes et al. 1979). Following primary infection, the virus persists latently throughout life. Repression of reactication is due, in part, to T lymphocytes: Thorley-Lawson et al. (1978) have shown that T cells suppress the outgrowth of B cells infected by EBV in vitro. The suppression of EBV infection occurs after infection but before transformation of the cell (Thorley-Lawson 1980). Perhaps the same subpopulations of T cells prevents the long-term establishment of LCL from seropositive persons (Moss and Pope 1975; Moss et al. 1978; Rickinson et al. 1979). Regression of LCL is probably due to long-term T cell immunity to EBV (Moss et al. 1979; Rickinson et al. 1980).

While cellular immune responses to EBV combat B cell proliferation, antibodies to EBV-specific antibodies neutralize virus and/or kill infected B cells through antibody-dependent cellular cytotoxicity (ADCC). Henle et al. (1979) have recently reported that ADCC activity correlated poorly with the clinical course of IM. Our studies of patients with the X-linked lymphoproliferative syndrome (XLP) have identified affected males, chronically infected by EBV and lacking antibody to EBV, who show relatively normal lymphocytotoxicity (Purtilo et al. 1978a,b,c). Thus, antibodies to EBV do not appear to be required in surviving EBV infection. How ADCC participates to end the proliferative state in immunocompetent persons is not yet determined.

An array of EBV-specific antibody responses occur in normal persons following primary infection (Henle et al. 1974) (Fig. 1). Such antibody determinations have greatly enhanced our understanding of the immunopathology of IM and facilitate differential diagnosis, especially in heterophile negative IM. The latter group accounts for 10% of EBV-induced IM (Evans 1978). Three major antibody responses to EBV deserving mention are EA, VCA, and EBNA. Following infection by EBV, transient IgM antibody responses to VCA appear which later switch to the IgG class and persist for life. Another transient antibody response is against EA. The high titer anti-EA of children with BL shows the restricted (R) component (Henle et al. 1974). In contrast, anti-EA of IM has the diffuse (D) component; recurrent or chronic IM also has the R component (Horwitz et al. 1975). Antibodies to EBNA appear late, after partial destruction of infected B cells, and persist for life (Henle et al. 1974).

The EBV antibodies and cellular cytotoxicity directed specifically against EBV antigens serve to stop B cell proliferation, but immunoregulatory mechanisms often short circuit during the chaotic immune struggle of IM, and thus, a hoard of autoantibodies can erupt in IM (Sutton et al. 1974; Thomas 1972; McKinney and Cline 1974; Carter 1975; Steele and Hardy 1970; Purtilo 1980; Langhorne and Feizi 1977). The atuoimmune reactions and misdirected lymphocytes are devisive and they injure tissues, as in graft-versus-host response (GVHR) (Purtilo 1980).

D. Immunopathology of the X-Linked Lymphoproliferative Syndrome

During the decade since I autopsied an 8-year-old boy in the Duncan kindred who had died of infectious mononucleosis, research efforts have revealed immunopathogenetic mechanisms of EBV-induced fatal lymphoproliferative disorders (Purtilo et al. 1974a,b, 1975, 1977a,b, 1978a,b,c, 1979a,b; Purtilo 1976a,b, 1977). XLP thus serves as a prototype for studying persons at high risk for fatal EBV infection, expecially opportunistic malignant lymphomas in immune deficient patients.

Our international registry of XLP has registered more than 25 kindreds involving 100 male patients (Purtilo 1979). Approximately 50% of the affected males thus far have succumbed to IM (Fig. 2) and 15% to IM complicated by immunoblastic sarcoma; 19% have survived IM but acquired agammaglobulinemia or developed dysgammaglobulinemia, and 25% have experienced malignant lymphoma (Hamilton et al. 1980). Only 20 of the 100 affected males survive (Purtilo et al. 1979a,b).

The clinical and pathologic manifestations of the XLP syndrome mimic GVHR, especially in the IM phenotype. Following EBV infection, lymphoid tissues initially undergo hyperplasia followed by depletion and occasionally by malignant lymphoma, as in experimental murine GVHR (Purtilo 1980). In addition, tropism of aggressor lymphocytes in XLP for epithelial tissues – thymic, skin, liver, and gut – resemble GVHR (Seemayer et al. 1977). The acquired aproliferative phenotypes following EBV have consisted of aplastic anemia and hypo- or agammaglobulinemia. In the latter phenotype profound necrosis in lymph nodes and other lymphoid tissues is found (Purtilo 1980; Purtilo et al. 1979a,b). The differential diagnosis of XLP can be achieved by pedigree analysis and laboratory studies, as discussed elsewhere (Purtilo 1980).

We have attempted, in addition to our hematophathology studies, to characterize comprehensively the immunologic, virologic, and genetic defects in the 20 surviving males and 25 carrier females.

E. Chromosomal Breakage

Our cytogenetic studies of families with XLP have revealed differences in various kindreds with XLP. The initial two families with the syndrome have not shown appreciable defects. In contrast, a recent kindred has shown extensive aneuploidy in both peripheral lymphocytes and in early passage LCL (Paquin et al. 1980). Carrier females as well as affected males have shown a propensity to chromosomal damage. We have tentatively concluded that cytogenetic changes may be a phenotype of XLP and that increased clastogenic activity could predispose to induction of fatal lymphoproliferative disorders induced by EBV. Other environmental carcinogens could also initiate the lymphoreticular malignancies; however, none have been found.

F. Immune Deficiency of XLP

Immunologic studies of 14 affected males with XLP show relatively normal numbers of T and B cells. However, significantly depressed ($P < 0.05$ compared to controls) lymphocyte transformation responses to phytohemagglutinin, conconavalin A, pokeeweed, and strepto-

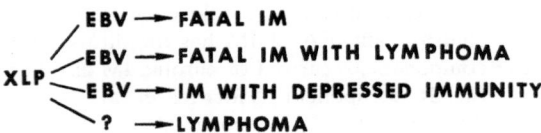

Fig. 2. Phenotypic expression of X-linked lymphoproliferative syndrome following infection by Epstein-Barr virus (reproduced with permission of C.V. Mosby Company, United States

lysin 0 antigens are found, and mixed leukocyte responses are diminished (Sullivan et al. 1980). Carrier females often show diminished responses to plant mitogens, but the magnitude of the depression is usually less than their sons. Affected males fail to develop a secondary IgG antibody response to ΦX 174 (a bacteriophage). This diminished responsiveness indicates that the immunodeficiency of XLP is not limited to EBV (Purtilo et al. 1979a,b) and that helper T cells may be defective. However, most surviving males have dysgammaglobulinemia. We are presently studying several affected males with relatively normal Ig Levels. Profound hypogammaglobulinemia has occurred in six surviving males who had a well-documented antecedent history of IM. Other survivors have shown selective IgA deficiency with or without elevated IgM (Purtilo et al. 1979a,b). Our preliminary studies of NK cells in XLP reveal defective activity in 80% of the patients who survive EBV infection but have other immune defects. Our studies indicate defective T lymphocytes and NK cell subsets which allow uncontrolled EBV-induced lymphoproliferation (Sullivan et al. 1980).

G. EBV-Specific Antibodies in XLP

Antibody studies for EBV in the 15 affected males reveal variable responses. Four patients entirely lacked antibodies to VCA, EA, and EBNA (Sakamoto et al. 1980). A second group of six XLP patients show normal anti-VCA titers but lack anti-EBNA and EA. In contrast, carrier females show a fourfold higher VCA antibody titer than do our normal adult controls; all carriers have anti-EBNA. EA antibodies were found in 11 of the 21 carriers, suggesting active infection. One carrier exhibited low grade, chronic lymphoproliferation (D. Purtilo, unpublished observations).

These serologic studies suggest that the B target cells of XLP are permissive of EBV infections. The lack of antibodies against EBNA in infected males suggests they have T cell defects against EBV. These latter findings corroborate our in vitro assays of defective T lymphocyte function and the hematopathologic findings of depletion of T cell zones in lymphoid tissues. Alternatively, helper T cell populations are lacking. In contrast,

the carrier females have approximately one-half defective B cells which are apparently permissive of EBV infection. Evidence substantiating this speculation is that their markedly high anti-VCA and normal anti-EBNA titers indicate vigorous response by normal lymphocytes to EBV infection. The elevated anti-EA activity in several carriers indicates chronic active infection. Thus, the women defend against the EBV infections and only manifest the XLP immunodeficiency in vitro.

H. Malignant Lymphomas in XLP

Documentation of EBV infection in immune deficient patients requires EBV antibody studies, transformation of peripheral blood lymphocytes or cells from lymphoid tissues, transformation of cord lymphocytes by throat washings in vitro, or demonstration of the genome in tissue by EBV DNA hybridization (Purtilo 1980). Employment of these techniques has resulted in the identification of EBV in numerous patients with inherited or acquired immunodeficiency who died of lymphoproliferative disease. In patients with XLP we have evidence suggesting that IM can progress to malignant lymphoma in immune deficient patients. We hypothesize that for the polyclonal proliferation characteristic of IM to become a monoclonal proliferation, a karyotypic abnormality appears which leads to a malignant monoclonal tumor cell. For example, the 14q+ marker chromosome of Burkitt lymphoma (Purtilo 1980) may be present. We are testing this hypothesis by testing affected males over many years (Fig. 1).

The malignant lymphomas in males with XLP have ranged the spectrum of B cell lymphomas (Paquin et al., to be published). In many cases, IM and immunoblastic sarcoma have occurred concurrently. Regrettably, cell surface marker studies for clonality and EBV DNA hybridization studies have not been possible on fresh lymphomas. However, EBV DNA hybridization of 7 cases of the fatal IM phenotype has revealed 7–20 EBV genome equivalents per cell in patients who lacked EBV antibody responses (Purtilo et al. 1981). Similar attempts to document EBV in opportunistic lymphomas in children with immunodeficiency (Kersey and Spector et al. 1978) and in renal transplant recipients ought to be attempted (Hanto et al. 1981).

I. Summary

We have developed a registry and laboratory of XLP dedicated to conducting multidisciplinary studies to provide:

1. Consultation to clinicians, families, and pathologists seeking diagnosis, treatment, evaluation, and genetic counseling;
2. Collection of data to define diagnostic criteria;
3. Further delineation of the diverse immune deficiencies and the basic genetical-immunologic defects responsible for the various phenotypic expressions;
4. The establishment of lymphoblastoid cell lines from patiens with XLP and related lymphoproliferative disorders which occur on genetic or sporadic bases for comparative studies;
5. Testing of the hypothesis that the common ubiquitous EBV can produce lethal lymphoproliferative diseases in individuals with inherited or acquired (renal and cardiac transplant recipients) immunodeficiency; and
6. Development of rational immunoprophylaxis (high titer EBV-specific gammaglobulin) and therapy (interferon and/or antiviral drugs) against EBV-induced oncogenesis.

References

Bausher JC, Smith RT (1973) Studies of the Epstein-Barr virus-host relationship: autochthonous and allogeneic lymphocyte stimulation by lymphoblast cell lines in mixed cell culture. Clin Immunol Immunophathol 1:270–281 – Berard C, O'Conor GT, Thomas LB, Torloni H (1979) Histophathological definition of Burkitt's tumor. Bull WHO 40:601–607 – Beverly P, Knight D (1979) News and Views: Killing comes naturally. Nature 278:119–120 – Borzy MS, Hong R, Horowitz S et al. (1979) Fatal lymphoma after transplantation of cultured thymus in children with combined immunodeficiency disease. N Engl J Med 301:565–568 – Burkitt DP (1958) A sarcoma involving the jaws in African children. Br J Surg 46:218–223 – Carter RL (1975) Infectious mononucleosis: Model for self-limiting lymphoproliferation. Lancet 11:846–849 – Carter RL, Penman HG (1969) Histopathology of infectious mononucleosis. In: Carter RL, Penman HG (eds) Infectious mononucleosis. Blackwell, Oxford Edinburgh, pp 146–161 – Dameshek W, Gunz F (1964) Leukemia. Grune & Stratton, New York, p 556 – Epstein MA, Achong BG, Barr YM (1964) Virus particles in cultured lymphoblasts from Burkitt's lymphoma. Lancet i:702–703 – Evans AS (1978) Infectious mononucleosis and related syndromes. J Med Sci 276:325–339 – Hamilton JK, Paquin LA, Sullivan JL, Maurer HS, Cruzi FG, Privisor AJ, Steuber CP, Hawkins E, Yawn D, Cornet JA, Clausen K, Finkelstein JZ, Landing B, Grunnet M, Purtilo DT (1980) X-linked lymphoproliferative syndrome registry report. J Pediatr 96:669–673 – Hanto D, Frizzera G, Purtilo D, Sakamato K, Sullivan JL, Saemundsen AK, Klein G, Simons RL, Najarian JS (1981) Lymphoproliferative disorders in renal transplant recipients. II. A. clinical spectrum and evidence for the role of Epstein-Barr virus. Cancer Res, in press – Haynes B, Schooley RT, Payling-Wright CR, Grouse JE, Dolin R, Fauci AS (1979) Emergence of suppressor cells of immunoglobulin synthesis during acute infectious mononucleosis. J Immunol 123:2095–2101 – Heberman RB, Djeu JY, Kay HD, Ortaldo JR, Riccardi C, Bonnard GD, Holden HT, Fagnani R, Santoni A, Puccetti P (1979) Natural killer cells: characteristics and regulation of activity. Immunol Rev 44:43–70 – Henle W, Henle G, Horwitz CA (1974) Epstein-Barr virus-specific diagnostic tests in infectious mononucleosis. Human Pathol 5:551–565 – Henle G, Lennette ET, Alspaugh MA, Henle W (1979) Rheumatoid factor as a cause of positive reactions in tests for Epstein-Barr virus-specific IgM antibodies. Clin Exp Immunol 36:415–422 – Horwitz CA, Henle W, Henle G, Schmitz H (1975) Clinical evaluations of patients with infectious mononucleosis and development of antibodies to the R component of the Epstein-Barr virus-induced early antigen complex. Am J Med 58:330–338 – Hutt LM, Huang YT, Discomb HE, Pagano LS (1975) Emhanced destruction of lymphoid cell lines by peripheral blood leukocytes taken from patients with acute infectious mononucleosis. J Immunol 115:243–248 – Junge U Hoekstra J, Deinhardt F (1971) Stimulation of peripheral lymphocytes by allogeneic and autochthonous mononucleosis lymphocyte cell lines. J Immunol 106:1306–1315 – Klein G (1975) The Epstein-Barr virus and neoplasia N Engl J Med 293:1353–1357 – Klein G, Svedmyr E, Jondal M, Person PO (1976) EBV-determined nuclear antigen (EBNA)-positive cells in the peripheral blood of infectious mononucleosis patients. Int J Cancer 17:21–26 – Klein E, Masucci MG, Masucci G, Vanky F (to be published) Natural and activated lymphocyte killers which affect tumor cells. In: Heberman R (ed) Natural cell-mediated immunity against tumors. Academic, New York – Langhorne J, Feizi T (1977) Studies on heterophile antibodies of infectious mononucleosis. Clin Exp Immunol 30:354–363 – McKinney AA, Cline WS (1974) Annotation: infectious mononucleosis. Br J Haematol 27:367 – Moss DJ, Pope JH (1975) EB virus-associated nuclear antigen production and cell proliferation in adult peripheral blood leukocytes inoculated with the QIMR-WIL strain of EB virus. Int J Cancer 15:503–511 – Moss DJ, Rickinson AB,

Pope JH (1978) Long-term T cell-mediated immunity to Epstein-Barr virus in man. I. Complete regression of virus-induced transformation in cultures of seropositive donor leukocytes. Int J Cancer 22:662–668 – Moss DJ, Rickinson AB, Pope JH (1979) Long-term T cell-mediated immunity to Epstein-Barr virus in man. III. Activation of cytotoxic T cells in virus-infected leukocyte cultures. Int J Cancer 23:618–625 – Pagano JS, Okasinski GF (1978) Pathogenesis of infectious mononucleosis, Burkitt's lymphoma and nasopharyngeal carcinoma: a unified scheme. In: de-Thé G, Henle W, Rapp F (eds) Oncogenesis and herpesvirus III. International Agency for Research on Cancer, Lyon, pp 687–697 – Papermichael M, Scheldon PJ, Holoboro EG (1974) T & B cell populations in infectious mononucleosis. Clin Exp Immunol 18:1–11 – Paquin LA, Maurer HS, Purtilo DT (to be published) Chromosomal abnormalities in the X-linked lymphoproliferative syndrome. – Pattengale PK, Smith RW, Perlin E (1974) Atypical lymphocytes in acute infectious mononucleosis. Identification by multiple T and B lymphocyte markers. N Engl J Med 291:1145–1148 – Purtilo DT (1976a) Hypothesis: Pathogenesis and phenotypes of an X-linked lymphoproliferative syndrome. Lancet ii:883–885 – Purtilo DT (1976b) Prevalence of Burkitt's lymphoma in males. N Engl J Med 295:1484 – Purtilo DT (1977) Non-Hodgkin's lymphoma in the X-linked recessive immunodeficiency and lymphoproliferative syndromes. Semin Oncol 4:335–343 – Purtilo DT (1980) Epstein-Barr virus-induced oncogenesis in immune definicent individuals. Lancet i:300–303 – Purtilo DT (1980) Immunopathogenesis and complications of infectious mononucleosis. In: Sommers S, Rosen PP (ed) Pathology Annual 1980. Appleton-Century-Crofts pp 253–299 – Purtilo DT, Sullivan JL (1979) Immunological bases for superior survival of females. Am J Dis Child 133:1251–1253 – Purtilo DT, Cassel C, Yang JPS (1974a) Fatal infectious mononucleosis in familial lymphohistiocytosis. N Engl J Med 291:736 – Purtilo DT, Hutt L, Cassel C (1974b) X-linked recessive familial lymphohistiocytosis. Clin Res 22:705A – Purtilo DT, Cassel C, Yang JPS, Stephenson SR, Harper R, Landing BH, Vawter GF (1975) X-linked recessive progressive combined variable immunodeficiency (Duncan's disease). Lancet i:935–941 – Purtilo DT, DeFlorio D, Hutt LM, Bhawan J, Yang JPS, Otto R, Edwards W, Rosen FS, Vawter G (1977a) Variable phenotypic expression of X-linked recessive lymphoproliferative syndrome. N Engl J Med 297:1077–1081 – Purtilo DT, Yang JPH, Allegra S, DeFlorio D, Hutt L (1977b) The pathogenesis and hematopathology of the X-linked recessive lymphoproliferative syndrome. Am J Med 62:225–233 – Purtilo DT Bhawan J, DeNicola L et al. (1978a) Epstein-Barr virus infections in a X-linked recessive lymphoproliferative syndrome. Lancet i:798–802 – Purtilo DT, Hutt LM, Allegra S, Cassel C, Yang JPS (1978b) Immunodeficiency to the Epstein-Barr virus in the X-linked recessive lymphoproliferative syndrome. Clin Immunol Immunopathol 9:147–156 – Purtilo DT, Paquin LA, Gindhart T (1978c) Genetics of neoplasia: Impact of ecogenetics on oncogenesis. Am J Pathol 91:609–688 – Purtilo DT, Hamilton J, Sullivan J, Paquin L, – Bhawan J, Sakamoto K (1979a) Epstein-Barr virus-induced oncogenesis in immunodeficient patients. Lab Invest 40:296 – Purtilo DT, Paquin LA, DeFlorio D, Virzi F, Sahkuja T (1979b) Diagnosis and immunopathogenesis of the X-linked recessive lymphoproliferative syndrome. Semin Hematol 16:309–343 – Purtilo DT, Sakamoto K, Saemundsen AK, Sullivan JL, Synnerholm A-C, Anvret M, Pritchard J, Seiff C, Pincott J, Pachman L, Rich K, Cruzi F, Cornet JA, Collins R, Barnes N, Knight J, Sandstedt B, Klein G (1981) Documentation of Epstein-Barr virus infection in immunodeficient patients with life-threatening lymphoproliferative diseases by clinical, virological and immunopathological studies. Cancer Res, in press – Purtilo DT, Sullivan JL, Paquin LA (to be published b) Biomarkers in immunodeficiency syndromes predisposing to cancer. In: Lynch H, Guirgis H (eds) Biological markers in cancer. Van Nostrand, New York – Reedman BM, Klein G (1973) Cellular localizations of an Epstein-Barr vjrus (EBV)-associated complement-fixing antigen in producer and nonproducer lymphoblastoid cell lines. Int J Cancer 11:499–520 – Rickinson AB, Moss DJ, Pope JH (1979) Long-term T-cell-mediated immunity to Epstein-Barr virus in man. II. Components necessary for regression in virus-infected leukocyte cultures. Int J Cancer 23:610–617 – Rickinson AB, Moss DJ, Pope JH, Ahlberg N (1980) Long-term T-cell-mediated immunity to Epstein-Barr virus in man. IV. Development of T-cell memory in convalescent infectious mononucleosis patient. Int J Caner 25:59–65 – Royston I, Sullivan JL, Periman PO, Perlin E (1976) Cell-mediated immunity in acute infectious mononucleosis. Bibl Haematol 43:278–280 – Sakamoto K, Freed H, Purtilo DT (1980) Antibody responses to Epstein-Barr virus in families with the X-linked lymphoproliferative syndrome. J Immunol 125:921–925 – Saksela E, Timonen T, Virtanen I, Cantell K (to be published) Regulation of human natural killer activity by interferon. In: Heberman R (ed) Natural cell-mediated immunity against tumors. Academic, New York – Seemayer TA, Lapp WS, Bolande RP (1977) Thymic involution in murine graft-versus-host reaction. Am J Pathol 88:119–134 – Spector BD, Perry GS, Kersey JH (1978) Genetically determined immunodeficiency diseases (GDID) and malignancy: Report from the Immuno-deficiency-Cancer Registry. Clin Immunol Immunopathol 11:12–29 – Stebbing N (1979) Interferons and inducers in vivo. Nature 279:581–582 – Steel CM, Hardy DA (1970) Evidence of altered antigenicity in cultured lymphoid cells from patients with infectious mononucleosis. Lancet i:1322–1323 – Sullivan JL, Byron K, Brewster F, Purtillo DT (1980)

Deficient natural killer (NK) cell activity in patients with the x-linked lymphoproliferative syndrome. Science 210:543–545 – Sutton RNP, Emond TD, Thomas DB, Doniach D (1974) The occurrence of autoantibodies in infectious mononucleosis. Clin Exp Immunol 17:427–436 – Svedmyr E, Jondal M (1975) Cytotoxic effector cells specific for B cell lines transformed by Epstein-Barr virus are present in patients with infectious mononucleosis. Proc Natl Acad Sci USA 72:1622–1626 – Thomas DB (1972) Antibodies to membrane antigens common to thymocytes and a subpopulation of lymphocytes in infectious mononucleosis sera. Lancet i:399–403 – Thorley-Lawson DA (1980) The suppression of Epstein-Barr virus infection in vitro occurs after infection, but before transformation of the cell. J Immunol 124:745–751 – Thorley-Lawson DA, Chess L, Strominger JL (1978) Suppression of in vitro Epstein-Barr virus antigens: a new role for adult T lymphocytes. J Exp Med 146:495–508 – Tosato G, Magrath I, Koski I, Dooley N, Blaese M (1979) Activation of suppressor T cells during Epstein-Barr virus-induced infectious mononucleosis. N Engl J Med 301:1133–1137

Haematology and Blood Transfusion Vol. 26
Modern Trends in Human Leukemia IV
Edited by Neth, Gallo, Graf, Mannweiler, Winkler
© Springer-Verlag Berlin Heidelberg 1981

Surface Characteristics of the U-937 Human Histiocytic Lymphoma Cell Line: Specific Changes During Inducible Morphologic and Functional Differentiation In Vitro

K. Nilsson, K. Forsbeck, M. Gidlund, C. Sundström, T. Tötterman, J. Sällström, and P. Venge

A. Introduction

A number of human hematopoietic cell lines representative of the neoplastic cell clone in vivo have been established in vitro during the last decade (for recent reviews see Minowada et al. 1980a, Nilsson 1979). Lymphoid leukemia and lymphoma lines all seem to be arrested at a particular stage of lymphoid differentiation (Nilsson 1978). Attempts to induce differentiation with mitogens have generally been unsuccessful. Only in the promyelocytic leukemia cell line HL-60 has spontaneous terminal differentiation been documented (Collins et al. 1977; Gallagher et al. 1979). Recently, however, inducible differentiation in vitro has been demonstrated in three non-lymphoid hematopoietic cell lines using substances known to induce differentiation in animal cell systems. Thus, dimethyl-sulfoxide (DMSO) and 12-tetradecanoyl-phorbol-13-acetate (TPA) will differentiate HL-60 cells (Collins et al. 1978; Gahmberg et al. 1979; Huberman and Callaham 1979; Rovera et al. 1979), butyric acid or hemin will induce the erythroleukemic K-562 cells (Andersson et al. 1979; Rutherford et al. 1979), and TPA or supernatant from mixed lymphocyte cultures (MLC), the histiocytic lymphoma U-937 cells (Koren et al. 1979; Nilsson et al. 1980a).

The phenotypic features of the U-937 cells (Sundström and Nilsson 1976) suggest that they represent immature monocytoid cells. When induced to differentiate, such cells will undergo a stepwise morphologic and functional maturation similar to that described for differentiating normal monocytic cells (Koren et al. 1979; Nilsson et al. 1980a). It was therefore suggested that the U-937 cells, although neoplastic, may be used as a model in studies of various biologic aspects of cells in the normal monoblast-macrophage differentiation lineage (Nilsson et al., to be published a).

The present paper summarizes our studies so far of inducible differentiation in U-937 and deals mainly with surface changes during treatment with MLC supernatant of TPA but also demonstrates that the U-937 may be induced to display functional features of mature monocytic cells.

B. Materials and Methods

I. Cells

The U-937 cell line was established in 1975 from a patient with a "true" histiocytic lymphoma (Sundström and Nilsson 1976). The line is Epstein-Barr virus negative and its neoplastic nature is demonstrated by its aneuploidy (Zech et al. 1976) and tumorigenic potential in nude mice (Nilsson, unpublished work). The morphology, the cytochemical features, and the surface and functional characteristics of U-937 are summarized in Table 1. Taken together the phenotype of U-937 cells is unique, without resemblence to any other published hematopoietic cell line, and suggests that the U-937 cells represent monocytic cells arrested at a fairly immature stage in the monocyte differentiation lineage.

All experiments with U-937 cells were performed as follows: Cells were harvested from optimally growing stock cultures and were incubated under standard culture conditions at an initial cell concentration of 2×10^5 cells/ml. The medium was F-10 supplemented by 10% foetal calf serum from a selected batch (GIBCO) and antibiotics (penicillin 100 IU/ml, streptomycin 50 µg/ml, gentamycin 50 µg/ml and amphotericin B 1.25 mg/ml). The medium was not changed during the incubation periods of 24–96 h: TPA was purchased from Sigma (United States); MLC supernatant was harvested from six day cultures as described (Gidlund et al., to be publi-

Table 1. Selected properties of U-937

Characteristics	Reference
Monocytoid morphology	Sundström and Nilsson 1976
Monocytoid-myeloid cytochemical profile	Nilsson et al. 1980a, Sundström and Nilsson 1977
Expression of Fc and C3 receptors, β_2-microglobulin, HLA, and Ia-like antigen	Huber et al. 1976; Nilsson et al., to be published
Absence of Helix Pomatia A agglutamin receptor	Nilsson et al., to be published
Monocyte-like surface glycoprotein pattern	Nilsson et al. 1980b
Capacity for lysozyme secretion	Ralph et al. 1976; Sundström and Nilsson 1976
Capacity (weak) for phagocytosis	Sundström and Nilsson 1976
Activity (weak) as effector cell in ADCC	Nilsson et al. 1980a
Tumorigenicity in nude mice	Nilsson, unpublished work
Aneuploid karyotype	Zech et al. 1976

shed). Monocytes were idolated from fresh human buffy coats on a two step Percoll gradient according to Pertoft et al. (1980).

II. Cell Surface Studies

The Fc and C3 receptors were quantitated using rosette assays (Huber et al. 1976; Sjöberg and Inganäs 1979). Expression of Ia-like antigen (HLA-DR), HLA, and B₂-microglobulin was quantitated by a single cell Zeiss cytophotometer as described (Nilsson et al. 1974). Indirect immunofluorescence was performed using the following antisera: rabbit anti-HLA-DR (Klareskog et al. 1978) rabbit anti-HLA (gift from Dr. P. Peterson, Uppsala), rabbit anti-B₂-microglobulin (Dakopatts, Copenhagen), and fluoresceinisothiocyanate labeled swine anti-rabbit serum (Dakopatts, Copenhagen).

The expression of major surface glycoprotein was studied by the galactoseoxidase tritiated sodium borohydride surface labeling technique of Gahmberg and Hakamori (Gahmberg and Hakomori 1973). The methodology used to study the sensitivity to natural killer (NK) cells have been detailed in Gidlund et al. (Gidlund et al., to be published).

III. Functional Assays

The activity as effector cell in an antibody-dependent cellular cytotoxicity (ADCC) assay with antibody-coated chicken erythrocytes (CRBC) as targets was studied as described (Gidlund et al., to be published). The phagocytic activity of immunoglobulin coated latex particles was quantitated under phase contrast after incubation of the cell particle mixture for 30 min at +37°C. The capacity for

lysozyme secretion was quantitated by a radioimmunoassay (Venge et al. 1979).

C. Results

Morphologic and functional changes may be induced in U-937 cells by addition of $10^{-12}-10^{-7}$ M TPA or 20%-30% of MLC supernatant to the culture medium (Nilsson et al. 1980a). Comparative studies on the effect of TPA and MLC supernatants showed that the induced changes in morphology, expression of nonspecific esterases, and activity as effector cells in ADCC were similar (Gidlund et al., to be published; Nilsson et al. 1980a). In the following the presentation will focus on our results with TPA as inducer, since this substance has the advantage over the MLC supernatant of being well defined.

I. Alterations of Growth Properties, Morphology, and Cytochemical Profile After Exposure to TPA

The optimal concentrations for the induction of the morphologic and functional changes listed in Table 2 was $1.6 \times 10^{-9}-1.6 \times 10^{-7}$ M. After addition of TPA increased cell clustering and the appearance of a small fraction of adherent cells (glass or plastic surfaces) was noted within 1 h. The adherent fraction increased with time to a maximum of 60%-80% during the first 24 h of incubation. After 24

Characteristic	Reference (if not this paper)
Morphologic maturation	Nilsson et al. 1980a
Increased content of nonspecific esterase (NASDAE, ANAE)	Nilsson et al. 1980a
Increased expression of Fc receptors	
Increased expression of Ia-like antigen, β_2-microglobulin, and HLA antigen	
Specific changes in the surface glycoprotein pattern	
Decreased sensitivity to natural killer (NK) cells	Gidlund et al, to be published
Increased activity as effector cell in ADCC	Gidlund et al., to be published
Increased phagocytic activity	
Increased secretion of lysozyme	
Concomitant inhibition of growth and DNA synthesis	

Table 2. Phenotypic changes in U-937 cells after exposure to TPA or MLC supernatant

h detachment of cells was noted, but 10%–20% of the cells remained on the surface during the observation time of up to 8 days. These cells spread out and acquired a macrophage-like morphology as described (Nilsson et al. 1980a) (Fig. 1). Also in free-floating clusters the individual cell size increased. Suface attachment of TPA-treated cells could be prevented by covering the petri dishes with agarose. Such cells clumped to form large aggregates.

Comparative studies on the various properties (Table 2) in U-937 of cells grown in petri dishes with and without an agarose bottom overlayer showed that the acquisition of macrophage-like features in U-937 cells after TPA treatment was not surface dependent. The cell clustering and increased adhesiveness induced by TPA seem to be reversible within 2 h. However, so far the reversibility of the simultaneous functional changes has not been studied.

The growth of U-937 cells was partially inhibited by TPA as evidenced by growth curves and a decreased uptake of ^{3}H-thymidine (Forsbeck, to be published). The cytochemical profile, as tested by the panel of cytochemical stains described by Sundström and Nilsson (1977) changed within 24 h after treatment of TPA. The expression of the nonspecific esterases naphtol AS-D esterase (NASDAE) and acid α-naphtyl-acetate esterase

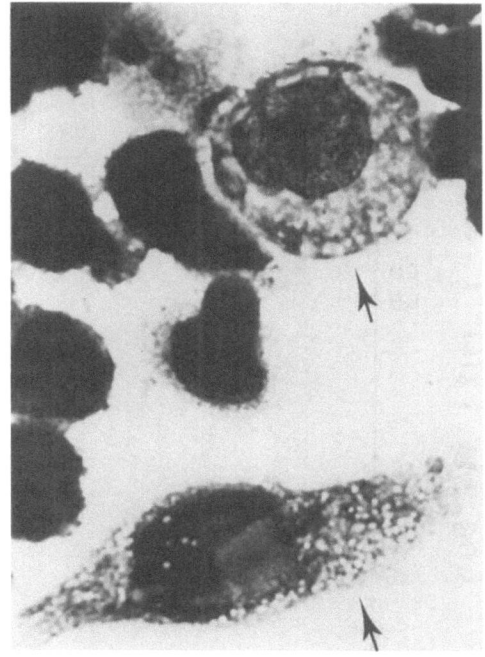

Fig. 1. U-937 cells exposed to 1.6×10^{-9} M TPA for 4 days in plastic petri dishes. Note the two macrophage-like cells *(arrows)* which contrast to the remaining, essentially morphologically unaltered cells

217

increased, with the most notable change found for NASDAE. The latter staining reaction could also be inhibited by NaF, a feature considered to be specific for the NASDAE of monocytic cells.

II. Surface Changes Induced by TPA

The composition of the major surface glycoproteins (SGP) of U-937 cells underwent characteristics changes after incubation with TPA or MLC supernatant (Fig. 2). The SGP of U-937 cells was characteristically different from that of other human hematopoietic cell lines (Nilsson et al. 1977). The most prominently labeled SGP had an apparent mol. w. of 160,000–145,000 daltons (160–145K). Less strongly labeled bands had apparent mol. wts. of 210K, 200K, 190K and 90K. After TPA treatment the following major changes in the SGP were found: the 200K band disappeared and the 145K-160K and the 90K bands were more strongly labeled. The "new" bands of apparent mol. wts. of 180K, 140K and 85K respectively, appeared. The MLC supernatant treated U-937 cells underwent essentially similar SGP changes with TPA treatment. Taken together the changes induced by TPA or MLC supernatant in the SGP in the U-937 cells made them resemble mature blood monocytes more closely than before.

The change in the expression of Fc receptors after TPA treatment varied from experiment to experiment, although culture conditions were strictly standardized. In most experiments, however, the percentage of rosetting cells increased from around 25% to 50%. In contrast the frequency of C3 receptor positive cells remained unchanged.

The amount of Ia-like antigen increased

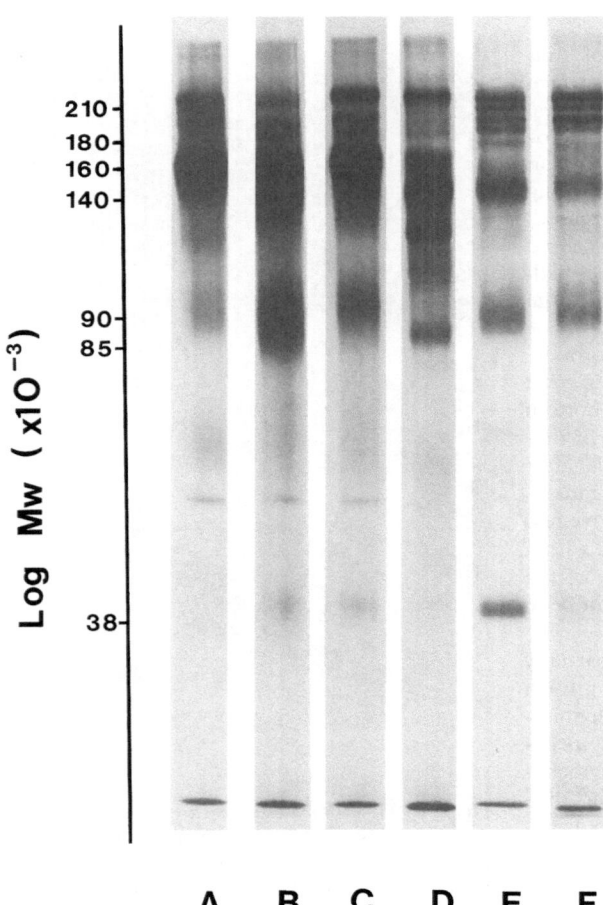

Fig. 2. Fluorography patterns of labeled surface glycoprotein obtained by SDS slab gel electrophoresis. Gel contration 7.5%. **A,** Untreated U-937 cells; **B,** TPA-treated U-937 cells; **C,** MLC-supernatant treated U-937; **D,** Untreated blood monocytes; **E,** TPA-treated blood monocytes; and **F,** MLC-supernatant treated blood monocytes. Molecular weights *(Mw)* calculated on basis of the following markers: myosin (200 KD), phosphorylase a (100 KD), albumin (66 KD), and ovalbumin (43 KD)

after TPA-induction (Table 3). The mean increase was twofold by day 2 and threefold by day 4. In a fraction (15%) of the cells, however, the change was 4–10-fold on day 2.

Table 3. Expression of Ia-like antigen on the surface of U-937 cells

	Day 2		
	No.	Mean fluorescence intensity (rel. units)	S.D.
Control	30	3.75	2.24
TPA-treatment	31	7.31	3.98
	Day 4		
	No.	Mean fluorescence intensity (rel. units)	S.D.
Control	30	3.74	1.65
TPA-treatment	32	10.50	6.33

The amount of HLA antigen and B_2-microglobulin also increased in four of five experiments. However, as for the expression of Fc receptors considerable variability was found in the different experiments (maximal increase on day 4 for HLA-antigen was two-fold and for B_2-microglobulin, five-fold).

The fact that TPA and MLC supernatant-induced differentiation of U-937 cells is associated with surface changes is also reflected by the dose-time dependent decrease in the sensitivity to human natural killer (NK) cells as has been reported (Gidlund et al., to be published).

III. Functional Changes Induced by TPA

Three functions (activity as effector cell in ADCC, secretion of lysozyme, and phagocytic activity) assumed to be typical for macrophages were studied. As is detailed by Gidlund et al. (to be published) U-937 acquired the capacity to kill antibody-coated CRBC. Even uninduced U-937 cells have a weak activity (<4% lysis) in ADCC against CRBC but only at a comparatively high effector to target cell ratio (Nilsson et al. 1980a). After exposure to TPA or MC supernatant the effectivity of the U-937 cells as killers increased as evidenced by a pronounced lysis (10%–20%) even at a very

low (2:1) effector to target cell ratio. The activity of TPA-induced U-937 cells as ADCC effectors was both time and dose dependent, being maximal after 4 days treatment with 1.6×10^{-8}–1.6×10^{-7} M TPA.

The secretion of lysozyme has been studied onyl in a limited number of experiments using MLC supernatant of 1.6×10^{-9} M TPA treatment for 24 h. However, the results demonstrated a clear increase (three-fold) in the rate of lysozyme secretion.

The capacity for phagocytosis was regularly found in TPA-treated cultures but not in the control cultures. The fraction of phagocytic cells in TPA-treated cultures ranged from 10%–20%.

D. Discussion

When exposed to TPA or MLC supernatant the histiocytic lymphoma U-937 cells undergo multiple changes of their phenotype (Table 2). Taken together the alterations are those expected to occur when immature monocytic cell differentiate. It is not yet clear whether the induced differentiation is restricted only to a fraction of the cells or whether all cells repond to the inductive signals of TPA or MLC supernatant. The morphologic studies and the quantitative analyses of the expression of Ia-like antigen would favor the former possibility, while studies on the ADCC activity of various fractions of TPA stimulated cells obtained a 1 g gradient separation procedures (Gidlund, personal communication) would indicate that all cells may differentiate. If the latter suggestion is true, the finding of only 10%–20% strongly Ia-like antigen positive cells and a fraction (10%–20%) of surface adherent macrophage-like cells could be explained by the fact that the induced U-937 cells traverse different lengths along the presumed monocyte differentiation pathway. Be that as it may, the U-937 seems to be a satisfactory clonal model for studies of various aspects of the monocyte differentiation lineage in vitro.

The results from the cytoplasmic assays for esterases and expression of surface Fc and C3 receptors and Ia-like, HLA and B_2-microglobulin molecules have been variable for unknown reasons. We interpret this as due to a marked sensitivity of the differentiating U-937 system to factors in the culture and assay systems which we have been unable to control. This variability for U-937, when induced to differentiate, has been noted before by Koren et al. (1979) using MLC supernatants to induce differentiation and concomitant increase in Fc receptor expression and activity in ADCC. A similar variability has been found also in differentiation experiments with the K-562 and HL-60 lines (Andersson, personal cummunication; Nilsson, unpublished work).

The functional assays alway gave reproducible results and leave room for no other interpretation than that the U-937 cells, after exposure to TPA or MLC supernatant, acquire the presumed typical functional features of mature monocytesmacrophages (increased capacity for phagocytosis, lysozyme secretion, and activity as effector cell in ADCC). We therefore suggest that the surface changes simultaneously recorded are associated with a change in the stage of monocytic differentiation of U-937 cells and therefore useful markers in studies of monoblast-macrophage differentiation. Of particular interest seems to be the possibility of using some of the major SGP, as detected by tritiated sodium borohydride labeling, as differentiation markers. The major SGP hallmarks for mature monocytic cells seems to be the 180K, 140K, and 85K SGP. All these are strongly labeled both in blood monocytes and TPA stimulated U-937 cells. Specific changes in the SGP compositions have previously been found in the HL-60 (Gahmberg et al. 1979) and in the K-562 cell lines (Nilsson et al. 1980a) during induced differentiation and thus further strenthens the usefulness of certain SGP as differentiation markers.

It is not yet clear whether "terimal" differentiation occurs at all in the U-937. Neither is the concomitant change in growth and DNA synthesis fully analyzed. Our studies so far indicate that at least partial inhibition of growth and DNA synthesis accompany TPA treatment and the induced phenotypic alterations. It is thus possible that TPA may induce a cell cycle block similar to what has been described by Rovera et al. (1979) for HL-60 cells.

D. Concluding Remarks

We conclude that the human histiocytic lymphoma cell line U-937 may be induced by TPA or MLC supernatant to undergo morphologic and functional differentiation in vitro which resembles the stepwise maturation events described for normal monocytic cells. The cell line may, therefore, be useful as a model for controlled in vitro studies of various aspects of monocytic differentiation. The observed specific changes in the composition of the major SGP suggest that such GP might be useful differentiation markers.

Acknowledgements

This study was supported by the Swedish Cancer Society and the Fortia Fund. The skillful technical assistance of Mrs. Ingela Stadenberg is gratefully acknowledged.

References

Andersson LC, Jokinen M, Gahmberg CG (1979) Induction of erythroid differentiation in the human leukaemia cell line K-562. Nature 278:364–365 – Collins SJ, Gallo RC, Gallagher RE (1977) Continuous growth and differentiation of human myeloid leukemic cells in suspension culture. Nature 270:347–349 – Collins SJ, Ruscetti FW, Gallagher RE, Gallo RC (1978) Terminal differentiation of human promyelocytic leukemia cells induced by dimethyl sulfoxide and other polar compounds. Proc Natl Acad Sci USA 75:2458–2462 – Forsbeck K (to be published) – Gahmberg CG, Hakomori S (1973) External labeling of cell surface galactose and galactosamine in glycolipid and glycoprotein of human erythrocytes. J Biol Chem 248:4311–4317 – Gahmberg CG, Nilsson K, Andersson LC (1979) Specific changes in the surface glycoprotein pattern of human promyelocytic leukemic cell line HL-60 during morphologic and functional differentiation. Proc Natl Acad Sci USA 76:4087–4091 – Gallagher R, Collins S, Trujillo J, McCredie K, Ahearn M, Tsai S, Metzgar R, Aulakh G, Ting R, Ruscetti F, Gallo F (1979) Characterization of the continuous differentiating myeloid cell line (HL-60) from a patient with acute promyelocytic leukemia. Blood 54:713–733 – Gidlund M. Örn A, Pattengale P, Wigzell H, Jansson M, Nilsson K (to be published) Induction of differentiation in two human tumor cell lines is paralleled by a decrease in NK susceptibility. Nature – Huber C, Sundström CC, Nilsson K, Wigzell H (1976) Surface receptors on human haematopoietic cell lines. Clin Exp Immunol 25:367–376 – Huberman E, Callaham MF (1979) Induction of terminal differentiation in human promyelocytic leukemia cells by tumor-promoting agents. Proc Natl Acad Sci USA 76:1293–1296 – Klareskog L, Trägårdh L, Lindblom JB, Peterson

PA (1978) Reactivity of a rabbit antiserum against highly purified HLA-DR antigens. Scand J Immunol 7:199–208 – Koren HS, Anderson SJ, Larrick JW (1979) In vitro activation of a human macrophage-like cell line. Nature 279:328–331 – Minowada J, Sgawa K, Lok MS, Kubonishi I, Nakazawa S, Tatsumi E, Ohnuma T, Goldblum N (1980) A model of lymphoid-myeloid cell differentiation based on the study of marker profiles of 50 human leukemia cell lines. In: Serrou B, Rosenfeld C (eds) International Symposium on new trends in human immunology and cancer immunotherapy. Doin éditeurs, Paris pp 180–199 – Nilsson K (1978) Established human lymphoid cell lines as models for B-lmphocyte differentiation. Human lymphocyte differentiation. Its application to cancer. In: Serrou B, Rosenfeld C (eds) INSERM Symposium No 8. Elsevier/North Holland Biomedical Press, pp 307–317 – Nilsson K (1979) The nature of lymphoid cell lines and their relationship to EB virus. In: Epstein MA, Achong BG (eds) The Epstein-Barr-virus. Springer, Heidelberg – Nilsson K, Evrin PE, Welsh KI (1974) Production of B_2-microglobulin by normal and malignant human cell lines and peripheral lymphocytes. Transplant Rev 21:53–84 – Nilsson K, Andersson C, Gahmberg CG, Wigzell H (1977) Surface glycoprotein patterns of normal and malignant human lymphoid cells. II. B-cells, B-blasts and Epstein-Barr virus (EBV) positive and negative B-lymphoid cell lines. Int J Cancer 20:708–718 – Nilsson K, Andersson LC, Gahmberg CG, Forsbeck K (1980a) Differentiation in vitro of human leukemia and lymphoma cell lines. In: Serrou B, Rosenfeld C (eds) International Symposium on new trends in human immunology and cancer immunotherapy. Doin éditeurs, Paris pp 271–282 – Nilsson K, Andersson LC, Gahmberg CG (1980b) Cell surface characteristics of human histiocytic lympho-

ma lines. I. Surface glycoprotein patterns. Leuk Res 4:271–277 – Nilsson K, Kimura A, Klareskog L, Andersson LC, Gahmberg CG, Hammarström S, Wigzell H (to be published) Cell surface characteristics of histiocytic lymphoma cell lines. II. Expression of Helix Pomatia A-hemagglutinin binding surface glycoproteins and Ia-like antigens. Leuk Res – Pertoft H, Johnsson A, Wärmegård B, Seljelid R (1980) Separation of human monocytes on density gradients of Percoll^R. J Immunol Methods 33:221–229 – Ralph P, Moore MAS, Nilsson K (1976) Lysozyme synthesis by established human and murine histiocytic lymphoma cell lines. J Exp Med 143:1528–1533 – Rovera G, Santoli D, Damsky C (1979) Human promyelocytic leukemia cells in culture differentiate into macrophage-like cells when treated with a phorbol diester. Proc Natl Acad Sci USA 76:2779–2783 – Rutherford TR, Clegg JB, Weatherall DJ (1979) K-562 human leukemic cells synthesize embryonic haemoglobin in response to haemin. Nature 280:164–165 – Sjöberg O, Inganäs M (1979) Detection of Fc receptor-bearing lymphocytes by using IgG-coated latex particles. Scand J Immunol 9:547–552 – Sundström C, Nilsson K (1976) Establishment and characterization of a human histiocytic lymphoma cell line (U-937). Int J Cancer 17:565–577 – Sundström C, Nilsson K (1977) Cytochemical profile of human haematopoietic biopsy cells and derived cell lines. Br J Haematol 37:489–501 – Venge P, Hällgren R, Stålenheim G, Olsson I (1979) Effect of serum and cations on the selective release of granular proteins from human neutrofils during phagocytosis Scand J Haematol 22: 317–326 – Zech L, Haglund U, Nilsson K3 Klein G (1976) Characteristic chromosomal abnormalities in biopsies and lymphoid cell lines from patients with Burkitt and non-Burkitt lymphomas. Int J Cancer 17:47–56

Haematology and Blood Transfusion Vol. 26
Modern Trends in Human Leukemia IV
Edited by Neth, Gallo, Graf, Mannweiler, Winkler
© Springer-Verlag Berlin Heidelberg 1981

Enzyme Polymorphism as a Biochemical Cell Marker: Application to the Cellular Origin and Homogeneity of Human Macrophages and to the Classification of Malignant Lymphomas*

H. J. Radzun, M. R. Parwaresch, and K. Lennert

The polymorphism of enzyme systems can be ascribed to four different mechanisms. *Physicochemical heterogeneity* ensues from free combination of subunits constituting the quaternary structure of enzyme proteins. The so-called *microheterogeneity* is caused by the presence of nonpeptide groups in the enzyme molecules. Furthermore, genetic activity leads to the appearance of molecular enzyme variants called *isoenzymes*. Finally, the phenotypical expression of genetic variations is usually obscured by the inductive and repressive influences exerted during ontogenesis and differentiation. This is referred to as *balanced polymorphism* (Ford 1940).

There is ample evidence that the pattern of enzyme variants remains constant within a homogeneous cell population and reveals a stable feature specific to this cell cohort (Li et al. 1970). We have used isoelectric focusing on polyacrylamide gels for investigation of the lysosomal acid esterase (EC 3.1.1.6) and lysosomal acid phosphatase (EC 3.1.3.2) polymorphism in purified human blood cell types (Radzun et al. 1980, to be published). It could be shown that clear differences in the pattern of enzyme variants were detectable between platelets, red blood cells, granulocytes, monocytes, and T and B lymphocytes.

The unique distribution pattern of acid esterase in human blood monocytes with four minor and one major anodic band within a pH range of 6.25–5.70 was used to detect the homogeneity and cellular origin of human peritoneal macrophages. Purified unstimulated sessile peritoneal macrophages, obtained

from noninflammatory peritoneal cavity, showed in addition to the five isoenzymes of acid esterase which are specific for blood monocytes, two further enzyme variants (Fig. 1). Exposure of blood monocytes to an uncoated glass surface led to the appearance of these two bands on the third day of culture. From these results we deduce that sessile peritoneal macrophages, like exudate peritoneal macrophages, represent a monocytic cell cohort. Thus, all macrophages of the peritoneal cavity constitute a homogeneous cell population. This contradicts the opinion of other authors, who hold the view that sessile peritoneal macrophages are self-sustaining (Daems et al. 1973).

Another example for the application of cell-specific polymorphism of enzymes is its employment in the characterization of tumor cells. On the basis of morphological conventions and enzyme cytochemical and immunocytochemical methods, human malignant lymphomas have been successfully classified (Lennert et al. 1978). It has been shown that the four lymphoma entities – chronic lymphocytic leukemia of B-cell type, follicular lymphoma, lymphoplasmacytic/lymphoplasmacytoid lymphoma, and plasmacytoma – represent B lymphocyte neoplasias, imitating various stages of activity and differentiation of normal B lymphocytes. In line with these considerations all four lymphoma entities shared the isoenzyme pattern of lysosomal acid phosphatase observed in normal human B lymphocytes (Fig. 2). Furthermore, the stepwise rise in enzyme activity from one lymphoma entity to the next was at least partly due to the appearance of additional isoenzymes (Schmidt et al., to be published). These results show that it is possible to classify a tumor as B lymphocytic in origin on the basis of its typical isoenzyme

* This work was supported by the Deutsche Forschungsgemeinschaft, programs CL3 and CN2

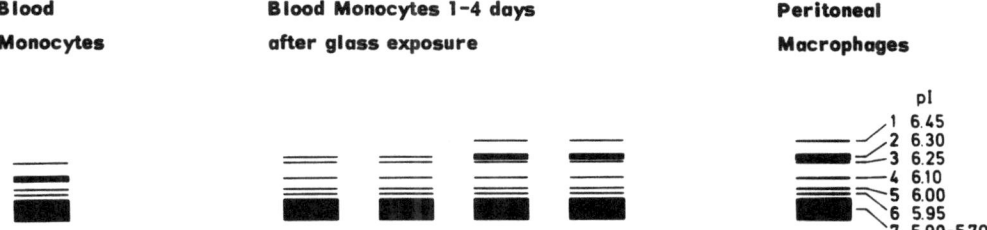

Fig. 1. Polymorphism of lysosomal acid esterase in normal human blood monocytes and sessile peritoneal macrophages. Prolonged exposure of blood monocytes to uncoated glass surface showed a gradual transition of the monocytic pattern of acid esterase into that of peritoneal macrophages. *pI*, isoelectric point

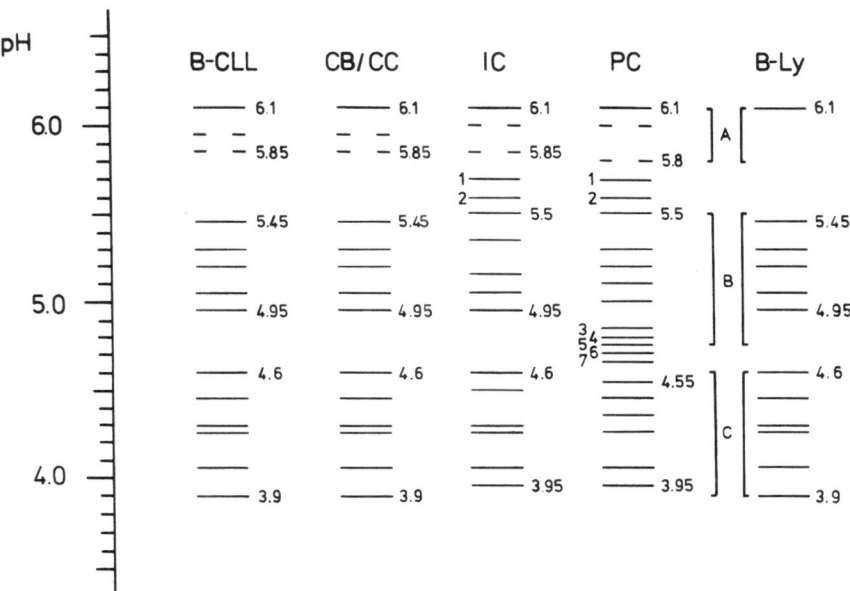

Fig. 2. Polymorphism of lysosomal acid phosphatase in chronic lymphocytic leukemia of B-cell type *(B-CLL)*, follicular lymphoma *(CB/CC)*, lymphoplasmacytic/lymphoplasmacytoid lymphoma *(IC)*, and plasmacytoma *(PC)* in comparison with normal human B lymphocytes *(B-Ly)*

pattern as long as pure populations of tumor cells are provided.

The examples mentioned above document the new perspectives of using enzyme polymorphism as a biochemical marker for the characterization of maturational stages, functional derivatives, and neoplastic variants of a certain cell line.

References

Daems WT, Poelman RE, Brederoo P (1973) Peroxidatic activity in resident peritoneal macrophages and exudate monocytes of the guinea pig after ingestion of latex particles. J. Histochem Cytochem 21:93–95 – Ford EB (1940) In: Huxley J (ed) The new systematics. Clarendon, Oxford, pp 493–513 – Lennert K, Stein H, Mohri N, Kaiserling E, Mueller-Hermelink KH (1978) Malignant lymphomas other than Hodgkin's disease. Springer, New York Berlin Heidelberg – Li CY, Yam LT, Lam KW (1970) Studies of acid phosphatase isoenzymes in human leucocytes. Demonstration of isoenzyme cell specificity. J Histochem Cytochem 18:901–910 – Radzun HJ, Parwaresch MR, Kulenkampff C Staudinger M, Stein H (1980) Lysosomal acid esterase: Activity and isoenzymes in separated normal human blood cells. Blood 55:891–897 – Radzun HJ, Parwaresch MR, Kulenkampff C,

Stein H (1980) Lysosomal acid phosphatase: Activity and isoenzymes in separated normal human blood cells. Clin Chim Acta 102:227–235 – Schmidt D, Radzun HJ, Schwarze E, Stein H, Parwaresch MR (1980) Activity and isoenzymes of acid phosphatase in human B-cell lymphoma of low grade malignancy. A novel aid in the classification of malignant lymphoma. Cancer 46:2676–2681

Haematology and Blood Transfusion Vol. 26
Modern Trends in Human Leukemia IV
Edited by Neth, Gallo, Graf, Mannweiler, Winkler
© Springer-Verlag Berlin Heidelberg 1981

Human Leukemic Lymphocytes – Biochemical Parameters of the Altered Differentiation Status

K. Wielckens, M. Garbrecht, G. Schwoch, and H. Hilz

A. Introduction

Deviation from normal differentiation is a general phenomenon of tumor cells. To study the misprogramming of normal gene function adequately, systems should be analyzed that are not complicated by concomitant changes in cell proliferation rates. A cell system in which the normal and the corresponding neoplastic cells do not proliferate at all is represented by normal human blood lymphocytes and lymphocytes from patients with chronic lymphocytic leukemia. Both cell types exhibit very low (^{3}H)thymidine incorporation (Wielckens et al. 1980), confirming that both types of lymphocytes are in the G_0 phase of the cell cycle. Thus, the leukemic lymphocyte is characterized exclusively by differentiation defects as represented by delayed or missing response to phytohemagglutinin and extended life span (cf. Havemann and Rubin 1968; Bremer 1978).

Altered differentiation of neoplastic cells should relate to alterations in cellular regulation. We therefore studied two parameters of posttransscriptional protein modification: the proteinphosphorylation system as represented by the protein kinase and the ADP ribosylation of nuclear proteins.

B. Protein Kinases and Regulatory Subunits

In recent years isolation of human lymphocytes has usually been performed with the aid of Ficoll/Metrizamide gradients. This procedure appears to induce marked changes of biochemical parameters. Using Percoll (Pharmacia) instead lymphocytes could be obtained with excellent preservation of the biochemical integrity (Wielckens et al. 1980). When normal human lymphocytes isolated by the Percoll-procedure were analyzed for protein kinases, about equal activities of histone kinase and casein kinase were found (Table 1). Of the total histone kinase activity, the cAMP-dependent enzyme comprised about 50% in both normal and leukemic lymphocytes as shown by immunotitration and by the use of the heat stable inhibitor. However, leukemic lymphocytes exhibited drastically reduced values of all three protein kinase activities, the most pronounced decrease (to 7% of the normal control) being observed with casein kinase.

The cAMP-dependent protein kinases in mammalian cells represent tetrameric structures composed of two catalytic and two regulatory subunits. When total regulatory subunits R were analyzed again, a reduction in leukemic lymphocytes to <20% of normal lymphocytes was found. These changes in the protein kinase system are paralleled by comparable alterations of basal cAMP levels. The data show that the functional aberrations of leukemic lymphocytes are associated with marked alterations in an important pathway of cellular regulation that uses multiple protein kinases to effect functional changes in proteins by phosphorylation.

C. ADP Ribosylation of Nuclear Proteins

Adenosine diphosphate ribosylation is a mechanism of covalent modification of nuclear proteins by enzymatic transfer of the ADP-ribose moiety from NAD, leading to the formation of mono (ADP-ribose)-protein and poly (ADP-ribose)-protein conjugates. Histones

Table 1. Protein kinases, total regulatory subunits R, and basal cAMP levels in normal and leukemic lymphocytes.[a]

Parameter	Normal		Leukemic		Leukemic / Normal
Protein Kinase (pmol incorp./min × 10⁶ cells)					
"Casein kinase"	145	±29	10	±8	0.07
Histone kinase	174	±29	32	±3	0.18
– cAMP independent	87	± 3	16	±1	0.18
– cAMP dependent	87	± 3	16	±1	0.18
Total regulatory subunits R (pmol binding sites/10⁶ cells)	123.3	±40.2	23.0	±5.7	0.19
cAMP level (pmol/10⁶ cells)	6.02±	2.46	0.31±	0.21	0.05

[a] For experimental details see Hilz et al. (1981, in press)

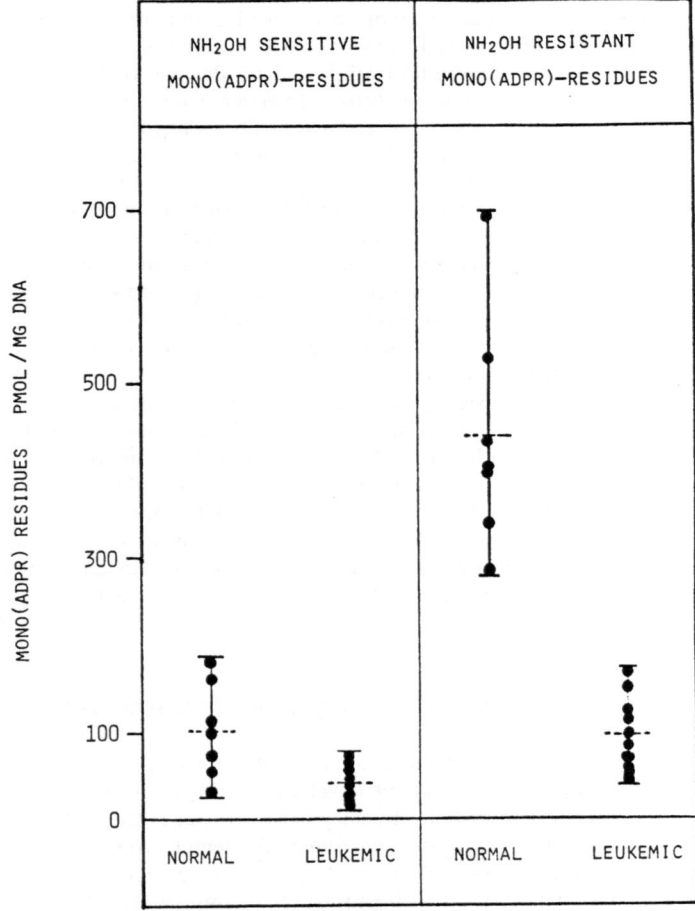

Fig. 1. Levels of hydroxylamine (NH₂OH) sensitive and resistant mono(ADPR)-in normal and leukemic lymphocytes. Taken from Hilz et al. (1980). For experimental details see Wielckens et al (1980)

and nonhistone proteins can serve as acceptors. Recent data suggest that poly ADP ribosylation of protein is involved in DNA repair processes while modification by mono (ADP-ribose)-residues of nuclear proteins appears to be involved in the maintenance of cellular differentiation (Juarez-Salinas et al. 1979; Hilz et al. 1980). Therefore, quantitation of mono (ADP-ribose)-protein conjugates was of special interest. Using a sensitive radioimmunological procedure, two types of mono(ADP-ribose) protein conjugates could be determined that differ in their sensitivity towards neutral NH_2OH. From analyses in the cell cycle (Wielckens et al. 1979), it had

become evident that the two subfractions of the mono(ADP-ribose)-conjugates are independently synthesized and therefore may serve independent functions in the chromatin. Determination of these conjugates in differentiating Dictyostelium discoideum (Bredehorst et al. 1980) and during liver development (Hilz et al. 1980) had indicated that it is primarily the subfraction of the NH_2OH resistant mono-(ADP-ribose)-conjugates that correlated with the degree of (normal) differentiation.

When normal and leukemic lymphocytes were analyzed for the extent of protein modification by mono(ADP-ribose)-residues, a marked reduction was noticed in the chronic

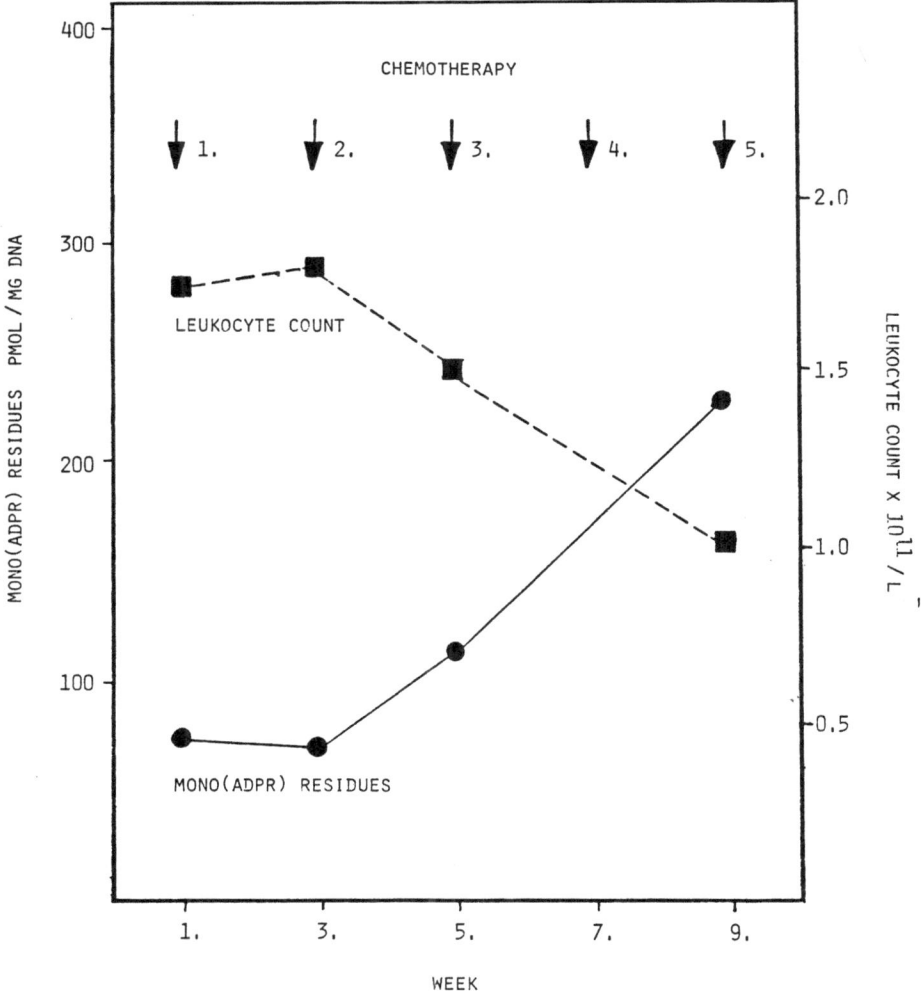

Fig. 2. Time course of ADP ribosylation under combination chemotherapy with chlorambucil/prednisone. Data from one patient with CLL. For experimental details see Wielckens et al. (1980)

lymphocytic leukemia (CLL) cells. This low level of mono(ADP-ribose)-protein conjugates, however, retained the NH_2OH sensitive subfraction only to a limited degree, the main loss being due to a pronounced diminution of the NH_2OH resistant conjugates. (Fig. 1). In all patients so far tested the values of this subfraction were well below the normal range.

The low degree of ADP ribosylation found in leukemic lymphocytes is not the consequence of chemotherapy, because patients with and without chemotherapeutic treatment were studied. Moreover, in a case of effective treatment, a progressive decrease in leukocytes was associated with increasing levels of ADP-ribose residues (Fig. 2).

The marked alterations of the ADP ribosylation status in lymphocytes from patients with CLL is characteristic for that disease and not the result of a shift to a lymphocyte population rich in B-type cells: Isolated B-lymphocytes from normal donors exhibited the same degree of mono(ADP)-ribosylation as total blood lymphocytes with their preponderance of T lymphocytes (Wielckens et al. 1980).

D. Conclusions

Marked reductions in various protein kinases, including the cAMP-dependent enzyme and its regulatory subunits, represent a for-reaching restriction of the specific functions of CLL lymphocytes compared to normal blood lymphocytes. This expression of dedifferentiation may be the consequence of a modified chromatin function as indicated by the altered extent of nuclear protein modification by mono(ADP-ribose)-residues. Since CLL cells represent a G_0 type tumor cell, the alterations

in nuclear mono (ADP)-ribosylation appear to be characteristic of tumors independently of their growth rate. Therefore, quantitation of the NH_2OH resistant protein conjugates may become a general tool to determine the degree of differentiation in tumor cells.

Acknowledgments

This work was supported by the Stiftung Volkswagenwerk.

References

Bredehorst R, Klapproth K, Hilz H, Scheidegger C, Gerisch G (1980) Protein-bound mono(ADP-ribose) residues in differentiating cells of dictyostelium discoideum. Cell Differ 9:95–103 – Bremer K (1978) Cellular renewal kinetics of malignant non-Hodgkin's lymphomas. Recent Results Cancer Res 65:5–11 – Havemann K, Rubin A (1968) The delayed response of chromic lymphocytic leukemia lymphocytes to phytohemagglutinin in vitro. Proc Soc exp Biol Med 127:668–671 – Hilz H, Adamietz P, Bredehorst R, Wielckens K (1980) Covalent modification of nuclear proteins by ADP-ribosylation: Marked differences in normal and tumor tissues. In: Wrba H, Letnansky K (eds) Kugler, Amsterdam, pp 409–414 – Hilz H, Schwoch G, Weber W, Gartemann A, Wielckens K (1981) Eur J Biochem (in press) – Juraz-Salinas H, Sims JL, Jacobson MK (1979) Poly (ADP-ribose) in carcinogen treated cells. Nature 282:740–742 – Wielckens K, Sachsenmaier W, Hilz H (1979) Protein-bound mono(ADP-ribose) levels during the cell cycle of the slime mold physarum polycephalum. Hoppe-Seylers Z Physiol Chem 360:39–43 – Wielckens K, Garbrecht M, Kittler M, Hilz H (1980) ADP-ribosylation of nuclear proteins in normal lymphocytes and low-grade non-Hodgkin lymphoma cells. Eur J Biochem 104:279–287

Haematology and Blood Transfusion Vol. 26
Modern Trends in Human Leukemia IV
Edited by Neth, Gallo, Graf, Mannweiler, Winkler
© Springer-Verlag Berlin Heidelberg 1981

Lymphoproliferation and Heterotransplantation in Nude Mice: Tumor Cells in Hodgkin's Disease*

V. Diehl, H. H. Kirchner, M. Schaadt, C. Fonatsch, and H. Stein

A. Summary

In the last 3 years we were able to establish four long-term cultures from Hodgkin-derived material [pleuraleffusions (2), bone marrow (1), and peripheral blood (1)], consisting of cells which represent morphologic and cytochemical as well as cytogenetic features of their in vivo ancestors. Two of these cell lines are described in this paper.

These two lines share the same features: non-B-T lymphocytes, non-macrophages, non myeloid cells, EBV genome negative, monoclonality, multiple numerical and structural chromosome aberrations, and tumor formation upon intracranial xenotransplantation in nude mice.

The two remaining lines are being characterized at the moment. The common characteristics expressed synonymously in the two described lines suggest that the Hodgkin tumor cell does not seem to share the features of marker-carrying lymphocytes, macrophages, or myeloblasts. The cellular origin of these cells is not clear. The loss of cellular differential markers during the process of possible dedifferentiation is discussed.

B. Introduction

The "Sternberg-Reed" (SR) and "Hodgkin" (H) cells are considered to be the neoplastic cells in Hodgkin's disease. Their cellular origin

is still subject of considerable controversy. There are arguments for a histiocytic origin of SR and H cells (Rappaport 1966; Mori and Lennert 1969) as well as for their lymphoid origin (Dorfman et al. 1973; Papadimitriou et al. 1978).

Because of the fragility of freshly isolated H and SR cells and the contamination with numerous reactive cells the precise analysis of their cell type is difficult. These limitations can be overcome by the establishment of in vitro proliferating cell populations with neoplastic properties from patients with Hodgkin's disease. The present report describes the features of two established in vitro cell lines from the pleural effusions of two patients with histologically proven Hodgkin's disease.

C. Patients, Material, and Methods

The pleural effusions were obtained from a 37-year-old woman (E.M.) with histologically proven Hodgkin's disease, which was of the nodular sclerosing type, stage IV B, and was primarily diagnosed in 1972 (L 428), and from a 36-year-old man (HR.) with Hodgkin's disease, nodular sclerosing type, which was diagnosed in 1976 from an inguinal lymph node biopsy (L 439).

I. Establishment of the In Vitro Cultures

The heparinized pleural effusion fluid was centrifuged at 150 g for 10 min and the pellet was resuspended in an 0.84% NH_4Cl solution to desintegrate the remaining erythrocytes. After two washings cells were incubated in RPMI 1640 medium supplemented with 20% fetal calf serum, glutamin, and penicillin/streptomycin at 37° C in a 5% CO_2 air atmosphere.

* This work was supported by the Deutsche Forschungsgemeinschaft Bad Godesberg (Di 184–5/6)

II. Cytochemistry

The following enzyme staining methods were performed: Naphthol-AS-D.chloracetate-esterase, peroxidase, acid-α-naphthyl acetate esterase, and alkaline posphatase.

III. Surface Markers

Membrane-bound immunoglobulins were investigated as described earlier. Ia-like antigen and lysozyme was detected by specific antisera in an indirect immunofluorescence procedure.

1. Rosette Assays

The E-rosette technique is described by Jondal et al. (1972). Rosette assays to demonstrate C3b and C3d receptors (EAC rosette assays) and IgG receptors were performed as described by Stein (1978). Intracellular antigens were demonstrated by immunostaining for k, λ, and lysozyme by means of the PAP technique (Stein and Kaiserling 1974).

2. Immune Phagocytosis

From the L 428 and L 439 line 1×10^6 cells were mixed with either IgG-E_{ox}A or EAC 3b, pelleted by centrifugation at 200 g for 5 min, and incubated at 37° C for 2 h. The pellet was resuspended by gentle shaking and centrifuged onto glass slides. The slides were stained with Grünwald Giemsa and the proportion of cells with ingested indicator cells was counted.

IV. EBV-Specific Antigens (EBNA, EA, and VCA)

The detection of EBV-associated nuclear antigen (EBNA) was performed according to Reedman and Klein (1973). For the demonstration of the viral capsid antigen (VCA) and the early antigen (EA) the method described by Henle and Henle (1966) was applied.

V. Cytogenetic Studies

The cytogenetic techniques are described elsewhere (Hellriegel et al. 1977). For a detailed analysis of metaphases the Giemsa-banding method was performed (Sumner et al. 1971).

VI. Heterotransplantation in Nude Mice

Details of breeding and colony maintenance of the Balb C nu/nu mice have been described previously (Krause et al. 1975). Cell suspension of $1 \times 10^6/0.01$ ml were injected intracranially or subcutaneously into 4-week-old mice. Transplantation of cells embedded in a plasma clot was performed according to the technique described by Lozzio et al. 1976.

D. Results

From the pleural effusions both cell lines (428, L 439) could be established after a lag phase of 4 to 6 weeks. Morphologically the L 428 cultures varied greatly in size and structure (Fig. 1). Beside large (50–80μm) multinucleated cells with smooth membrane surfaces, medium sized (30–50 μm) mono- or binucleated cells with "hairy" membrane protrusions became obvious. A third variant consisted of rather small cells (15–30 μm).

The second culture (L 439) contained round mono- or multinucleated cells with prominent nucleoli and few villi on the surface membrane.

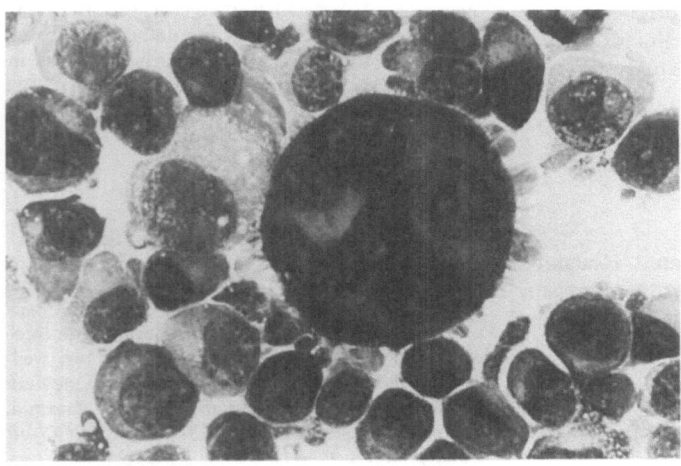

Fig. 1. L 428 cultures using Pappenheim. ×613

The findings of the evaluation of surface membrane and cytoplasmic constitutents are summarized in Table 1. The only structurally defined surface antigen demonstrable in both lines was the Ia-like antigen. Membrane receptors capable of binding T-lymphocytes were formed in more than 90% of the L 428 and L 439 cells. By enzyme cytochemistry the reactions for acid phophatase and acid esterase were found positive in two cell lines.

The L 428 and L 439 cells did not exhibit EBV-specific antigens (EBNA, VCA, EA). EBV-receptors could be demonstrated on the L 428 cells.

Cytogenetic evaluation revealed various structural and numerical chromosome aberra-

Table 1. Characteristics of the Hodgkin cell lines L 428 and L 439

Properties/reagents	L 428 cells	L 439 cells
Surface staining for:		
Polyvalent Ig	Neg.	Neg.
IgM	Neg.	Neg.
IgA	Neg.	Neg.
IgG	Neg.	Neg.
K	Neg.	Neg.
λ	Neg.	Neg.
Ia-like antigen	Pos. (60%–80%)	Pos. (70%–95%)
Lysozyme	Neg.	Neg.
Binding of aggr. IgG	Neg.	Neg.
Rosette assays with:		
EAC3b	Neg.	Neg.
EAC3d	Neg.	Neg.
IgG-EA	Neg.	Neg.
Sheep E[a]	Neg.	Neg.
Human T – cells	Pos. (90%)	Pos. (90%)
Cytoplasmic Staining for:		
IgG	Neg.	Neg.
K	Neg.	Neg.
λ	Neg.	Neg.
Lysozyme	Neg.	Neg.
Immunophagocytosis of:		
C3b-coated E	Neg.	Neg.
IgG-coated E	Neg.	Neg.
Enzyme cytochemical staining		
Naphthol chloracetate esterase	Neg.	Neg.
Peroxidase	Neg.	Neg.
Acid α-naphthyl acetate esterase	Pos.	Pos.
Alkaline phosphatase	Neg.	Neg.
Epstein-Barr virus specific antigens		
EBNA	Neg.	Neg.
EA	Neg.	Neg.
VCA	Neg.	Neg.
EBV receptors	Pos.	Not tested
Heterotransplantation in nude mice		
Primary material		
Intracranial	2/2	Not tested
Cultured cells		
Intracranial	5/6	4/4
Subcutaneous (suspension)	0/1	0/3
Subcutaneous (plasma clot)	2/2	Not tested

[a] Untreated and neuraminidase-treated sheep erythrocytes

231

	L 428	L 439
Cell size (mean diameter)	15–80 μm	40–60 μm
Growth pattern	Single cells	Single cells with small clumps
Doubling time	42–46 H	38–72 H
Max. concentration (cells/ml)	1.56×10^6	0.72×10^6

Table 2. Growth characteristics of cell lines L 428 and L 439 in vitro

tions in both lines. In the L 428 line the total number of chromosomes per cell amounted to 48–50. The monoclonal origin was ascertained by identifying several identical marker chromosomes: 1 p+, 2 p+, 6 q+, 7 q+, 9 p+, 11 q-, 13 p+, and 21 q-. Each metaphase evaluated showed an extra chromosome No. 12 and lacked one chromosome 13. Some cells exhibited a 14 q+ marker.

In the L 439 line likewise a variety of identical marker chromosomes could be shown which indicated its monoclonal origin: 1 p+, 1 q-, 1 p-, 2 q+, 10 p-, 15 p+, 18 q+, and 21 q-. In addition an extra chromosome No. 5 and No. 12 was constantly detected.

Intracranial heterotransplantation of L 428 and L 439 cells into nude mice resulted in tumor formation. Intracerebral tumor growth could be histologically confined (Fig. 2).

After subcutaneous inoculation both lines failed to induce tumors. When the L 428 cells (1×10^6) were embedded in a fibrin clot prior to transplantation, infiltrative tumor growth could be induced subcutaneously (Fig. 3).

Detailed growth characteristics are shown in Table 2.

E. Discussion

The L 428 line as well as the L 439 line have been obtained from the pleural effusion of two patients with histologically proven Hodgkin's disease. The monoclonal origin of the culture cells was demonstrated by identical marker chromosomes in each metaphase, despite the morphologic variations among individual cells. An additional argument for the malignant nature of both lines is the lack of EBV specific antigens, since hitherto EBV-negative lymphoid cell lines of a nonneoplastic nature have not been described.

The tumorigenicity of L 428 and L 439 cells after intracranial heterotransplantation in nude mice does not provide proof of the neoplastic nature, since this is a common feature of LCL and lymphoma lines (Schaadt et al. 1979). Tumor formation after subcutane-

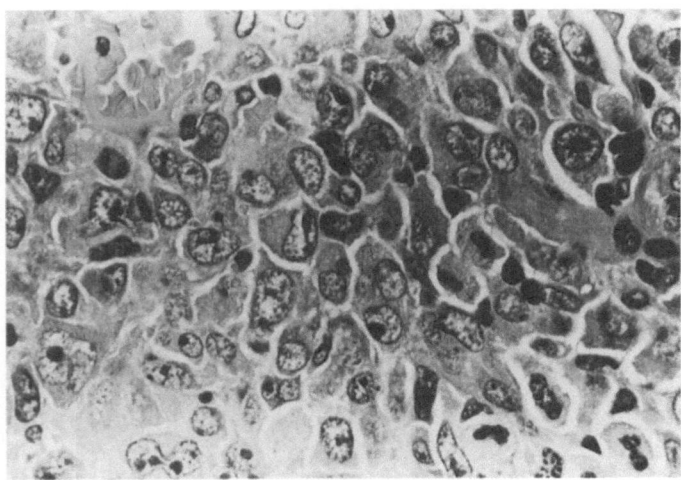

Fig. 2. Intracerebral tumorgrowth of the cell line L 428. Giemsa. ×244

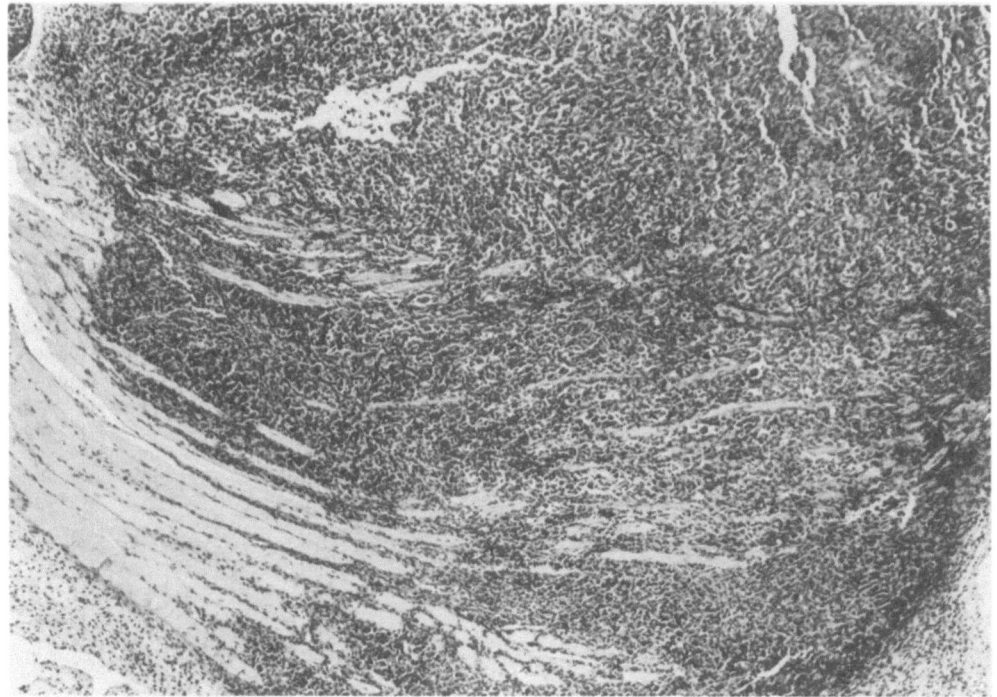

Fig. 3. Tumor growth of L 428 cells after transplantation in a fibrin clot into the subcutaneous tissue. Giemsa ×32

ous transplantation, which seems to be more strongly correlated to other markers of malignancy (Diehl et al. 1977), did not occur after inoculation of a cell suspension from the cell lines but did occur after embedding of L 428 cells in a fibrin clot before subcutaneous transplantation.

The histologic sections of the mouse tumors derived from the L 428 and the L 439 lines showed cell individuals representing a morphology very similar to that of "Sternberg-Reed" and "Hodgkin" cells. The immunologic and biologic characterization of both Hodgkin lines revealed the identical pattern observed in freshly obtained H and SR cells (Papadimitriou et al. 1978): they lack SIgG, HTLA, and receptors for C3b, C3d, IgFc, mouse E, and sheep E; are devoid of lysozyme, peroxidase, and chloracetate esterase; and they express Ia-like antigens and receptors for T cells and contain acid phosphatase and acid esterase. The origin of the cultured cells thus far is still obscure. These cells, however resemble very closely features of cultured Hodgkin cells described by Kaplan et al. (personal communication).

Acknowledgments

The skilful technical assistence of Ms. Anke Gleser, Mrs. Elvira Lux, Mrs. Cristina Boie, and Ms. Gabriele Seifert is gratefully acknowledged.

References

Diehl V, Krause P, Hellriegel KP, Busche M, Schedel J, Laskewitz E (1977) Lymphoid cell lines: in vitro cell markers in correlation to tumorigenicity in nude mice. In: Thierfelder S, Rodt H, Thiel E (eds) Haematology and blood transfusion: Immunological diagnosis of leukemias and lymphomas, vol 20. Springer, Berlin Heidelberg New York pp 289–296 – Dorfman RF, Rice DF, Mitchel AD, Kempson RL, Levine G (1973) Ultrastructural studies of Hodgkin's disease. Natl Cancer Inst Monogr 36:221–238 – Hellriegel KP, Diehl V, Krause PH, Meider S, Blankenstein M, Busche W (1977) The significance of chromosomal findings for the differentiation between lymphoma and lymphoblastoid cell lin es. In: Thierfelder S, Rodt H, Thiel E (eds) Haematology and blood transfusion: Immunological diagnosis of leukemias and lymphomas, Vol 20. Springer, Berlin Heidelberg New York,

233

p 307 – Henle G, Henle W (1966) Immunofluorescence in cells derived from Burkitt's lymphoma. J Bacteriol 91:1248–1256 – Jondal M, Holm G, Wigzell H (1972) Surface markers on human T- and B-cells. J Exp Med 136:207 – Krause P, Schmitz R, Lindemann M, Georgii A (1975) Xenotransplantation etablierter Tumorzellen auf congenital thymuslose "nude"-Mäuse. Z Krebsforsch 83:177 – Lozzio BB, Lozzio CB, Machado E (1976) Brief Communication: Human myelogenous (Ph 1 +) leukemia cell line: Transplantation into athymic nude mice. J Natl Cancer Inst 56 3:627–629 – Mori Y, Lennert K (1969) Electron microscopic atlas of lymph node cytology and pathology. Springer, Berlin Heidelberg New York, pp 29–30 – Papadimitriou CS, Stein H, Lennert K (1978) The complexity of immunohistochemical staining pattern of Hodgkin and Sternberg-Reed cells – Demonstration of immunoglobulin, albumin α_1-antichymotrypsin and lysozyme. Int J Cancer 21:531–541 – Rappaport H (1966) Tumors of the hematopoetic system. Atlas of tumor pathology Sect 3, Fasc 8. Armed Forces Institute of Pathology, Washington DC – Reedman BM, Klein G (1973) Cellular localisation of an Epstein-Barr virus (EBV)-associated complementfixing antigen in producer and non-producer lymphoblastoid cell lines. Int J Cancer 11:499–520 – Schaadt M, Kirchner HH, Fonatsch Ch, Diehl V (1979) Intracranial heterotransplantation of human hematopoetic cells in nude mice. Int J Cancer 23:751–761 – Sumner AT, Evans HJ, Buckland RA (1971) New technique for distinguishing between human chromosomes. Nature [New Biol] 232:31–32 – Stein H (1978) The immunologic and immunochemical basis for the Kiel classification. In: Lennert K (ed) Malignant lymphomas other than Hodgkin's disease. Springer, Berlin Heidelberg New York (Handbuch der speziellen pathologischen Anatomie und Histologie, vol I/3B, pp 529–657) – Stein H, Kaiserling E (1974) Surface immunoglobulins and lymphocyte – specific antigens on leukemic reticuloendotheliosis cells. Clin Exp Immunol 18:63–71

**Cell biological and
Immunological Aspects**

Haematology and Blood Transfusion Vol. 26
Modern Trends in Human Leukemia IV
Edited by Neth, Gallo, Graf, Mannweiler, Winkler
© Springer-Verlag Berlin Heidelberg 1981

Genetic and Oncogenic Influences on Myelopoiesis

M. A. S. Moore

A Introduction

An increased understanding of hemopoietic regulation has provided insight into the pathophysiology of leukemia in man and other species. This may be illustrated if we consider the use of leukemic cell lines as models pointing to specific defects which may confer a malignant phenotype. An additional consequence of studying such cell lines has been the insight obtained into the regulatory biology of normal hemopoiesis. I have elected to document this thesis by considering information we have obtained by studying the murine myelomonocytic leukemic cell line, WEHI-3. This myelomonocytic leukemia was detected in a Balb/c mouse which had undergone mineral oil (parrafin) injections intended to induce plasma cell tumor development. (Warner et al. 1969; Metcalf et al. 1969). The tumor was composed of a mixed population of monocytic and granulocytic cells. On transplantation of the tumor, four distinct sublines developed, two of which retained the original chloroma appearance and were distinguishable by karyotype (one diploid and one tetraploid). The other two nonchloroma sublines were also distinguishable karyologically, because one had a hypodiploid 39 stemline. Chromosome marker studies in vivo and DNA-content studies on cells from mice carrying the tetraploid subline confirmed that in this leukemia both the monocytic and granulocytic cells are neoplastic, indicating the existence of a neoplastic stem cell capable of differentiation into both cell series. Serum and urine samples from mice carrying this tumor contained high levels (frequently over 200 µg/ml) of muramidase, and cell suspensions of the solid tumor also contained this enzyme. This tumor therefore fulfills all the criteria applied to human myelomonocytic leukemia and proved a useful laboratory model for this type of leukemia. Tumor cells could proliferate in agar to form mixed colonies of granulocytes and macrophages, and both colony size and plating efficiency were significantly increased in the presence of an exogenous source of colony stimulating factor (Metcalf et al. 1969; Metcalf and Moore 1970). Individual colonies were capable of self renewal upon in vitro recloning and can be considered as leukemic stem cells, since individual colonies implanted in vivo into the spleen or kidney produced progressively growing tumors with the same morphology as the original WEHI-3 tumor (Metcalf and Moore 1970). Recent studies have shown that pure GM-CSF consistently increased the proportion of colonies exhibiting partial or complete differentiation in agar culture (Metcalf 1979). Serial recloning of WEHI-3 colonies in the presence of GM-CSF showed that the colonies differentiated completely and self replication of colony forming cells was suppressed; however, clonal instability was evident, since even in the continuous presence of GM-CSF many colony forming cells still generated cells able to form undifferentiated colonies. The primary tumor and early passage generations could be considered as in a conditioned state due to the dependence of in vitro proliferation upon endogenous or exogenous provision of CSF. The former characteristic of endogenous production of CSF by WEHI-3 cells was evident both in vivo and in vitro (Metcalf and Moore 1970) and has provided one of the most valuable features of this leukemic model. The subsequent history of WEHI-3 follows its adaptation to culture as a continuous cell line and the derivation of this cell line merits

237

consideration. Sanel (1973) obtained the WEHI-3 subline B (the hypodiploid line) at the 35th in vivo passage and maintained this by intraperitoneal passage in NIH Balb/c mice, reporting that it did not deviate from the original description through a further 50 passages. It is also of interest that Sanel (1973) reported a preponderance of immature C-type particles in WEHI-3 by electron microscopy with high titers of infectious NB-tropic virus of the Friend-Moloney-Rauscher subgroup. (It should be noted that the present WEHI-3 B cell line appears to be devoid of detectable C-type virus). A cell line was developed by Ralph et al. (1976) from the WEHI-3 B subline of Sanel at the 125th passage and all subsequent reports are based on the properties of this cell line which has been maintained in our laboratories at Sloan-Kettering since 1975.

A number of properties of this cell line are shown in Table 1, and what is most striking is the retention of the capacity to produce a wide spectrum of biologically relevant molecules that influence hemopoiesis and immune responses. While it may be argued that production of these various regulatory macromolecules reflects oncogenic transformation, it should be noted that all the features of the cell line are features displayed by subpopulations of macrophages under appropriate stimulation. Indeed, the most neoplastic feature of the cell line is that most of the factors are produced constitutively rather than as a result of lymphokine or adjuvant induction.

B. Properties of G-CSF and M-CSF Produced by WEHI-3

Activities in WEHI-3-conditioned medium (WEHI-3 CM) stimulated granulocyte and macrophage colony formation over an approximately 100-fold dilution of an eight fold concentrate of serum-free conditioned medium, and with optimal concentrations of CM approximately 40–50 granulocyte-macrophage colonies could be stimulated per 10^4 cells plated. Partial separation of the activities stimulating the formation of granulocyte and macrophage colonies can readily be obtained by passing concentrated WEHI-3 CM through a DEAE Sephadex (A-25, Pharmacia) column. One type of colony stimulating activity is found in the break through volume and another in the bound fraction which is eluted with 1 M NACl in equilibrating buffer (Williams et al. 1978). The morphology of colony cells stimulated by increasing dilutions of the break through fraction was exclusively macrophage. In contrast, high percentages (greater than 90%) of purely granulocytic colonies were stimulated using low concentrations of the break through fraction. When the break through fraction and eluate were mixed, dose-response curves identical to the unfractionated material were obtained, suggesting that the two entities acted independently in stimulating colony formation. In subsequent studies we have used this semipurified neutrophil colony stimulating activity and will refer to it as "G-CSF".

Prostaglandins of the E Series (PGE) inhibit myeloid colony formation (Kurland et al. 1979; Kurland and Moore 1977), and biosynthesis of PGE by normal or neoplastic macrophages and monocytes may be of significance to hemopoietic regulation. Using WEHI-3 CM as a source of CSF, we have shown that PGE inhibition is selective and that physiologically relevant suppression is restricted to colonies

Table 1. Properties of the WEHI-3 myelomonocytic cell line

1. Partial retention of ability to differentiate to macrophage and granulocyte.
2. Fc and C receptor positive, phagocytic (Ralph et al. 1977). Thy-1 positive.[a]
3. Produces lysozyme (Ralph et al. 1976) and plasminogen activator.[a]
4. Growth inhibited 50% by 0.004 µg/ml LPS (Ralph and Nakoinz 1977), by $10^{-9}M$ prostaglandin E (Kurland and Moore 1977), and by 5 µg/ml tumor necrosis factor (Shah et al. 1978).
5. Produces GM-CSF (Ralph et al. 1978), macrophage (M) – CSF, neutrophil (G) – CSF (Williams et al. 1978), and eosinophil CSF (Metcalf et al. 1974).
6. Produces megakaryocyte-CSF (Williams et al. 1980) and Burst-promoting activity.[a]
7. Produces LAF (Interleukin I). (Lachman et al. 1977).
8. Produces endogenous pyrogen (Interleukin I?) (Bodel 1978).
9. Produces prostaglandin E (Kurland et al. 1979).
10. Produces mast cell growth factor (Yung et al., to be published).
11. Has receptors for and responds to lactoferrin inhibition (Broxmeyer and Ralph 1977).

[a] Unpublished observations

PGE$_1$ (Concentration)	Colonies % of control			
	Total	Macrophage[a]	GM-mixed	Neutrophil
$10^{-5}M$	41%	8%	30%	74%
$10^{-6}M$	59%	16%	55%	89%
$10^{-7}M$	76%	41%	85%	95%
$10^{-8}M$	85%	50%	95%	95%
$10^{-9}M$	96%	58%	100%	100%
$10^{-10}M$	94%	83%	100%	100%

Table 2. Effects of prostaglandin E$_1$ on proliferation and morphology of CFU-c stimulated by WEHI-3 CM

[a] Single colony morphology of 50 sequential colonies

with an exclusively or predominantly macrophage-monocyte differentiation, whereas colonies of an exclusively neutrophil morphology (and dependent on G-CSF) are PGE insensitive (Pelus et al. 1979). Table 2 shows that PGE inhibition of WEHI-3 CM stimulated mouse bone marrow colony formation was selectively directed at macrophage and mixed colony types. Since the biosynthesis of prostaglandin E by normal and neoplastic macrophages is intrinsically linked to their synthesis of and exposure to myeloid colony-stimulating factors (Kurland et al. 1979), we addressed the question of the extent to which different CSF species possessed the capacity to induce macrophages to synthesize PGE. Adherent peritoneal macrophages were exposed to unfractionated WEHI-3 CM and to its DEAE breakthrough (G-CSF) and eluate (M-CSF) fractions. As can be seen in Table 3, WEHI-3 CM induced a striking increase in macrophage PGE biosynthesis within 24 h, and this inducing activity resided in the M-CSF and not in the G-CSF-containing fractions of WEHI-3 CM.

Thus WEHI-3 displays the capacity to synthesize PGE constitutively, but this basal level can be increased 5–10 times by exposing the leukemic cells to an exogenous source of CSF (Kurland et al. 1979). The leukemic cells also produce one CSF species (M-CSF) which stimulates normal and leukemic macrophage PGE synthesis and macrophage colony formation, the latter being sensitive to PGE inhibition. Leukemic cell-derived G-CSF stimulates PGE-insensitive neutrophil colony formation and lacks the capacity to induce macrophage PGE synthesis (Pelus et al. 1979). Finally, WEHI-3 leukemic cells are particularly sensitive to PGE inhibition (Kurland and Moore 1977) which may reflect the preponderance of monocytoid rather than granulocytic differentiation of the cell line.

C. Genetic Restrictions in Response to WEHI-3 CSF

Our laboratory has extensively used WEHI-3 CM as a source of CSF and in doing so we have some striking strain differences in marrow CFU-c incidence which were not apparent when other types of CSF, such as L cell or

CSF dilution	PGE[a]		
	WEHI-3CM	DEAE breakthrough (G-CSF)	DEAE elute (M-CSF)
Control	65± 11	65± 11	65± 11
1:2[b]	2030± 12	186±112	4093±711
1:4	1504±180	19±16	2485± 78

Table 3. Production of PGE by resident murine peritoneal macrophages after stimulation by WEHI-3 colony stimulating activities

[a] Radioimmunoassay measurements of PGE in cell-free 24-h supernates. The results are expressed as mean concentration of PGE (picograms/milliliter)±SE elaborated by adherent macrophages derived from cultures of 2.5×10^5 BDF$_1$ peritoneal exudate cells
[b] Concentrations of CSF which maximally stimulates CFU-c proliferation

endotoxin serum, were used. A particular abnormality was evident in NZB marrow cultures, since with unfractionated WEHI-3 CM, CFU-c numbers were consistently low over a broad age span, and when this material was partially purified by passage over DEAE, an even lower response was measured in these mice (Kincade et al. 1979, see also Table 4). In contrast, when either media conditioned by L cells or endotoxin serum were used, NZB marrow cells not only responded well but the plateaus of colony numbers seen with normal mice were not obtained. The incidence of WEHI-3 CSF-responsive cells in NZW mice was normal, and (NZB×NZW)F_1 had an intermediate CFU-c incidence that reflected the influence of both the parental strains (Table 4). Certain other strains besides NZB are very poor responders to WEHI-3 CSF, for example, the NZC strain, which unlike the NZW shares a common origin with the NZB. The C58/J strain also has a low incidence of CFU-c and like NZB produces xenotropic virus and has a high incidence of spontaneous leukemia (Kincade to be published). Horland et al. (1980) recently reported that the RF strain of mice which has a very high spontaneous incidence of granulocytic leukemia also had a marked defect in CFU-c numbers (<1 colony per 10^5 marrow cells). It is of interest that they used WEHI-3 CM as their exclusive source of CSF.

The possible relationship of the defective WEHI-3 CSF response in certain mouse strains to a more fundamental lesion at the pluripotential stem cell level was suggested by published evidence of CFU-s defects in NZB and NZC mice (Warner and Moore 1971) and in RF mice (Horland et al. 1980). To investigate this possibility, we attempted to establish long marrow cultures using a single femoral inoculum of marrow from NZB, NZW, and (NZB×NZW) F_1 mice. The technique was as described by Dexter et al. (1977) with cultures subjected to weekly demidepopulation of suspension cells. Cultures were assayed for CFU-s by injection into lethally irradiated syngeneic or allogeneic DBA/2 mice. (Note that NZB-irradiated recipients are not suitable for CFU-s assay due to their abnormally high incidence of endogenous spleen colonies). CFU-c were assayed using both WEHI-3 CM and L cell conditioned medium. Table 4 shows that CFU-c and CFU-s were produced for 3–4 months at high levels in NZW and F_1 cultures with a normal pattern of myelopoiesis. In contrast, NZB marrow failed to support myelopoiesis. CFU-c responding to either WEHI-3 CM or L cell CSF disappeared rapidly from culture, and CFU-s could not be detected by the 2nd week. Mast cells develop in long-term marrow cultures of most strains, generally some weeks after initiation of cultures. In the present study such cells appeared in NZW and F_1 cultures at 11 weeks but were not observed in NZB cultures at any stage. Refeeding of NZB marrow cultures with a second inoculum of NZB marrow was also unsuccessful in establishing sustained stem cell replication and myelopoiesis in culture.

In order to further define the level of the lesion in NZB bone marrow, marrow coculture studies were undertaken. We have previously shown that bone marrow from genetically

Table 4. Defective response of NZB marrow to WEHI-3 CM and associated defects in continuous marrow culture

Strain	CFU-c/10^5 marrow[a]	Continuous marrow cultures[b]		
		Duration of production (wks)		Mast cells Produced
		CFU-c	CFU-s	
NZB	1± 1	4.5±1.3	1	—
NZW	220±10	12 ±3	11	+
(NZB×NZW) F_1	152±11	15.5±2	12	+

[a] Stimulated by semipurified WEHI-3 G-CSF. L Cell CSF stimulated 290±11 colonies with NZB marrow

[b] Continuous marrow cultures established with a single inoculation of bone marrow without refeeding using conditions as described by Dexter et al. (1977). The maximum duration of CFU-c production determined in cultures stimulated with L cell CSF

anemic WW^v and S1/S1^d mice was defective in vitro, and long-term bone marrow cultures could not be established (Dexter and Moore 1977). However, the addition of S1/S1^d marrow (with normal stem cell function) to adherent bone marrow monolayers of WW^v (with a normal hemopoietic environment) resulted in normal long term hemopoeisis. Coculture studies were undertaken involving NZB bone marrow with either WW^v or S1/S1^d marrow. The results clearly indicated that coculture of NZB and S1/S1^d marrow did not augment the in vitro replication of stem cells of either genotype, whereas coculture of NZB with WW^v marrow showed long-term maintenance of stem cell production and myelopoiesis significantly in excess of that observed with marrow from either strain when cultured alone. These results point to a defect in a regulatory cell population in NZB marrow, and a defect in macrophage function has been proposed (Warner 1978).

D. Conclusion

The linked production of a wide spectrum of hemopoietic growth regulatory factors, as displayed by the WEHI-3 cell line, can be duplicated by pokeweed mitogen stimulation of murine spleen cells (Metcalf et al. 1978). A mitogenic stimulus, T lymphocytes, and adherent cells are required for multifactor production by spleen cells suggesting that induced lymphokines may in turn induce macrophages to elaborate the growth factors. The feature of the WEHI-3 myelomonocytic cells is their ability to produce factors constitutively and thus circumvent control networks implied by mitogen-lymphocyte-macrophage interactions. A second feature is that the leukemic cells produce factors (G$^-$, GM$^-$, M$^-$ CSF) to which the leukemic cells can respond by proliferation and differentiation (Metcalf and Moore 1970; Metcalf 1979). Under normal conditions the myelomonocytic progenitor cells respond to GM-CSF but do not produce it; in contrast the neoplastic myelomonocytic CFU-c of WEHI-3 (50%–100% cloning efficiency) both produce and respond to GM-CSF. In this context normal monocytes and macrophages can be induced to produce CSF and can be shown to possess receptors for CSF, since macrophage proliferation and prostaglandin synthesis can be induced by exposure

of the cells to exogenous CSF (Kurland et al. 1979. Pelus et al. 1979). Individual WEHI-3 leukemic cells would appear to possess a combination of features possessed by the earliest committed progenitor cells (CFU-c) and their differentiated progeny. The association of growth factor production with the presence of growth factor receptors on the cell surface is rare among tumor cells but has been reported in the case of nerve growth factor and human melanoma cells (Sherwin et al, 1979). It is possible that this represents an opportunity for "autostimulation" of tumor cells by growth factors and may be more universally applicable as we better understand the characteristics of specific growth factors required for different tissues. The model developed by Todaro and De Larco (1978) to explain the mechanism of sarcoma virus transformation mediated by endogenous polypeptide growth stimulatory factors may equally be applicable to leukemogenesis. In this model growth factors are produced by cells that normally do not respond to their own product. Inappropriate production by a target cell of an active factor for which it also has receptors may be sufficient to stimulate cell division, and the persistent production of a growth factor may serve as a continuous endogenous stimulus leading to continued inappropriate cell growth.

The inability of CFU-c from certain mouse strains to respond to G-CSF of a WEHI-3 origin may involve a defect in the CSF molecule, i.e., WEHI-3 G-CSF is a leukemic product similar but not identical to normal G-CSF. Alternatively, or perhaps in addition, an impaired G-CSF response reveals a broader defect involving growth factor receptors back as far as the pluripotential stem cell. Certainly the associated abnormality of NZB, NZC, and C58 mice involving impaired stem cell replication in long term marrow culture would suggest a broader defect. This is supported by the in vivo evidence of multiple defects in G-CSF-unresponsive mouse strains variously involving autoimmunity, endogenous xenotropic virus expression, and high leukemia incidence.

References

Bodel P (1978) Spontaneous pyrogen production by mouse histiocytic and myelomonocytic tumor cell lines in vitro. J Exp Med 147:1503 – Broxmeyer HE, Ralph P (1977) Regulation of a mouse myelomonocytic leukemia cell line in culture. Cancer Res 37:3578 – Dexter M, Moore MAS (1977) In vitro duplication and "cure" of hemopoietic defects in genetically anemic mice. Nature 269:412 – Dexter TM, Allen TD, Lajtha LG (1977) Conditions controlling the proliferation of hemopoietic stem cells in vitro. J Cell Physiol 91:335 – Horland AA, McMarrow L, Wolman SR (1980) Growth of granulopoietic bone marrow cells of RF mice. Exp Hematol 8:1024 – Kincade PW (to be published) Hemopoietic abnormalities in New Zealand Black and Motheaten mice. In: Gershwin ME, Merchant B (eds) Laboratory animals. Plenum, New York – Kincade PW, Lee G, Fernandes G, Moore MAS, Williams N, Good RA (1979) Abnormalities in clonable B lymphocytes and myeloid progenitors in autoimmune NZB mice. Proc Natl Acad Sci USA 76:3464 – Kurland J, Moore MAS (1977) Modulation of hemopoiesis by prostaglandins. Exp Hematol 5:357 – Kurland J, Pelus L, Bockman R, Ralph P, Moore MAS (1979) Synthesis of prostaglandin E by normal and neoplastic macorohages is dependent upon colony stimulating factors (CSF). Proc Natl Acad Sci USA 76:2326 – Lachman LB, Hacker MP, Blyden GT, Handschumacher T (1977) Preparation of lymphocyte-activating factor from continuous murine macrophage cell lines. Cell Immunol 34:416 – Metcalf D (1979) Clonal analysis of the action of GM-CSF on the proliferation and differentiation of myelomonocytic leukemic cells. Int J Cancer 24:616 – Metcalf D, Moore MAS (1970) Factors modifying stem cell proliferation of myelomonocytic leukemic cells in vitro and in vivo. J Natl Cancer Inst 44:801 – Metcalf D, Moore MAS, Warner N (1969 Colony formation in vitro by myelomonocytic leukemic cells. J Natl Cancer Inst 43:983 – Metcalf D, Parker J, Chester HM, Kincade PW (1974) Formation of eosinophiliclike granulocyte colonies by mouse bone marrow cells in vitro. J Cell Physiol 84:275 – Metcalf D, Russell S, Burgess AW (1978) Production of hemopoietic stimulating factors by pokeweed-mitogen stimulated spleen cells. Transplant Proc 10:91 – Pelus LM, Broxmeyer HE, Kurland JI, Moore MAS (1979) Regulation of macrophage and granulocyte proliferation. J Exp Med 150:277 – Ralph P, Nakoinz I (1977) Direct toxic effects of immunopotentiators on monocytic, myelomonocytic and histiocytic or macrophage tumor cells in culture. Cancer Res 37:546 – Ralph P, Moore MAS, Nilsson K (1976) Lysozyme synthesis by human and murine histiocytic lymphoma cell lines. J Exp Med 143:1528 – Ralph P, Nakoinz I, Broxmeyer HE, Schrader S (1977) Immunologic functions and in vitro activation of cultured macrophage tumor lines. Natl Cancer Inst Monogr 48:303 – Ralph P, Broxmeyer HE, Moore MAS, Nakoinz I (1978) Induction of myeloid colony-stimulating activity in murine monocyte tumor cell lines by macrophage activators and in a T-cell line by concanavalin A. Cancer Res 38:1414 – Sanel FT (1973) Studies of neoplastic myelomonocytic cells in Balb/c mice producing infectious C-type virus. Cancer Res 33:671 – Shah RG, Green S, Moore MAS (1978) Colony-stimulating and inhibiting activities in mouse serum after corynebacterium Parvum-endotoxin treatment. J Reticuloendothel Soc 23:29 – Sherwin SA, Sliski AH, Todaro GJ (1979) Human melanoma cells have both nerve growth factor and nerve growth factor-specific receptors on their cell surface. Proc Natl Acad Sci USA 76:1288 – Todaro GJ de Larco JE (1978) Cancer Res 38:4147 – Warner NL (1978) Genetic aspects of immunologic abnormalities in New Zealand mouse strains. Arthritis Rheum 21:5106 – Warner NL, Moore MAS (1971) Defects in hematopoietic differentiation in NZB and NZC mice. J Exp Med 134:313 – Warner N, Moore MAS, Metcalf D (1969) A transplantable myelomonocytic leukemia in BALB/c mice: Cytology, karyotype and muramidase content. J Natl Cancer Inst 43:963 – Williams N, Eger RR, Moore MAS, Mendelsohn N (1978) Differentiation of mouse bone marrow precursor cells into neutrophil granulocytes by an activity separated from WEHI-3 cell-conditioned medium. Differentiation 11:59 – Williams N, Jackson HM, Eger RR, Long MW (to be published) The separate roles of factors in murine megakaryocyte colony formation. In: Levine R, Williams N, Evatt B (eds) Megakaryocytes in vitro. Elsevier North Holland, New York Oxford – Yung YP, Eger R, Tertian G, Moore MAS (1981) Long term culture of mouse mast cells. II. Purification of mast cell growth factor and its dissociation from T cell growth factor. J Imunol, in press

Haematology and Blood Transfusion Vol. 26
Modern Trends in Human Leukemia IV
Edited by Neth, Gallo, Graf, Mannweiler, Winkler
© Springer-Verlag Berlin Heidelberg 1981

Acidic Isoferritins as Feedback Regulators in Normal and Leukemic Myelopoiesis*

H. E. Broxmeyer, J. Bognacki, M. H. Dörner, M. deSousa and L. Lu

A. Background on Leukemia-Associated Inhibitory Activity

The absence of normal hematopoiesis during acute leukemia not in remission and the recovery of apparently normal blood cells during chemotherapy-induced remission suggest that suppressive cell interactions may be involved in the pathogenesis of acute leukemia. Others have shown inhibition of normal progenitor cell proliferation and differentiation by cells from patients with leukemia, but little or no information was provided regarding the actual characterization of the inhibitory cells or the mechanisms of action (Broxmeyer and Moore 1978). We have demonstrated the existence of an S-phase specific inhibitory activity [leukemia-associated inhibitory activity (LIA)] against normal granulocyte-macrophage progenitor cells (CFU-GM) which was produced by bone marrow, spleen, and blood cells from patients with acute and chronic myeloid and lymphoid leukemia and "preleukemia" (Broxmeyer et al. 1978a,b, 1979a,b). Greater concentrations of LIA were found during acute leukemia (newly diagnosed and untreated, or on therapy but not in remission) than during chronic leukemia (Broxmeyer et al. 1978a,b). Remission of acute leukemia was associated with low levels of LIA (Broxmeyer et al. 1978b, 1979a), and LIA at that time was not found in hemopoietic cells from normal donors (Broxmeyer et al. 1978a,b, 1979a,b). In contrast to its action on normal CFU-GM,

LIA was not effective in suppressing the growth of normal CFU-GM from patients with acute leukemia who were not in remission and from many patients with acute leukemia during remission and with chronic leukemia (Broxmeyer et al. 1978b, 1979a,b). We postulated that LIA may thus confer a proliferative advantage to abnormally responsive cells (Broxmeyer et al. 1978b).

We have now documented these inhibitory interactions in neonatal and adult Balb/c mice infected with Abelson virus (Broxmeyer et al. 1980). Within 2–4 days after virus infection, the CFU-GM from bone marrow and spleen became insensitive to inhibition by human LIA and by mouse LIA-like material, even though colony morphology appeared normal. Shortly after or simultaneously with the detection of the colony forming cell resistance phenomenon LIA was found in bone marrow, spleen, and thymus cells. The abnormal interactions appeared to be related to induction of lymphoma in Balb/c neonates and to a lymphoproliferative disease in adult Balb/c mice. In contrast, normal cellular interactions were noted in adult C57B1/6 mice which were not susceptible to Abelson disease after virus inoculation and in untreated neonatal and adult Balb/c and adult C57B1/6 mice. Their CFU-GM were sensitive to inhibition by LIA and no LIA-like material was detected in their bone marrow, spleen, and thymus cells. We have also noted LIA interactions in mice given Friend virus (SFFV plus helper) (L. Lu and H. E. Broxmeyer, unpublished work) and others have developed a model for LIA based on induction of leukemia in mice with the RFV strain Friend virus, the spontaneous regression of the disease and its recurrence (Marcelletti and Furmanski 1980).

* Supported by Public Health service grants CA 23528 and CA 08748 from the National Cancer Institute and by the Tumorzentrum Heidelberg–Mannheim, the H. Margolis Fund and the Gar Reichman Foundation

B. Isolation, Characterization and Identification of LIA as Acidic-Isoferritins

After isolating and characterizing LIA (Bognacki et al. 1981) we noted that it was similar to a subclass of ferritins (Drysdale et al. 1977). The LIA to be purified was pooled from more than 5000 samples of extracts from bone marrow, spleen, and blood cells collected over a 5-year period from more than 1000 different patients with all types of acute and chronic leukemia and at all stages of disease progression. LIA was isolated by a combination of procedures including ultracentrifugation, Sephadex G-200, carboxymethyl cellulose, SDS-polyacrylamide gel electrophoresis, analytical and preparative isoelectric focusing, and Concanavalin A Sepharose (Bognacki et al. 1981). LIA had an apparent molecular weight of $\sim 550{,}000$ and a pI of 4.7 and copurified with the acidic isoferritins. LIA was detected in all the ferritin preparations tested (Broxmeyer et al. 1981). Additionally, purified preparations of LIA were composed almost entirely ($>90\%$) of acidic isoferritins as determined by radioimmunoassay and isoelectric focusing, and the inhibitory activity in the LIA and ferritin samples was inactivated by a battery of antisera specific for ferritins, including those prepared against acidic isoferritins from normal heart and spleen tissues from patients with Hodgkin's disease (Broxmeyer et al. 1981). LIA and the acidic isoferritin-inhibitory activity had similar physico-chemical characteristics as treatment with trypsin, chymotrypsin, pronase, and periodate, and breakdown of the ferritin into subunits by reduction inactivated the inhibitory activity. DNase, RNase, neuraminidase, lipase, phospholipase C, iron depletion, and heat treatment (75°C for 20 min) did not inactivate the activity (Broxmeyer et al. 1981). Inhibitory activity was detected at concentrations as low as 10^{-17} to 10^{-19}M and all samples were inactive against CFU-GM from patients with nonremission acute leukemia. A similar curve of inhibition was noted when mouse ferritin was assayed against mouse CFU-GM. The human and mouse acidic isoferritin inhibitory activity suppressed colony formation of cells giving rise to colonies containing purely granulocytes, macrophages, eosinophils, or mixtures of granulocytes and macrophages (L. Lu and H. E. Broxmeyer, unpublished work).

We were not able previously to detect LIA in bone marrow and blood cells from normal donors, but we have now found it in heart, spleen, placentae, and liver ferritin isolated from normal individuals (Broxmeyer et al. 1981) and mice. This was probably due to a combination of factors. Acidic isoferritins are elevated in leukemia and lymphoma but are in very low concentrations in bone marrow, blood cells, and serum from normal donors. Additionally, we now have evidence that medium conditioned by normal human bone marrow and blood monocytes, placental cells, mouse macrophages and WEHI-3 cells, which are used to stimulate colony formation, contain acidic isoferritins. Removal of the ferritins by preincubation with antisera to acidic isoferritins or by passing the material over Sepharose 6B columns or over columns to which ferritin antibodies have been fixed to Sephadex beads by CNBr enhances the stimulatory capacity of the conditioned medium by 50% to 100%. Not surprisingly, acidic isoferritins (LIA) demonstrate greater inhibition of colony and cluster formation (e.g., 60% inhibition vs 40%) when the preparations free of ferritin are used to stimulate CFU-GM. The relevance in vivo of acidic isoferritins as regulators of myelopoiesis is still to be determined, but the low concentrations needed for activity on the progenitor cells in vitro (10^{-17} to 10^{-19}M) suggest that they may be of importance as physiologic regulators, a role we have postulated previously for lactoferrin (Broxmeyer et al. 1979c), an iron-binding glycoprotein which acts on factor production rather than on the progenitor cells.

References

Bognacki J, Broxmeyer HE, LoBue J (1981) Isolation and biochemical characterization of leukemia-associated inhibitory activity that suppresses colony and cluster formation of cells. Biochim Biophys Acta 672:176 – Broxmeyer HE, Moore MAS (1978) Communication between white cells and the abnormalities of this in leukemia. Biochim Biophys Acta 516:129 – Broxmeyer HE, Jacobsen N, Kurland J, Mendelsohn N, Moore MAS (1978a) In vitro suppression of normal granulocyte stem cells by inhibitory activity derived from leukemia cells. J Natl Cancer Inst 60:497 – Broxmeyer HE, Grossbard E, Jacobsen N, Moore MAS (1978b) Evidence for a proliferative advantage of human leukemia colony forming cells (CFU-c) in vitro. J Natl Cancer Inst 60:513 – Broxmeyer HE,

Grossbard E, Jacobsen N, Moore MAS (1979a) Persistence of leukemia inhibitory activity during remission of acute leukemia. N Engl J Med 301:346 – Broxmeyer HE, Ralph P, Margolis VB, Nakoinz I, Meyers P, Kapoor N, Moore MAS (1979b) Characteristics of bone marrow and blood cells in human leukemia that produce leukemia inhibitory activity (LIA). Leuk Res 3:193 – Broxmeyer HE, Smithyman A, Eger RR, Meyers PA, deSousa M (1979c) Identification of lactoferrin as the granulocyte-derived inhibitor of colony stimulating activity (CSA)-production. J Exp Med 148:1052 – Broxmeyer HE, Ralph P, Gilbertson S, Margolis VB (1980) Induction of leukemia associated inhibitory activity and bone marrow granulocyte-macrophage progenitor cell alterations during infection with Abelson virus. Cancer Res 40:3928 – Broxmeyer HE, Bognacki J, Dorner MM, deSousa M (1981) Identification of leukemia-associated inhibitory activity as acidic isoferritins: a role for acidic isoferritins in the regulation of the production of granulocytes and macrophages. J Exp Med, in press – Drysdale JW, Adelman TG, Arosio P, Casareale D, Fitzpatrick P, Hazard JI, Yokota M (1977) Human isoferritins in normal and disease states. Semin Hematol 14:71 – Marcelletti J, Furmanski P (1980) A murine model system for the study of the human leukemia associated inhibitory activity. Blood 56:134

Haematology and Blood Transfusion Vol. 26
Modern Trends in Human Leukemia IV
Edited by Neth, Gallo, Graf, Mannweiler, Winkler
© Springer-Verlag Berlin Heidelberg 1981

Assessment of Human Pluripotent Hemopoietic Progenitors and Leukemic Blast-Forming Cells in Culture*

H. A. Messner, A. A. Fauser, R. Buick, L. J-A. Chang, J. Lepine, J. C. Curtis, J. Senn, and E. A. McCulloch

A. Introduction

Myeloproliferative diseases such as acute myeloid leukemia (AML), chronic myeloid leukemia (CML), and polycythemia vera (PV) are now generally considered to be clonal disorders originating in abnormal stem cells (Wiggans et al. 1978; Fialkow et al. 1967, 1977; Adamson et al. 1976; McCulloch and Till 1977; McCulloch 1979). A growth advantage typically displayed by the abnormal clone appears to be responsible for the increased production of phenotypically normal or abnormal cells. The underlying mechanisms for the altered growth rate are presently not understood. Further investigations of this phenomenon are dependent upon the development of assays that facilitate assessment of normal human pluripotent stem cells and permit identification of members of the abnormal clone present in these disorders.

We have recently described such an assay for human pluripotent progenitors (Messner and Fauser 1978; Fauser and Messner 1978, 1979a). They can be readily identified in culture by their ability to form mixed hemopoietic colonies that contain components of all myeloid lineages. Blast-forming cells in patients with acute myeloid leukemia are also accessible for studies in culture (Dicke et al. 1976; Park et al. 1977; Buick et al. 1977). They give rise to colonies of cells with leukemic phenotype. In addition, blast colonies from patients with cytogenetic markers displayed the same chromosomal abnormality as that

observed for primary blast cell populations (Izaguirre and McCulloch 1978). These assays permitted investigations directed to examine mechanisms of increased proliferation by utilizing the following principle approaches: The proliferative state of clonogenic cells can be directly assessed by comparing the plating efficiency in controls with that observed after short-term exposure to H_3TdR. Recloning experiments of colonies are instrumental in examining the proliferative potential of cells with respect to self-replication.

It is the purpose of the present communication to review the currently available information about proliferative parameters of human pluripotent progenitors and leukemic blast colony-forming cells and to demonstrate their potential use for the assessment of individual patients.

B. Methodology

I. Culture Conditions for CFU-GEMM and Blast Colony-Forming Cells

The culture assays for CFU-GEMM and blast colony forming cells followed well established principles for hemopoietic progenitors. CFU-GEMM in bone marrow and peripheral blood specimens of normal individuals (Messner and Fauser 1978; Fauser and Messner 1978, 1979a) and patients with leukemia or PV were grown with α-medium or modified Dulbecco's MEM, fetal calf serum, erythropoietin, and medium conditioned by leukocytes in the presence of phytohemagglutinin (PHA-LCM) (Aye et al. 1974). After 12 to 14 days of culture in humidified atmosphere supplemented with 5% CO_2, colonies of 500 to 10,000

* Supported by the Medical Research Council of Canada and the Leukemic Research Foundation, Toronto

cells could be identified that contained granulocytes, erythroblasts, megakaryocytes, and macrophages.

Identical culture conditions led to the development of blast cell colonies in peripheral blood specimens of patients with acute myeloid leukemia (Buick et al. 1977). These colonies develop within 5 to 7 days of culture and grow to a size of 20 to 200 cells with blast cell morphology. Numerical assessment of colonies in primary cultures yielded the primary plating efficiency (PE1) (Buick et al. 1979).

II. Cycle State Analysis

The proliferative state of CFU-GEMM and blast colony-forming cells was examined as previously described (Becker et al. 1965; Minden et al. 1978).

III. Assessment of Self-Renewal

Individual mixed hemopoietic colonies were sufficiently large to be removed from the cultures by micropipette for redispersion into a single cell suspension (Messner and Fauser 1979) and subsequent replating in Linbro micro titer wells. Some colonies were seeded under conditions identical to those employed for primary colonies; others were, in addition, exposed to the feeder effect of 2×10^4 irradiated mononuclear peripheral blood cells from normal individuals. Secondary colonies were scored after 12 to 14 days of culture.

Primary blast cell colonies within individual plates were pooled and redispersed. These cells were counted prior to replating with 2×10^4 irradiated normal peripheral blood cells (Buick et al. 1979). The results were expressed as secondary plating efficiency (PE2).

IV. Separation of PHA-LCM

Isoelectric focusing in a density gradient was used to separate PHA-LCM (Scandurra et al. 1969; Fauser and Messner 1979b). Each fraction was dialyzed, reconstituted with DMEM, and examined for stimulatory activity for CFU-GEMM, BFU-E, CFU-C in normal individuals and blast colonyforming cells in patients with acute leukemia.

C. Results

I. Comparison of the Culture Conditions for CFU-GEMM and Blast Colony Forming Cells

Almost identical culture conditions are employed for both clonal assays. The addition of PHA-LCM is essential for the development of mixed hemopoietic colonies and blast cell colonies in the majority of the examined specimens; only occasionally can mixed colonies (Messner et al., to be published) or blast cell colonies be observed without the addition of this stimulatory material. With the exception of PV, erythropoietin is required for the maturation of erythroid cells within mixed colonies. Attempts were not successful to alter the cellular composition of blast cell colonies and induce erythroid differentiation with erythropoietin.

Some information is now available that the stimulatory activity for both colony types present in PHA-LCM may be associated with different molecules (Fauser and Messner 1979b). Separation of PHA-LCM by isoelectric focusing yielded the stimulatory activity for CFU-GEMM, BFU-E, and CFU-C in fractions of Ph 5 to 6.5. In contrast, stimulatory activity for leukemic blast cells was observed in fractions of Ph 5.5 to 7.5. This information suggests that molecules responsible for the stimulation of CFU-GEMM and blast colony forming cells are not completely identical.

II. Assessment of the Proliferative State of CFU-GEMM and Blast Colony Forming Cells

The proliferative state of CFU-GEMM was assessed by short term exposure to H_3TdR for patients with different clinical conditions: normal individuals in steady state and during bone marrow regeneration and patients with various clonal hemopathies such as PV, CML AML and acute myelofibrosis. CFU-GEMM were found to be quiescent under steady state conditions. They proliferate actively during bone marrow regeneration, for instance after bone marrow transplantation (Fauser and Messner 1979c). A reduction of the plating efficiency to 50% of control values was regularly observed during the early phase of engraftment. CFU-GEMM in patients with clonal hemopathies generally displayed a similar increase in proliferative activity. Data are available for six patients with PV (Fauser and Messner 1979d), seven patients with CML (Messner et al. 1980; Lepine and Messner, unpublished work), one patient with AML and acute myeolofibrosis (Messner et al. 1980) that demonstrate a reduction of the plating efficiency ranging from 20% to 60%. The results for patients with PV suggest that the proliferative state of individual patients was independant of the clinical condition or therapeutic modulation. Similar examinations are in progress for patients with CML and AML.

The cycle state of blast colony forming cells was assessed for patients with acute myeloid leukemia and patients with preleukemia that contained blast colony forming cells in their peripheral circulation (Senn et al. 1979). Minden et al. (1978) demonstrated that blast colony forming cells in all examined patients with acute myeloid leukemia were found to be in cycle as documented by a 50% reduction of their plating efficiency with short-term exposure to H_3TdR. This observation was confirmed for three of four patients with preleukemia (Senn et al. 1979). Studies are in progress on patients with long-lasting remissions that have not been subjected to recent chemotherapeutic interventions.,

III. Recloning of CFU-GEMM and Blast Colony Forming Cells

Mixed hemopoietic colonies were removed from the cultures by micropipette, redispersed to yield a single cell suspension, and replated in Linbro micro titer plates. These experiments were performed using mixed colonies grown from bone marrow samples of four normal individuals. Of the 107 mixed colonies 26 gave rise to 13 mixed, 192 pure granulocytic, and 195 erythroid secondary colonies. This observation supports the view that clones derived from various pluripotent progenitors are heterogeneous. While 75% of primary mixed colonies contained only mature elements, some primitive progenitors were identified in 25%.

Recloning experiments of blast cell colonies derived from various patients with acute myeloid leukemia demonstrated that secondary colonies of blast cell phenotype can be observed (Buick et al. 1979). The frequency may vary greatly. Morphologically, the secondary colonies appear to be rather homogeneous. However, functional assessment of pooled blast colonies as feeder cells indicated that cells within blast cell colonies may elaborate stimulators that promote growth of blast cell colonies (Taetle, personal communication).

1. Clinical Correlations

It was attempted to assess the clinical value of these culture studies by correlating the recloning efficiency of primary blast cells with the response of patients to chemotherapy. In 44 patients, a significant association was found between low PE2 values and successful remission induction (Buick et al. 1979; Buick et al. 1981).

2. Modulation of Cloning Efficiency In Vitro

Since the recloning efficiency may represent an important prognostic parameter to predict the responsiveness of patients to chemotherapy, the question of whether the recloning efficiency represents an invariable determinant for each patient or whether it can be modulated was asked. This was tested in three different experimental approaches: primary blast colonies were grown after exposure to adriamycin and cytosine aribinoside (ARA-C) and surviving colonies replated. While dose-dependent reduction of PEl was regularly observed for both drugs, PE2 was not influenced by adriamycin but was decreased for ARA-C. In addition, tumor promotors such as TPA enhanced the recloning efficiency (PE2) (Chang and McCulloch 1979). Taetle and McCulloch (1979) reported that interferon was capable of inhibiting PE2.

D. Conclusions

Assays are now available that permit the identification of human pluripotent hemopoietic progenitors in culture and facilitate assessment of leukemic cell populations that form colonies of blast cell phenotype. Both colonies develop under almost identical culture conditions and require stimulatory molecules that are provided by PHA-LCM. Preliminary evidence suggests that these molecules may not be identical and may be separable by procedures such as isoelectric focusing. CFU-GEMM of normal individuals under steady state conditions appear to be quiescent. This contrasts with results obtained for the proliferative state of CFU-GEMM during regeneration and for patients with various clonal hemopathies. It was feasible to study patients with PV and CML prior to and subsequent to therapeutic interventions without demonstrating changes in the proliferative state. The increased proliferative rate of CFU-GEMM may adequately explain the increased number of cells observed in these disorders. The active proliferation of leukemic blast colony forming cells is consistent with the interpretation of a growth advantage of blast cells observed under these clinical conditions. This was further documented by assessing the recloning ability of blast colony forming cells. In addition, it becomes apparent that chemotherapeutic intervention in patients with acute myeloid leukemia is complex and may include, beside cytoreduction, changes in the recloning ability of blast colony forming cells. It is thus conceivable to select drugs with differing biological effects for patients with specific cell culture prognostics.

Our studies thus far have not succeeded in identifying the relationship of pluripotent hemopoietic progenitors and blast-forming cells. One of the main difficulties is related to the low frequency of mixed colonies observed during phases of relapse and the greatly reduced number of blast cell colonies at the time of remission. The observation that CFU-GEMM as well as blast cell colonies can be recloned may provide a powerful tool to be employed in the future, particularly if specific fractions of PHA-LCM become available to facilitate selective cloning.

References

Adamson JW, Fialkow PJ, Murphy S, Prchal JF, Steinmann E (1976) Polycythemia vera: Stem cell and probable clonal origin of the disease. N Engl J Med 295:913–916 – Aye MT, Niho Y, Till JE, McCulloch EA (1974) Studies of leukemic cell populations in culture. Blood 2/205:219 – Becker AJ, McCulloch EA, Siminovitch L, Till JE (1965) The effect of differing demands for blood cell production on DNA synthesis by hemopoietic colony forming cells of mice. Blood 26:296–308 – Buick RN, Chang LJ-A, Messner HA, Curtis JE, McCulloch (1981) Self-renewal capacity of leukemia blast progenitor cells. Cancer, in press – Buick RN, Till JE, McCulloch EA (1977) Colony assay for prolife-

rative blast cells circulating in myeloblastic leukemia. Lancet I:862–863 – Buick RN, Minden MD, McCulloch EA (1979) Self renewal in culture of proliferative blast progenitor cells in acute myeloblastic leukemia. Blood 54:95–104 – Chang LJ-A, McCulloch EA (1979) A tumor promotor increases the self renewal of blast progenitors in acute myeloblastic leukemia. Blood [Supp I] 54/5: p 169a – Dicke KA, Spitzer G, Ahearn MJ (1976) Colony formation in vitro by leukemic cells in acute myelogenous leukaemia with phytohaemagglutinin as stimulating factor. Nature 259:129–130 – Fauser AA, Messner HA (1978) Granuloerythropoietic colonies in human bone marrow, peripheral blood and cord blood. Blood 52:1243 – Fauser AA, Messner HA (1979a) Identification of megakaryocytes, macrophages and eosinophils in colonies of human bone marrow containing neutrophilic granulocytes and erythroblasts. Blood 53:1023 – Fauser AA, Messner HA (1979b) Separation of stimulating activity in PHA-LCM by isoelectric focusing for leukemic blast cell colonies and colonies of normal hemopoietic progenitors. Blood [Supp I] 54: p 107 – Fauser AA, Messner HA (1979c) Proliferative state of human pluripotent hemopoietic progenitors (CFU-GEMM) in normal individuals and under regenerative conditions after bone marrow transplantation. Blood 54/5:1197 – Fauser AA, Messner HA (1979d) Pluripotent hemopoietic progenitors in peripheral blood of patients with polycythemia rubra vera. Blood [Supp I] 54: p 138 – Fauser AA, Messner HA (submitted to Blood) Pluripotent hemopoietic progenitors (CFU-GEMM) in polycythemia vera: Analysis of erythropoietin requirement and proliferative activity – Fialkow PJ, Gartler SM, Yoshida A (1967) Clonal origin of chronic myelogenous leukemia in man. Proc Natl Acad Sci USA 58:1468–1471 – Fialkow PJ, Jacobson RJ, Papayannopoulou TH (1977) Chronic myelocytic leukemia: Clonal origin in a stem cell common to the granulocyte erythrocyte, platelet and monocyte/macrophage. Am J Med 63:125–130 – Izaguirre CA, McCulloch EA (1978) Cytogenetic analysis of leukemic clones. Blood [Supp 1] 52:287 – McCulloch EA (1979) Abnormal myelopoietic clones in man. J Natl Cancer Inst 63:883–891 – McCulloch EA, Till JE (1977) Stem cells in normal early hemopoiesis and certain clonal hemopathies. In: Hoffbrant AV, Brain M, Hersh J (eds) Recent advances in hematology, vol 2. Churchill-Livingston, London, pp 85–110 – Messner HA, Fauser AA (1978) Distribution of fetal hemoglobin in individual colonies by RIA: A lead towards human stem cells. In: Stamatoyannopoulos, Nienhuis (eds) Cellular and molecular regulation of hemoglobin switching. Grune & Stratton, pp 379 – Messner HA, Fauser AA (1979) Human pluripotent hemopoietic progenitors (CFU-GEMM) in culture. In: NIH Conference on Aplastic Anemia, San Francisco. – Messner HA, Fauser AA, Lepine J, Martin M (1980) Properties of human pluripotent hemopoietic progenitors. Blood Cells 6:595–607 – Minden MD, Till JE, McCulloch EA (1978) Proliferative state of blast cell progenitors in acute myeloblastic leukemia. Blood 52:592–600 – Park C, Savin MA, Hoogstrated B, et al. (1977) Improved growth of the in vitro colonies in human acute leukemia with the feeding culture method. Cancer Res 37:4594–4601 – Scandurra R, Cannella C, Elli R (1969) Use of isoelectric focusing in the purification of L-glutamate – phenylpyruvate aminotransferase. Sci Tools 16:17 – Senn JS, Pinkerton PH, Messner HA, McCulloch EA (1979) Detection of blast cell colonies in preleukemic states. Blood [Suppl I] 54/5: p 175a – Taetle R, Buick RN, McCulloch EA (1980) Effect of Interferon on colony formation in culture by blast cell progenitors in acute myeloblastic leukemia. Blood 56:549–552 – Wiggans RG, Jacobson AJ, Fialkow PJ, et al. (1978) Probable clonal origin of acute myeloblastic leukemia following radiation and chemotherapy of colon cancer. Blood 52:659–663

Haematology and Blood Transfusion Vol. 26
Modern Trends in Human Leukemia IV
Edited by Neth, Gallo, Graf, Mannweiler, Winkler
© Springer-Verlag Berlin Heidelberg 1981

Proliferation and Maturation of Hemopoietic Cells in Adult Patients with Different Forms of Acute Leukemia and Chronic Myeloid Leukemia in Agar and Liquid Cultures

B. V. Afanasiev, E. Elstner, M. A. Saidali, and T. S. Zabelina

The cloning of haemopoietic cells in semi-solid agar medium makes it possible to evaluate their response to the colony-stimulating factor (CSF). The response to CSF suggests that target cells are of myeloid origin. However, the lack of response to CSF does not exclude the possibility of myeloid origin of target cells, since the blast cells of some patients with acute myeloid leukaemia (AML) do not respond to CSF in agar culture. The cultivation of the haemopoietic cells in liquid cultures (Golde and Cline 1973) makes it possible to investigate the maturation of blast cells, and the origin of blast cells can be determined by the analysis of morphologically distinguishable daughter cells.

A. Material and Methods

A total of 183 patients were investiged (Table 1). The morphological type of blast crisis (BC) and acute-leukemia (AL) was identified using common morphological and cytochemical methods (Giemsa, Sudan black, myeloperoxidase, PAS). Janossy revealed a good correlation between cytomorphological and immunological division of BC into "myeloid" and "lymphoid" types (M- and L-type).

The cloning of hemopoietic cells was performed in the double layer agar culture by Pike and Robinson (1970) with slight modification (Afanasiev et al. 1976). Colonies (>20 cells) and clusters (3–20 cells) were scored at day 6–7. It was possible to characterize four types of growth patterns in bone marrow cell cultures: hypoplastic, normal, hyperplastic and leukaemic (Fig. 1).

In patients with AL the response of haemopoietic cells to CSF was designated when the leukaemic type of growth was seen in agar culture and in patients with CML when leukaemic or hyperplastic growth was seen. The maturation of blood and/or bone marrow blast cells (acute lymphoblastic leukaemia [ALL] – 6, acute non-lymphoblastic leukaemia [ANLL] – 16, acute undifferentiated leukaemia [AUL] – 4, and CML-BC – 11 patients) was studied in the liquid culture system by Golde and Cline. Morphological investigation was performed at 7–14 days.

Table 1. Patients studied

Diagnosis	Number of patients
Acute lymphoblastic leukaemia (ALL)	31
Acute non-lymphoblastic leukaemia (ANLL)	45
Acute undifferentiated leukaemia (AUL)	10
Haemopoietic dysplasia (HD) (Smouldering leukaemia)	9
Chronic myeloid leukaemia-blast crisis (CML-BC)	26
Chronic myeloid leukaemia-chronic stage (CML-CS)	43
Chronic myeloid leukaemia-accelerated stage (CML-AS)	16
Myelofibrosis-blast crisis (MMM-BC)	3
Control group	72

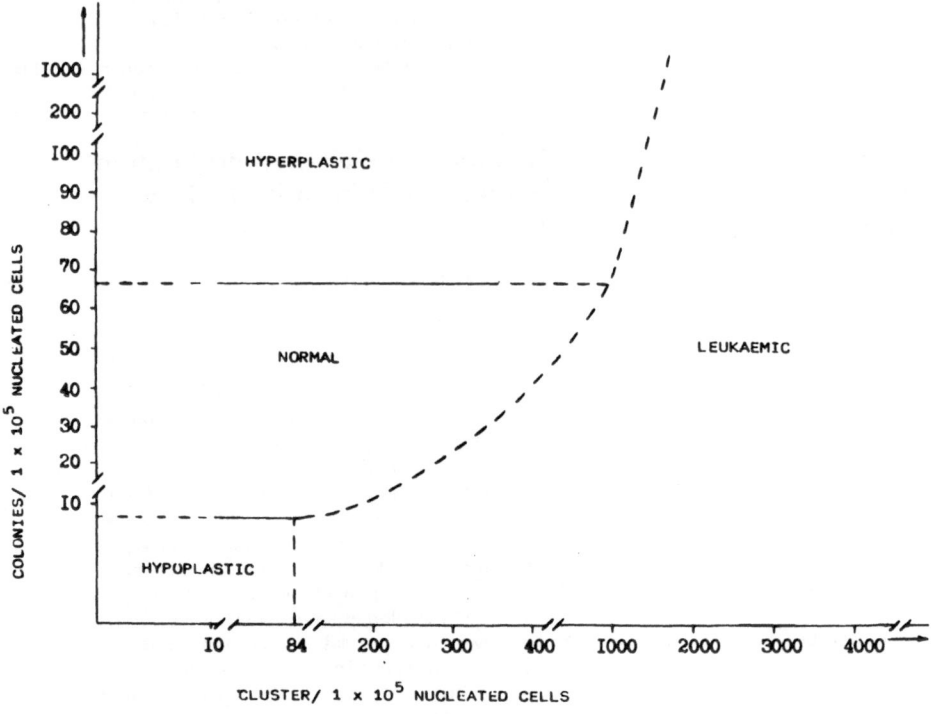

Fig. 1. Picture of zones from different growth patterns of bone marrow cells and the criteria for definition of growth types of bone marrow cells in double layer agar system. *normal,* colony count from 8 to 67, normal size of colonies, cluster: colony<12; *hypoplastic,* colony count<8, and cluster count<84; *hyperplastic,* colony count>67, and cluster: colony<12; *leukaemic,* cluster: colony>12, small size of colonies (20–40 cells) and consisting of single cells

B. Results

The results of the study of haemopoietic cell growth type in patients with AL in agar cultures are presented in Fig. 2. The leukaemic type of growth (response of leukaemic cells to CSF; a myeloid cell property) has been observed in 6% of ALL, 67% of ANLL, 50% of AUL and 56% of haemopoietic dysplasia (smouldering leukaemia). In 6 of 16 patients with ANLL (non-maturation group) the blast cells had an absolute arrest of maturation at the level of blasts-promyelocytes and blasts-promonocytes in liquid culture. In ten patients (maturation group) the blast cells possessed the ability to mature to monocytes-macrophages and/or immature granulocytes. In patients of this group the ability of blast cells to mature was more pronounced in the monocytes-macrophages cell line than in granulocytes. In patients with AUL and ALL we have observed

an intensive granulomonocytopoiesis in a 7-day-old liquid culture. The results of the study of the growth type of haemopoietic cells in patients with different stages of CML are presented in Fig. 3. In 75% of the patients with the L-type of CML-BC and 82% with the M-type haemopoietic cells responded to CSF in double layer agar culture. In most of the patients with both L-type (five of seven) and M-type (three of four) of blast crisis the blast cells possessed the ability to mature to granulocytic and monocytic cells in the liquid culture system. This finding has been observed in two patients with both the L-type of CML-BC and neuroleukaemia.

C. Discussion

The results obtained confirm the data that the patients with AL are a very different group in

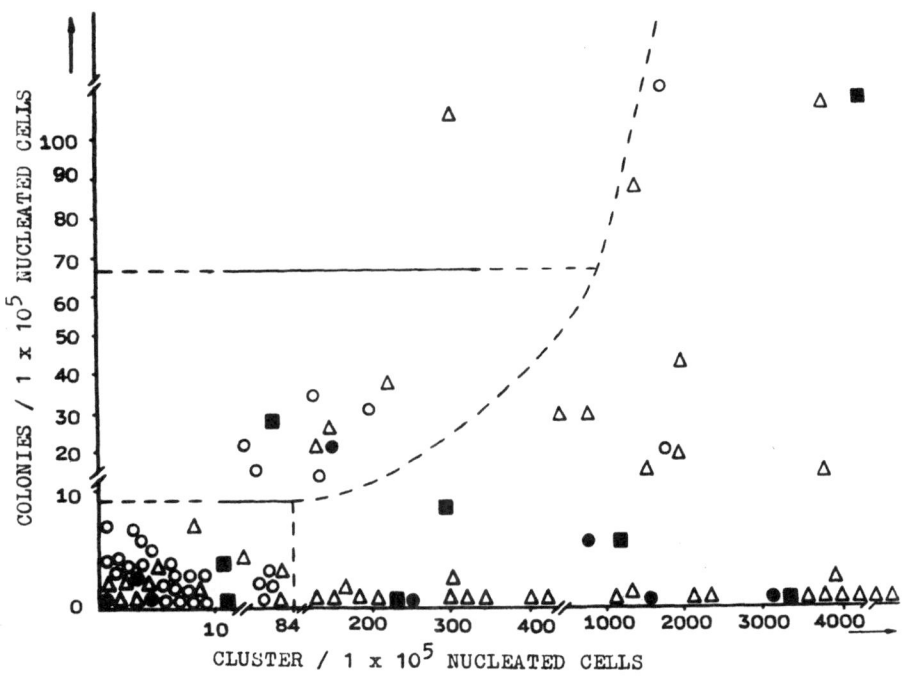

Fig. 2. Growth patterns of bone marrow cells in patients with different forms of acute leukemia (double layer agar technique). ○, ALL; △, ANLL; ●, AUL; and ■, HD

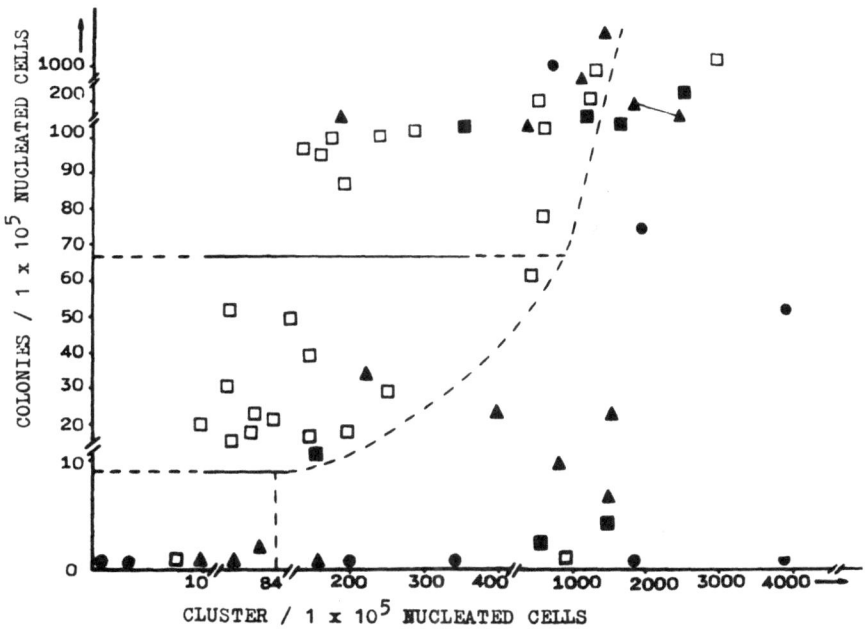

Fig. 3. Growth patterns of bone marrow cells in patients with CML (double layer agar technique). □ CML (chronic stage), ■ CML (accelerated stage), ● CML (blast crisis, "lymphoid type"), and ▲ CML (blast crisis, "myeloid type")

their haemopoietic cells' ability to proliferate and mature in vitro. In ANLL patients haemopoetic cells responded to CSF much more frequently than in ALL. Only in 6% of ALL patients there was a typical leukaemic type of growth patterns in agar culture. These data are in agreement with Spitzer et al. (1976) who have discovered a leukaemic type of growth pattern in agar culture of haemopoietic cells in some patients with AL. The origin of these clusters and colonies in agar culture has not been determined. The leukaemic type of growth pattern observed in the agar cultures in 56% of the haemopoietic dysplasia (HD) patients indicates that most of the cases could be considered as patients with true leukaemia.

Our results of cultivating in the liquid culture system indicate that in most of the ANLL patients the ability of blast cells to mature was more pronouced in the monocytes-macrophages cells line than in granulocytes. Cultivation of haemopoietic cells in patients with CML-BC in liquid and agar culture suggests that the type of blast cells is not always determinable in the light microscope by morphological and cytochemical tests. Most of our patients with L-type of BC have blast cells of myeloid origin (response to CSF and ability to mature to granulomonocytic cells). These data are in agreement with Marie et al. (1979) who have discovered that in 9 of 12 patients with BC the blasts contained peroxidase activity detectable only by electron microscope.

References

Afanasiev BV, Zaritsky AJu, Zabelina TS (1976) Colony forming ability of the bone marrow in haematologically healthy individuals in agar culture. Fisiol Čeloveka (Moskva) 2:301–307 – Golde DW, Cline MJ (1973) Growth of human bone marrow in liquid culture. Blood 41:45–57 – Marie JP, Vernant JP, Dreyfus B, Breton-Gorius J (1979) Ultrastructural localization of peroxidases in "undifferentiated" blasts during the blast crisis of chronic granulocytic leukaemia. Br J Haematol 43:549–558 – Pike BL, Robinson WA (1970) Human bone marrow colony growth in agar-gel. J Cell Physiol 76:77–84 – Spitzer G, Dicke KA, Gehan EA, Smith T, McCredie KB, Barlogie B, Freireich EY (1976) A simplified in vitro classification for prognosis in adult acute leukemia: The application of in vitro results in remission-predictive models. Blood 48:795–807

Haematology and Blood Transfusion Vol. 26
Modern Trends in Human Leukemia IV
Edited by Neth, Gallo, Graf, Mannweiler, Winkler
© Springer-Verlag Berlin Heidelberg 1981

Cytological and Cytochemical Analysis of Plasma Clot Cultures and Peripheral Granulocytes Related to Long Term Survival in Childhood ALL and Cancer Patients Under Cytostatica Therapy

E. Burk, L. Chennaoui-Antonio, H. Beiersdorf, H. H. Hellwege, K. Winkler, B. Heinisch, G. Küstermann, U. Krause, H. J. Kitschke, H. Voigt, and R. Neth

Colony number and cytology, the cluster/colony ratio, and the peroxydase reaction were investigated in plasma clot cultures (Stephenson et al. 1971; Hellwege et al. 1978; Biermann et al. 1979) of 45 normal persons and 250 patients with childhood AL (Neth et al. 1980).

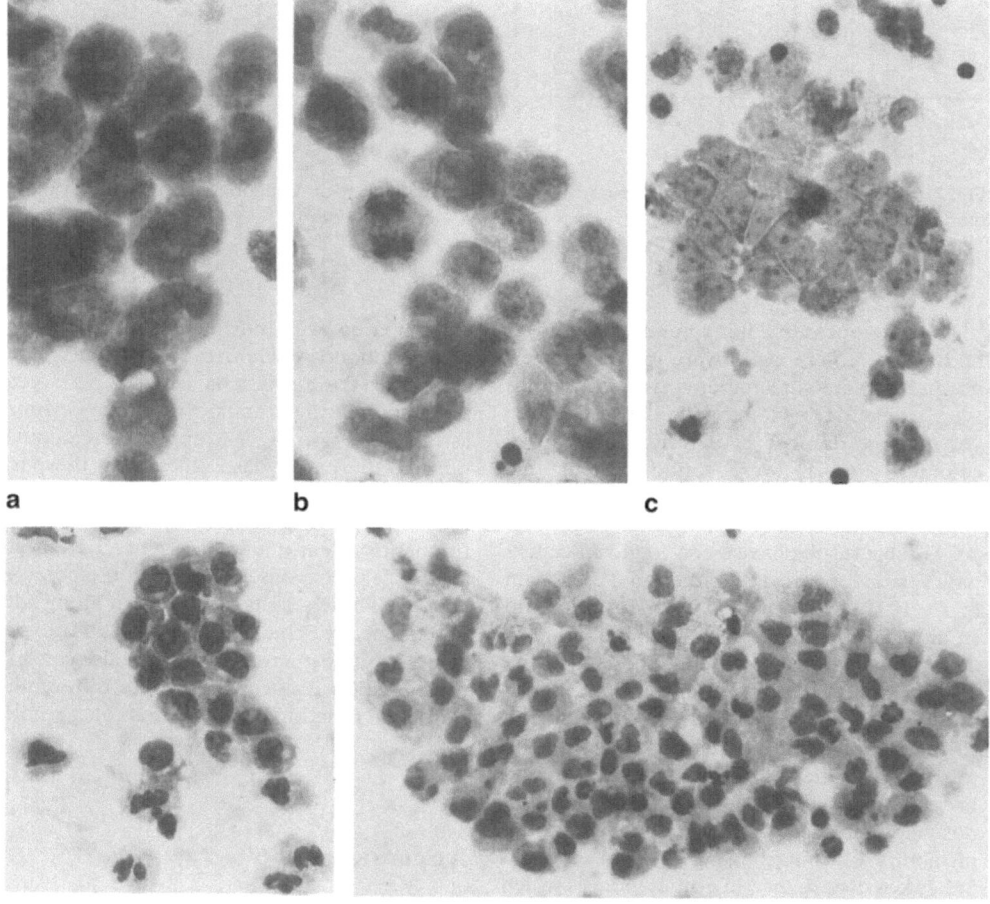

Fig. 1a—e. Plasma clot colonies. **a** peroxydase positive; **b** weak peroxydase positive; **c** peroxydase negative; **d** weak peroxydase positive small colony; **e** weak peroxydase positive large colony

normal persons $n=11$	normal persons $n=19$	ALL 2.5 years after therapy	ALL 3.5 years after therapy	ALL 2.5 years after therapy
100	100	100	100	100
100	100	92	100	95
100	100	92	100	88
100	100	77	94	81
95	100	68	83	71
94	100	40	38	13
92	100	15	0	0
88	100	0		0
86	100			0
78	100			
55	98			
	95			
	95			
	88			
	86			
	82			
	70			
	59			
	48			
$\overline{X}$ 90	90	60	74	50

Fig. 2. % Peroxydase positive colonies in normal persons and patients with childhood leukemia (ALL) in long time remission

No differences in colony number, cytology, and cluster/colony ratio were found between normal persons and patients with childhood ALL except during leukemic relapses. However, a large number of peroxydase negative colonies (Fig. 1) were found in leukemic patients even in remission after as many as 2–6 years without therapy (Neth et al. 1980, Fig. 2). Similar results have been found in cancer patients under cytostatica therapy (Biermann et al. 1979; Neth et al. 1980). In follow up studies for up to 2 years in bone marrow cultures of patients with childhood ALL the colony number cluster/colony ratio, and the peroxydase reaction varied to a high degree (Fig. 3). For technical reasons there are no follow up studies of normal persons, but as bone marrow cultures of normal persons did not show a high degree of variation, the instability of childhood ALL cultures could indicate a disturbance in granulopoiesis which could result in a relaps if an additional noxa occurs.

Compared with normal persons, patients with childhood ALL and cancer patients under cytostatica therapy also have a weak peroxydase reaction in the granulocytes of the peripheral blood (Figs. 4–6). Comparable examinations of the peroxydase reaction in the peripheral blood showed that the peroxydase reaction in the peripheral granulocytes was frequently clearly decreased in contrast to a normal peroxydase reaction in the colonies (Fig. 6) These results indicate that along with pathologically changed stem cells morbid changes of the microenvironment also can lead to regulation disturbances in the differentiation and functional maturation of granulocytes.

Acknowledgments

Supported by the Deutsche Forschungsgemeinschaft and the Tumorzentrum Hamburg

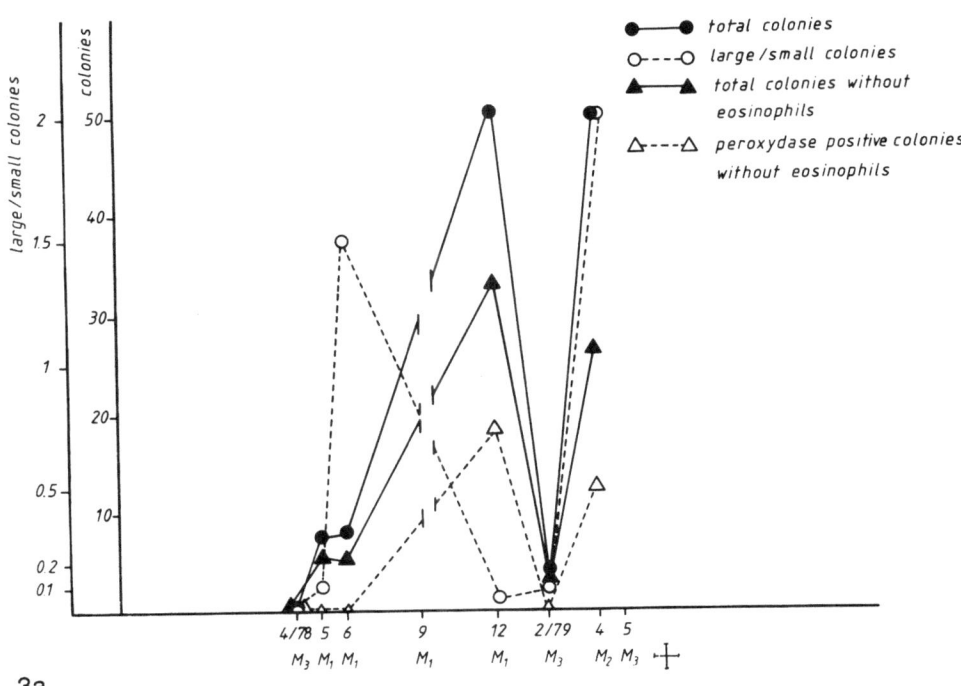

3a

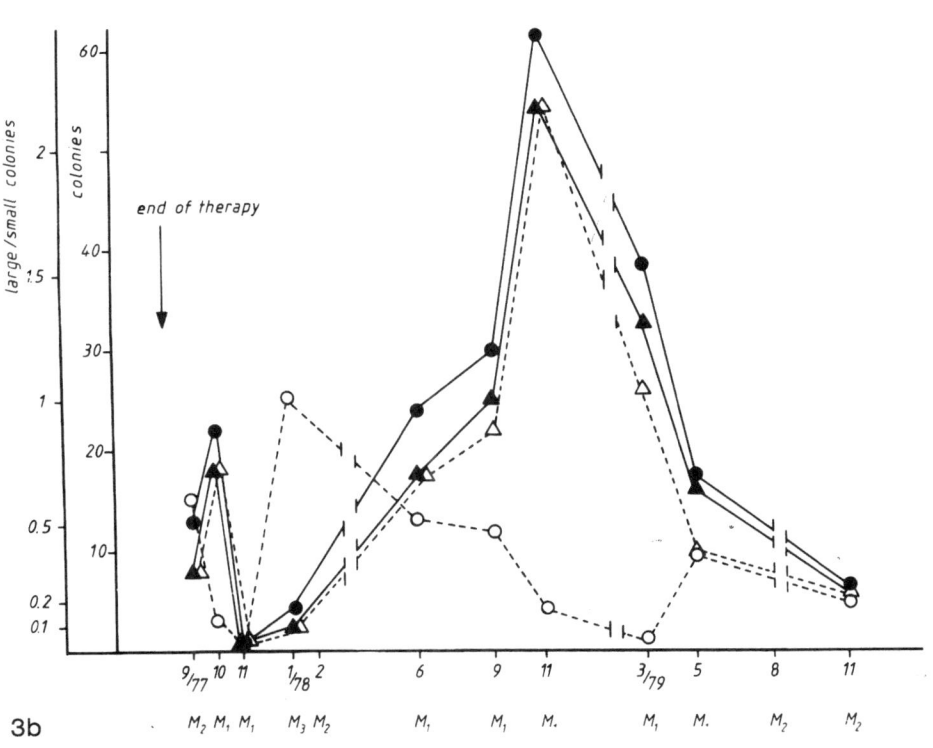

3b

257

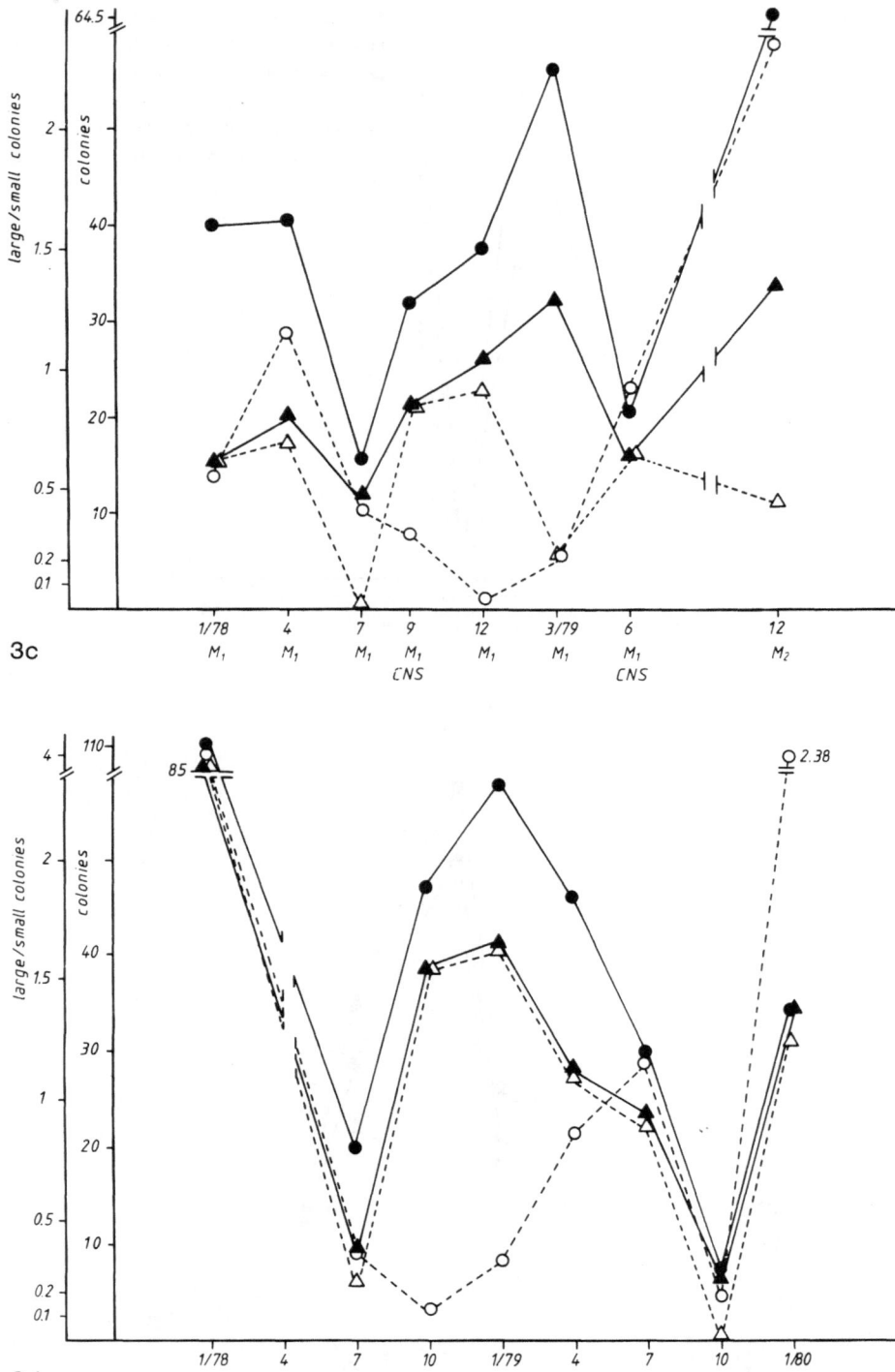

Fig. 3a–d. Follow up studies of patients with childhood ALL; **a,b,c** in therapy; **d** without therapy. M_1, remission; M_2, partial remission; M_3, relapse.

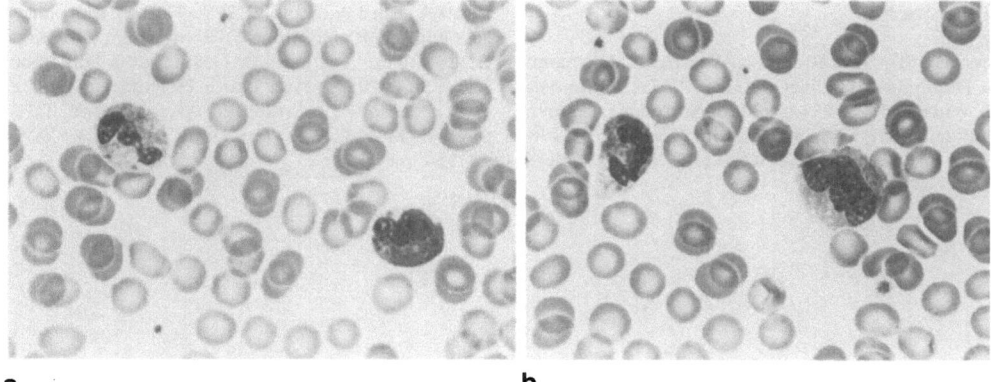

a   **b**

Fig. 4.a *Left* peroxydase negative granulocyte, *right* peroxydase positive granulocyte, **b** *Left* weak peroxydase positive granulocyte, *right* peroxydase negative monocyte

normal persons	I	II	III	IV	V	VI
100	100	99	97	97	100	99
100	99	96	96	97	99	95
99	97	95	92	94	95	94
98	96	89	91	93	92	89
97	94	88	90	88	90	88
97	93	85	88	87	90	85
96	92	84	88	76	88	84
95	89	82	85	76	85	80
95	87	75	80	75	80	79
91	85	70	77	74	70	68
90	83	66	72	73		31
89	80	64	69	47		0
88	74	36	51	43		
59	70		49	26		
$\overline{X}$ 92	82	79	80	75	89	74

Fig. 5. % Peroxydase positive peripheral granulocytes in patients with melanom in DTIC-therapy

months after therapy	% peroxydase pos. colonies	% peroxydase pos. peripheral granulocytes
14	100	58
28	97	16
31	97	70
12	96	31
5	94	62
46	90	92
45	88	76
27	86	83
20	79	93
30	6	1

Fig. 6. Peroxydase positive colonies in plasma clot cultures and peroxydase positive peripheral granulocytes in patients with childhood leukemia (ALL) in long time remission

References

Biermann E, Neth R, Grosch-Wörner I, Hausmann K, Heinisch B, Hellwege HH, Kötke A, Skrandies G, Winkler K (1979) In: Modern trends in human leukemia III. Springer, Berlin Heidelberg New York, pp 211–215 – Hellwege HH, Bläker F, Neth R (1978) Eur J Pediatr 129:279 – Neth R, Biermann E, Heinisch B, Hellwege HH, Marsman G, Burk E (1980) in: Advances in Comparative leukemia research 1979. Elsevier/North Holland, pp 39–40 – Stephenson JR, Axelrad AA, McLeod DL, Streeve MM (1971) Proc natl Acad Sci USA 68:1542

Haematology and Blood Transfusion Vol. 26
Modern Trends in Human Leukemia IV
Edited by Neth, Gallo, Graf, Mannweiler, Winkler
© Springer-Verlag Berlin Heidelberg 1981

Maturation of Blast Cells in Acute Transformation of Chronic Myeloproliferative Syndrome* **

D. Hoelzer, E. B. Harriss, and F. Carbonell

In recent years, data have accumulated which demonstrate that the failure of human leukaemic blast cells to differentiate is not an inherent defect, but rather one that can be overcome under in vitro culture conditions. This has been established both for cell lines and for fresh human leukaemic blast cells (LBC). The differentiation of human LBC into different cell pathways is possible. Differentiation to more mature stages has been demonstrated, into granulopoietic cells for the K60 human promyelocytic line (Collins et al. 1977) and for the K61 cell line (Koeffler et al. 1978), into cells with erythropoietic features for the K562 cell line (Anderssen et al. 1979), and even into lymphopoiesis, as for the Reh cell line (Lau et al. 1979).

The maturation of fresh human LBC from some cases of acute myeloid leukaemia (AML) into granulopoietic cells or macrophages has also been observed during in vitro culture as a liquid suspension or in a agar system. When AML blast cells are cultured in diffusion chambers (DC), a terminal differentiation into mature granulocytes is observed in half of the patients, and these cells show partially normal function when tested for phagocytosis or by nitrotetrazolium blue reduction (Hoelzer et al. 1980).

In the present study, blast cells from patients in the blast crisis of chronic myelocytic leukaemia (CML) were investigated for their ability to differentiate in diffusion chamber culture. The aim was to see whether terminal differentiation into mature granulocytes occurs, as in AML, and whether differentiation into other haemotological cell lines is also possible, which might indicate that blast cells in CML blast crisis are primitive cells and therefore able to differentiate into haemopoietic pathways other than granulopoiesis.

A. Materials and Methods

The material was provided in a cooperative study on the pathophysiology of CML blast crisis by the Süddeutsche Hämoblastosegruppe. The blast cells in CML blast crisis were characterized by cytochemistry (PAS, POX, esterase) and by immunological cell surface markers. The findings presented in this paper relate to cells from 24 patients showing the myeloid type of blast crisis.

Peripheral blood cells were separated by centrifugation on an Isopaque-Ficoll gradient resulting in an enrichment of blast cells to over 80% in most cases. The diffusion chamber technique was carried out as described previously (Hoelzer et al. 1977). In brief, DC were filled with 5×10^5 nucleated cells, implanted into host mice pre-irradiated with 750 rad and cultured for up to 8 weeks. The chambers were removed every week, cleaned with sterile gauze to remove the host cells coating the membranes and re-implanted into fresh, irradiated hosts. Chamber contents were harvested at weekly intervals and investigated for total and differential cell counts and for cytochemical tests, including peroxidase, PAS, naphthol-AS-acetate esterase and leucocyte alkaline phosphatase, and for CFU-C content cytogenetics, phagocytosis and NTB reduction.

B. Results

When leukaemic blood cells from patients with blast crisis in CML were cultured in diffusion

* Supported by the Deutsche Forschungsgemeinschaft, Sonderforschungsbereich 112, Zellsystemphysiologie, Project B3.
** A cooperative study of the Süddeutsche Hämoblastosegruppe

chambers, the growth pattern observed was quite distinct from that for cells from the chronic phase of CML and also from that for normal peripheral blood cells. For most of the patients in blast crisis, there was a net increase in total cell number which was almost continuous, reaching values greatly in excess of normal. This rise in cellularity was due to proliferation of blast cells and a considerable degree of maturation of DC cells into proliferating and non-proliferating granulopoiesis As shown in Fig. 1, the increase in proliferating granulopoietic cells, i.e. promyelocytes and myelocytes, was immediate. Mature granulopoietic cells decreased initially in most cases, most probably owing to death. A rise in mature granulopoietic cells was delayed, usually for about 1 week, until cells newly developed from the immature stages appeared (Fig. 2). In 22 of 24 cases the values reached for granulopoietic cells were well above the levels for normal peripheral blood cells cultured in DC, as well as above the levels for CML in the chronic phase.

Development of megakaryocytes was observed in 16 of the 24 patients studied who had

CML blast crisis. New erythropoietic cells were seen in 13 of the 24 cases. Lymphocytes were fewer and plasma cells scarce in comparison with those found in cultures of mononuclear blood cells from normal persons.

C. Discussion

The experiments described here show that when blast cells from patients with blast crisis in CML are cultured in diffusion chambers for periods of up to 8 weeks, there is a marked proliferation of blast cells and a new development of granulopoietic cells together with some megakaryocytes and erythropoietic cells. The differentiation into granulopoietic cells is not restricted to the immature forms, but terminal differentiation into mature granulocytes could also be observed in 80% of the patients studied. The origin of these differentiated cells is a crucial point. They might be derived from the implanted blast cells, from Ph' positive stem cells typical of the chronic phase of CML or even from remaining normal stem cells. Arguments in favour of an at least

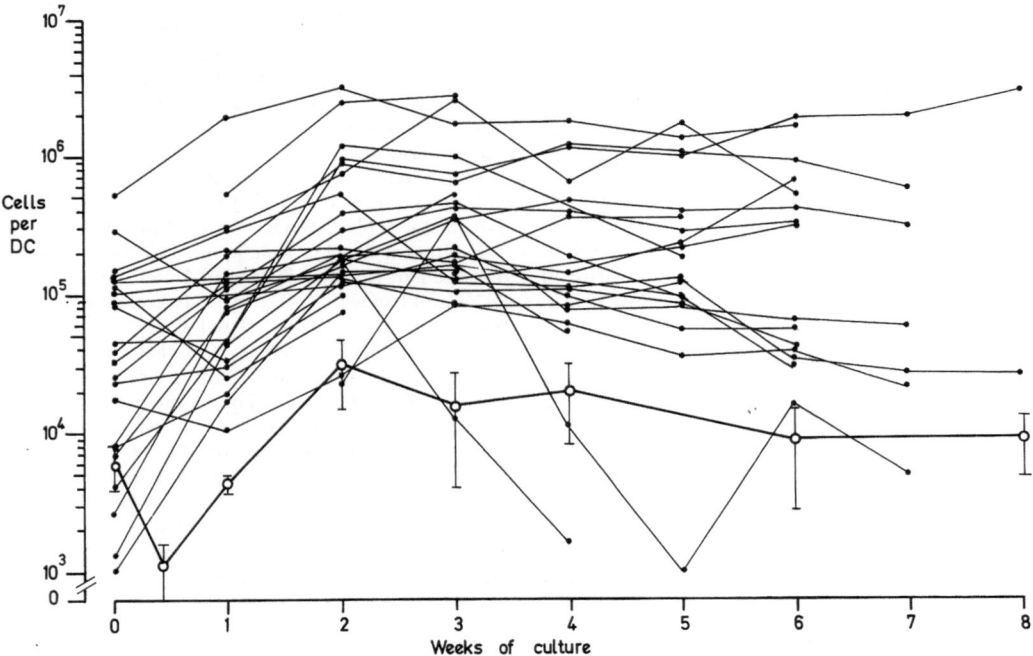

Fig. 1. Change in number of proliferating granulopoietic cells harvested from diffusion chambers at weekly intervals. Results from 24 patients with blast crisis in chronic myeloid leukaemia. *Open Circles* and *bars* denote mean values ±S.E.M. for *DC* growth of mononuclear blood cells from normal persons

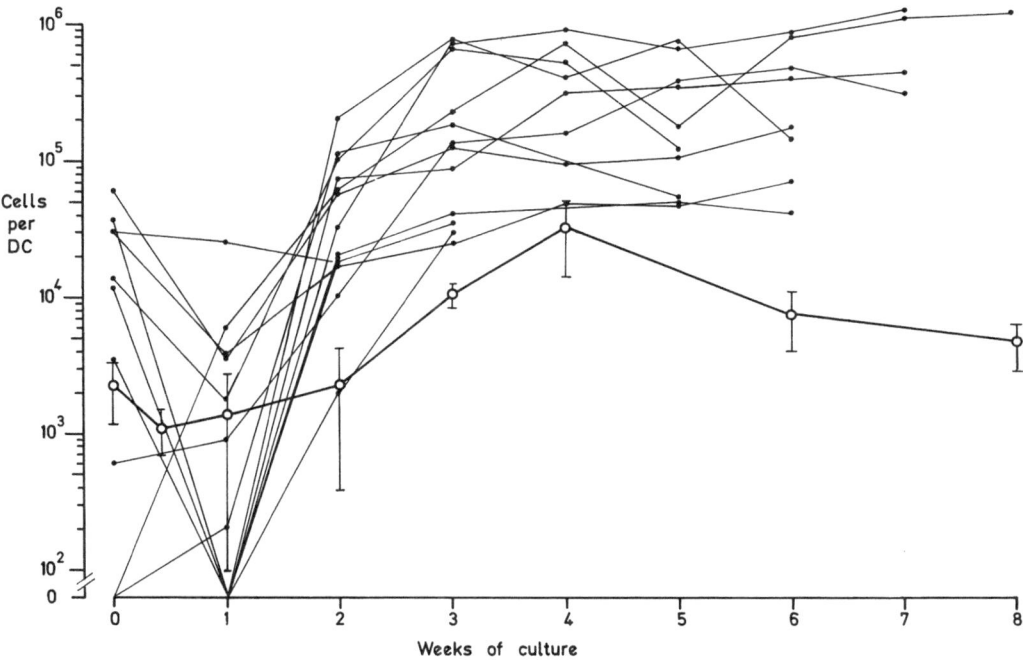

Fig. 2. Change in number of non-proliferating granulopoietic cells. Details as in Fig. 1

partial origin from blast cells are the fact that the cell suspension used for culture consisted of more than 90% blast cells in some cases, the growth pattern of the cells in culture and the results of cytogenetic analysis.

The growth pattern for CML blast crisis cells in DC culture with continuous proliferation and differentiation resulting in a progressive increase in total cell number, in some cases for the whole 8-week culture period, differs strikingly from the growth pattern for CML cells from the chronic phase. In the latter, although proliferation and differentiation into granulopoietic cells were also observed, the constant decline in total cellularity, as found also by Chikkappa et al. (1973), indicated that Ph' positive stem cells in the chronic phase apparently do not possess the potential for unlimited proliferation under these culture conditions.

In the patients studied who had CML blast crisis, the cells harvested from DC and subjected to cytogenetic analysis were Ph' positive and some cases also showed additional chromosome aberrations characteristic of acute transformation in CML. There were, however, five cases of CML blast crisis in which *all* the

DC cells tested had, as well as the Ph' chromosome, an additional clonal aberration, indicating that the proliferating cells in these DC cultures were derived from that abnormal clone. It might, therefore be concluded that the mature cells are also descendants of these clones.

A noteworthy finding is the proportion of newly developed megakaryocytes and erythropoiesis from CML blast crisis cells, which was much higher than that developing from chronic phase cells in DC. Although it seems likely, there is as yet no certain proof that either the megakaryocytes or erythropoietic cells are descendants of the blast cells in CML blast crisis and are not descendants from remaining chronic phase cells. From the former possibility one could speculate that blast cells in the myeloid type of blast crisis possess a greater potential for differentiation into different cell lines than do AML cells. This in turn would mean the transformation of an early precursor cell, similar to that known from studies of CML in the chronic phase, where involvement of granulopoiesis, erythropoiesis and megakaryocytopoiesis has been demonstrated (Fialkow, 1979).

References

Anderssen LC, Jokinen M, Gahmberg CG (1979) Induction of erythoid differentiation in the human leukaemia cell line K 562. Nature 278:364–365 – Chikkappa G, Boecker WR, Borner G, Carsten AL, Conkling K, Cook L, Cronkite EP, Dunwoody S (1973) Return of alkaline phosphatase in chronic myelocytic leukemia cells in diffusion chamber cultures. Proc. Soc. exp. Biol. Med. 143:212–217 – Collins SJ, Gallo RC, Gallagher RE (1977) Continuous growth and differentiation of human myeloid leukaemic cells in suspension culture. Nature 270:347–349 – Fialkow PJ (1979) Use of glucose-6-phosphate dehydrogenase markers to study human myeloproliferative disorders. In: Neth R, Gallo RC, Hofschneider HP, Mannweiler K (eds) "Modern Trends in Human Leukemia III". Springer-Verlag, Berlin Heidelberg New York, pp 53–58 – Hoelzer D, Kurrle E, Schmücker H, Harriss EB (1977) Evidence for differentiation of human leukemic blood cells in diffusion chamber culture. Blood 49:729–744 – Hoelzer D, Harriss EB, Bültmann B, Fliedner TM, Heimpel H (1980) Differentiation into granulopoiesis in human acute leukaemia and blast crisis in chronic myelocytic leukaemia. In: Cronkite EP, Carsten AL (eds) Diffusion Chamber Culture. Springer-Verlag, Berlin Heidelberg New York, pp 242–250 – Koeffler HP, Golde E (1978) Acute myelogenous leukemia: A human cell line responsive to colony-stimulating activity. Science 200:1153–1154 – Lau B, Jäger G, Thiel E, Rodt H, Huhn D, Pachmann K, Netzel B, Böning L, Thierfelder S, Dörmer P (1979) Growth of the Reh cell line in diffusion chambers. Evidence for differentiation along the T- and B-cell pathway

Haematology and Blood Transfusion Vol. 26
Modern Trends in Human Leukemia IV
Edited by Neth, Gallo, Graf, Mannweiler, Winkler
© Springer-Verlag Berlin Heidelberg 1981

Patterns of Cell Surface Differentiation of cALL Positive Leukemic Blast Cells in Diffusion Chamber Culture

B. Lau, G. Jäger, E. Thiel, K. Pachmann, H. Rodt, S. Thierfelder, and P. Dörmer

A. Introduction

The majority of acute lymphoblastic leukemias (ALL) can be characterized by the presence of the common ALL antigen (cALLA) (Greaves et al. 1977). Since this cell marker is only rarely found on bone marrow cells of healthy individuals, the normal cellular equivalent of leukemic cALL positive blasts still remains unknown. However, some observations support the hypothesis that these cells might represent a common stem cell of the T- and B-cell lineage (Janossy et al. 1976). In order to explore a possible relationship between the cALLA and a certain developmental stage during lymphatic ontogeny, peripheral cALL blasts from four children and cells of the Reh line were cultured in diffusion chambers (DC). During the culture period membrane markers were investigated to determine differentiation in either the T- or B-cell axis.

B. Material and Methods

Peripheral blood samples obtained from four untreated ALL patients between 4–11 years of age were separated on an Isopaque-Ficoll gradient. In all cases, leukemic blasts constituted at least 95% of these mononuclear cell fractions, the rest being normal lymphoid cells. The Reh cells were taken from the continuously maintained line which originally had been established from an ALL of the "non-T, non-B" type (Rosenfeld et al. 1977).

Diffusion chambers were filled with 5×10^5 cells of the respective material as already described previously (Lau et al. 1979). Two chambers were inserted into the peritoneal cavity of each CBA mouse preirradiated with 700 rad. At different instances during a 13- or 16-day culture DC were removed and were shaken in an 0.5% pronase solution. In case of the Reh line two experiments of this type were conducted, each lasting 20 days.

Besides total and differential counts the majority of the chamber harvest was processed for cell surface characterization with specific antisera (Rodt et al. 1975). Direct immunofluorescence was performed after the cells had been labeled with polyvalent anti-human immunoglobulin (AIg) or the F(ab)₂ fragment of AIg, anti-cALL globulin (AcALLG), and anti-T-cell globulin (ATCG). For double labeling two different antisera were mixed simultaneously with the cells. Cytoplasmic Ig (cIg) was investigated after sedimentation of the cells onto glass slides and fixation in ice cold methanol followed by incubation with antibodies in a moist chamber. In addition, we tested the ability of the cells to form E-rosettes (Bentwich and Kunkel 1973) as well as rosettes with mouse erythrocytes (Forbes and Zalewski 1976).

C. Results and Conclusions

After 6 days of ALL culture, the chamber content had dropped considerably. No further increase of the total cell number was observed throughout the culture period. Cells of the Reh line, on the other hand, grew exponentially from day 3 until the end of both experiments. The types of cells observed during ALL cultivation were mainly leukemic blasts and, to a smaller extent, normal appearing lymphoid cells, macrophages, and granulocytic cells. The morphology of Reh cells resembling that of undifferentiated blast-like cells remained unchanged.

Cell marker analysis revealed remarkable surface changes (Fig. 1). In two patients, T.H. and V.M., the cells had the typical appearance of a cALL on day 0 (Jäger et al. 1979). In both cases the cells developed surface Ig (sIg), mostly in combination with the cALLA

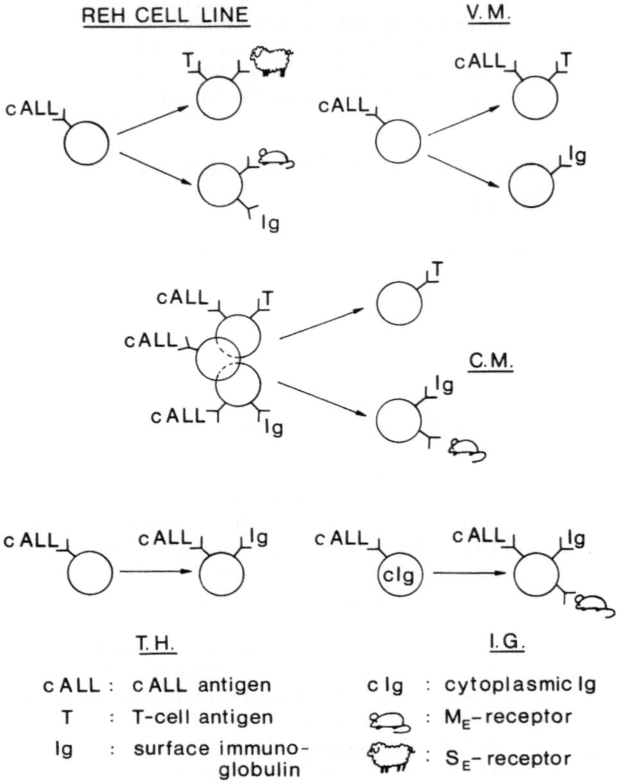
REH CELL LINE
V.M.
cALL
T
Ig
cALL
T
Ig
cALL
T
cALL
C.M.
T
Ig
cALL
Ig
cALL
cALL
Ig
cALL
cALL
Ig
clg
T.H.
I.G.
cALL : cALL antigen
T : T-cell antigen
Ig : surface immuno-globulin
c Ig : cytoplasmic Ig
: M_E-receptor
: S_E-receptor

Fig. 1. Changes in the membrane phenotypes of cALL positive blasts from four children and of the Reh cells during culture in DC

(70%/75/%). Furthermore, a fairly constant portion of cells (24%) carrying the cALLA together with the T-cell antigen was seen from day 6 on in V.M.

In addition to 50% of the chamber input showing the cALLA alone, 28% of the cells in patient C.M. could already be characterized by double labelling with AcALLG and AIg(Fab)$_2$ on day O (Jäger et al. 1979). At the same time 23% of the cells expressed the cALLA together with the T-cell antigen. More mature descendants of these cells with only sIg or the T-cell antigen were already seen early in the culture. A receptor for mouse erythrocytes known to be a B-cell characteristic (Forbes and Zalewski 1976) was detected in this case in 6% of the cells on day 0 and increased up to 30% on day 9.

No change in the percentage of cALL positive cells could be registered during the whole culture period in patient I.G. (25%–33%); cIg was demonstrated in more than 90% of the blast cells already on day 0. At the end of the culture, sIg was found together with the cALLA in 30% of the cell harvest. This change was accompanied by the occurance of 33% of mouse rosette forming cells (M-RFC). With regard to the phenotypic characteristics of the Reh line cells (Lau et al. 1979) the cALLA was the only membrane marker found at the beginning of both experiments (10%/70%). Towards the end of the first culture period 70% T-positive cells developed along with 14% E rosetting cells. In the course of the second culture Reh cells could onyl be classified as belonging to the T-cell series according to their expression of the T-cell antigen. In this instance, M-RFC appeared on day 9 in 27% and on day 16 in 7% of the cell yield. During two further experiments performed with thymectomized mice as DC recipients a considerable portion of Reh cells (22% vs. 65%) was found to stain positively with AIg(Fab)$_2$ (unpublished observations).

Although a rise in the number of apparently normal lymphoid cells was evident in all ALL cases, two observations support the view that the cALL positive leukemic blasts were truly responsible for lymphatic differentiation: (1) At the onset of the culture the leukemic cells of I.G. contained cIg which enabled us to identify these cells as B-lymphocyte precursors. During cultivation the cells expressed sIg and a receptor for mouse erythrocytes. (2) Cells of the Reh line fulfilling all criteria of a leukemic cell line developed membrane markers of T-lymphocytes as well as characteristics of B-cells. The process of differentiation was accompanied by neither a change in morphology nor in the karyotype (Lau et al. 1979). On the basis of these findings we conclude that leukemic cALL blasts represent arrested early lymphatic progenitors. Under the environmental conditions of the DC culture the block in differentiation was at least partially released, and the cells were induced to further mature, mimicking a development into either the B- or T-cell series.

References

Bentwich Z, Kunkel HG (1973) Specific properties of human B and T lymphocytes and alterations in disease. Transplant Rev 16:29–50 – Forbes IJ, Zalewski PD (1976) A subpopulation of human B lymphocytes that rosette with mouse erythrocytes. Clin Exp Immunol 26:99–107 – Greaves MF, Janossy G, Roberts M, Rapson NT, Ellis RB, Chessels J, Lister TA, Catowsky D (1979) Membrane phenotyping: Diagnosis, monitoring and classification of acute lymphoid leukemias. In: Thierfelder S, Rodt H, Thiel E (eds) Immunological diagnosis of leukemias and lymphomas. Springer, Berlin Heidelberg New York, p 61 – Jäger G, Lau B, Pachmann K, Rodt H, Netzel B, Thiel E, Huhn D, Thierfelder S, Dörmer P (1979) Cell surface differentiation of acute lymphoblastic cALL-type leukemias in diffusion chambers. Blut 38:165–168 – Janossy G, Roberts M, Greaves MF (1976) Target cell in chronic myeloid leukemia and its relationship to acute lymphoid leukemia. Lancet II:1058–1060 – Lau B, Jäger G, Thiel E, Rodt H, Huhn D, Pachmann K, Netzel B, Böning L, Thierfelder S, Dörmer P (1979) Growth of the Reh cell line in diffusion chambers: Evidence for differentiation along the T- and B-cell pathway. Scand J Haematol 23:285–290 – Rodt H, Thierfelder S, Thiel E, Götze B, Netzel B, Huhn D, Eulitz M (1975) Identification and quantitation of human T-cell antigen by antisera purified from antibodies crossreacting with hemopoietic progenitors and other blood cells. Immunogenetics 2:411–430 – Rosenfeld C, Goutner A, Choquet C, Venuat AM, Kayibanda B, Pico JL (1977) Phenotypic characterization of a unique non-T, non-B acute lymphoblastic leukemia cell line. Nature 267:841–843

Haematology and Blood Transfusion Vol. 26
Modern Trends in Human Leukemia IV
Edited by Neth, Gallo, Graf, Mannweiler, Winkler
© Springer-Verlag Berlin Heidelberg 1981

Maturation of Human Peripheral Blood Leukemic Cells in Short-Term Culture

P. Forbes, D. Dobbie, R. Powles, and P. Alexander

A. Summary

This work is a continuation of earlier studies in this laboratory (Palú et al. 1979) in which two populations of cryopreserved acute myelogenous leukaemia (AML) cells were whown to undergo progressive maturation in vitro. Twelve other populations of AML cells have since been studied and three distinct patterns of in vitro behaviour have been observed:

1. Cells which did not mature.
2. Cells which matured to the polymorph series and
3. Cells which matured to the macrophage series.

Six populations of AML cells were studied both before and after cryopreservation to demonstrate that exposure to the cryopreservative agent dimethylsulphoxide (DMSO) does not influence the patterns of maturation observed. The effect of thioproline and prostaglandins A1 and A2 on maturation was also studied. It is too early to say whether any correlation between the prognosis of the AML patients and the maturation pattern of their AML cells can be established.

B. Materials and Methods

The AML cells were collected using an NCI/IBM continuous flow blood cell separator (Powles et al. 1974), cryopreserved (Chapuis et al. 1977), and stored in the vapour phase of liquid N_2 below $-150°C$.

Ampoules of AML cells were thawed rapidly in a 37°C water bath as required and diluted dropwise with 20 ml culture medium. The culture medium used throughout the procedure was RPMI 1640 (Gibco) with 25mM Hepes, 100 units/ml penicillin, 100 ng/ml streptomycin, 600 mg/l L-glutamine and 15% V/V foetal calf serum (FCS). After three min centrifugation at 400 g the cell pellet was resuspended in 10 ml culture medium and layered onto an equal volume of a sodium metrizoate-Ficoll density gradient (Lymphoprep. Nyegaard). The cell suspension was separated at 400 g at the interface for 15 min. The leucocytes lighter than 1.077 g/ml were collected at the interface and washed twice. The viable cells were counted in a haemocytometer by method of Trypan blue exclusion.

Cultures were established in 35 mm tissue culture dishes (Corning 2.500) at a concentration of 5×10^6 or 10^7 viable cells in 3 ml culture medium. The cultures were incubated at 37°C in a moist atmosphere containing 5% CO_2. Every two to three days 1 ml medium was exchanged by gentle aspiration for 1 ml fresh culture medium.

The following tests, selected from those used by Palú et al. (1979), were applied at regular intervals during the 2 to 3 week culture period:

1. Cell proliferation: An estimation was made by using a haemocytometer to count a 1/4 dilution of the non-adherent cell suspension in trypan blue. The adherent cells were lysed by the method of Currie and Hedley (1977) and the nuclei counted;
2. Morphology and cytochemistry: Slides of the non-adherent cultured cells were fixed and stained with Geimsa for morphology purposes and for the enzymes non-specific esterase (NSE) and chloracetate esterase (CAE) to show monocyte and polymorph differentiation, respectively (Li et al. 1973). Adherent cells were fixed and stained directly in the culture dishes; and
3. Fc receptors: The percentage of EA rosette-forming cells was estimated by the technique of Frøland and Wisløff (1976).

C. Results

Figure 1 shows a typical example of each of the three different patterns of maturation seen in the AML cell cultures. Three populations of

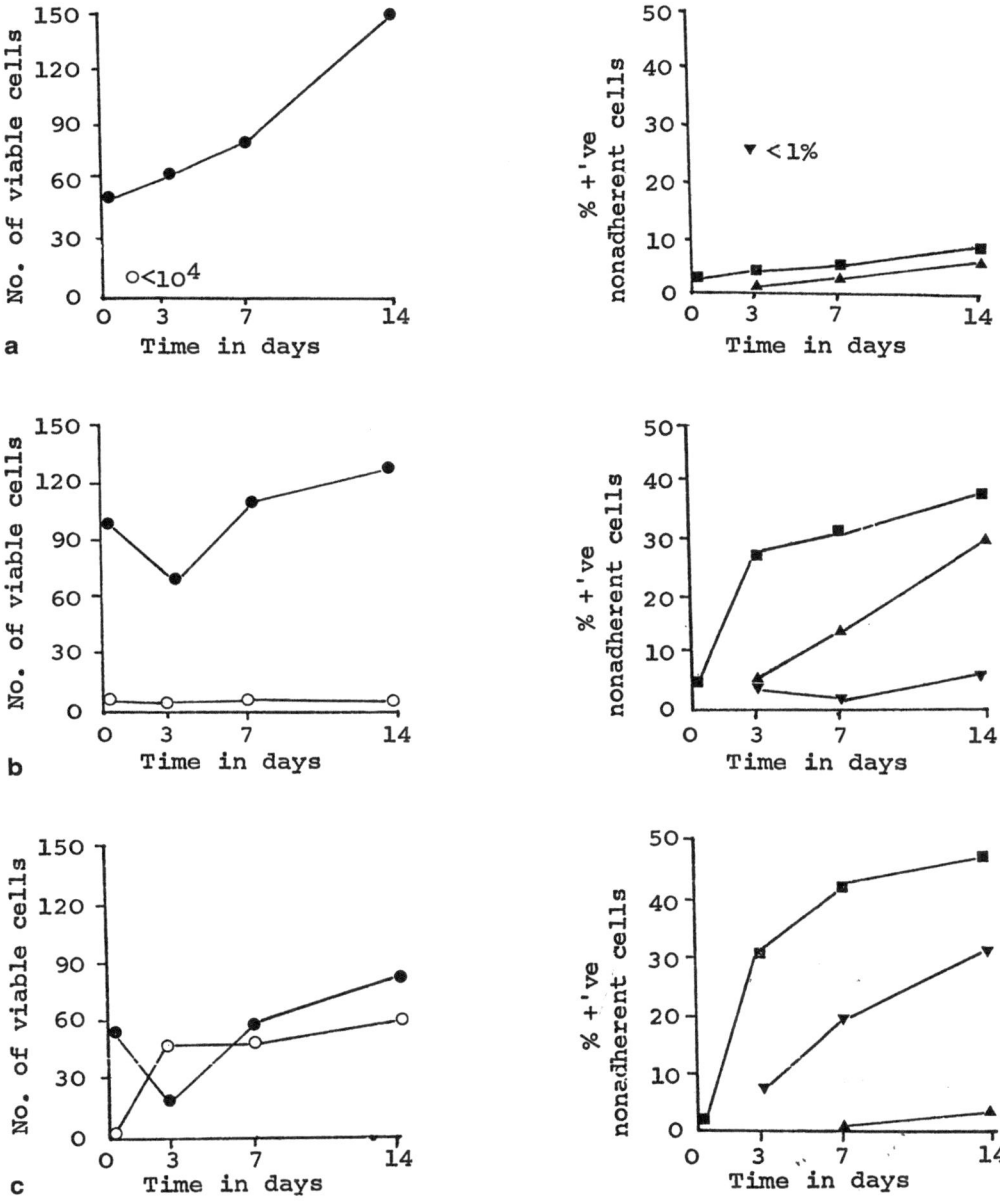

Fig. 1a–c. A typical example of the growth and maturation behaviour of each of the three types observed in vitro. **a** No maturation; **b** maturation to polymorphs; **c** maturation to macrophages. ● non-adherent cells × 10⁵. ○ adherent cells × 10⁴. ■ Fc+'ve cells. ▲ CAE+'ve cells. ▼NSE+'ve cells.

cells did not mature, although they proliferated in vitro. These three populations had very few adherent cells and the non-adherent cells had very low percentages of Fc positive, NSE positive and CAE positive cells. Six populations showed progressive maturation to the polymorph series in which the fraction of the adherent and the non-adherent cells which were positive for Fc and CAE increased, whilst the percentage of NSE positive cells remained low throughout the culture period. Five populations showed progressive maturation towards the macrophage series in which the proportion of non-adherent cells which were positive for Fc and NSE increased and more than 90% of the adherent cells were NSE positive. Both adherent and non-adherent cells had low percentages of CAE positive cells.

Six populations of cells were cultured prior to cryopreservation before and after the addition of 5% DMSO and subsequently cultured after cryopreservation to see whether the maturation pattern of the cells was altered in the presence of DMSO. No difference in maturation pattern was seen in any of the three types of pattern described.

Figure 2 shows the effect of prostaglandins A1 and A2 on the percentage of CAE positive cells in the cells of one patient (J.B.) which matured to the polymorph series when cultured in the absence of prostaglandins A1 and A2. The figure illustrates that increasing the amounts of prostaglandins A1 and A2 increased the percentage of CAE positive cells seen.

The prostaglandins raised the percentage of Fc positive (i.e. EA rosetting) cells by day 12 to 60% as compared to 40% in the FCS control cultures. The numbers of adherent and non-adherent cells were unaffected by the prostaglandins. No significant effect was seen in the cultures containing thioproline. None of the three chemical agents tested had any effect on the one non-maturing population CP in which they were studied.

Table 1 summarises the clinical state of the 14 patients whose AML cells were studied in vitro. As yet it is too early to determine whether the in vitro behaviour of the cells is related to the prognosis of the patients.

References

Chapuis B, Summersgill B, Cocks P, Howard P, Lawler S, Alexander P, Powles R (1977) Test for cryopreservation efficiency of human acute myelo-

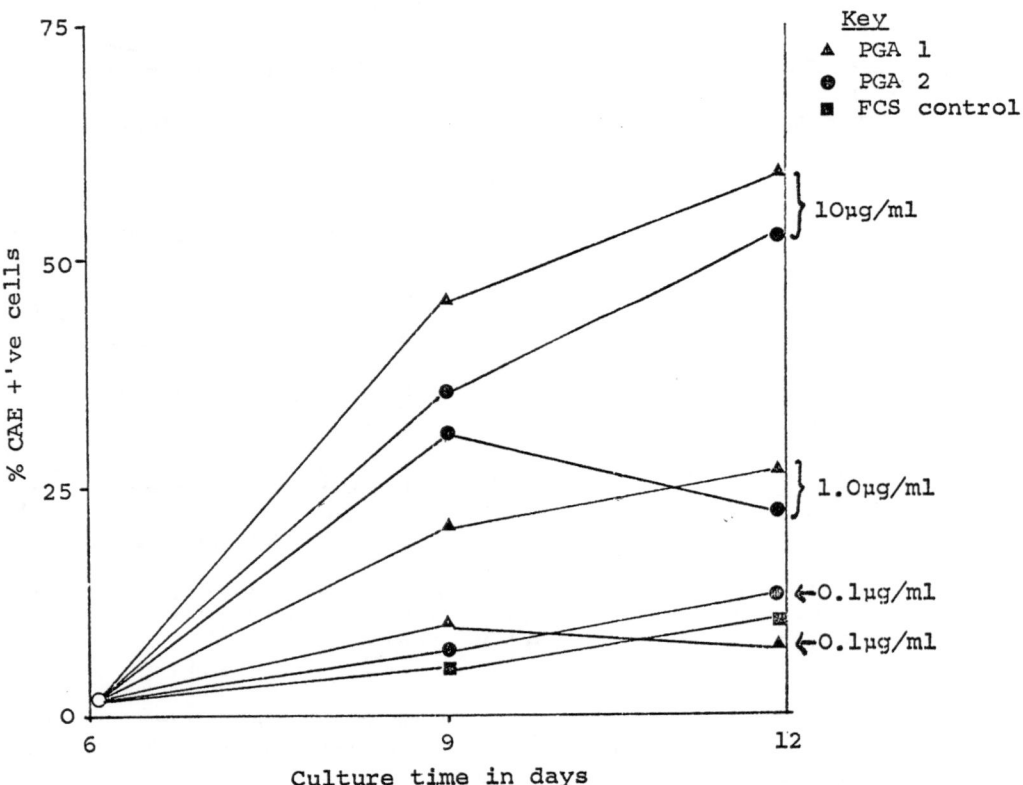

Fig. 2. Percentage of CAE+'ve non-adherent cells in patient J.B. cultured cells in 3 concentrations of prostaglandins A1 and A2

Table 1. Clinical status of patients whose AML cells were studied in vitro

Patient	Maturation type	Diagnosis	Obtained 1st remission	Length of 1st remission	Survival time
No maturation					
E.K.		AMML	no	–	5 months
C.P.		AMbL	yes	6 months	9 months
V.S.		AMML	not yet	–	5 weeks→
Maturation to polymorphs					
J.B.		AMbL	yes	9 months	24 months
D.H.		AMoL	no	–	3 months
G.J.		AMbL	yes	2 months→	3 months→
C.Pr.		AMbL	yes	15 months	27 months
J.S.		AMML	not yet	–	4 months→
E.W.		AMML	yes	15 monts	25 months
Maturation to macrophages					
R.H.		AMoL	yes	2 weeks→	8 weeks→
I.I.		AMbL	not yet	–	7 months→
F.L.		AMML	yes	4 weeks→	2 months→
C.S.		AMML	no	–	1 month
J.W.		AMb	yes	8 months	17 months

genous leukaemia cells relevant to clinical requirements. Cryobiology 14:637–648 – Currie GA, Hedley DW (1977) Monocytes and macrophages in malignant melanoma. 1) Peripheral blood macrophage precursors. Br J Cancer 36:1 – Frøland SS, Wisløff F (1976) A rosette technique for identification of human lymphocytes with Fc receptors. In: Bloom and David (eds) In vitro methods in cell-mediated and tumour immunity. Academic Press, London, p 137 – Li CY, Lam KW, Yam LT (1973) Esterases in human leucocytes. J Histochem Cytochem 21:1 – Palú G, Powles R, Selby P, Summersgill B, Alexander P (1979) Patterns of maturation in short-term culture of human acute myeloid leukaemic cells. Br J Cancer 40:719 – Powles RL, Lister TA, Oliver RTD (1974) Safe method of collecting leukaemia cells from patients with acute leukaemia for use as immunotherapy. Br Med J 4:375

Haematology and Blood Transfusion Vol. 26
Modern Trends in Human Leukemia IV
Edited by Neth, Gallo, Graf, Mannweiler, Winkler
© Springer-Verlag Berlin Heidelberg 1981

Regulator-Dependent Haemopoiesis and Its Possible Relevance to Leukemogenesis

T. M. Dexter

A. Introduction

Haemopoiesis is regulated by a variety of factors determining proliferation, differentiation, amplification and maturation of stem cells and their committed progeny, the myeloid and lymphoid precursor cells. Investigation of putative regulatory molecules has been facilitated by the development of clonogenic in vitro systems whereby restricted progenitor cells are induced to undergo clonal expansion and maturation in soft gel media, resulting in discrete colonies of mature cells. Using these systems, most committed precursor cells can be grown in culture (Reviewed in Metcalf 1977). Furthermore, haemopoietic stem cells can now be maintained in vitro for many months, continuously generating myeloid and lymphoid restricted cells (Dexter et al. 1977a; Dexter et al. 1978). In all aspects so far studied the haemopoietic cells produced in such long-term culture are apparently normal and possess characteristics in common with their counterparts present in freshly isolated bone marrow (Dexter et al. to be published a). Using these cultures we have heen investigating the regulation of stem cell proliferation and differentiation and the effects of a variety of RNA C-type leukaemia viruses on in vitro haemopoiesis (Dexter et al. 1977b; Teich and Dexter 1979; Teich et al. 1979; Dexter and Teich 1979; Testa et al. 1980).

B. Isolation of Normal and Leukaemic Cell Lines and Their Response to Haemopoietic Regulators

Several cell lines have been isolated from long-term cultures infected with Friend leukaemia virus (FLV):

1. In one experiment, cells isolated from long-term cultures 14 days after FV infection showed GM-CSF independent colony growth in soft agar. When individual colonies were isolated, it was found that the cells grew antonomously in suspension and that injection of the cells in vivo produced a rapidly progressing myelomonocytic leukaemia (Testa et al. 1980). This cell line, designated 427E, was aneuploid with a mean of 78 chromosomes and a constitutive producer of GM-CSF. When plated in soft agar, colony formation occurred in the absence of added stimulatory molecules. However, if the cells were plated in the presence of excess exogenous GM-CSF, it was found that although the initial colony forming efficiency was not altered, the self-renewal ability of the colony forming cells (measured by re-plating ability) was dramatically reduced. These leukaemia cells, therefore, show at least some biological response when cultured in the presence of excess GM-CSF – a proposed regulator of granulopiesis. Similar effects of GM-CSF have been observed in other myelomonocytic leukaemia cell lines (Metcalf et al. 1969; Ichikawa 1969; Fibach et al. 1972).

Infection of marrow culture with FBJ osteosascoma virus has similarly led to the rapid emergence of a malignant myelomonocytic clone of cells (426-C) with characteristics similar to those described above.

2. Long-term cultures treated with Abelson leukaemia virus readily undergo malignant transformation to produce poorly differentiated B-cell leukaemia cell lines (Teich et al. 1979; Teich and Dexter 1978). The cells grow autonomously in suspension and in soft agar and are inducible for intracytoplasmic IgM production by various reagents.

3. The infection of marrow cultures with FLV can also lead to the production of apparently normal, non-leukaemic cell lines which possess characteristics of either stem cells or committed granulocyte progenitor cells (Dexter et al. 1979; Dexter and Teich 1979; Dexter et al. 19780b). These cell lines are characteristically isolated only from long-term cultures which have been maintained for several months. 416B cells were isolated from a culture more than 5 months after infection with FLV and were established as a continuous cell line, growing in suspension independently of added stimulatory molecules. Upon isolation the cells were initially bipotential (Dexter et al. 1979) when injected into irradiated mice and formed spleen colonies containing granulocytes and megakayocytes, although they grew in suspension (in vitro) as an undifferentiated cell population. The cells had a normal diploid karyotype and were non-leukaemic. Colony formation in soft agar was only seen in the presence of exogenous GM-CSF (Dexter et al. 1978a). Eventually, karyotype instability was seen, the cells became restricted to erythroid development when injected in vivo and colony formation in soft agar occurred in the absence of added GM-CSF. However, the cells were still non-leukaemic.

Another cell line, 458C, was isolated more than 5 months after FLV infection (Dexter et al. 1980b), also grew autonomously in suspension culture, maintained a diploid karyotype and was non-leukaemic. Colony formation in soft agar initially occurred only in the presence of added GM-CSF, and the colonies produced consisted of neutrophil granulocytes. Presently, this cell line also has aquired the ability to undergo clonal expansion in soft agar in the absence of GM-CSF, and a karyotype investigation is in progress.

4. It has recently been reported by Greenberger et al. (1979) that infection of susceptible long-term bone marrow cultures with FLV is followed consistently by the generation of promyelocytic leukaemia cell lines. For their continued growth such cells must be sub-cultured in medium conditioned by the growth of WEHI-3CM. Since one component of WEHI-3CM is GM-CSF, it was assumed that this moiety acted as the growth promoter for the proliferation of these cells (Greenberger et al. 1979). According to this report, WEHI-3CM dependent cell lines could not be obtained from control (non-infected) cultures. However in recent work we have shown that cells from uninfected long-term marrow cultures will consistently generate cell lines in the presence of either WEHI-3CM or pokeweed-mitogen spleen cell conditioned medium (Dexter et al. 1980c). Such cell lines are non-leukaemic, maintain a diploid karyotype and from colonies containing . granulocytes when plated in soft agar. Growth in suspension culture or in soft agar is absolutely dependent upon the continued presence of WEHI-3CM or SCM. Other GM-CSF containing conditioned media or highly purified GM-CSF preparation did not support the growth of these cells (Dexter et al. 1980c). This suggests that GM-CSF is not the regulatory molecule involved in the maintenance of proliferation. We have further suggested that such cells represent a population of committed granulocyte progenitor cells which are capable of extensive self renewal and which are responding to a hitherto unrecognised regulator. Thus far cell lines have been produced from marrow cultures of strain DBA/2, C57BL/6, BDF$_1$ and Swiss mice. No evidence of viral replication can be found in these cell lines, which are designated Factor-Dependent Continuous cell lines, Paterson Labs (FDC-P).

A summary of these cell lines is given in Table 1. FDC-P lines produced from untreated cultures demonstrate factor dependency for growth in suspension and in soft agar. Initial isolates of 416B and 458C showed independent growth in suspension but dependent growth in soft agar. These cell lines are characterised by being diploid and non-leukaemic and apparently undergo normal differentiation. Karyotype changes occurring in 416B are associated with a restriction in development potential and acquisition of factor-independent growth in soft agar.

Other cell lines produced from virus infected long-term cultures show a restricted developmental potential, are aneuploid, leukaemic and are independent of the addition of exogenous factors for growth in suspension or in soft agar. The Ml cells represent a line derived from cultures treated with the carcinogen methylnitrosourea (MNU). These cells are also factor independent, aneuploid and leukaemic with restricted differentiation ability.

Table 1. Production of factor dependent and independent cell lines from long-term marrow cultures[a]

Cell Line	Treatment	Factor dependence		Karyotype	Differentiation	Leukaemogenic
		Suspension	Agar			
FDC-P (Several)	—	+	+	Diploid	Mature grans	No
458-C	FLV	—	+	Diploid	Mature grans	No
416-B	FLV	—[b]	+	Diploid	E+G+Meg	No
416-B	FLV	—[b]	—	Aneuploid (41 chromosomes)	Erythroid	No
AB-1	Abelson	—	—	?	IgM production	Yes
426-C	FBJ virus	—[c]	—[c]	Aneuploid	Metamyelocytes	Yes
427-E	FLV	—[c]	—[c]	Aneuploid	Metamyelocytes	Yes
M1	MNU	—	—	Aneuploid	TdT production	Yes

[a] MNU = methylnitrosourea
[b] No response to Fraction IV (CFU inhibitor) (Lord et al. 1976)
[c] Constitutive producers of GM-CSF

C. Do the Cell Lines Represent Different Stages in Leukaemic Transformation?

Treatment with a leukaemogen may have diverse effects one or more of which is important in leukaemogenesis. In one case there may be a direct transformation of a haempoietic "target cell", leading as a result to regulator-independent growth or to an altered response to the regulator. Such a leukaemogen may be expected to produce a rapid disease such as that seen with Friend Leukaemia virus infection, where the growth of erythroid progenitor cells becomes independent of the requirement for erythropoietin, Abelson disease may also fall into this category.

Alternatively, tratment with leukaemogens may result in alterations in the level of the various regulatory molecules, such as the factors specifically controlling stem cell proliferation (Lord et al. 1977) or GM-CSF or BPA production, or in the levels of factor required for the sustained proliferation of FDC-P cells. In this case there would be population changes in the factor dependent but normal cells – presumably leading to hyperplasia or aplasia of one or more cell lineages. The next stage in leukaemogenesis may be represented by a mutation event leading to the generation of cells which have acquired proliferative autonomy (i.e. grow independently of growth factors) but which none the less still respond to differentiation stimuli. Cells in this category would include 416B and 458C cell lines, which may

be regarded as "pre-leukaemic" cells. The final stage would be the generation of clones which do not, or only partially, respond to differentiation signals – such as the ABl, 426C, 427E and Ml cells. These are characteristically aneuploid cells. The generation of such cell lines having a multi-step process, would take a relatively long time as is seen after treatment with most viruses, X-rays and chemicals.

Using the long-term cultures, the hypothesis presented can be tested in some detail. Not only can the levels of regulators be monitored in the cultures, but the cell lines produced (particularly FDC-P cells) represent a model for transformation studies including a variety of leukaemogens and analysis of the subsequent response of the cells to the various regulators. Such studies are now in progress.

Acknowledgments

This work was supported by the Medical Research Council and the Cancer Research Campaign. The author is a Fellow of the Cancer Research Campaign.

References

Dexter TM, Teich NM (1979) Modification of the proliferative and differentiation capacity of stem cells following treatment with chemical and vival leukaemogens. In: Neth R, Galls RC, Hofschneider PH Mannweiler K (eds) Modern trends in human leukaemia III. Springer, Berlin Heidelberg New York, pp 223–229 – Dexter TM, Allen TD, Lajtha LG (1977a) Conditions controlling the proliferation of hemopoietic stem cells in vitro. J Cell Physiol 91:335–344 – Dexter TM, Scott D, Teich NM (1977b) Infection of bone marrow cell proliferation, differentiation and leukaemogenic capacity. Cell 12:355–364 – Dexter TM, Allen TD, Lajtha LG, Krizsa F, Testa NG, Moore MAS (1978). In vitro analysis of self-renewal and committment of hemopoietic stem cells. In: Clarkson B, Marks PA, Till JE (eds) Differentiation of normal and neoplastic hemopoietic cells. Cold Spring Harbor Press, New York, pp 63–80 – Dexter TM, Allen TD, Scott D, Teich NM (1979) Isolation and characterisation of a bipotential hemopoietic cell line. Nature 277:471–474 – Dexter TM, Spooncer E, Toksoz D, Lajtha LG (to be published a) The role of cells and their products in the regulation of in vitro stem cell proliferation and granulocyte development. J Supramol Struct – Dexter TM, Allen TD, Teich NM (to be published b) Production of 'normal' stem cell lines following treatment of long-term marrow cultures with Friend murine leukaemia viruses. – Dexter TM, Garland J, Scott D, Scolnick E, Metcalf D (1980c) Growth of factor dependent hemopoietic precursor cell lines. J Exp Med 152:1036–1047 – Fibach E, Landau T, Sachs L (1972) Normal differentiation of myeloid leukaemic cells induced by a differentiation inducing protein. Nature 237:276–279 – Greenberger JS, Gans PJ, Davisson PB, Maloney WC (1979) In vitro induction of continuous acute promyelocyte leukaemia cell lines by Friend or Abelson murine leukaemia viruses. Blood 53:987 – Ichikawa Y (1969) Differentiation of a cell line of myeloid leukaemia. J Cell Physiol 74:223–234 – Lord BI, Mori KJ, Wright EG, Lajtha LG (1976) An inhibitor of stem cell proliferation in normal bone marrow. Br J Haematol, 34:441–445 – Lord BI, Mori KJ, Wright EG, Lajtha LG (1977) A stimulator of stem cell proliferation in regenerating bone marrow. Biomed Express (Paris) 27:223–226 – Metcalf D (1977) Hemaopoietic colonies. Springer, Berlin Heidelberg New York, p 277 – Metcalf D, Moore MAS, Warner NL (1969) Colony formation in vitro by myelomonocytic leukaemic cells. J Natl Cancer Inst 43:983–1001 – Teich NM, Dexter TM (1978) Effects of murine leukaemia virus infection on differentiation of hemapoietic cells in vitro. In: Clarkson B, Marks PA, Till JE (eds) Differentiation of normal and neoplastic hemapoietic cells. Cold Spring Harbor Press, New York, pp 657–670 – Teich NM, Dexter TM (1979) Interaction between murine leukaemia viruses and differentiating hemopoietic cells. In: Oncogenic viruses and host cell genes. Academic Press, New York, pp 263–276 – Teich N, Boss M, Dexter TM (1979) Infection of mouse bone marrow cells with Abelson murine leukaemia virus and establishment of producer cell lines. In: Neth R, Callo RC, Hofschneider PH, Mannweiler K (eds) Modern trends in human leukaemia III. Springer, Berlin Heidelberg New York, pp 487–490 – Testa NG, Dexter TM, Scott D, Teich NM (1980) Malignant myelomonocytic cells after in vitro infection of marrow cells with Friend leukaemia virus. Br J Cancer 41:33–39

Haematology and Blood Transfusion Vol. 26
Modern Trends in Human Leukemia IV
Edited by Neth, Gallo, Graf, Mannweiler, Winkler
© Springer-Verlag Berlin Heidelberg 1981

Long-Term Culture of Normal and Leukemic Human Bone Marrow

S. Gartner and H. S. Kaplan

A. Introduction

Clonal culture systems using semisolid media for the detection of granulocyte-macrophage (Bradley and Metcalf 1966; Pike and Robinson 1970; Pluznik and Sachs 1966), erythroid (Stephenson et al. 1971), lymphoid (Fibach et al. 1976; Metcalf et al. 1975a; Sredni et al. 1976) and megakaryocytic (Metcalf et al. 1975b) progenitors have contributed greatly to investigations of hematopoiesis. Unfortunately, such systems possess two major limitations: (1) observations are restricted to relatively short time intervals and (2) the interaction between different kinds of cells cannot easily be studied.

More recently, liquid culture systems have also been investigated. Golde and Cline (1973) described the short-term liquid culture of human marrow using an in vitro diffusion chamber in which cells grew both in suspension and on a dialysis membrane. Proliferation and maturation of granulocytes and macrophages in these chambers persisted for 4 weeks. Dexter et al. (1973) reported the development of a liquid system for the cocultivation of mouse thymus and bone marrow in which CFU$_c$s (granulocyte-macrophage progenitor cells) were generated for at least 10 weeks and CFU$_s$s (pluripotent stem cells) were present for 14 days. The same group (Dexter and Lajtha 1974; Dexter and Testa 1976; Dexter et al. 1977) later developed a method for the long-term culture of mouse bone marrow cells alone in liquid medium. Such cultures produce both CFU$_c$s and CFU$_s$s for several months. Hematopoiesis in this system is dependent upon the presence of a marrow-derived adherent population consisting of three cell types: phagocytic mononuclear cells, endothelial cells, and giant lipid-laden adipocytes. Initially, only certain lots of horse serum had the ability to stimulate the growth of these essential adipocytes. Greenberger (1978) reported that "deficient" lots of horse serum could be reconstituted with corticosteroids.

Long-term liquid culture systems for the cultivation of human bone marrow cells are urgently needed. Moore and Sheridan (1979) reported the establishment of human marrow cultures using conditions similar to those described by Dexter et al., but CFU$_c$ production was limited to 6–8 weeks. More recently, Moore et al. (1979) reported sustained long-term hematopoiesis in liquid cultures of marrow from a subhuman primate, the tree shrew *(Tupaia glis)*. We now present additional information concerning a recently described method (Gartner and Kaplan 1980) for the long-term culture of human marrow cell populations based on modifications of the murine system.

B. Materials and Methods

I. Media

Fischer's complete growth medium consisted of Fischer's medium (Gibco #320–1735) supplemented with 10^{-7} M hydrocortisone sodium succinate (Upjohn) and either 25% horse serum (HoS; Flow Labs), 25% fetal bovine serum (FBS; Microbiological Associates), or 12.5% each of HoS and FBS. McCoy's complete growth medium consisted of the following: McCoy's 5a medium, modified, (Gibco #430–1500), 10^{-7} M hydrocortisone, 1% sodium bicarbonate solution (Gibco #670–5080), 1% MEM sodium pyruvate solution (Gibco 320–1360), 1% MEM vitamin solution (Gibco #320–1120), 0.8% MEM amino acids solution (Gibco

#320–1135), 0.4% MEM nonessential amino acids solution (Gibco #320–1140) 1% L-glutamine, 200mM solution (Gibco 320–5030), 1% penicillin-streptomycin solution, 10,000 u pen/ml, 10,000 mcg strep/ml (Gibco #600–5140), and either 25% HoS, 25% FBS, or 12.5% of each. Only freshly prepared medium was used for the initiation and maintenance of cultures. All serum was heat inactivated at 56°C for 1 h and stored frozen prior to use. In the presence of 10^{-7} M hydrocortisone, all lots of HoS tested were able to support the development of a good stromal layer. Only those lots of FBS which sustained the growth of our fastidious human lymphoma cells (Epstein and Kaplan 1974; Kaplan et al. 1979) were used for these cultures.

II. Initiation and Maintenance of Cultures

Normal marrow specimens were obtained from resected ribs of patients undergoing thoracotomy. Immediately after removal from the patient, the rib was cut into segments 2–3 cm in length and immersed in cold, Ca + +-free Dulbecco's phosphate-buffered saline (PBS; Gibco) supplemented with 1% pen-strep solution and beef lung sodium heparin (Upjohn), 10 μ/ml final concentration. All extraneous connective tissue was cut away from the segments and they were gently rinsed with fresh Ca + +-free Dulbecco's PBS. Care was taken not to flush the marrow from the segments at this step. Using two 6" blunt-ended forceps, the rib segments were pried apart longitudinally. With the tip of a forcep, the marrow was scraped into a 100 mm glass or plastic petri dish containing 20 ml cold complete growth medium (two dishes were used for the marrow from each resected rib.) The medium containing the marrow clumps was then transferred to a 50 ml centrifuge tube (Corning) and pipetted moderately vigorously to break apart the cell clumps and create a single cell suspension. (In our hands, cultures initiated from single cell suspensions have consistently proven superior to those in which cell clumps were seeded). Viable cell counts were performed using 0.04% trypan blue; viability was consistently 98%–100%. Wright-Giemsa-stained slides of the fresh specimens were also prepared to insure that the marrow was normal. Between $1–2 \times 10^9$ nucleated cells were usually recovered from a rib. Two $\times 10^7$ viable nucleated cells in 10 ml of complete growth medium were seeded into plastic T-25 flasks (Corning) or 1×10^7 nucleated cells were seeded into Cluster[6] 35 mm wells (Costar) containing glass coverslips (Corning.) Cultures were incubated at 33°C in 5% CO_2 in air. (Our early experiments demonstrated the superiority of 33°C over 37°C in terms of supporting long-term hematopoiesis, although 37°C accelerated the development of the stromal layer. In contrast, Moore and Sheridan (1979) reported that 37°C was superior for their human marrow cultures.) Weekly feedings consisted of removal of 5 ml spent medium containing nonadherent cells and addition of 5 ml fresh medium. The nonadherent cells were counted, used for morphologic and cytochemical studies, and assayed for CFU_c.

Aspirates of normal sternal marrow were obtained from patients undergoing cardiovascular surgery. Aspirates were also obtained from the iliac crests of patients with acute myeloid leukemia (AML) before treatment, while in remission, and during relapse. These specimens were drawn into heparinized syringes and immediately transferred to tubes containing 2 ml of the previously described complete McCoy's growth medium. Wright's Giemsa-stained preparations of the leukemic aspirates were examined to estimate the seeding density required for the development of the stromal microenvironment in culture. Specimens comprised almost exclusively of myeloid blasts required greater seeding densities for development of the stromal microenvironment. Cell counts were also performed. With the leukemic specimens, between 5×10^6 and 2×10^7 nucleated cells were seeded per T-25 flask, depending on the total number of nucleated cells available. From the normal marrow aspirates, $1–2 \times 10^7$ nucleated cells were seeded per T-25 flask. Two to five days after the initial seeding of the aspirate suspensions, the nonadherent cells were removed from each flask independently and separated on individual "mini" Ficoll-Hypaque gradients (Boyum 1968) using 8 ml cell suspension in PBS plus 3 ml Ficoll-Hypaque solution. The cells at the gradient interface were washed three times in Dulbecco's PBS and returned to the original flasks which contained some adherent cells. Aspirate cultures were fed weekly as described for rib-derived cultures.

III. CFUc Assay

One million human peripheral blood mononuclear cells were suspended in 1 ml volumes of 0.5% Noble agar (Difco) in McCoy's 5a medium supplemented with 15% FBS as described by Pike and Robinson (1970) and seeded into 35 mm wells of cluster[6] plates (Costar). 1×10^5 viable bone marrow cells in 1 ml volumes of 0.3% Noble agar in McCoy's 15% FBS medium were overlayed on the 0.5% agar layer. Only 0–1-day-old underlayers were used. Clusters and colonies were scored at day 12–14. Clusters contained 20–50 cells and colonies contained more than 50 cells. CFU_c values represent the average of at least three cultures, and three wells per culture were assayed.

IV. Cytochemical stains

For morphologic characterization nonadherent cells and coverslip cultures were stained with Wright's-Giemsa; cytochemical tests were also performed for the presence of nonspecific esterase and myeloperoxidase activity (Yam et al. 1971).

Table 1. Characteristics of the adherent population

Cutture medium[a]	Serum		Length of time to confluence (days)	Longevity (months)	Presence of adipocytes[b]
	FBS %	HoS %			
Fischer's		25	14–21	>12	3+ − 4+
Fischer's	25		12–14	> 6	0 − 1+
Fischer's	12.5	12.5	12–14	> 6	3+ − 4+
McCoy's		25	14–21	> 6	3+ − 4+
McCoy's	25		7–12	> 6	0 − ±
McCoy's	12.5	12.5	7–10	> 6	3+ − 4+

[a] All cultures were supplemented with 10^{-7}M hydrocortisone
[b] Stromal layers of very old cultures were composed almost exclusively of adipocytes

C. Results

Table 1 demonstrates that adipocyte-containing confluent stromal layers could be initiated and maintained for periods of at least 5 months in either Fischer's or McCoy's medium when supplemented with both horse serum and hydrocortisone. The stromal layers of very old cultures (greater than 6 months), especially those grown in Fischer's medium, were comprised almost exclusively of adipocytes (Fig. 1). Greenberger (1979) also reported the induction by corticosteroids of lipogenesis in adipocytes in human marrow cultures. In the absence of horse serum, either medium, despite supplementation with hydrocortisone and FBS, failed to support the development of significant numbers of lipid-laden adipocytes. In such cultures almost no nonadherent cells were recovered after 6–8 weeks. Cultures grown in McCoy's medium supplemented with FBS with or without HoS developed confluent

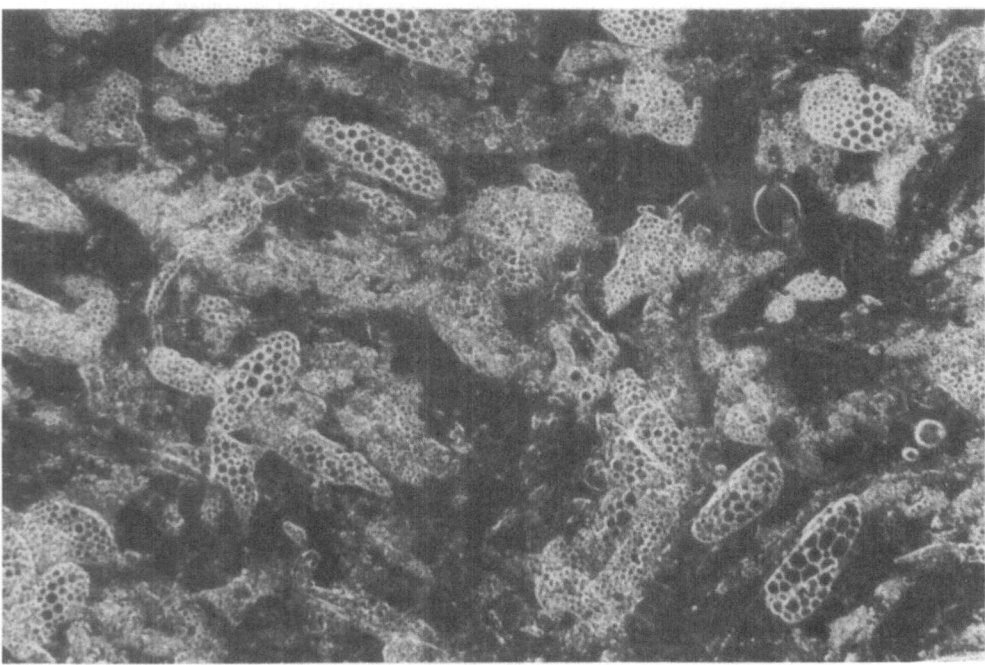

Fig. 1. A human marrow culture at 6 months illustrating abundant adipocytes. ×20

stromal layers earlier than those supplemented with HoS alone or grown in Fischer's medium.

Fischer's growth medium supplemented with hydrocortisone and 25% HoS or 12.5% HoS and 12.5% FBS was able to support the generation of CFU_c-forming cells for up to 12 weeks in some cases. However, the number of colony-forming cells recovered from such cultures was usually less than 50 per 10^5 cells assayed. In contrast, McCoy's complete growth medium supplemented with both FBS and HoS not only provided adequate nutrition for the early development and maintenance of stromal layers containing abundant adipocytes but also contributed either directly or indirectly (through the stromal microenvironment) to longterm hematopoiesis and significantly greater yields of CFU_c.

Figure 2 illustrates the appearance of a typical culture at day 14. A confluent stromal layer can be seen underneath the nonadherent cells. A most important feature of these long-term cultures is the presence of "cobblestone"-like areas, presumably regions of hematopoiesis from which the nonadherent cells arise. Figures 3 and 4 illustrate such cobblestone-like areas in cultures at 6 weeks and 16 weeks,

respectively. At higher magnification (Fig. 5), the flattened polygonal cells in such areas are seen to be so tightly packed together that their boundaries may be difficult to discern. With time some of these cells become more rounded granules can be seen to appear within their cytoplasms and ultimately they become non-adherent.

When coverslip cultures were gently washed extensively to remove nonadherent cells and stained for myeloperoxidase activity, it was observed that cobblestone areas did indeed contain both myeloid and monocytoid cells. Coverslip cultures stained for nonspecific esterase activity revealed monocytoid cells scattered throughout the stromal layer, in islands of hematopoiesis, and sometimes in large, tight clusters within the stromal layer. In general, nonspecific esterase-positive cells were much more intensely stained outside of the cobblestone areas.

The kinetics of the generation of cells with colony-forming ability in these long-term cultures appeared to follow two different patterns, designated the "hyperproliferative" and "homeostatic" patterns. The hyperproliferative pattern describes cultures in which the

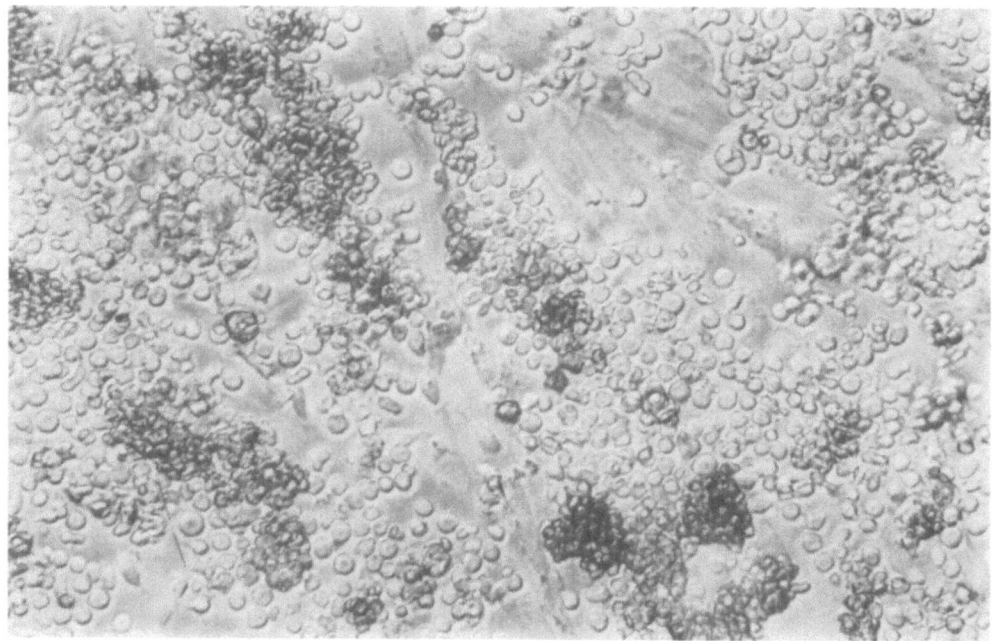

Fig. 2. A human marrow culture at 14 days. ×81

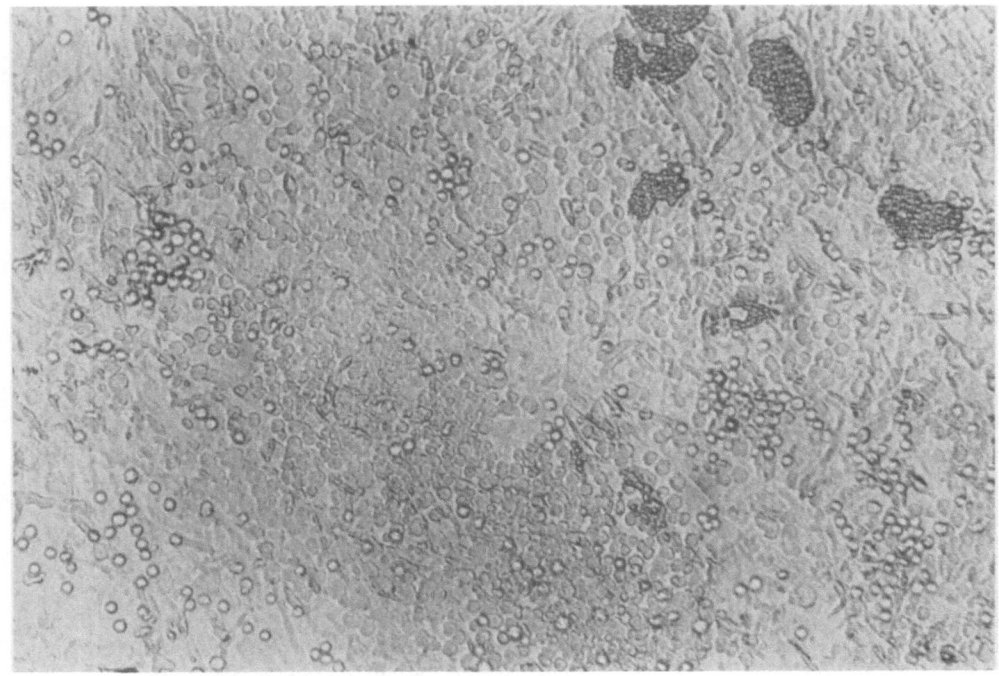

Fig. 3. A human marrow culture at 6 weeks illustrating adipocytes and cobblestone areas of active hematopoiesis. ×50

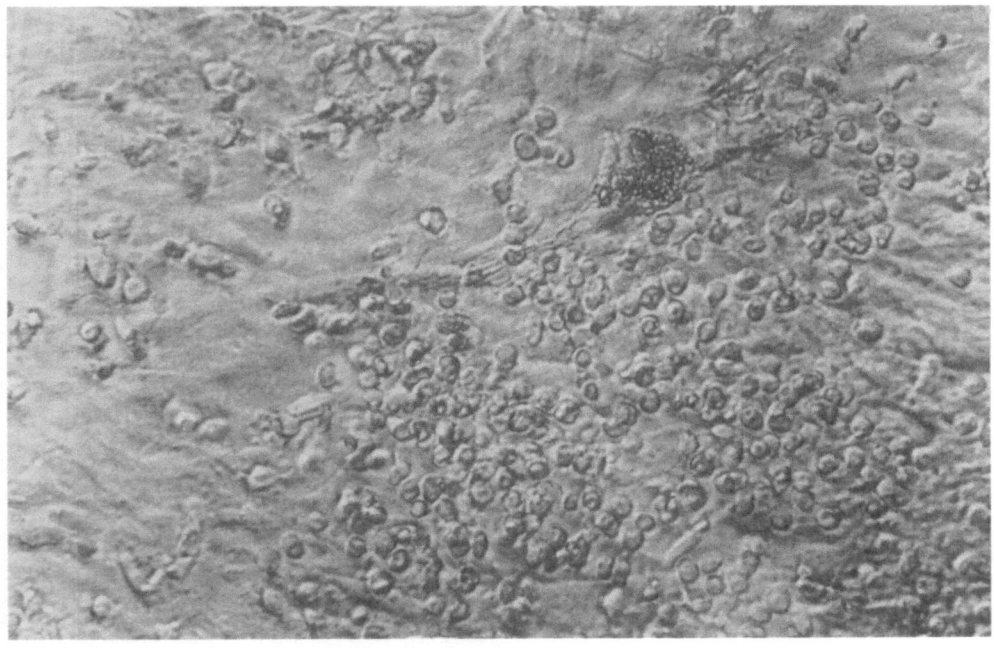

Fig. 4. A human marrow culture at 16 weeks illustrating a cobblestone area. ×77

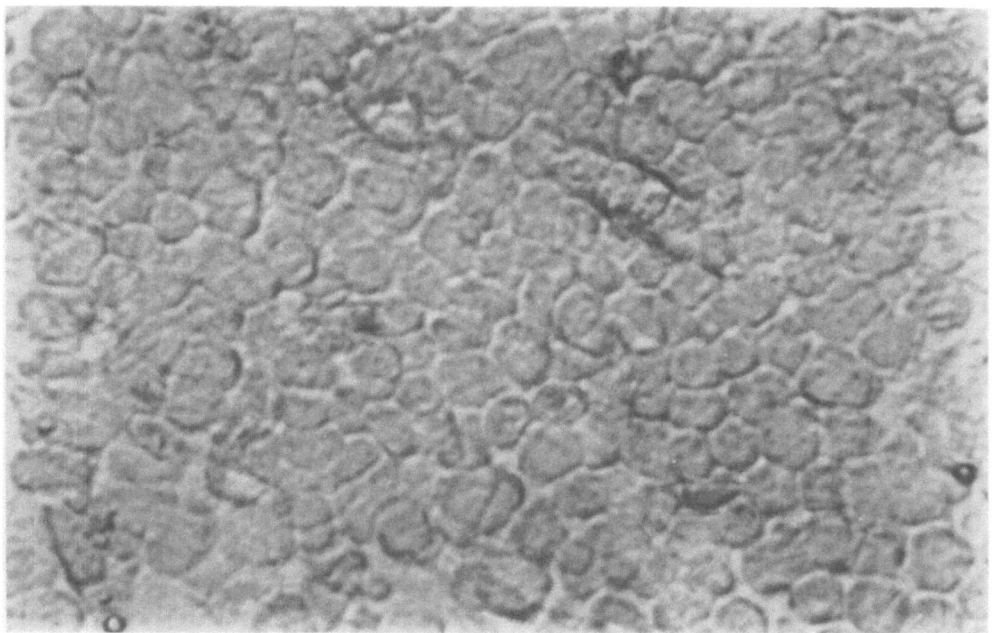

Fig. 5. A human marrow culture at 14 weeks illustrating a very early cobblestone area. ×324

number of CFU_cs generated exceeds 100 per 10^5 cells in serial assays over several weeks. In contrast, the homeostatic pattern describes a steady-state situation in which a lower level of CFU_cs, usually between 25–75 per 10^5 cells, is continuously present in the cultures. An example of each pattern is shown in Fig. 6. Of nine different rib specimens incubated in McCoy's complete growth medium supplemented with both FBS and HoS, four showed the hyperproliferative pattern and five the homeostatic pattern. With the other growth media only the homeostatic pattern was observed, and only in rare instances were CFU_c detected beyond 12 weeks. With all growth media and at all time intervals most colonies were very large, containing more than 500 cells. An example is shown in Fig. 7. Adipocyte colonies were also occasionally seen in the agar cultures. After approximately 8 weeks the numbers of nonadherent cells recovered weekly usually varied between 2×10^5 and 2×10^6 per culture. Before 7–8 weeks, between 1×10^6 and 1.5×10^7 cells were routinely recovered. Such recovery frequencies were common to both the hyperproliferative and homeostatic patterns.

The numbers of CFU_cs did not increase during the first 4 weeks of culture (Fig. 6). In the murine system Dexter et al. (1977) described the "recharging" of cultures at 4 weeks by the addition of fresh marrow. Addition of fresh cells was found to be unnecessary for prolonged hematopoiesis in *Tupaia glis* marrow cultures (Moore et al. 1979; Moore and Sheridan 1979). We have found that recharging did not enhance the production of CFU_cs in our human marrow cultures and in some cases proved deleterious either by destroying the stromal microenvironment or by decreasing the number of CFU_cs recovered. In the absence of recharging, the numbers of CFU_cs began to increase between 4–6 weeks. In most normal marrow cultures, CFU_c production continued for at least 20 weeks.

Table 2 indicates the relative abundance of different morphologic cell types in the nonadherent populations. Figs. 8 and 9 illustrate the nonadherent population from cultures at 9 weeks and 12 weeks, respectively. In older (greater than 8 weeks) cultures grown in Fischer's or McCoy's medium with FBS only, relatively small numbers of nonadherent cells were recovered, the vast majority of which

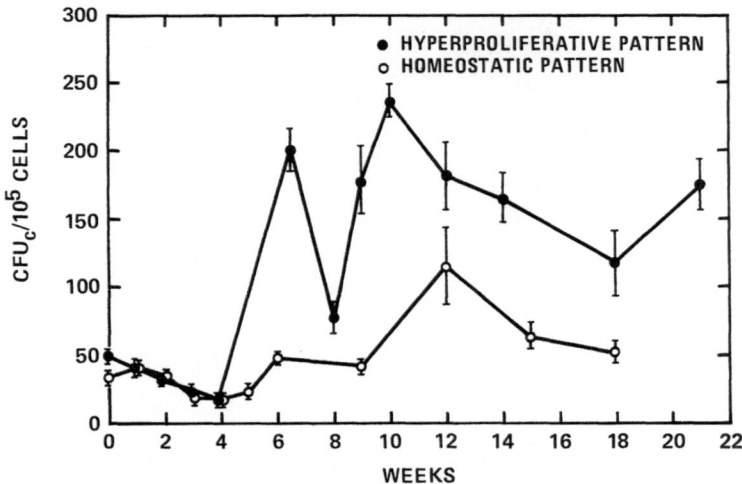

Fig. 6. Serial CFU$_c$ production in long-term human marrow liquid cultures. The results represent the means ± SEM of three wells for each of three cultures

were mature macrophages. This finding is in agreement with that of Moore and Sheridan (Moore and Sheridan 1979; Moore et al. 1979) in long-term human marrow cultures grown in Fischer's medium with HoS. With Fischer's medium plus 25% HoS or 12.5% HoS and 12.5% FBS, some immature monocytoid and both immature and mature myeloid cells were also present but in small numbers. In contrast, cultures grown in McCoy's FBS plus HoS growth medium contained many more immature monocytoid and myeloid cells as well as mature myeloid cells. Spontaneous mitotic figures were also seen in stained preparations of these nonadherent cells. The numbers of myeloid cells often exceeded the

numbers of mature macrophages in the McCoy's FBS plus HoS cultures, unlike the situation in Fischer's medium. In younger cultures (less than 6–8 weeks) monocytoid and myeloid cells at various stages of differentiation were generally observed, and fewer differences were detected between the different growth media.

Aspirates of normal sternal marrow taken from patients during cardiovascular surgery and of leukemic marrow from the iliac crests of AML patients were also cultured. The probability of successful establishment of cultures from such specimens appeared dependent upon the quality of the aspirate and, in the case of the leukemic specimens, the previous medi-

Table 2. Characteristics of the nonadherent population

Culture medium[a]	Serum		Monocytoid[b]		Myeloid[b]		CFU[c]-forming Capacity
	FBS %	HoS %	Immature	Mature	Immature	Mature	
Fischer's		25	1+	4+	1+–2+	1+–2+	1+
Fischer's	25		0–±	4+	0–±	0–±	0–±
Fischer's	12.5	12.5	1+	4+	1+	1+–2+	0–1+
McCoy's		25	1+	3+	1+	1+–2+	1+
McCoy's	25		0–±	2+	0–±	0–±	NT[c]
McCoy's	12.5	12.5	1+–2+	3+	2+–4+	2+–4+	2+–4+

[a] All cultures supplemented with 10^{-7}M hydrocortisone
[b] Based on Wright's-Giemsa, nonspecific esterase, and myeloperoxidase staining characteristics
[c] NT = not tested; too few nonadherent cells were recovered after 8 weeks

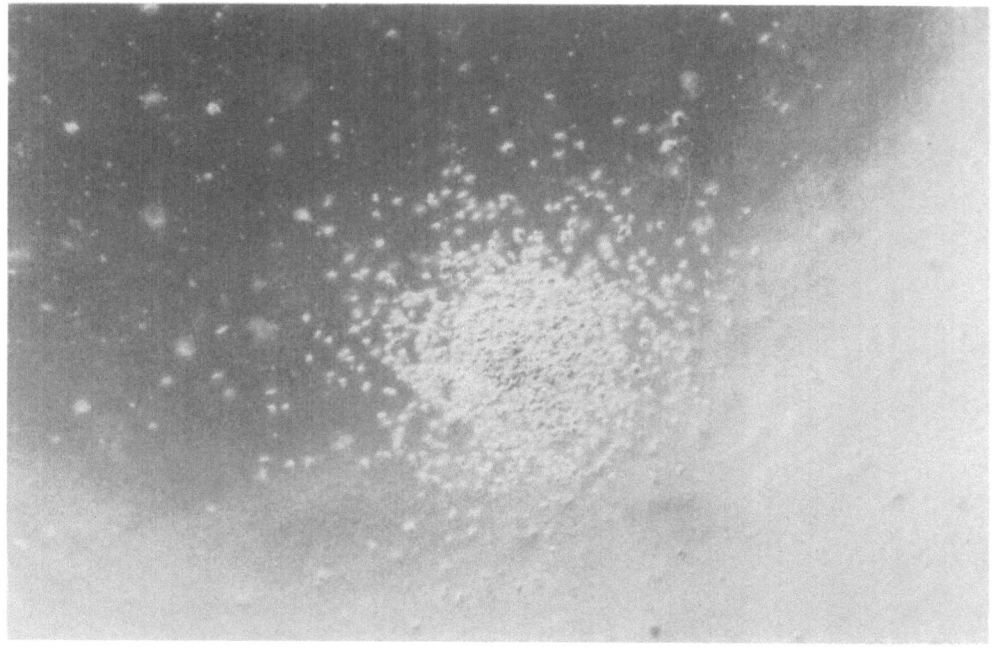

Fig. 7. Agar culture colony arising from a CFU$_c$ harvested from a 14-week-old human marrow culture in liquid medium. ×19

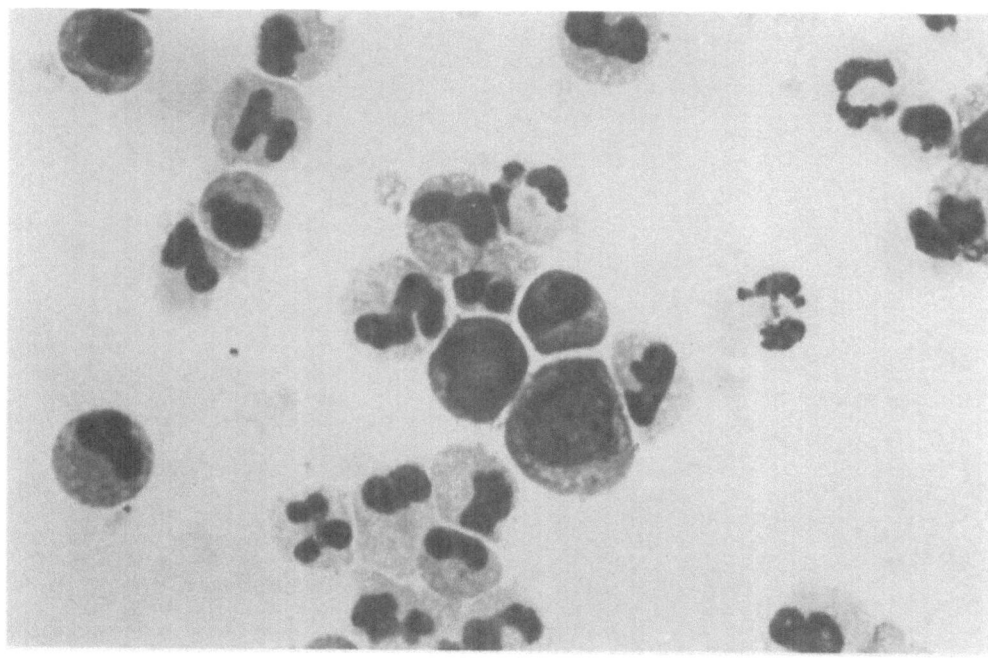

Fig. 8. Nonadherent population from a 9-week-old human marrow culture. ×310

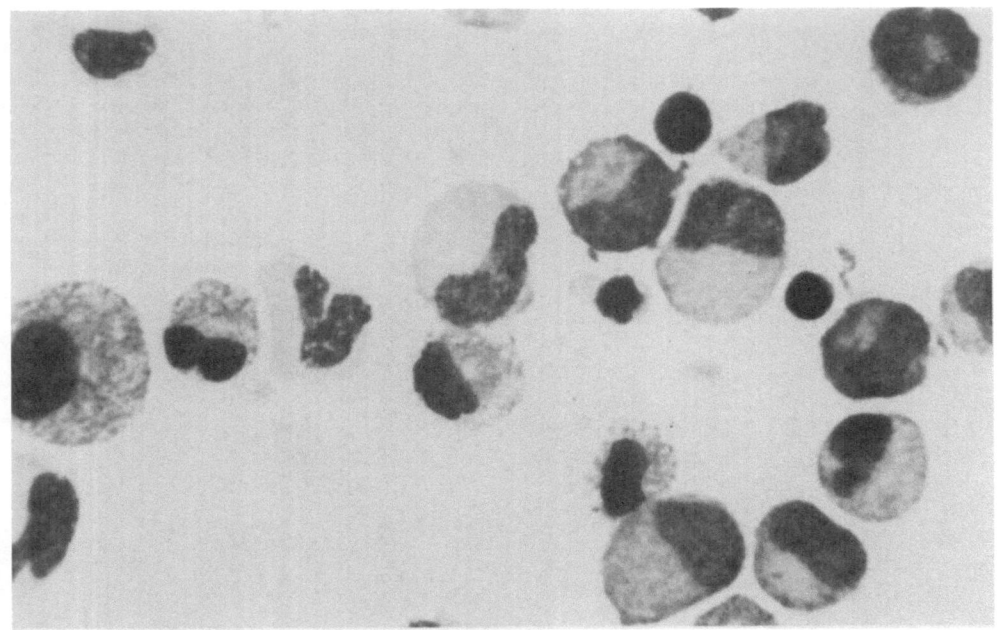

Fig. 9. Nonadherent population from a 12-week-old human marrow culture. ×324

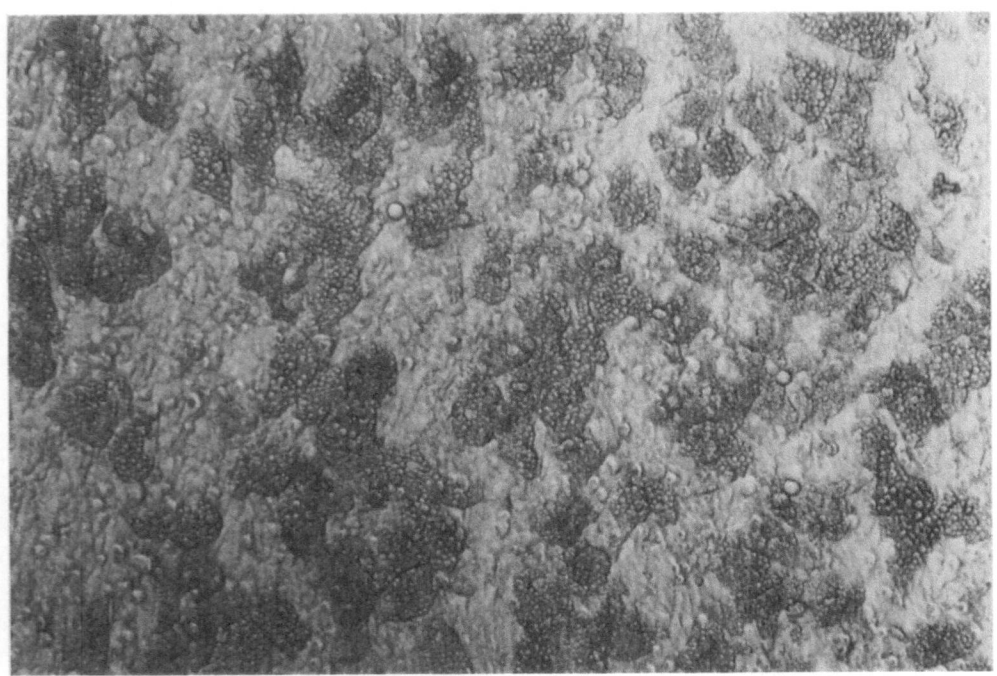

Fig. 10. A 1-month-old human marrow culture from an aspirate from AML patient T. H. ×50

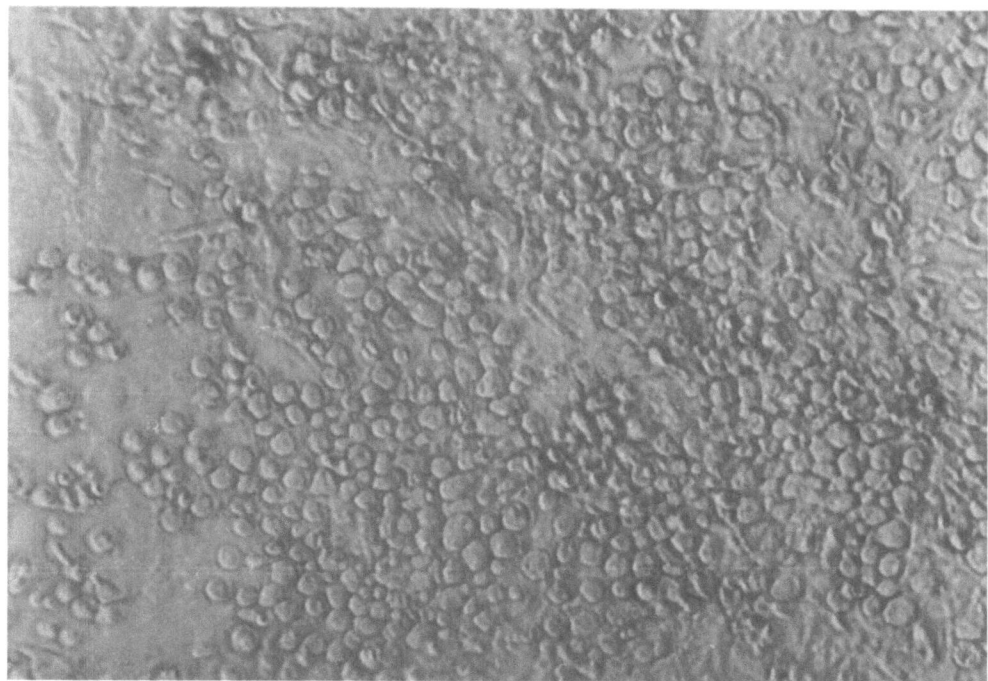

Fig. 11. A 1-month-old human marrow culture from a second aspirate from AML patient T. H. ×80

cal treatment of the patient. Cultures in which cobblestone areas were observed were established from both normal and leukemic aspirates. Figure 10 illustrates such a culture at 4 weeks from an AML patient in remission. Faint cobblestone-like areas can be seen sandwiched between the abundant adipocytes. Figure 11 illustrates a 4 week culture from the same patient established from an additional aspirate taken 1 month later. Although we have been able to recover colony-forming cells from cultures of normal aspirate specimens for at least 8 weeks, the duration of granulopoiesis has been much more variable than that observed in cultures from rib specimens.

D. Discussion

It has been demonstrated that hematopoiesis in long-term liquid cultures of murine (Allen and Dexter 1976) and *Tupaia glis* (Moore et al. 1979) marrow is dependent upon the presence of lipid-laden adipocytes. Our results suggest that this is also the case for human marrow. Horse serum in conjunction with hydrocortiso-

ne appears to be essential for the initial growth and/or differentiation of the adipocytes. In limited studies cultures grown in the presence of freshly collected pooled human serum and $10^{-7} M$ hydrocortisone, with or without the addition of FBS, failed to develop mature adipocytes.

The numbers of lipid-containing adipocytes in cultures from different specimens varied tremendously, especially in younger cultures (less than 8 weeks). Interestingly, some cultures established from AML marrow aspirates often possessed extremely large numbers of adipocytes within 2 weeks after initiation of the cultures. In contrast, occasionally other AML marrow cultures completely failed to develop any adipocytes. In those cases where more than 1 aspirate was obtained at different time intervals from the same AML patient considerable variation was also seen between specimens with regard to the numbers of adipocytes observed in the cultures, without any evident correlation with the patient's clinical condition or the status of the disease. The culture of additional leukemic specimens may elucidate this problem.

The cobblestone areas were often not seen immediately adjacent to the adipocytes, especially in younger cultures. This suggests that direct cell-to-cell contact between granulocytemacrophage committed progenitors and well-differentiated adipocytes may not be required for the maturation of the progenitors.

It seems clear that the successful maintenance of long-term hematopoiesis in these cultures is crucially dependent upon the development and preservation of an intact, competent stromal layer. Factors which affect the integrity of the adherent layer, such as increased acidity of the culture medium or sometimes the addition of an extraneous cell population to the culture, resulted in a decrease in hematopoiesis as measured by CFU$_c$ production. The regeneration of the stromal population in the original culture vessel has not occurred to any significant degree in our cultures. (This is unlike the situation reported for cultures of tree shrew marrow where hematopoiesis was restored along with the regeneration of the stromal layer [Moore et al. 1979]). Thus, great care must be taken to preserve the integrity of the stromal micro-environment.

Our recent efforts to subculture stromal populations have met with limited success. When adherent cells trypsinized from old cultures of normal marrow were reseeded into new culture vessels, we have again observed the growth of an adherent population to confluence. Lipid-laden adipocytes are lost during trypsinization, so that subcultured layers are initially comprised only of large, polygonal or fibroblastoid cells and macrophages. In some cases, lipid-containing cells have appeared some time later in these cultures, suggesting that adipocyte precursors are trypsinizable or that the lipid droplets are lost during trypsinization and require considerable time to be regenerated. The restoration of long-sustained hematopoiesis in such trypsinized cultures has been generally unsuccessful, though cobblestone areas have occasionally been observed.

Trypsinization has proven valuable in generating confluent stromal layers in cultures from AML patients. With some such specimens, very few adherent cells (other than macrophages) were present in the cultures and confluence of an adherent population was never reached. Such cultures were later trypsinized and the recovered cells seeded at higher cell densities.

Confluence of an adherent layer was thus ultimately obtained in many cases.

An additional problem in the culture of leukemic specimens was the lack of an appropriate assay system to monitor granulopoiesis in these cultures. In the case of some of the specimens from patients in remission, the nonadherent cells recovered from the cultures did not form colonies in soft agar, although such nonadherent cell populations morphologically resembled those recovered from cultures of normal marrow.

We believe that both the hyperproliferative and homeostatic patterns described for CFU$_c$ production reflect the actual de novo generation of granulocyte-macrophage progenitor cells in the cultures. It appears that the numbers of CFU$_c$ detected over time in such cultures exceed the numbers of granulocyte-macrophage committed progenitor cells initially seeded. Moreover, serial CFU$_c$ assays would have been expected to reveal a rapid depletion of CFU$_c$ as weekly samples were withdrawn, if CFU$_c$ were merely persisting rather than proliferating in the cultures. This interpretation is further supported by the observation of mitotic figures and by the fact that production of CFU$_c$ did not begin to increase in the hyperproliferative pattern until about 4 weeks. Myeloperoxidase-stained preparations have demonstrated that cobblestone areas do contain myeloid cells. The alternative possibility that granulocyte-macrophage committed progenitors remain dormant and undetectable within the stromal matrix for long periods of time until they receive appropriate signals for proliferation and maturation or until they are sloughed off as the culture ages seems less likely in the face of these observations. The differences between the two growth patterns may be attributable to age and other constitutional factors affecting individual hematopoietic activity; they may have been more readily apparent because most of our rib specimens came from older patients. Greenberger et al. (to be published) have demonstrated that the capacity for long-term hematopoiesis in murine marrow cultures differs considerably from strain to strain. Studies of the stromal microenvironment of these cultures are currently underway which may provide a better understanding of the source of CFU$_c$s.

Sampling problems have been encountered during attempted recovery of nonadherent cells from these cultures. The nonadherent cells tend to "hover" closely over the stromal layers. Phase contrast observations immediately following feeding of the cultures reveal that even with gentle agitation of the culture vessel, large numbers of nonadherent cells remain close to the stromal layer. Possibly the viscosity of the growth medium enhances this effect. Therefore, we believe that the numbers of nonadherent cells harvested in the aliquots of spent medium may not accurately reflect the numbers of nonadherent cells present in the cultures. More vigorous agitation of the culture vessel results in some destruction of the delicate stromal microenvironment and cessation of hematopoiesis. We are presently attempting to improve our methods of quantitation.

Erythroid (BFU-E) (Testa and Dexter 1977) and megakaryocytic (CFU-M) (Williams et al. 1978) progenitors are also produced in long-term murine cultures. The persistence for at least 16 weeks of pre-T cells in murine cultures has also been recently reported (Jones-Villeneuve et al. 1980). To date we have not attempted to assay for such populations in our cultures of human marrow. However, we have established three permanent, polyclonal cell lines of Epstein-Barr virus transformed B-lymphoblastoid cells from marrow cultures of different nonleukemic specimens. All three arose from what appeared to be hematopoietically exhausted stromal layers, one developing at 3 months, one at 4 months, and one at 6 months after initiation of the cultures. All were derived from cultures in Fischer's medium with 25% HoS and hydrocortisone. In the case of the 6-month-old stromal layer, no cobblestone areas remained, and no nonadherent cells had been recovered for 2 months prior to the appearance of the B cells. Moore and Sheridan (1979) reported the conversion of 10% of their human cultures to a lymphoblastoid morphology by the 6th week of culture. We are at present uncertain as to whether our observations represent the generation of B cells from immature precursors in these old cultures or the delayed outgrowth of long-lived EBV-transformed mature B cells. Given the complexity of the stromal microenvironment, it is quite possible that small numbers of mature B cells could have survived undetected.

Methods for the culture of human bone marrow are essential for furthering our understanding of normal hematopoiesis and of hematopoietic disease states as well as the effects of therapeutic regimens on marrow subpopulations. Although there are still many improvements to be made in the application of the liquid phase murine culture system to human marrow, we believe the modifications we have described allow for the routine establishment of such cultures in a reproducibly successful way.

Acknowledgments

This work was supported by research contract N01-CP-91044 from the National Cancer Institute, National Institute of Health, U.S. Dept. of Health, Education, and Welfare (DHEW). Suzanne Gartner is the holder of a predoctoral traineeship in a Cancer Biology Training Program supported by training grant CA-09302 awarded by the National Cancer Institute, DHEW. We thank Dr. James B. D. Mark for providing the rib specimens, Dr. Stuart Jamieson for providing the normal sternal marrow aspirates, and Drs. Peter Greenberg, Richard Hornes, Robert Feiner, and Ms. Betty Reitsma for providing the leukemic marrow specimens. We are also grateful to Ms. Glenda Garrelts for the nonspecific esterase tests, Dr. Werner Henle for the EBNA determinations, and Dr. Joel Greenberger for helpful discussions.

References

Allen TD, Dexter TM (1976) Cellular Interrelationships during in vitro Granulopoiesis. Differentiation 6:191–194 – Bradley TR, Metcalf D (1966) The growth of mouse bone marrow cells in vitro. Aust J Exp Biol Med Sci 44:287–300 – Böyum A (1968) Isolation of mononuclear cells and granulocytes from human blood. Scand J Clin Lab Invest [Suppl 21] 77: – Dexter TM, Lajtha LG (1974) Proliferation of hematopoietic stem cells in vitro. Br J Hematol 28:525–530 – Dexter TM, Testa NG (1976) Differentiation and proliferation of hematopoietic cells in culture. In: Methods in cell biology, vol 14. Academic Press, New York, pp 387–405 – Dexter TM, Allen TD, Lajtha LG, Schofield R, Lord BI (1973) Stimulation of differentiation and proliferation of hematopoietic cells in vitro. J Cell Physiol 82:461–470 – Dexter TM, Allen TD, Lajtha LG (1977) Conditions controlling the proliferation of hematopoietic stem cells in vitro. J Cell Physiol 91:335–344 – Epstein AL, Kaplan HS (1974) Biology of the human malignant lymphomas. I. Establishment in continuous cell culture and heterotransplantation of diffuse histiocytic lymphomas. Cancer 34:1851–1872 – Fibach E, Gerassi E, Sachs

L (1976) Induction of colony formation in vitro by human lymphocytes. Nature 259:127–129 – Gartner S, Kaplan HS (1980) Long-term culture of human bone marrow cells. Proc Natl Acad Sci USA 77:4756–4759 – Greenberger JS (1978) Sensitivity of corticosteroid-dependent insulin-resistant lipogenesis in marrow preadipocytes of obese diabetic (db/db) mice. Nature 275:752–754 – Greenberger JS (1979) Corticosteroid-dependent differentiation of human marrow preadipocytes in vitro. In Vitro 15:823–828 – Greenberger JS, Sakakeeny MA, Berndtson K (to be published) Longevity of hematopoiesis in mouse long-term bone marrow cultures demonstrates significant mouse genotypic variation. J Supramol Struct – Golde D, Cline M (1973) Growth of human bone marrow in liquid culture. Blood 41:45–57 – Jones-Villeneuve EV, Rusthoven JJ, Miller RG, Phillips RA (1980) Differentiation of Thy 1-bearing cells from progenitors in long-term bone marrow cultures. J Immunol 124:597–601 – Kaplan HS, Goodenow RS, Gartner S, Bieber MM (1979) Biology and virology of the human malignant lymphomas: 1st Milford D. Schultz Lecture. Cancer 43:1–24 – Metcalf D, Warner NL, Nossal GJV, Miller JFAP, Shortman K, Rabellino F (1975a) Growth of B lymphocyte colonies in vitro from mouse lymphoid organs. Nature 255:630–632 – Metcalf D, MacDonald HP, Odartchenko N, Sordat LB (1975b) Growth of mouse megakaryocyte colonies in vitro. Proc Natl Acad Sci USA 72:1744–1748 – Moore MAS, Sheridan APC (1979) Pluripotent stem cell replication in continuous human, prosimian and murine bone marrow culture. Blood Cells 5:297–311 – Moore MAS, Sheridan APC, Allen TD, Dexter TM (1979) Prolonged hematopoiesis in a primate bone marrow culture system: characteristics of stem cell production and the hematopoietic microenvironment. Blood 54:775–793 – Pike B, Robinson W (1970) Human bone marrow colony growth in agar-gel. J Cell Physiol 76:77–84 – Pluznik DH, Sachs L (1966) The induction of clones of normal mast cells by a substance from conditioned medium. Exp Cell Res 43:553–563 – Sredni B, Kalechman Y, Michlin H, Rozenszajn LA (1976) Development of colonies in vitro of mitogen-stimulated mouse T lymphocytes. Nature 259:130–132 – Stephenson JR, Axelrad AA, McLeod DL, Shreeve MM (1971) Induction of colonies of hemoglobin-synthesizing cells by erythropoietin in vitro. Proc Natl Acad Sci USA 68:1542–1546 – Testa NG, Dexter TM (1977) Long-term production of erythroid precursors (BFU) in bone marrow cultures. Differentiation 9:193–195 – Williams N, Jackson H, Sheridan APC, Murphy MJ, Elste A, Moore MAS (1978) Regulation of megakaryopoiesis in long-term murine bone marrow cultures. Blood 51:245–255 – Yam LT, Li CY, Crosby WH (1971) Cytochemical identification of monocytes and granulocytes. Am J Clin Pathol 55:283–290

Haematology and Blood Transfusion Vol. 26
Modern Trends in Human Leukemia IV
Edited by Neth, Gallo, Graf, Mannweiler, Winkler
© Springer-Verlag Berlin Heidelberg 1981

Corticosteroid Dependence of Continuous Hemopoiesis In Vitro with Murine or Human Bone Marrow

H. M. Greenberg, L. M. Parker, P. E. Newburger, J. Said, G. I. Cohen, and J. S. Greenberger

A. Introduction

Continuous mouse bone marrow cultures (Dexter and Testa 1977) have been used to study in vitro normal marrow hemopoiesis and viral or chemical leukemogenesis (Dexter et al. 1977; Greenberger 1978; Greenberger 1979b; Greenberger et al., to be published a; Greenberger et al. 1980; Greenberger et al., to be published b; Greenberger et al., to be published c). Modifications in culture technique, including elimination of a second marrow inoculum ("recharging") and weekly addition of fresh 17-hydroxycorticosteroid (hydrocortisone), have lengthened the period of produc-

tion of pluripotent hemopoietic stem cells (CFUs) and committed granulocyte-macrophage progenitor cells (GM-CFUc) in vitro (Greenberger et al. 1979a, to be published a). Mouse strain genotype influences the longevity of hemopoiesis in corticosteroid-supplemented cultures (Greenberger et al. 1979c) and is emphasized by the comparison of marrow cultures from AKr/J and NZB mice (Table 1).

We now report a system for continuous hemopoiesis using human marrow. Weekly addition of $10^{-7} M$ hydrocortisone was required; however, other conditions were found necessary for human marrow culture.

Table 1. Influence of mouse strain genotype on the duration of hemopoiesis in corticosteroid-supplemented long-term bone marrow cultures

Mouse strain[a]	Added hydrocortisone concentration (M)	Duration of hemopoiesis in 25% fetal calf serum		
		Longest duration production of:[b]		
		GM-CFUc (wks)	Immature granulocytes (wks)	Mature granulocytes wks
AKr/J	10^{-7}	61	61	63
AKr/J	None	3	4	6
NZB	10^{-7}	14[c]	14	16
NZB	None	2	3	3

[a] Contents of one tibia and one femur from 6–8-week-old female mice were inoculated into each 10.0 ml flask and medium changed weekly by removal of all nonadherent cells and medium. Cultures were not recharged with additional marrow

[b] Results are the mean of at least 16 flasks for each strain. GM-CFUc were scored at 7 days in 0.3% agar with 10% L929 cell CSF (Greenberger et al. 1979b). There were <5% toluidine blue positive mast cells detected in AKr/J cultures at 63 weeks or NZB cultures at 16 weeks

[c] Difference from AKr/J highly significant $P < 1001$

B. Materials and Methods

I. Tissue Culture

McCoy's 5A, Dulbecco's modified Eagle's, RPMI 1640, and Fisher's medium were obtained from Gibco. Horse serum and fetal calf serum were obtained from Flow Laboratories, Rockville, Maryland; human serum was obtained from the Blood Products aboratory Sidney Farber Cancer Institute. All media were supplemented with 100 µg/ml penicillin and 100 µg/ml streptomycin (Gibco). Marrow from AKr/J or NZB mice was prepared as described (Greenberger et al. 1979b). Human marrow biopsy specimens were obtained intraoperatively from femur or rib, and fragments dissected in McCoy's 5A medium. A single cell suspension was prepared by crushing marrow fragments, filtering through gauze to remove bone spicules, drawing cells through successively smaller gauge needles to a 26-gauge needle, washing several times in McCoy's 5A medium, and transferring at $2.0-4.0 \times 10^7$ nucleated cells in 10.0 ml to 40 cm^2 Corning plastic flasks. Cultures were compared by depopulation using several feeding schedules. The methods for detection of mouse and human GM-CFUc (Greenberger et al. 1979b) and detection of myeloid-esterase (ASD chloroacetate substrate-specific) and nonspecific esterase (alpha-naphthol-buterate substrate) have been described (Greenberger et al. 1979c).

C. Results

I. Method for Growth of Human Long-Term Bone Marrow Cultures

The methods for mouse marrow culture applied to human bone marrow result in poor longevity (Greenberger 1979a; Greenberger, et al., 1979l). Growth of 2.0×10^7 nucleated bone marrow cells in hydrocortisone-supplemented Fisher's medium or Dulbecco's modified Eagle's medium with 25% horse serum or 25% fetal calf serum produced no detectable GM-CFUc after 4 weeks (Table 2). Cultures grown in these media supplemented with hydrocortisone and either 12.5% horse serum plus 12.5% human serum or 12.5% fetal calf plus 12.5% human serum were also ineffective. In marked contrast cultures grown in McCoy's 5A medium supplemented with 12.5% horse serum, 12.5% fetal calf serum, and $10^{-7} M$ hydrocortisone generated GM-CFUc and $>10^5$ granulocytes weekly for over 10 weeks. The ultrastructure of adherent cell areas detected at 14 days after initiation (Fig. 1) was similar to those in mouse cultures (Fig. 2). Twice weekly or once weekly feeding with removal of all nonadherent cells was

Table 2. Results at 10 weeks for hemopoiesis in unrecharged human long-term marrow cultures in McCoy's 5A medium with $10^{-7} M$ hydrocortisone using a single donor femur marrow (amputation specimen) and varying serum combination

Serum combination tested[a]	No. cells per culture ($\times 10^5$)	Mean results at week 10 Percentage immature granulocytes	GM-CFUc per 10^5 cells
1. Horse serum (25%)	0.4	2	0
2. Fetal calf serum (25%) FCS	0.5	6	0
3. Horse serum (25%) switch to FCS (25%) at wk 4	0.2	3	0
4. Fetal calf serum (25%) switched to horse serum (25%) at week 4	0.3	2	0
5. Human serum (pooled) 25%	0.6	2	0
6. Human serum (25%) to wk 4, then horse serum 25%	0.2	3	0
7. Human serum (25%) to wk 4, then FCS 25%	0.7	2	0
8. *Horse serum 12.5% + fetal calf serum 12.5%*	*6.3*	*15*	*17*
9. Horse serum 12.5% + human serum 12.5%	0.2	2	0
10. Human serum 12.5% + FCS 12.5%	0.3	1	0

[a] 2.4×10^7 nucleated marrow cells were seeded to each of triplicate 10.0 ml flasks and kept at 33°C, 3% CO$_2$ pH 7–7.5. All media and nonadherent cells were removed each 7th day and fesh medium added. Weekly total cell counts, differential cell counts, and assay for GM-CFUc were performed. Results are the mean of at least three culture flasks for each point. McCoy's 5A medium was supplemented with the additives described previously (Greenberger et al. 1980)

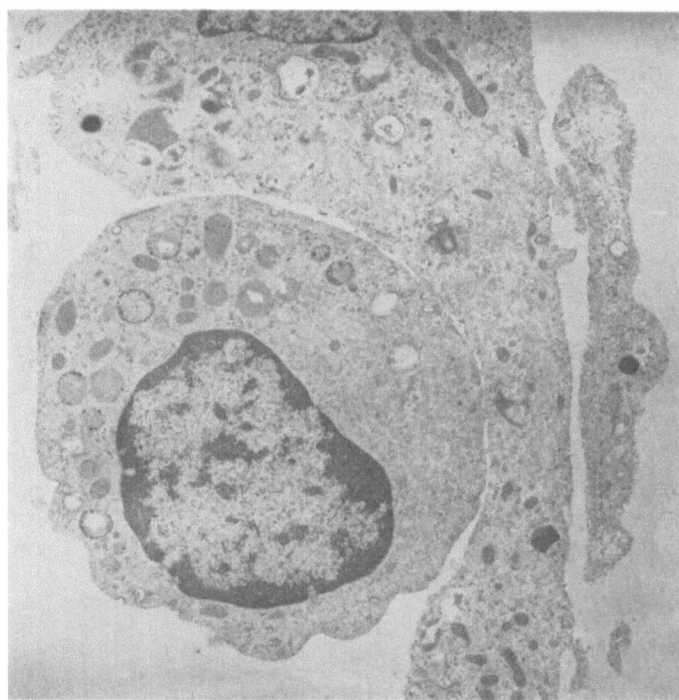

Fig. 1. Ultrastructural appearance of adherent cell microenvironment of human continuous bone marrow culture at 12 weeks prepared as described in the Fig. 1 legend. Note close apposition of early granulocyte and fibroblastic cells (×27,000)

associated with loss of human GM-CFUc by 10–12 weeks. In contrast, cultures depopulated twice weekly of all nonadherent cells with replacement of fresh medium and 50% of the washed nonadherent cells generated GM-CFUc past 15 weeks. Delayed removal of red blood cells 3–5 days after culture initiation (Gartner and Kaplan, see this vol p 276) resulted in a further improvement with GM-CFUc produced for over 18 weeks and in three samples for over 20 weeks. Using the optimal conditions, 3 of 50 amphoteracin-B (fungazone; 0.25 µg/ml) treated cultures established a functional "cobblestone" monolayer that produced GM-CFUc for at least 6 weeks and in 15 beyond 10 weeks. Thus, amphoteracin-B was toxic to human marrow cultures. Granulocytes generated after 10 weeks from each of 42 human donor marrow cultures were positive for myeloperoxidase and ASD-chloroacetate-specific esterase. There were on average 1% erythroid, 10% early granulocyte, 70% late granulocyte, 2%–13% monocytes, 2%–5% lymphocyte, and <1% eosionophils, mast cells, or megakaryocytes detected in nonadherent cells removed weekly between weeks 10–20.

II. Fluctuation in Generation of GM-CFUc in Human Long-Term Marrow Cultures

Weekly assay of GM-CFUc in nonadherent cells harvested over 10–20 weeks revealed differences in the numbers of colony-forming cells within each specimen as well as between individuals. Results with a representative specimen are shown in Fig. 3. Fluctuation in GM-CFUc has been observed in mouse long term bone marrow cultures (Dexter et al. 1977; Greenberger et al. 1980) and fluctuation in CFUs has been shown to occur through a process of clonal succession (Mauch et al. 1980).

D. Discussion

An in vitro culture technique is described for generation of human granulocyte-macrophage progenitor cells and mature granulocytes in excess of 20 weeks in continuous marrow culture. The requirement of freshly added hydrocortisone for continuous human marrow cultures was similar to that for murine cultures; however, major differences included de-

291

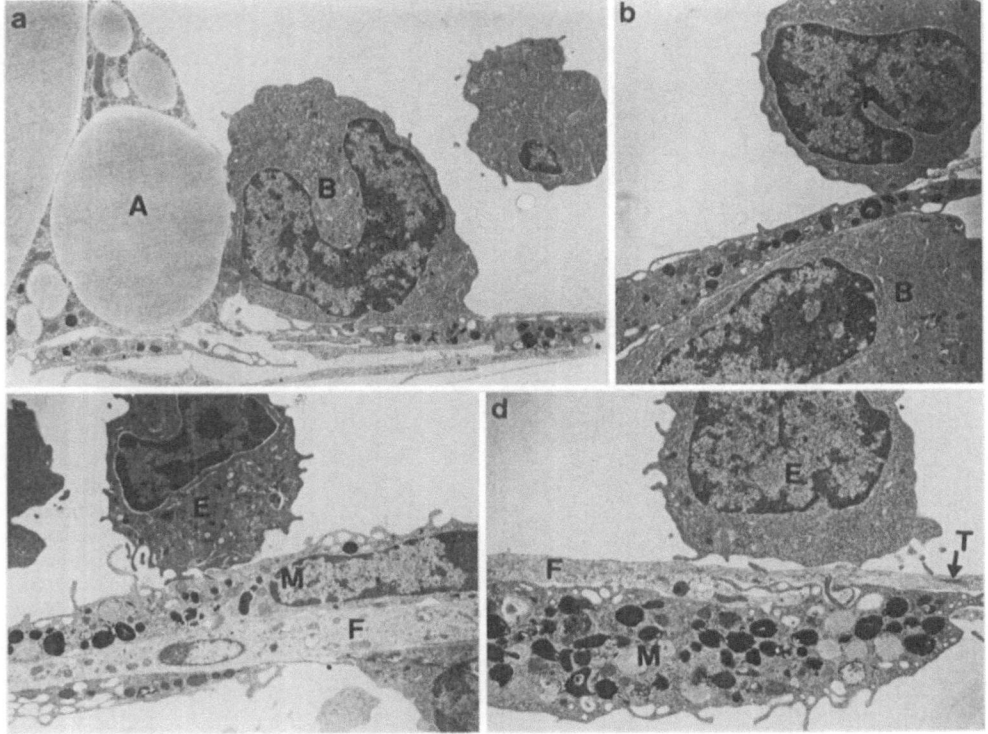

Fig. 2. Ultrastructural appearance of 8 week culture from C3H/HeJ marrow grown in 25% horse serum with $10^{-7}M$ hydrocortisone fixed in glutaraldehyde, postfixed in osmium, and poststained with uranyl acetate and lead citrate. **a–d** interaction between myeloid cells and the cells of the adherent layer. *A*, adipocyte, *B*, band neutrophil, *E*, early myelocyte, *F*, fibroblast, *M*, macrophage, *P*, promonocytic cell, and *T*, tight junction. (×26,400)

layed red blood cell removal and pH 7.0–7.5 with PCO_2 at between 3%–5%. The morphology of the adherent microenvironment in human cultures showed more fibroblastic proliferation, but groups of flat, tightly packed cells termed "cobblestone areas" for mouse cultures were enmeshed within fibroblasts and macrophages in the stroma. Granulocytes produced in human continuous marrow cultures were normal in morphology and synthesized esterase and myeloperoxidase. Individually removed GM-CFUc contained both granulocytes and macrophages in >80% of the colonies tested. Furthermore, granulocytes generated in these cultures have normal physiologic functions including ingestion, respiratory burst activity, degranulation, and bacterial killing (Greenberg et al., unpublished work). Application of human long-term marrow cultures is now feasible for study of the cell biology of hematological diseases.

Acknowledgments

Supported by Research Grants CA-254202, CA-26033, CA-26506, and CA-26785–01, and a Basal O'Connor tarter Research Grant from the March of Dimes Birth Defect Foundation.

References

Dexter TM, Testa NG (1976) Differentiation and proliferation of hemopoietic cells in culture. Methods Cell Biol 14:387–405 – Dexter TM, Scott D, Teich NM (1977) Infection of bone marrow cells in vitro with FLV: Effects on stem cell proliferation, differentiation, and leukemogenic capacity. Cell: 12:355–364 – Greenberger JS (1978) Sensitivity of

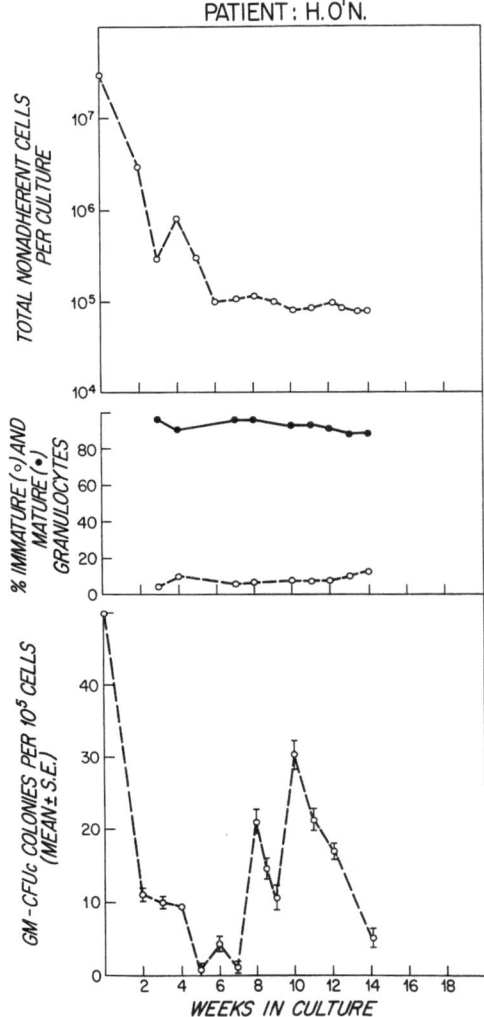

PATIENT: H.O'N.

Fig. 3. Kinetics of generation of granulocytes and GM-CFUc in vitro over 14 weeks in a representative human continuous marrow culture. Results are the mean of at leat four cultures at each time point. Cultures were established in McCoy's 5A medium supplemented with $10^{-7}M$ hydrocortisone, 12.5% FCS, and 12.5% horse serum, with delayed removal of red blood cells after 5 days

corticosteroid-dependent, insulin-resistant lipogenesis in marrow preadipocytes of mutation diabeticobese mice. Nature 275:752–754 – Greenberger JS (1979a) Corticosteroid-dependent differentiation of human bone marrow preadipocytes. In vitro 15:823–828 – Greenberger JS (1979b) Phenotypically-distinct target cells for murine sarcoma virus and murine leukemia virus marrow transformation in Vitro. J Nat Cancer Inst 62:337–348 – Greenberger JS, Davisson PB, Gans PJ (1979a) Murine sarcoma viruses block corticosteroid-dependent differentiation of bone marrow preadipocytes associated with long-term in vitro hemopoiesis. Virology 95:317–333 – Greenberger JS, Donahue D, Sakakeeny MA (1979c) Induction of ecotropic endogenous murine leukemia virus in long-term bone marrow cultures from mouse strains of varying natural leukemia incidence. J. Reticuloendothel Soc 26:839–853 – Greenberger JS, Gans PJ, Davisson PB, Moloney WC (1979c) In vitro induction of continuous acute promyelocytic cell lines in long-term bone marrow cultures by Friend or Abelson leukemia virus. Blood 53:987–1001 – Greenberger JS, Sakakeeny MA, Parker LM (1979l) In vitro proliferation of hematopoietic stem cells in long-term marrow cultures: Principals in mouse applied to man. Exp Hematol (Suppl 5) 7:135–148 – Greenberger JS, Newburger PE, Lipton JM, Moloney WC, Sakakeeny MA, Jackson PL (1980) Virus and cell requirements for Friend virus granulocytic leukemogenesis in long-term bone marrow cultures of NIH swiss mice. J Natl Canc Inst 64:867–878 – Greenberger JS, Eckner RJ, Ostertag W, Colletta G, Boshetti S, Nagasawa H, Karpas A, Weichselbaum R, Moloney WC (to be published a) Release of spleen focus-forming virus (SFFV) from differentiation inducible promyelocytic leukemia cell lines transformed in vitro by Friend leukemia virus. Virology – Greenberger JS, Newburger P, Sakakeeny MA (to be published b).Phorbol myristate acetate stimulates macrophage proliferation and differentiation and alters granulopoiesis and leukemogenesis in long-term bone marrow cultures. Blood – Greenberger J, Wroble LM, Sakakeeny MA (to be published c) Murine leukemia viruses induce macrophage production of granulocyte-macrophage colony stimulating factor in vitro. J Natl Çanc Inst – Mauch P, Greenberger JS, Botnick LE, Hannon EC, Hellman S (1980) Evidence for structured variation in self-renewal capacity within long-term bone marrow cultures. Proc Natl Acad Sci USA 77:2927–2930.

Haematology and Blood Transfusion Vol. 26
Modern Trends in Human Leukemia IV
Edited by Neth, Gallo, Graf, Mannweiler, Winkler
© Springer-Verlag Berlin Heidelberg 1981

Cloning Cells of the Immune System

N. A. Mitchison

The purpose of this introductory note is to explain why the immunological papers in this collection concentrate on cloning. There are three good reasons for choosing cloning as an appropriate subject at the present time. One is that cloning provides a valuable means of acquiring information about the working of the immune system. Another is that several of the technical problems which prevented satisfactory cloning have just been solved, so that rapid progress can and is being made. The third is that application of the new procedures is providing insight into leukaemia.

The value of cloning follows from the way in which the immune system is arranged as a loose population of cells which traffic from place to place interacting through transient contacts and soluble factors. In consequence cells are differentiated from one another not by their anatomical position and connections but by their genetic and epigenetic makeup. There is a strong contrast here between the nervous and immune systems, the two most complex and highly integrated systems of the body which otherwise share many features in common. No doubt clones from the nervous system can provide interesting information about such topics as receptor function and metabolic control, but they cannot be expected to tell us directly how neurones work. This is not true of lymphocytes and to a lesser extent, of antigen-presenting cells: here we can expect clones to express all major functions.

The major technical problem has been to find ways of keeping cells alive and multiplying outside the body. The first step forward was to maintain clones of B cells under antigenic stimulation in irradiated mice (Askonas and Williamson 1972). For B cells the in vitro problem has now largely been solved by the

hybridoma technique (Köhler and Milstein 1976). Monoclonal antibodies produced by this technique turn out to be immensely powerful tools in biochemistry, cell biology, and medicine. Their application is well exemplified by Beverley's study of stem cell surface markers described in this volume. The hybridoma revolution is sweeping all before it, leaving only little room for alternatives such as the immortalization of human immunoglobulin-secreting cells by Epstein-Barr virus infection (Steinitz et al. 1977).

For T cells, hybridomas have thus for proved less successful. Our own experience has been that immunoregulatory activity can be maintained in this way for a while, but tends to decline in an unpredictable and uncontrollable way (Kontiainen et al. 1978). Other laboratories find the same decline. On the other hand, T cells are proving highly amenable to less drastic cloning procedures.

One such procedure is to maintain them on T cell growth factor (TCGF). Another is to restimulate cultures with antigen at intervals. Both of these procedures are discussed and evaluated in detail at the International Congress of Immunology this year, and the latter is well exemplified by Hengartner's study described here.

Our approach (Czitrom et al. 1980) has been to generate allospecific helper T cells by stimulation in vitro. Our previous work had shown that the adoptive secondary response in mice could be successfully adapted for the study of helper T cells directed at cell surface antigens. We generate helper T cells by alloantigen-induced proliferation in vitro directed at I^k (A.TH anti-A.TL) and test for their ability to help in vivo primed B cells directed at D^b (A.TH anti-B10) in an adoptive secondary response with 2000-R irradiated boosting antigen – a cell carrying both the I^k and the D^b antigens [B10.A(2R)]. Helper T cells did increase the anti-D^b response, as judged by Cr^{51} cytotoxicity titrations 9 days after cell transfer. The in vitro generated specific helper T cells in primary and repeatedly stimulated mixed lymphocyte cultures were more effective in helping these B cell responses than equivalent helper T cells induced by in vivo priming.

Similar results have been obtained with helper T cells boosted in vitro and directed at H-minor antigens (CBA anti-B10.Br) in helping in vivo primed B cells directed at Thy.1 (CBA anti-AKR). Thus, we are still at an early stage in our attempt to generate clones. The point of our approach is that it utilizes a powerful and important group of antigens, the murine alloantigens, at the expense of having to use a rather cumbersome assay for function.

How far will these approaches take us with leukaemia? The use of TCGF for growing leukaemic and normal lymphocytes in vitro are just beginning to be explored and will be made easier by the purification of the agent as here described by Gallo. TCGF is itself both a candidate agent and a target for therapy in immunological diseases, including leukaemia. Lymphocytes can be generated in vitro with the capacity to kill MHC-identical human leukaemic cells (Sondel et al. 1976). There are still many questions about these cells, such as their relationship with natural killer (NK) cells. These can surely best be answered by cloning.

On the B cell side, the main application of monoclonal antibodies to leukaemia thus far has been in (1) the identification of markers on lymphocyte subsets and their use in defining leukaemic phenotypes, topics discussed here by Greaves and (2) the characterization of transformation proteins such as $ppSRC^{60}$ (for references see Mitchison and Kinlen 1980).

Some fascinating questions are beginning to arise in ontogeny as one attempts to relate the stages of lymphocyte development to events affecting immunoglobulin genes. At what stage, for instance, do V_H and V_L genes move to their "differentiated" position close to J and C genes? If, as seems likely in the mouse at least, V_H genes are expressed (as idiotypes) earlier than V_L genes, why does the intervening interval (the pre-B cell) last so long? Could it be that movement of V_H is a difficult and dangerous process for the cell, as the evidence of mistaken movements on the unexpressed chromosome suggests; if so, may not the rapid proliferation of pre-B cells represent a mechanism for expanding a premium cell before it has to undergo the equally costly business of moving a V_L gene? Such speculations may at least begin to explain why so many ALLs are of pre-B types (this discussion of pre-B cells draws on M. Cooper's unpublished data and is derived from discussion with him).

References

Askonas BA, Williamson AR (1972) Factors affecting the propagation of a B cell clone forming antibody to the 2,4-dinitrophenyl group. Eur J Immunol 2:487–493 – Czitrom AA, Yeh Ming, Mitchison NA (1980) Allospecific helper T cells generated by alloantigenic stimulation in vitro. In: Preud'homme JL, Hawken VAL (eds) Abstracts the 4th international congress of immunology, Paris, 1980, Academic Press, New York – Köhler C, Milstein C (1976) Derivation of specific antibody-producing tissue culture and tumour lines by cell fusion. Eur J Immunol 6:511–519 – Kontiainen S, Simpson E, Bohrer E, Beverley PCL, Herzenberg LA, Fitzpatrick WC, Vogt P, Torano A, McKenzie IFC, Feldmann M (1978) T cell lines producing antigen-specific suppressor factor. Nature 274:477–480 – Mitchison NA, Kinlen L (1980) Present concepts in immune surveillance. In: Fougereau M, Dausset J (eds) Immunology 1980 (Proceedings of the 4th international congress of immunology, Paris, 1980). Academic Press, New York pp 641–650 – Sondel PM, OBrien C, Porter L, Schlossman SF, Chess L (1976) Cell-mediated destruction of human leukaemic cells by MHC identical lymphocytes: requirement for a proliferative trigger in vitro. J Immunol 117:2197–2203 – Steinitz M, Klein G, Koskimies F, Mäkelä O (1977) EB virus induced B lymphocyte cell lines producing specific antibody. Nature 269:420–422

Haematology and Blood Transfusion Vol. 26
Modern Trends in Human Leukemia IV
Edited by Neth, Gallo, Graf, Mannweiler, Winkler
© Springer-Verlag Berlin Heidelberg 1981

Comparative Antigenic Phenotypes of Normal and Leukemic Hemopoietic Precursor Cells Analysed with a "Library" of Monoclonal Antibodies

M. F. Greaves, J. B. Robinson, D. Delia, J. Ritz, S. Schlossman, C. Sieff, G. Goldstein, P. Kung, F. J. Bollum, and P. A. W. Edwards

A. Introduction

A dominant paradigm of cancer research is that alterations in the cell surface are of paramount importance to tumour cell behavior (Wallach 1978; Marchesi 1976). It is widely held that this is in part reflected in the regular expression of neo-antigens resulting from gene derepression [or "retrogressive differentiation" (Coggin 1978)], mutation (Baldwin 1974) or altered processing [e.g. glycosylation (Hakomori 1975)]. The search for novel antigens or other cell surface features of human tumour cells has an obligatory control demand which is frequently ignored or inadequately dealt with, i.e. that the appropriate cellular controls be analysed in parallel. Since most epithelial carcinomas and acute leukemias probably arise from tissue stem cells and, moreover, frequently have a maturation arrest imposed upon them, it should be self-evident that (a) many or most of the consistent phenotypic features of leukemic cells (and tumour cells in general) will be a reflection of their immature cell origins and (b) the significance of potentially unique biochemical or molecular features of tumour cells cannot be interpreted until we have access to normally infrequent tissue precursor cells.

The latter demand may be satisfied in the future by the development of new culture methods (see Dexter, this volume); in the meantime one of the most incisive approaches we have to the analysis of tumour cell phenotypes is the serological characterization of cell surface antigen expression on individual leukemic cells, particularly by monoclonal antibodies. The crucial advantages of leukemia in this context are that "equivalent" normal tissue is available in a physical form that is amenable to

"cell surface" serology (i.e. single cell suspensions) and that stem cells and progenitor cells, whilst not morphologically recognisable, can be detected by functional assays in vitro. By the same token, acute leukemias offer an opportunity to discover antigenic and other characteristic marker features of hemopoietic stem cells which might be functionally relevant to the regulation of differentiation or at least be useful as "markers" for isolating these cells.

These arguments were in part developed in previous Wilsede symposia; here they are further explored with particular reference to two well-characterized cell surface glycoproteins – the gp 100 common ALL-associated antigen and the gp 28/33 Ia-like or HLA-DR antigens. In addition a systemic comparison of leukemic cells and their "presumed" equivalent normal counterparts using a panel of monoclonal antibodies is described.

B. The Terminal Transferase Positive "Lymphocyte" in Normal Bone Marrow has the Same Composite Cell Surface Phenotype as Common Acute Lymphoblastic Leukemia (cALL)

Rabbit antisera to non-T, non-B ALL have defined an antigen present on leukemic cells from 75% of children with ALL (common ALL) and on blast cells in some cases of AUL and CML in blast crisis (reviewed in Greaves and Janossy 1978; Greaves 1979a). The cell surface polypeptides (gp 100) reactive with anti-cALL have been isolated and characterized (Sutherland et al. 1978; Newman et al. 1981; Newman et al., this volume). Antisera with a similar if not identical specificity have now been produced by other laboratories

(Borella et al. 1977; Netzel et al. 1978; Pesando et al. 1979; Kabisch et al. 1979; LeBien et al. 1979), including a monoclonal antibody – J-5 (Ritz et al. 1980). Some of these sera, including the monoclonal J-5, also appear to precipitate a cell surface glycoprotein of 95–100,000 daltons (Billing et al. 1978; Pesando et al. 1980); however, several of these authors were unable to find normal bone marrow cells reacting with their reagents and therefore concluded that the latter could be identifying an antigen(s) unique to leukemic cells.

We have documented elsewhere the evidence that the cALL antigen as detected by our particular rabbit antibodies is present on small numbers of "lymphoid" cells in normal bone marrow and particularly in regenerating marrows of pediatric patients (Greaves et al. 1978; 1980; Janossy et al. 1979). Furthermore, a gp 100 molecule can be isolated from these sources with anti-ALL sera (Newman et al. 1981 and this volume).

Although some one-third of cALL have a "pre-B" (μ chain positive) phenotype (Vogler et al. 1978; Brouet et al. 1979; Greaves et al. 1979), the majority express no markers of mature T and B cells and presumably represent hemopoietic precursor cells in maturation arrest (Greaves and Janossy 1978); whilst they are likely to be lymphoid, i.e. precursors committed to T and/or B lineages, this is not formally proven. These leukemias also express the nuclear enzyme TdT which can be identified by fluorescent antibodies (Bollum 1979). A small proportion of normal lymphoid cells in bone marrow (as well as most cortical thymocytes) contain TdT (Bollum 1979); this enzyme, therefore, provides a very convenient single cell marker against which cell surface phenotype can be analysed. We reported previously that the TdT positive cell in normal bone marrow expressed the cALL and Ia-like antigens but not T cell antigens or Ig (Janossy et al. 1979). We have now assessed the composite antigenic phenotype of TdT-positive marrow cells using an extensive library of monoclonal antibodies (Greaves 1981a, b). The results (Table 1) indicate that the majority of TdT positive cells in bone marrow have a cell surface phenotype that is a replica of that seen in common ALL (Greaves 1981a, b; Greaves and Janossy 1978) and which includes no *exclusive* markers of either non-lymphoid lineages or mature T and B cells. The antigenic

determinant detected by monoclonal PI153/3 which is present on most normal TdT-positive cells is, however, present on normal B cells as well as pre-B cells and cALL (Greaves et al. 1980). It should also be noted that the majority (90%) of TdT-positive cells in normal bone marrow do not express any of the T lineage antigens detected by the OKT series of monoclonals, including those that are reactive with some or most TdT-positive T-ALL (Reinherz et al. 1979a, 1980). An exception to this is OKT10 which, though reactive with most T-ALL (Janossy et al. 1978a), is also present on the majority of cALL and AML (Greaves et al. 1981).

Of 25 marrows analysed (donors 2–41 years) with monoclonal (J-5) anti-ALL, 21 showed positive reactivity on 2%–39% positive cells. This was variable in intensity but occasionally quite bright (Fig. 1a). There was a high degree of concordance with the TdT-positive cells (Table 1, Fig. 1c) in pediatric samples as previously reported with rabbit antisera (Janossy et al. 1979). Since monoclonal J-5 gives completely concordant reactivity pattern on more than 200 leukemias assessed (Ritz et al. 1980; M.F. Greaves and J. Ritz, unpublished work) and co-redistributes with the cell surface with rabbit anti-ALL (Fig. 1d), then the simplest explanation is (a) that it can recognise the same structure (though possibly not the same determinants) as rabbit anti-ALL and (b) that this structure, or one similar to it [since a family of gp 100 molecules may exist (Pesando et al. 1980)], is present on normal TdT-positive lymphoid cells in bone marrow. More detailed biochemistry is now required to determine the degree of similarity between the gp 100 molecules from cALL and normal bone marrow cells.

Another monoclonal antibody reactive with cALL has recently been described [BA-2 (Kersey et al. 1981)]. In contrast to J-5 and rabbit anti-cALL, this antibody appears to identify a p 24 structure; it is also present on a small number of normal bone marrow cells.

This analysis indicates therefore that the composite antigenic phenotype of cALL mirrors that of a normal (TdT⁺) cell type in bone marrow. We presume therefore that (a) these determinants are most likely normal gene products of hemopoietic precursors that *continue* to be co-ordinately expressed in leukemia and (b) that the cALL⁺ TdT⁺ normal cell which is restricted to bone marrow (Greaves et

Table 1. Monoclonal antibody reactivity with TdT-positive bone marrow lymphocytes and cALL[a]

Selectivity	Designation	Ref.	Reactivity with TdT-positive cells in bone marrow	Reactivity with cALL
HLA associated:				
1. HLA-ABC "framework"	W6/32			
	PA 2.6			
2. HLA-DR "framework"	DA2	Brodsky et al. (1979)	+(85–95%)	+>95%
	OKI-1			
3. β_2 microglobulin	EC3			
	BB5			
T lineage associated:				
1. "Pan"-T	OKT11	[b]		
2. Mature T	OKT1	Reinherz et al. (1979b)		
	OKT3	Kung et al. (1979)		
	L17 F12	Levy (to be published)		
3. Functional subset				
(a) "Suppressor" T	OKT8	Reinherz et al. (1980)	−	−
(b) "Helper" T	OKT4	Reinherz et al. (1980)		
4. Intrathymic subset	OKT6	Reinherz et al. (1980)		
	NA134	McMichael et al. (1979)		
5. Thymic associated[c]	OKT9	Reinherz et al. (1980)		
	OKT10	Reinherz et al. (1980)	+(50–95%)	+
B lineage associated:				
1. Pan-B	FMC1	Brooks et al. (1980)	−	−
2. Pre-B, Pan-B/Neural	PI153/3	Greaves et al. (1980) Kennett and Gilbert (1979)	+(45–90%)	+
Common ALL/lymphocyte progenitor associated:				
	J-5	Ritz et al. (1980)	+(45–95%)	+
Other non-lymphoid lineages:				
1. Monocyte/Granulocyte	OKM-1	Breard et al. (1979)		
2. Erythroid:				
Glycophorin A	LICR.LON/R10	Edwards (1980)	−	−
Band III	1/6A	Edwards (1980)		
3. Platelet[d]	AN51	McMichael (to be published)		

[a] All monoclonals have been tested on 2–5 normal bone marrow suspensions and a minimum of 20 cALL

[b] A pan-T monoclonal antibody, reactive with the sheep erythrocyte receptor on T cells (W. Verbi, M. F. Greaves, G. Janossy, P. Kung and G. Goldstein in preparation)

[c] OKT9 reacts with approximately 10% of thymocytes and OKT10 with all thymocytes. However, neither monoclonal is T-lineage specific. OKT9 reacts with the receptor for transferrin which is ubiquitous in distribution and associated with cell proliferation (Sutherland et al. 1981). OKT10 reacts with almost all non-lymphoid acute leukemias (Greaves et al. 1981)

[d] Reacts selectively with platelets and possibly with megakaryocytes. −, less than 2 cells per 100 positive. With the exception of OKT6 and NA134, all monoclonals stained some cells in the marrow suspension tested. All reagents were titrated on the Fluorescence Activated Cell Sorter (FACS-I) to determine the maximum dilution giving 2× saturation on known positive control cells. Binding of mouse monoclonal antibodies to viable cells in suspension was followed by the addition of affinity-purified goat antibodies to mouse Ig which had been cross-absorbed with insolubilized human Ig digested with pepsin to give a f(b)$_2$ preparation and labelled with rhodamine isothiocyanate. Cells were then smeared (cytospin), fixed in methanol and stained with affinity purified rabbit anti-TdT followed by fluorescein isothiocyanate-labelled and affinity-purified goat f(ab')$_2$ anti-rabbit Ig

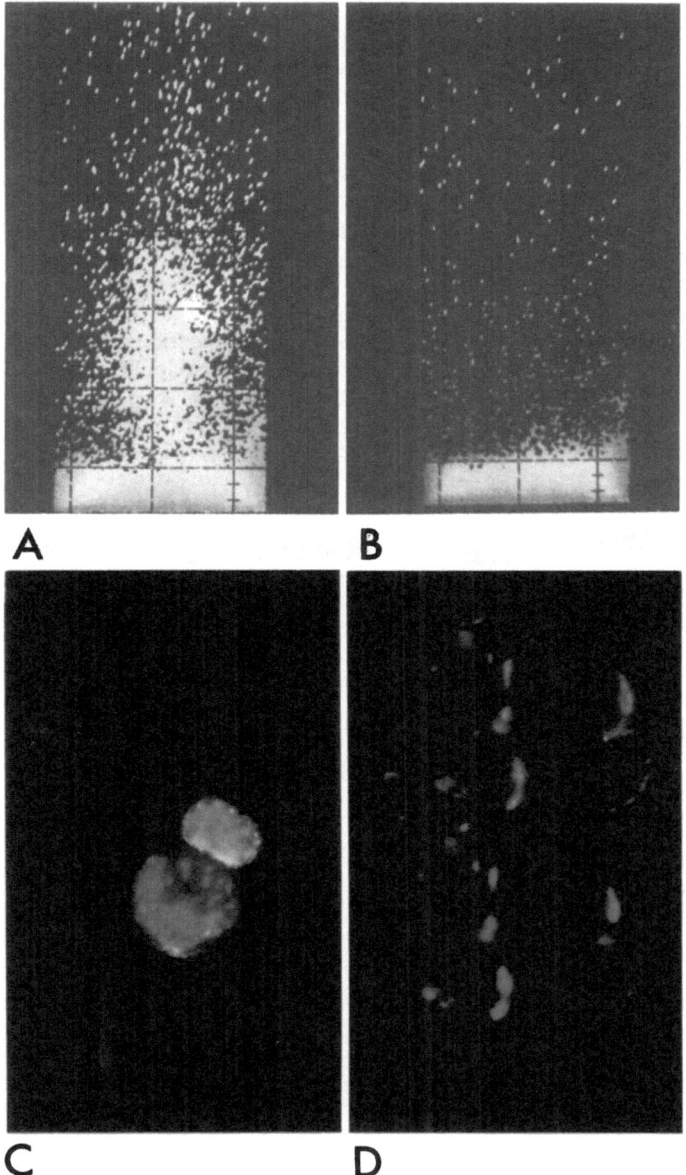

Fig. 1. Reactivity of normal and leukaemic cells with monoclonal J-5 anti-ALL (gp100) antigen. **A,B.** FACS analysis. Vertical axis, relative fluorescence intensity; horizontal axis, relative cell size (light scattering). Uninvolved bone marrow from a child with rhabdomyosarcoma was stained with J-5 anti-ALL (A) or control mouse ascites Ig (B). **C.** Normal paediatric bone marrow cells stained (in suspension) with monoclonal J-5 anti-cALL (gp100) plus (after cytospin preparation and fixation) rabbit anti-TdT. Cell surface stains green/yellow for the cALL antigen and nucleus red/orange for TdT. **D.** ALL cell line (Nalm-1) cells stained first with rabbit anti-cALL (gp100) under capping conditions rhodamine labelled goat anti-rabbit Ig added at 37° for 30 mins. Cells were then kept in the cold (4°) with sodium azide and stained with mouse monoclonal J-5 anti-ALL followed by fluorescein labelled goat anti-mouse Ig. Field of 4 cells was photographed using filters for rhodamine (upper half of picture) then moved slightly to re-expose same photograph frame for fluorescein (lower half of picture). Note complete co-incidence of red and green images indicates co-redistribution of the rabbit and mouse antibodies

299

al. 1979; Janossy et al. 1979) is either the major "target" population for cALL and/or represents a post-target developmental level of maturation arrest in ALL [as evidenced for example by cALL blast crises of CML (Greaves and Janossy 1978)].

C. The Cellular Selectivity of HLA-DR Expression in Leukemia Parallels Its Presence on Hemopoietic Progenitor Cells of the Myeloid and Erythroid Lineages

The Ia-like, p28,33 or HLA-DR antigens (Moller 1976) are present on pre-B cells, B lymphocytes, a T cell subset macrophages and different types of epithelia, e.g. thymic, intestinal and lactating mammary. Plasma cells, thymocytes and most T cells have no demonstrable cell surface HLA-DR. Hetero-antisera and allo-antisera to these molecules react with B cell leukemias (e.g. CLL) as well as almost all cases of non-T ALL (Greaves and Janossy 1978). More surprisingly, AML (Schlossman et al. 1976; Janossy et al. 1978b) and CML in "myeloid" blast crisis (Janossy et al. 1977) were found to express HLA-DR or Ia-like antigens. These observations have now been rationalized by reference to HLA-DR expression on normal hemopoietic precursors. Thus some normal immature myeloblasts may express Ia-like antigens (Ross et al. 1978; Winchester et al. 1977). CFU-GM activity in vitro can be inhibited by pretreating with anti-Ia-like reagents and complement, (Koeffler et al. 1979; Moore et al. 1980) and CFU-GM can be positively selected on the fluorescence-activated cell sorter (FACS) using rabbit antibodies to the p28,33, Ia-like or HLA-DR polypeptide complex (Janossy et al. 1978a).

These observations have now been confirmed and extended using a monoclonal antibody [DA2 (Brodsky et al. 1979)] to a monomorphic or conserved determinant of HLA-DR. Table 2 lists the leukemias that show reactivity with this antibody. Acute myeloblastic leukemias are usually but not invariably positive with anti-HLA-DR, whereas acute promyelocytic and chronic granulocytic leukemias are negative, which further emphasizes the inverse association between HLA-DR expression and granulocytic maturation.

Notice that erythroleukemias are consistently HLA-DR negative (Table 2). This observation is of some importance in relation to two other reported observations: (a) that both BFU-E and CFU-E can be inhibited by rabbit anti-p28/34 and complement (Moore et al. 1980; Winchester et al. 1978) and (b) that rabbit anti-glycophorin may detect "cryptic" early erythroid leukemias which would otherwise escape this differential identification (Andersson et al. 1979, 1980 and see also Andersson, this volume).

We have used both "conventional" antisera to glycophorin and a monoclonal antibody [LICR.LON.R10 (Edwards 1980)] to screen large numbers of different leukemias. To date we have detected three cases of glycophorin positive acute leukemias that were not overtly

Table 2. Reactivity of different leukemic cells with monoclonal anti-HLA-DR (DA2)[a]

ALL:	
cALL	201/203
T-ALL	0/53
"Null"-ALL	38/38
B-ALL	5/5
CGL-blast crisis ("L" type)	15/15
Chronic l. leukemias:	
B-CLL	26/26
B-PLL	5/5
T-PLL	0/6
T-CLL	1/7
T-Sezary	1/5
B-hairy cell leukemia	4/4
Myeloma/Plasma cell leukemias:	0/4
Myeloid leukemias:	
AML	83/110
AMML	20/28
AMonL	8/9
CGL	1/26
CGL blast crisis ("M" type)	17/21
APML	0/6
Erythro-leukemias:	0/11

[a] L, lymphocytic; ALL, acute lymphoblastic leukemia; CGL, chronic granulocytic leukemia; PLL, prolymphocytic leukemia; CLL, chronic lymphocytic leukemia; AML, acute myeloblastic leukemia; AMML, acute myelo-monocytic leukemia; AMonL, acute monocytic leukemia; APML, acute promyelocytic leukemia; "L" type, lymphoid (TdT[+]/cALL[+]) variety of blast crisis; "M" type, myeloid or non-lymphoid (TdT[-]/cALL[-]) variety of blast crisis

erythroid. Two were CML in blast crisis and one was a child with poorly differentiated acute leukemia (Greaves 1981a). In these cases a proportion of cells also reacted with monoclonal and polyclonal anti-HLA-DR; however, double labelling showed that glycophorin and HLA-DR were present almost exclusively on different cells.

To explore further the significance of erythroleukemic phenotypes in relation to normal early erythroid differentiation we have labelled normal bone marrow cells with various monoclonal antibodies, separated positive and negative cells under sterile conditions using the FACS and assayed for BFU-E and CFU-E activity. The details of these results are published elsewhere (Robinson et al. 1981) and summarized as a 'model' diagram in Fig. 2. BFU-E are predominantly HLA-DR$^+$, HLA-ABC$^+$, and glycophorin$^-$; CFU-E are predominantly HLA-DR$^-$, HLA-ABC$^+$, and glycophorin$^-$. All morphologically recognisable erythroid cell precursors are HLA-DR$^-$, HLA-ABC$^{+ or -}$, and glycophorin $^{+ or -}$. All erythroid progenitors (BFU-E and CFU-E) were in addition reactive with monoclonal anti-blood group A (in an A$^+$ donor) but unreactive with OKT1, OKT11 and J-5 (see Table 1). As an incidental observation in these experiments (since the cultures were all set up with erythropoietin) we noted that CFU-GM and CFU-Eo when present also localized predominantly in the HLA-DR$^+$, HLA-ABC$^+$, glycophorin$^-$ population.

These observations, therefore, establish as directly as is currently possible that HLA-DR antigens are indeed expressed on committed hemopoietic progenitor cells [although they may be absent from pluripotential stem cells (Basch et al. 1977; Moore et al. 1980) and raise the possibility that cell interactions involving HLA-DR or Ia-like antigens might play a role in early hemopoiesis as well as in immune responses (McDevitt 1978).

Since both covert and overt erythroleukemias are glycophorin$^+$, HLA-DR$^-$ we can place their likely dominant maturational arrest position close to the post-CFU cells. However, erythroleukemia can almost certainly originate in a pluripotential progenitor cell, since it regularly involves a granulocytic component or may indeed occur in Ph^1 positive CML. These studies with monoclonal antibodies confirm that glycophorin may provide a useful marker for cryptic early erythroleukemia (Andersson et al. 1979, 1980) but also indicates that many more HLA-DR$^+$ or HLA-DR$^-$ acute leukemias corresponding to BFU-E or CFU-E, respectively, might exist but remain undetected as such since no exclusive marker for these early erythroid cells yet exists.

D. Conclusions

Detailed serological analysis of leukemic cell surfaces using both conventional and monoclonal antibodies indicates that acute leukemic cells have composite antigenic phenotypes that appear to correspond to their lineage affiliation and "position" of maturation arrest. If leukemia specific antigens exist then they are not readily revealed by this type of investigation. Although leukemic cells appear to show a remarkable fidelity of phenotype, the degree

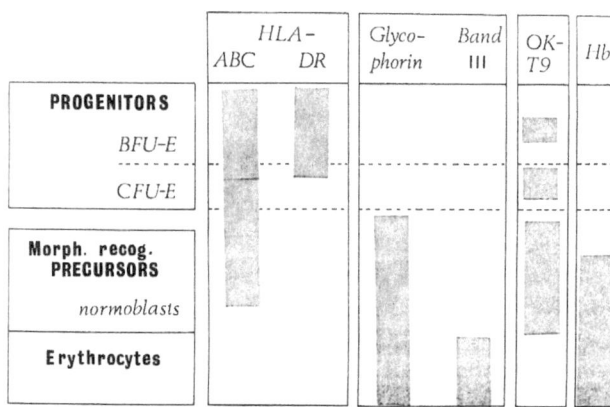

Fig. 2. Patterns of cell surface antigen expression during erythroid differentiation. *Hb*, haemoglobin

to which this is an exact replica of the normal counterpart is still open to question. Subsequent analyses with monoclonal antibodies could identify novel antigens perhaps restricted to individuals or small subsets of paients or occurring in association with particular chromosomal alterations (Rowley 1978). Karyotypic data suggest that gene dosage effects might have a critical bearing on leukemia (see G. Klein, this volume) and, similarly, quantitative rather than qualitative alterations in cell surface antigens might be important.

Finally, some putative anomalies in antigenic expression are encountered in studies on human leukemic cells (Shumak et al. 1975; Bradstock et al. 1980; Greaves 1979c, 1980), although it can be ruled out that these examples also reflect our ignorance of the heterogeneity of normal immature cell phenotypes. Since acute leukemia is generally regarded as a fairly high grade malignancy, it is of some interest to find that cell surface phenotypes are conserved or only marginally altered, suggesting an analogy with "minimally-deviated" hepatomas (Potter 1978). This permits some speculation about the contribution of the cell surface in malignancy (Greaves 1979b) and, as shown above, reveals characteristics of normal hemopoietic progenitors.

Acknowledgments

This work was supported by the Imperial Cancer Research Fund. We are grateful to those colleagues listed in the references in Table 1 who also supplied monoclonal antibodies used in part of this study.

References

Andersson L, Gahmberg CG, Teerenhovi L, Vuopio P (1979) Glycophorin A as a cell surface marker of early erythroid differentiation in acute leukemia. Int J Cancer 23:717–720 – Andersson LC, Wegelius R, Borgström GH, Gahmberg CG (1980) Change in cellular phenotype from lymphoid to erythroid in a case of ALL. Scand J Haematol 24:115–121 – Baldwin R (1974) Tumour specific antigens. In: The physiopathology of cancer. Vol. 1, pp 334–392 – Basch RS, Janossy G, Greaves MF (1977) Murine pluripotential stem cells lack Ia antigen. Nature, 270:520–522 – Billing R, Monowada J, Cline M, Clark B, Lee K (1978) Acute lymphocytic leukemia-associated cell membrane antigen. J Natl Cancer Inst 61:423–429 – Bollum F (1979) Terminal deoxynucleotidyl transferase as a hemopoietic cell marker. Blood 54:1203–1215 – Borella L, Sen L, Casper JT (1977) Acute lymphoblastic leukemia (ALL) antigens detected with antisera to E rosette-forming and non-E rosette-forming ALL blasts. J Immunol 118:309–315 – Bradstock KF, Janossy G, Bollum FJ, Milstein C (1980) Anomalous gene expression in human thymic acute lymphoblastic leukaemia (Thy-ALL). Nature 284:455–457 – Breard JM, Reinherz EL, Kung PC, Goldstein G, Schlossman SF (1979) A monoclonal antibody reactive with human peripheral blood monocytes. J Immunol 124:1943–1948 – Brodsky FM, Parham P, Barnstable CJ, Crumpton MJ, Bodmer WF (1979) Hybrid myeloma monoclonal antibodies against MHC products. Immunol Rev 47:3–61 – Brooks DA, Beckman I, Bradley J, McNamara PJ, Thomas ME, Zola H (1980) Human lymphocyte markers defined by antibodies derived from somatic cell hybrids. I. A hybridoma secreting antibody against a marker specific for human B lymphocytes. Clin Exp Immunol 39:477–485 – Brouet JC, Preud'homme JL, Penit C, Valensi F, Rouget P, Seligmann M (1979) Acute lymphoblastic leukaemia with pre-B characteristics. Blood 54:269–273 – Brown G, Biberfeld P, Christensson B, Mason D (1979) The distribution of HLA on human lymphoid, bone marrow and blood cells. Eur J Immunol 9:272–275 – Coggin JH (1978) Retrogressive differentiation in cancer. In: Castro J (ed) Immunological aspects of cancer. MTP, Lancaster, pp 89–100 – Edwards PAW (1980) Monoclonal antibodies that bind to the human erythrocyte-membrane glycoproteins glycophorin A and Band III. Biochem Soc Trans 8:334–335 – Greaves MF (1979a) Immunodiagnosis of leukaemia. In: Herberman RH, McIntire KR (Eds) Immunodiagnosis of cancer. Dekker, New York, pp 542–587 – Greaves MF (1979b) Tumour markers, phenotypes and maturation arrest in malignancy: A cell selection hypothesis. In: Boelsma E, Rümke P (eds) Tumour Markers. Elsevier, Amsterdam, pp 201–211 – Greaves MF (1979c) Cell surface characteristics of human leukaemic cells. In: Campbell PN, Marshall RD (eds) Essays in biochemistry. Academic Press, New York, pp 78–124 – Greaves MF (1980) Analysis of human leukaemic cell populations using monoclonal antibodies and the fluorescence activated cell sorter. In: Yohn DS, Lapin BA, Blakeslee JR (eds) Advances in comparative leukemia research 1979. Elsevier/North Holland, Amsterdam, New York, pp 235–242 – Greaves MF (1981b) Analysis of lymphoid phenotypes in acute leukaemia: Their clinical and biological significance. Cancer Res, in press – Greaves MF, Janossy G (1978) Patterns of gene expression and the cellular origins of human leukaemias. Biochim Biophys Acta 516:193–230 – Greaves MF, Delia D, Janossy G, Rapson N, Chessells J, Woods M, Prentice G (1980) Acute lymphoblastic leukaemia associated antigen. VI. Expression on non-leukaemic 'lymphoid' cells. Leuk Res 4:15–32 – Greaves MF, Janossy G, Francis GE, Minowada J (1978) Membrane phenotypes of human leukemic cells and leukemic cell lines. Clinical correlates and biological implications. In: Differentiation of normal and neoplastic hematopoietic cells. Cold Spring Harbor Laboratory, New York, pp 823–841 – Greaves MF, Verbi W, Vogler L, Cooper M, Ellis R, Ganeshaguru K, Hoffbrand V, Janossy G, Bollum FJ: Antigenic and enzymatic phenotypes of the pre-B subclass of acute lymphoblastic leukaemia. Leuk Res 3:353–362 – Greaves MF, Verbi W, Kemshead J, Kennett R (1980) A monoclonal antibody identifying a cell surface antigen shared by common acute lymphoblastic leukemias and B lineage cells. Blood 56:1141–1144 – Hakomori S (1975) Structure and organization of cell surface glycolipids: dependency on cell growth and malignant transformation. Biochim Biophys Acta 417:55–89 – Janossy G, Greaves MF, Sutherland R, Durrant J, Lewis C (1977) Comparative analysis of membrane phenotypes in acute lymphoid leukaemia and in lymphoid blast crisis of chronic myeloid leukaemia. Leuk Res 1:289–300 – Janossy G, Francis GE, Capellaro D, Goldstone AH, Greaves MF (1978a) Cell sorter analysis of leukaemia-associated antigens on human myeloid precursors. Nature 276:176–178 – Janossy G, Goldstone AH, Capellaro D, Greaves MF, Kulenkampff J, Pippard M, Welsh K (1978b) Differentiation linked expression of p28,33 (Ia-like) structures on human leukaemic cells. Br J Haematol 37:391–402 – Janossy G, Bollum F, Bradstock K, Rapson N, Greaves MF (1979) Terminal deoxynucleotidyl transferase positive human bone marrow cells exhibit the antigenic phenotype of common acute lymphoblastic leukaemia. J Immunol 123:1525–1529 – Kabisch H, Arndt R, Becker W-M, Thiele H-G, Landbeck G (1979) Serological detection and partial characterization of the common-ALL-cell associated antigen in the serum of cALL-patients. Leuk Res 3:83–91 – Kennett RH, Gilbert F (1979) Hybrid myelomas producing antibodies against a human neuroblastoma antigen present on fetal brain. Science 203:1120–1121 – Kersey JH, LeBien TW, Abramson CS, Newman R, Sutherland R, Greaves M (to be published) gp24: a human hemopoietic progenitor and acute lymphoblastic leukemia-associated cell surface structure identified with monoclonal antibody. J Exp Med 153:726–731 – Koeffler HP, Niskanen E, Cline M, Billing R, Golde D (1979) Human myeloid precursors forming colonies in diffusion chambers expresses the Ia-like antigen. Blood 54:1188–1191 – Kung PC, Goldstein G, Reinherz EL, Schlossman SF (1979) Monoclonal antibodies defining destinctive human T cell surface antigens. Science 206:347–349 – LeBien TW, Hurwitz RL, Kersey JH (1979) Characterization of a xenoantiserum produced against three molar KC1-solubilized antigens obtained from a non-T, non-B (pre-B) acute lymphoblastic leukemia cell line. J Immunol 122:82–88 – Levy

R (to be published) In: Cell markers and acute leukaemia. Cancer Treat Rep – Marchesi VT (ed) (1976) Membranes and neoplasia. Prog Clin Biol Res 9 – McDevitt HO (1978) Ia antigens and Ir genes. Academic Press, London New York – McMichael AJ, Pilch JR, Galfre G, Mason DY, Fabre JW, Milstein C (1979) A human thymocyte antigen defined by a hybrid myeloma monoclonal antibody. Eur J Immunol 9:205–210 – Moller G (ed) (1976) Transplant Rev 30 – Moore MAS, Broxmeyer HE, Sheridan APC, Meyers PA, Jacobsen N, Winchester RC (1980) Continuous human bone marrow culture: Ia antigen characterization of probable pluripotential stem cells. Blood 55:682–690 – Netzel B, Rodt H, Lau B, Thiel E, Haas RJ, Dörmer P, Thierfelder S (1978) Transplantation of syngeneic bone marrow incubated with leukocyte antibodies. II. Cytotoxic activity of anti-cALL globulin on leukemic cells and normal hemopoietic precursor cells in Man. Transplantation 26:157–161 – Newman RA, Sutherland R, Greaves MF (1981) The biochemical characterization of a cell surface antigen associated with acute lymphoblastic leukemia and lymphocyte precursors J Immunol, in press – Pesando JM, Ritz J, Lazarus H, Baseman Costello S, Sallan S, Schlossman SF (1979) leukemia-associated antigens in ALL. Blood 54:1240–1248 – Pesando JM, Ritz J, Levine H, Terhorst C, Lazarus H, Schlossman SF (1980) Human leukemia-associated antigen: Relation to a family of surface glycoproteins. J Immunol 124:2794–2799 – Potter VR (1978) Phenotypic diversity in experimental hepatomas: the concept of partially blocked ontogeny. Br J Cancer 38:1–23 – Reinherz EL, Kung PC, Goldstein G, Schlossman SF (1979a) Separation of functional subsets of human T cells by a monoclonal antibody. Proc Natl Acad Sci USA 76:4061–4065 – Reinherz EL, Kung PC, Goldstein G, Schlossman SF (1979b) A monoclonal antibody with selective reactivity with functionally mature human thymocytes and all peripheral human T cells. J Immunol 123:1312–1317 – Reinherz EL, Kung PC, Goldstein G, Levey RH, Schlossman SF (1980) Discrete stages of human intrathymic differentiation: Analysis of normal thymocytes and leukemic lymphoblasts of T lineage. Proc Natl Acad Sci USA 77:1588–1592 – Ritz J, Pesando JM, Notis-McConarty J, Lazarus H, Schlossman SF (1980) A monoclonal antibody to human acute lymphoblastic leukemia antigen. Nature 283:583–585 – Robinson J, Sieff C, Delia D, Edwards P, Greaves M (1981) Expression of cell surface HLA-DR, HLA-ABC and glycophorin during erythroid differentiation. Nature 289:68–71 – Ross GD, Jarowski GI, Rabellino EM, Winchester RJ (1978) The sequential appearance of Ia-like antigens and two different complement receptors during the maturation of human neutrophils. J Exp Med 147:730–744 – Rowley JD (1978) Chromosomes in leukaemia and lymphoma. Semin Haematol 15:301–319 – Schlossman SF, Chess L, Humphreys RE, Strominger JL (1976) Distribution of Ia-like molecules on the surface of normal and leukemic human cells. Proc Natl Acad Sci USA 73:1288–1292 – Shumak KH, Rachkewich RA, Greaves MF (1975) I and i antigens on normal human T and B lymphocytes and on lymphocytes from patients with chronic lymphocytic leukaemia. Clin Immunol Immunopathol 4:241–247 – Sutherland R, Smart J, Niaudet P, Greaves MF (1978) Acute lymphoblastic leukaemia associated antigen. II. Isolation and partial characterisation. Leuk Res 2:115–126 – Vogler LB, Crist WM, Bockman DE, Pearl ER, Lawton AR, Cooper MD (1978) Pre-B cell leukemia. N Engl J Med 298:872–878 – Wallach DFH (ed) (1978) Membrane anomalies of tumor cells. Karger, Basel – Winchester RJ, Ross GD, Jarowski CI, Wang CY, Halper J, Broxmeyer HE (1977) Expression of Ia-like antigen molecules on human granulocytes during early phases of differentiation. Proc Natl Acad Sci USA 74:4012–4016 – Winchester RJ, Meyers PA, Broxmeyer HE, Wang CY, Moore MAS, Kunkel HG (1978) Inhibition of human erythropoietic colony formation in culture by treatment with Ia antisera. J Exp Med 148:613–618

Haematology and Blood Transfusion Vol. 26
Modern Trends in Human Leukemia IV
Edited by Neth, Gallo, Graf, Mannweiler, Winkler
© Springer-Verlag Berlin Heidelberg 1981

Surface Antigens of Pluripotent and Committed Haemopoietic Stem Cells

G. van den Engh, B. Trask, and J. Visser

A. Introduction

Blood cells are formed from stem cells which occur in low numbers in the bone marrow and spleen. A certain fraction of the stem cells is capable of giving rise to all types of blood cells. These are defined as the "pluripotent stem cells". A more mature cell type which is still capable of extensive proliferation but which is restricted in its maturation to a single blood cell line is defined as the "committed stem cell".

In mice the two types of stem cells can be demonstrated in different assay system. The pluripotent cells are measured in the spleen colony assay or CFU-S assay (Till and McCulloch 1961). A number of in vitro culture systems are available to detect committed stem cells. These culture techniques depend on the addition of growth regulators for a particular blood cell line. In the experiments that are reported here in vitro colony forming cells (CFU-C) which grow upon exposure to CSF were studied (Bradley and Metcalf, 1965). These CFU-C are considered to represent stem cells which are committed to granulocyte/macrophage differentiation.

The differentiation from pluripotent into committed stem cells is not accompanied by a morphologic change. Cell separation studies have shown that CFU-S and CFU-C are very similar in their overall morphologic characteristics and that they cannot be separated by their physical properties.

In this paper some cell surface antigens are studied. The results show that the differentiation of pluripotent stem cells to committed cells is accompanied by changes in cell surface antigen density.

B. Materials and Methods

Details about the colony assays for haemopoietic stem cells and handling of the bone marrow cells in suspension are described elsewhere (Till and McCulloch 1961; Bradley and Metcalf 1966; Van den Engh 1974). The cytotoxicity of an antiserum was determined by incubating cells for 30 min with the serum at 0°C followed by incubation with rabbit complement for 30 min at 37°C. Cell sorting was done on a FACS II (Becton and Dickinson). The cells were labeled by incubating them with a DNP-labeled antibody followed by incubation with an FITC-labeled antibody against DNP. Except for the rabbit anti-mouse brain sera (Golub 1972), the sera were raised in congenic mouse strains (Trask and Van den Engh 1980).

C. Results

The expression of cell surface antigens on haemopoietic stem cells was investigated in two ways. In one method mouse bone marrow cells were treated with antisera and complement to see whether CFU-S and CFU-C would be affected by this treatment. Experiments of this type led to the conclusion that the CFU-S shared an antigen with mouse brain tissue. This antigen was not found on CFU-C (Golub 1972; Van den Engh and Golub 1974). The same procedure showed both CFU-S and CFU-C to be negative for the Thy-1 antigen. Thus, a potential differentiation antigen which discriminated between pluripotent and committed stem cells was described. Using the same methods, other antigenic differences between CFU-S and CFU-C were observed. K and D region antigens of the H-2 complex are abundantly expressed on the CFU-S and are present at much lower densities on CFU-C.

I region antigens were found to be absent on both cell types (Russell and Van den Engh 1979).

Some uncertainty about the proper interpretation of these results remained. The inhibition of spleen colony formation of pluripotent stem cells by antibody treatment also occurs in the absence of complement. Therefore, the failure to abolish in vitro colonies did not unequivocally demonstrate an antigenic difference.

In a second series of experiments the surface antigens of the CFU-S and CFU-C were studied by measuring the binding of fluorescent antibodies in a cell sorter. The results obtained with anti-H2 sera and anti-Thy-1 sera confirmed the conclusions which were drawn on the basis of the cytotoxic properties of the antisera. Figures 1 and 2 show the fluorescence distribution of mouse bone marrow cells after treatment with DNP-labeled α-H2 or α-Thy-1 followed by incubation with an FITC-labeled α-DNP antibody. The figures also sow the relative distribution of CFU-S that is observed after the cells are sorted into fractions of different fluorescence intensity. As in cytotoxicity studies, Thy-1 is not present in appreciable amounts on the CFU-S surface and H-2 antigens are present at high densities.

Similar experiments with rabbit anti-mouse brain serum fal to show a preferential binding of these sera to CFU-S. Figure 3 shows the fluorescence intensity profiles of bone marrow cells treated with an α-brain-DNP α-DNP-

FITC sandwich. Most bone marrow cells bind some amount of the antisera. Only a small proportion of cells can be considered to be strongly positive. When the cells are sorted according to fluorescence intensity, the CFU-S are found among the weakly positive cells. Therefore, CFU-S do bind some of the antibody, but this binding is by no means specific. The abolishment of the CFU-S in vivo must therefore be due to a particular property of the in vivo assay rather than specificity of the antiserum.

D. Discussion

The demonstration of surface antigens on pluripotent haemopoietic stem cells in the mouse (CFU-S) was found to be dependent on the method used. When the cytotoxic properties of the antisera were used to demonstrate binding of antibody, heterologous anti-mouse brain serum seemed to react specifically with CFU-S. However, in experiments in which the affinity of fluorescent-labeled anti-mouse brain serum was measured, no preferential binding to CFU-S was observed. Since the cytotoxic effect of anti-mouse brain serum does not depend on complement treatment, the most likely explanation is that CFU-S suppression is due to mechanisms which are particular for the CFU-S assay rather than due to the presence of a differentiation antigen specific for pluripotent stem cells (Trask and Van den Engh 1980).

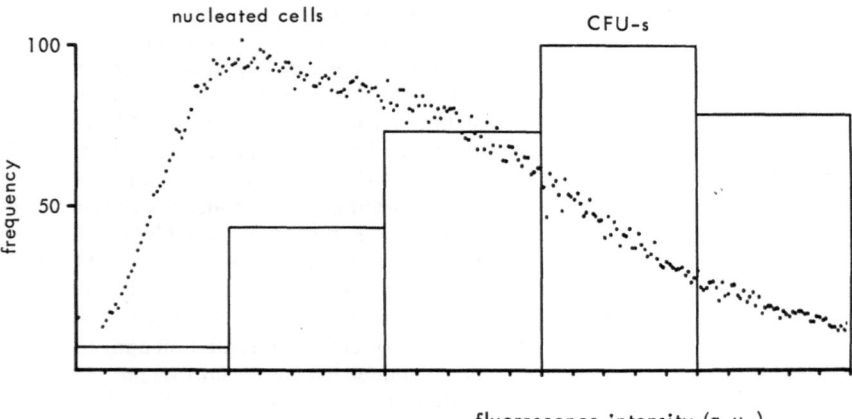

Fig. 1. Fluorescence distribution of CFU-S compared to that of viable bone marrow cells after treatment with anti-H-2-DNP-γG followed by anti-DNP-FITC. The *dots* give the fluorescent distribution of viable bone marrow cells. The *histogram* gives the numbers of CFU-S found in fractions of increasing fluorescence intensity (corrected to 100% peak value). *a.u.*, arbitrary units

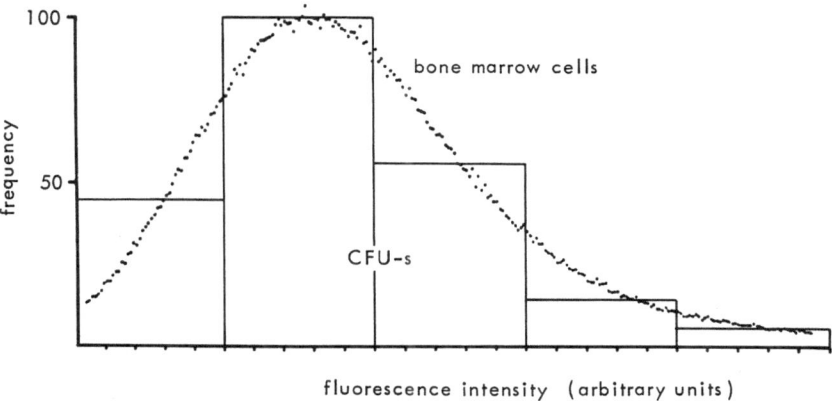

Fig. 2. Fluorescence distribution of CFU-S compared to that of viable bone marrow cells after treatment with anti-Thy-1.2-DNP-γG and 1/6 anti-DNP-FITC. The *dots* give the fluorescence of viable bone marrow cells. The *histogram* gives the numbers of CFU-S found in fractions of increasing fluirescence intensity (corrected to 100% peak value)

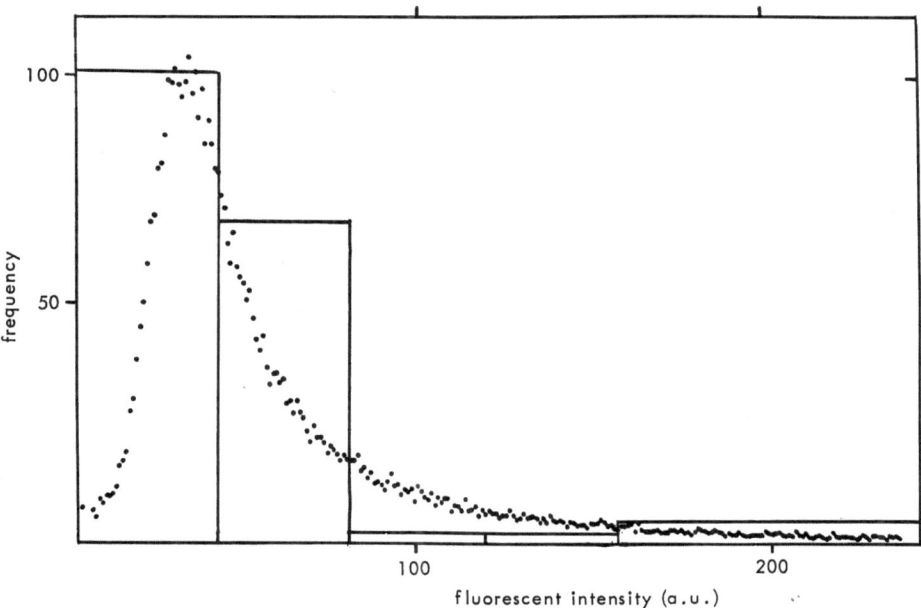

Fig. 3. Fluorescence distribution of CFU-S compared to that of viable bone marrow cells after treatment with RAMBR-DNP-γG followed by anti-DNP-FITC. The *dots* give the fluorescence distribution of viable bone marrow cells. The *histogram gives the numbers of CFU-S found in fractions of increasing fluorescence intensity (corrected to 100% peak value). a. u.,* arbitrary units

However, the results obtained with cytotoxicity test using congenic mouse sera were confirmed by flow cytometry in a cell sorter. These methods show that in the mouse Thy-1 is not present on CFU-S. CFU-S has a high density of H-2 KD antigens and are comparable in this property to spleen lymphocytes. H-2 I antigens are not yet expressed on these early cells. This pattern of antigen expression is probably species specific. Thy-1 has been reported to be expressed by the CFU-S in rat bone marrow (Goldschneider et al. 1978). This observation has been confirmed in our laboratory. In the human I region antigens have been reported to be present on CFU-C. The abundance of H-2 KD antigens may be of particular interest. Y. L. Weissman (personal communication) showed that this is also characteristic for thymic precursor cells and thus may be a common feature of the earliest blood cells of the mouse.

Acknowledgments

This work is supported in part by FUNGO.

References

Bradley TR, Metcalf D (1966) Aust J Exp Biol Med Sci 44:287–300 – Goldschreider I, Gordon LK, Morris RJ (1978) J Exp Med 148:1351–1366 – Golub ES (1972) J Exp Med 136:369 – Russell JL, van den Engh GJ (1979) Tissue Antigens 13:45–52 – Till JE, McCulloch EA (1961) Radiat Res 14:213–220 – Trask BJ, van den Engh GJ (1980) In: Baum SJ, Ledney GD (eds) Experimental hematology today. Karger, New York – Van den Engh GJ (1974) Cell Tissue Kinet 7:537–548 – Van den Engh GJ, Golub ES J Exp Med 139:1621–1627

Haematology and Blood Transfusion Vol. 26
Modern Trends in Human Leukemia IV
Edited by Neth, Gallo, Graf, Mannweiler, Winkler
© Springer-Verlag Berlin Heidelberg 1981

Human Leucocyte Antigens

P. C. L. Beverley, D. Linch, and R. E. Callard

A. Introduction

The analysis of leucocyte differentiation has been facilitated by developments in two areas of methodology: firstly, by the ability to identify and separate by surface markers cells of different lineages and stages of differentiation, and secondly, by the introduction of new functional assays, both for haemopoietic progenitor cells and mature leucocytes. In humans the production of monoclonal antibodies by somatic cell hybridisation has provided many markers for human leucocytes, whereas previously there was a paucity of reliable antisera.

We have used a number of such antisera to characterise human bone marrow progenitor cells and to trace various stages of human T lymphocyte differentiation.

B. Materials and Methods

I. Cell culture and hybridisation

Cell lines were maintained in RPMI 1640 medium supplemented with 2mM glutamine and pyruvate and 10% foetal calf serum (FCS). All fusions were carried out using the P3/NSI/1-Ag4-1 myeloma line. Hybridisation was carried out by a method slightly modified from that of Kohler and Milstein (1975) using 50% w/v polyethylene glycol (PEG 1500, BDH) in medium. Cells were cloned by limiting dilution on normal mouse peritoneal cell feeders.

II. Screening

Culture supernatants were screened on panels of target cells using an indirect I^{125} labeled antiglobulin binding assay (Beverley 1980).

III. Antisera

Serum 2A1 is an IgG1 monomorphic anti-HLA-A and anti-HLA-B serum. DA2 is a monomorphic anti-HLA-Dr serum of IgG-1 class (Brodsky et al. 1979). Anti-HLe-1 (2D1) is an IgG1 antibody derived from an immunisation with peripheral blood mononuclear cells and identifying a determinant present on T and B lymphocytes, monocytes and granulocytes (Beverley 1980, Bradstock et al, to be published). UCHT1 (T28) is an IgG1 antibody derived from an immunisation with thymocytes followed by Sezary cells.

The IgM antibody (TG-1) was derived from a mouse immunised with a thymus membrane glycoprotein fraction eluted from a Con A column (Sullivan and Beverrley, unpublished work). The antiserum stains peripheral blood neutrophils and eosinophils, but not T and B lymphocytes or thymocytes. It stains mature cells of the granulocyte lineage in the bone marrow.

Details of other monoclonal and conventional sera used are given elsewhere (Bradstock et al. to be published). Staining for TdT was kindly performed by Mr W. Verbi of the Membrane Immunology Laboratory, I.C.R.F. London.

IV. Indirect Immunofluorescence and Cell Sorting

Cells were incubated for 30 min on ice using saturating amounts (usually undilute culture supernatant) of monoclonal antiserum, washed twice in Hepes buffered RPMI 1640 with 5% FCS and stained with immunoabsorbent purified and human immunoglobulin absorbed, FITC sheep anti-mouse Ig. In some experiments an F(ab)₂ fragment of the anti-Ig was used. Controls included cells stained with second layer only or with culture supernatants from hybridomas of irrelevant specificity but of the IgG1 or IgM class. In some experiments normal sheep serum (10%) was included in the second layer to compete for Fc receptors. Cells were analysed and sorted on a Becton Dickinson FACS-I.

V. Functional Assays

Assays for PHA and Con A responsiveness were carried out in 96 well microtitre trays using 2×10^5 cells per well. Cultures were pulsed for 4 h on day 3 with I^{125} iododeoxyuridine and harvested with a MASH.

MLCs were carried out in a similar fashion using 2×10^5 2000R irradiated E rosette negative cells as stimulators. They were pulsed and harvested on day 5.

In vitro antibody responses to influenza virus were carried out as described previously (Callard 1979).

Assays for myeloid clusters and colonies and erythroid colonies and bursts were carried out as described by others (Pike and Robinson 1970; Burgess et al. 1977; Iscove 1978).

C. Results and Discussion

Because many leukaemias probably originate in the pool of bone marrow progenitor cells, even when the predominant cell type is of a more mature phenotype (Greaves and Janossy 1978), the regulation of this cell pool is clearly of interest. We have, therefore, attempted to develop a method for the isolation of these cells from bone marrow. Ficoll-hypaque separated bone marrow cells are first treated with anti-myeloid antibody (TG-1) and complement, which lyses approximately 50% of the cells, mainly the myelocytes and metamyelocytes.

The remaining cells are stained with anti-HLe-1 for cell sorting. A weakly staining fraction of cells containing less than 2% of the bone marrow nucleated cells is collected. The properties of this population are summarised in Table 1. In addition to containing the myeloid and erythroid progenitor activity, this

Table 1. Properties of cell sorted progenitor fraction

Stains weakly for HLE-1

Contains approximately 2% of marrow nucleated cells
40%–50% blast cells
3%–15% TdT+ cells
20–50× enrichment for myeloid clones[a]
20–50× enrichment for CFU-GM
20–100× enrichment for CFU-E
20–100× enrichment for BFU-E

[a] Compared to Ficoll-Hypaque isolated marrow cells

population contains significant numbers of cells with nuclear TdT (Beverley et al., unpublished work). It is likely that these are lymphoid progenitors (Greaves and Janossy 1978). Thus all these cells share a common phenotype, HLe-1±, TG-1−. Other data suggests that erythroid and myeloid progenitors are also HLA-A, -B, -C+ and HLA-DR+, although pluripotential stem cells may lack HLA-Dr (Moore et al. 1980). The ability to isolate the cells will enable us to study their heterogeneity and regulation in isolation from mature progeny.

Recent studies by us and others (Reinherz and Schlossman 1980) show that there are several phenotypically distinct populations within the thymus. Table 2 shows a speculative scheme for T cell differentiation based on double label fluorescence experiments, fluorescence activated cell sorting data and studies of tissue sections by indirect fluorescence.

We identify as the earliest step of intrathymic differentiation a small population (5%) of cells which are larger in size and lack the cortical thymocyte marker HTA-1 (McMichael et al. 1979) and the strong staining with anti-HLe-1 which is characteristic of the major cortical population. Provisionally these cells may also be equated with the earliest stage of differentiation identified by Reinherz and Schlossman (1980). In their scheme a sub-population lacking characteristic thymic antigens but carrying the OKT10 marker is detectable, though it is not yet known whether this cell is HLA− and TdT+ as is the early HTA-1−, HLe-1± cell (Bradstock et al., to be published). The exact location of these early cells within the thymus is not established, but it is suggestive that the cells found nearest to the cortical interlobular connective tissue strain most weakly with another antiserum (F10-89-4) which appears to recognise an antigen which is similar or perhaps identical to HLe-1 (Fabre, personal communication). It is provocative that our data shows that the earliest cortical cells have already lost HLA-A, -B, and -C antigens, whereas the presumed bone marrow progenitor carries these antigens. Whether this loss is the signal for emigration from the marrow or occurs after entry to the thymus is not known.

The major cortical population exhibits further heterogeneity, for example in the expression of TdT enzyme and the OKT9 marker which appears on a small sub-population of

Table 2. T cell differentiation

Antigens	Bone marrow progenitors	Early cortical cells	Late cortical cells	Medulla	Peripheral T cells
HLA	—————			—————	—————
Ia	–– ———				— — —
HLe-1	———————————————————————————————————				
TdT	———————————————————				
OKT10	———————————————————————————				
OKT9		–– ———————			
HTA-1			———————		
OKT6			———————		
OKT4[a]			———————————————————————————		
OKT5,8[a]			———————————————————————————		
OKT1,3				———————————————————	
UCHT1			· · · · · · · · · · ———————————————		

[a] In the cortex OKT 4,5 and 8 are present on all cells, while in the medulla and in the periphery T cells have either OKT 4 or OKT 5 and 8

what are probably early cells. A more dramatic difference in phenotype however is that between the cortical and medullary cells. In many respects the medullary cells approximate in phenotype peripheral T cells, having lost HTA-1 and TdT and regained HLA. With additional markers it is however possible both to distinguish medullary cells from peripheral T cells and furthermore to identify two separate lines of medullary cells which correspond to those identified in the peripheral T cell pool (Reinherz & Schlossman 1980). This is reminiscent of murine data suggesting an early commitment to different lines of T cell development. The heterogeneity of thymic phenotypes is reflected in the heterogeneity of T lineage leukaemia phenotypes which has been described (Reinherz et al. 1979). This heterogeneity also suggests that caution should be used in identifying a phenotype as not seen in normal differentiation, since small populations with rare phenotypes may have been overlooked.

I. Peripheral T Lymphocyte Differentiation

In the peripheral lymphoid system we have studied the properties of cells which carry the antigen defined by the UCHT1 monoclonal antiserum. Table 3 shows the tissue distribution of UCHT1 + cells which suggests that the antigen may be a mature T cell antigen. Additional evidence is provided by experiments in which peripheral blood mononuclear cells (PBM) were separated by sheep red blood

cell (E) rosetting into E+ and E-ve fractions before staining with UCHT1 antiserum. Table 4 shows such an experiment. While E+ cells always show high percentages of UCHT1 staining, the E− cells show few UCHT1 positive cells. More intriguingly, when PBM are separated by cell sorting into UCHT1+ and UCHT1− fractions, the unstained fraction always contains significant numbers (12%–30%) of E rosette forming cells (Table 4).

Table 3. Tissue distribution of UCHT1 positive cells

	UCHT1 (%)	E rosettes (%)
PBM (10)[a]	69	74
Thymus (5)	41	N.D.[b]
Tonsil (4)	31	24
Spleen (2)	36	25

[a] number of samples
[b] conventionally 100%

Table 4. Fractionation of peripheral blood mononuclear

	UCHT1 (%)	E rosettes (%)
Fraction		
E+	91	96
E−	5	7
UCHT1 +	98	91
UCHT1 −	<0.5	25

Functional studies of UCHT1 separated cells (Beverley & Callard in preparation) show that while the antigen positive cells provide help for an antibody response to influenza virus (Callard 1979) and respond in MLC and to PHA and Con A, the UCHT1 — cells, which include up to a third of E+ cells, fail to respond to mitogens. Thus the E+ UCHT1 — cells show as yet little evidence of mature T cell function. They may perhaps correspond to the subset of cells identified as E+, Fcγ+ and monocyte antigen positive (Reinherz et al. 1980), though we have no direct evidence for this.

On the other hand, recent data from studies of neutropenic patients suggests that a true Tγ subset does exist (Bom-van Noorloos et al. 1980). We have studied two similar patients and data from one of these are presented in Table 5. Significant numbers of the patients' PBM have the phenotype E+, UCHT1+, Fcγ+ HLA-Dr+. The presence of HLA-Dr is intriguing, since this has been shown to be expressed on a variety of activated T lymphocytes and in addition, evidence has been presented for the presence of a small subset of Fcγ and Dr+ T cells in normal individuals (Kaszubowski et al. 1980). We would thus suggest in agreement with Cooper (1980) that the E+ Fcγ+ subset includes both T and non-T cells. In the neutropenic patient described there appears to be an expansion of the Fcγ+ T cell subset. Whether the appearance of Fcγ receptors is a consequence of activation, as is that of HLA-Dr, is not yet clear.

At present our data suggest that UCHT1 is a marker for mature T cells, but it should be noted that the functional data is not yet exhaustive. In addition the studies presented here indicate that careful comparisons with existing markers (E and Fcγ receptors) of new monoclonal reagents may not only lead to new definitions for cells but allow clear identification of previously ambiguous cell types.

Acknowledgments

We should like to acknowledge the collaboration of Drs G. Janossy and J. Cawley and Mr C. Worman in this work. Mrs D. Boyle gave skilful technical assistance.

References

Beverley PCL (1980) Production and use of monoclonal antibodies in transplantation immunology. In: Touraine JL, Traeger J, Betuel H, Brochier J, Dubernard JM, Revillard JP, Triau R (eds) Transplantation and clinical immunology, vd XI. Excerpta Medica, Amsterdam, pp 87–94 – Bom-van Noorloos AA, Pegels HG, van Oers RJJ, Silberbusch J, Feltkamp-Vroom TM, Goudsmit R, Zeijlemaker WP, von dem Borne AEG, Melief CJM (1980) Proliferation of Tγ cells with killer-cell activity in two patients with neutropenia and recurrent infections. N Engl J Med 302:933–937 – Bradstock KF, Janossy G, Pizzolo G, Hoffbrand AV, McMichael A, Pilch JR, Milstein C, Beverley PCL, Bollum FJ (to be published) Subpopulations of normal and leukaemic human thymocytes: An analysis with the use of monoclonal antibodies. J Natl Cancer Inst – Brodsky FM, Parham P, Barnstaple CJ, Crumpton MJ, Bodmer WF (1979) Monoclonal antibodies for analysis of the HLA system. Immunol Rev 47:3–62 – Burgess AW, Wilson EMA, Metcalf D (1977) Stimulation by human placental conditioned medium of hemopoietic colony formation by human marrow cells. Blood 49:573–583 – Callard RE (1979) Specific in vitro antibody response to influenza virus by human blood lymphocytes. Nature 282:734–736 – Cooper MD (1980) Immunologic analysis of lymphoid tumours. N Engl J Med 302:964–965 – Greaves MF, Janossy G (1978) Patterns of gene expression and the cellular origins of human leukaemias. Biochim Biophys Acta 516:193–230 – Iscove N (1978) Regulation of proliferation and maturation at early and late stages of erythroid differentiation. In: Saunders GF (ed) Cell differentiation and neoplasia. New York, Raven, pp 195–209 – Kaszubowksi PA, Goodwin JS, Williams RC (1980) Ia antigen on the surface of a subfraction of T cells that bear Fc receptors for

Table 5. Phenotype of lymphocytes from a neutropenic patient

	Patient G.G.		Control E.Z. Whole PBM
	Whole PBM	E+ cells	
%E rosettes	80	N.D.	79
%UCHT1	80	91	68
%HLA-Dr	N.D.	62	15
%Fc γ	N.D.	70	N.D.

IgG. J Immunol 124:1075–1078 – Kohler G, Milstein C (1975) Continuous cultures of fused cells secreting antibody of predefined specificity. Nature 256:495–497 – McMichael AJ, Pilch JR, Galfre G, Mason DY, Fabre JW, Milstein C (1979) A human thymocyte antigen defined by a hybrid myeloma monoclonal antibody. Eur J Immunol 9:205–210 – Moore MAS, Broxmeyer HE, Sheridan APC, Meyers PA, Jacobsen N, Winchester RJ (1980) Continuous human bone marrow culture: Ia antigen characterization of probable pluripotential stem cells. Blood 55:682–690 – Pike BL, Robinson J (1970) Human bone marrow colony growth in agar gel. J Cell Physiol 76:77–84 – Reinherz EL, Schlossman SF (1980) The differentiation and function of human T lymphocytes. Cell 19:821–827 – Reinherz EL, Nadler LM, Sallan SE, Schlossman SE (1979) Subset derivation of T cell acute lymphoblastic leukaemia in man. J Clin Invest 64:392–397 – Reinherz EL, Moretta L, Roper M, Breard JM, Mingari MC, Cooper MD, Schlossman SF (1980) Human T lymphocyte subpopulations defined by Fc receptors and monoclonal antibodies: A comparison. J Exp Med 151:969–974

Haematology and Blood Transfusion Vol. 26
Modern Trends in Human Leukemia IV
Edited by Neth, Gallo, Graf, Mannweiler, Winkler
© Springer-Verlag Berlin Heidelberg 1981

Immunologic Subsets in Human B-Cell Lymphomas in Relation to Normal B-Cell Development

T. Godal, T. Lindmo, E. Ruud, R. Heikkilä, A. Henriksen, H. B. Steen, and P. F. Marton

A. Introduction

Human non-Hodgkin lymphomas represent a complex group of diseases with extremely varied clinical courses and a large number of histopathologic subtypes. Immunologic approaches to this group of diseases have clearly shown that a great majority of these neoplasias are derived from B-cells (see Lennert 1978). Moreover, as with other neoplasias (Fialkow 1976) they appear, with very few exceptions, to be of monoclonal origin as shown by light chain isotype restriction (Levy et al. 1977).

Various morphological entities are included in B-cell lymphomas. Although the details and the nomenclature of the histopathologic classification remain an issue of controversy, there is general agreement that some B-cell lymphomas are derived from cells of germinal centers, whereas others, such as immunoblastic lymphomas and lymphomas with plasmacytoid features, appear to be at a maturation stage close to plasma cells with high intracellular concentrations of immunoglobulin as demonstrated by immunohistochemistry (Taylor 1978). These observations suggest that B-cell lymphomas are derived from different stages of B-cell differentiation and maturation pathways.

In our laboratory we are trying to obtain more detailed information on the relationship between human B-cell lymphomas and normal B-cell differentiation and maturation pathways. The problem is approached in two ways. First, a more detailed multiparameter analysis of surface markers on human lymphomas has been undertaken. Second, attempts are being made to trigger these lymphomas to proliferate and differentiate in vitro. Data from both these approaches will be summarized in the present paper. Our studies clearly demonstrate that human B-cell lymphomas can be divided into immunologically distinct subsets. Moreover, such lymphomas may be triggered to proliferate and differentiate as measured by immunoglobulin (Ig) synthesis by anti-Ig, usually in combination with tumor promotor (TPA).

B. Materials and methods

I. Lymphoma Biopsies

The studies to be reported have been carried out on cell suspensions from lymphoma biopsies containing more than 50% B-cells staining monoclonally for surface immunoglobulin (sIg). Histologic classification was performed according to the Kiel classification system (Lennert 1978).

II. Surface Markers and Capping

For identification of sIg, anti human Ig sera labeled with fluorescein isothiocyanate (FITC) were obtained from Dakopatts (Copenhagen, Denmark), with the exception of FITC-labelled anti-δ which was obtained from Behringwerke (Marburg, West Germany) to be described elsewhere (Godal et al., to be published). Complement receptors (CR) were identified by standard procedures with C_5-deficient mouse serum in a blind fashion (Godal et al. 1978). Capping was carried out as described by Elson et al. (1973).

III. Single Cell Flow Cytometry

Two parameter flow cytometric measurements of light scatter and fluorescence from lymphocytes stained with FITC-conjugated antisera were performed with a laboratory-built flow cytometer (FCM) (Lindmo and Steen 1977). The method will be described in detail elsewhere (Godal et al., to be published).

IV. Cell and Nuclear Volumetry

For determination of the cellular volume distributions, the cells were suspended in 10 ml counting solution (isotone to Coulter electronics) and immediately measured by means of a modified Coulter counter (Steen and Lindmo 1978). Nuclear volume distributions were obtained by the same procedure using a counting solution which removes cytoplasm and fixes the nuclei in acid formaldehyde (Stewart and Ingram 1967).

V. Lymphocyte Stimulation

For stimulation with anti-Ig and/or TPA (12-O-Tetra-decanoyl-phorbol-13-acetate) (Midland Corporation, United States), cells were cultured in microtitration plates with 2×10^5 cells per well with RPMI 1640 medium and 10% fetal calf serum final concentration (Henriksen et al. 1980).

VI. Ion Flux

Cellular uptake of ^{86}Rb, which is assumed to reflect membrane transport of potassium, was carried out essentially as described elsewhere (Godal et al. 1978; Iversen 1976).

C. Results

I. Immunological Subsets in Human B-Cell Lymphomas

Surface concentration of Ig was determined by FCM analysis of cells stained under saturating conditions. The data were expressed as mean intensity for the positive cells as expressed relative to the mean intensity of unstained cells.

As shown in Table 1, different histologic and immunologic groups showed large variations

with regard to relative amounts of sIg. Thus, centroblastic/centrocytic lymphomas of the nodular type expressing IgG had only about one fifth of the sIg of lymphomas of the same histological type expressing IgM. Similarly, lymphocytic lymphomas or lymphoplasmacytoid lymphomas had clearly lower concentrations of sIgM. Similar findings were made with anti-light chains in a radioimmunoassay. Moreover, as shown in Fig. 1 the relative amounts of IgD to IgM on lymphoma cells expressing both these isotypes varied considerably from one lymphoma to the other, i.e., from a 1:1 ratio down to a 1:6 ratio. The variation was particularly striking within the nodular group.

Further evidence for immunological heterogeneity among human B-cell lymphomas was uncovered by CR and capping studies. Only 26 of 51 lymphomas expressed CR, and a very close association between the presence of CR and capping with anti-μ was found. Out of 45 lymphomas tested by both parameters, 42 could be allocated into groups positive or negative in both test systems, whereas only two were clearly positive in one test system and negative in the other. This relationship between expression of complement receptors and capping was specific to sIgM, as capping with anti-δ has been found positive irrespective of whether IgM was capped or not. Moreover, sIgG positive lymphomas revealed capping with anti-γ, whereas all these lymphomas tested so far lack CR.

Based on these combined data we can at present distinguish between five immunological subsets in B-cell lymphomas. The relationship between these groups and the histopathologic classification is shown in Table 2. All five immunologic groups were found among the

Histologic type	Mean intensity, positive subpopulation	
	μ	γ
Centroblastic/centrocytic (nodular type) (n=4)		4.8±0.5[a]
Centroblastic/centrocytic (nodular type) (n=4)	25 ±7	
Centroblastic/centrocytic (diffuse type) (n=3)	24 ±5	
Lymphoplasmacytoid (n=3)	10 ±4	
Lymphocytic (n=3)	6.4±0.8	

Table 1. The relative amounts of μ and γ heavy chains on lymphocytes from various histologic types of B-cell lymphomas by flow cytometric analysis

[a] ±s.e. (mean)

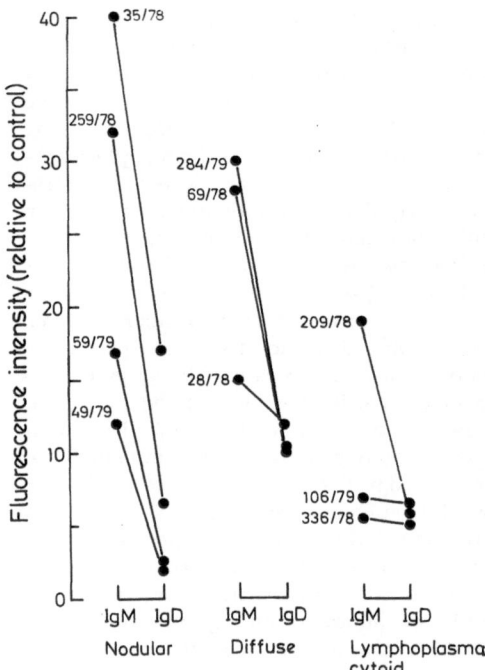

Fig. 1. The relative amounts of μ and δ heavy chains on lymphocytes from nodular and diffuse centroblastic/centrocytic lymphomas and lymphoplasmacytoid lymphomas as assessed by flow cytometric analysis. The *lines* connect the results with anti-μ and anti-δ on each lymphoma tested. Cell suspension (biopsy) number is shown

these two, indicating a more limited heterogeneity with regard to immunologic types, but the numbers are here too small to allow definite conclusions to be drawn.

II. Responses of Lymphoma Cells to TPA and Anti-Ig

Among various substances tested which are known to induce differentiation in erythroleukemia cells, such as di-methyl-sulphoxide, we have found that TPA (10^{-7} M) induced striking changes in a majority of lymphomas. These alterations include a rapid enlargement in cellular volumes which can be measured within hours after exposure and the induction of cytoplasmic protrutions). In about 50% of the lymphomas nuclear volume also increases after addition of TPA. When anti-Igs are added to TPA, mitogenic effects can be observed as measured by thymidine incorporation and FCM. The mitogenic effects have a clear dose-response relationship to anti-Ig, with peak responses ranging from 2.5 to 250 µg per ml final concentration. The response shows a sharp peak on day 2 or 3. Among anti-Igs anti-μ most commonly gave a positive proliferative response (8 out of 14 cases), whereas 4 out of 11 responded to anti-δ and only one out of five to anti-γ.

By FCM analyses simultaneously measuring DNA and Ig contents in cells it can be clearly shown that lymphomas also often start to synthesize Ig. Moderate increases were found with TPA alone, whereas this was greatly enhanced by anti-Ig. Cells staining most strongly for Ig are found both with a G_1 and G_2

nodular lymphomas, whereas in contrast all six lymphomas examined in the diffuse lymphocytic group belonged to one immunologic group. The other histopathologic groups fall between

Table 2. Relationship between immunologic subtypes and the histopathologic classification in human B-cell lymphomas

	Lymphocytic (diffuse)	Centroblastic/ centrocytic (diffuse)	Centroblastic/ centrocytic (nodular)	Centroblastic (diffuse)	Immunoblastic (diffuse)	Lymphoplasma cytoid (diffuse)	Total
IgM, IgD, CR[a]		4[c]	4			3	11 (22%)
IgM, IgD[b]			3				3 (6%)
IgM, CR[a]	6	1	4	1	1	2	15 (30%)
IgM[b]		2	4	3	2	4	15 (30%)
IgG		1[d]	5				6 (12%)
Total	6 (12%)	8 (16%)	20 (40%)	4 (8%)	3 (6%)	9 (8%)	50

[a] The great majority also positive for capping with anti-μ
[b] The great majority negative for capping with anti-μ
[c] One in addition expressing sIgG
[d] Also expressing sIgM

content of DNA, showing that at least in many cells DNA synthesis and Ig synthesis may occur simultaneously.

By studying ion flux with anti-Igs we have found that early ^{86}Rb uptake is closely associated with a proliferative response to anti-Ig plus TPA. This uptake can be measured within minutes after addition of anti-Ig and takes place without TPA, whereas there was no correlation between ^{86}Rb-uptake and anti-Ig induced capping.

D. Discussion

The present study demonstrates that human B-cell lymphomas can be subdivided into a number of distinct immunologic subsets. These subsets correspond only partially to the histopathologic classification. Some histologic groups comprise several distinct immunologic subsets. The prognostic significance of immunologic subclassification in B-cell lymphomas remains to be determined. The material is enlarged and will be followed up to answer this question.

Our findings raise a number of questions with regard to the B-cell maturation and differentiation processes. Of particular interest in this regard is sIgD. Studies based on cell sorting (Black et al. 1978; Zan-Bar et al. 1979) and parental administration of anti-IgD serum in mice (Dresser and Parkhouse 1978) have shown that IgD positive cells are involved in primary responses but that IgD becomes lost and is not present on mature memory cells. In our study IgD was found only on a proportion of nodular lymphomas derived from germinal center cells. Moreover, the mean amounts of IgD on those lymphomas which were positive were shown by FCM to vary from relatively strongly positive to almost negative. These findings suggest that IgD becomes lost during the B-cell maturation processes taking place in germinal centers. It is interesting to note that a dissociation between capping of IgM and IgD was also found on a distinct subset of nodular lymphomas, raising the possibility that IgD plays a distinct role in germinal centers.

The lymphomas were also found to be heterogenous with regard to CR. Thus, all lymphomas expressing sIgG only were CR negative, whereas CR positive and CR negative lymphomas were found both in the IgM + IgD and IgM groups. The most likely explana-

tion for these findings would be that CR may also be lost during B-cell maturation. This view is supported by experimental data from studies of thoracic duct lymphocytes, where Mason (1976) found 19S AFC precursors exclusively in the CR positive fraction, whereas 7S AFC precursors were found both in the CR positive and CR negative population. Since nodular lymphomas of germinal center cell origin showed this CR heterogeneity, our findings would indicate that CR may also be lost during B-cell maturation taking place in germinal centers. Thus, our data would be compatible with a differentiation (bifurcation) process taking place in germinal centers, by which B-cells loose IgD but retain CR for the generation of recirculating sIgM and CR positive memory cells, whereas the loss of CR may be an event along another maturation pathway involving a switch to sIgG.

Lymphocytic lymphomas would be candidates a neoplastic counterparts to recirculating sIgM and CR positive memory cells. These lymphoma cells are different from chronic lymphocytic leukemia (CLL) cells (Godal et al. 1978) because they cap with anti-IgM.

The role of CR negative B-cells remains unclear, but since CR negative cells are found in immunoblastic lymphomas which have high intracellular concentrations of Ig (Landaas et al., in press; Stein 1978; Taylor 1978) and also plasma cells are known to lack CR (Burns et al. 1979), these cells may represent precursors to antibody-producing cells. The lack of capping of sIgM in these cells is interesting. This would make them suitable as antigen-presenting cells to T-cells, which are essential for maturation to antibody secretion (Rohrer and Lynch 1979) and possibly to other B-cells for producing antibodies of higher affinity.

Plasma cell development must also take place by events not involving germinal center formation, because the appearance of antibody-producing plasma cells occurs before germinal center formation (White et al. 1975). In fact, the appearance of germinal centers coincides with the occurrence of circulating immune complexes (White et al. 1975), and immune complexes are highly effective in generating memory cells (Klaus 1979). The lymphoplasmacytoid group is interesting in this regard. Histopathologically, these lymphomas show morphologic evidence of maturation towards plasma cells. This can also be demonstrated with immunohistochemical methods (Landaas et al., in press; Stein 1978) by which cytoplasmic immunoglobulin can easily be detected. This group comprised 3 immunologic subsets (sIgM, sIgD, and CR positive; IgM and CR positive; only IgM positive), demonstrating that plasma cells may develop from different subsets of B-cells. The sIgM, sIgD, and CR positive cells have the surface characteristics of B-cells involved in a primary response and could reflect a plasma cell maturation pathway branching off prior to germinal center formation.

The present study revealed definite differences with regard to the concentration of sIg. The highest concentrations were found in positive lymphomas of follicular center cell origin, whereas positive lymphomas within the same category had a substantially lower sIg concentration. Similarly, low concentrations were also present on lymphocytic lymphomas. As has been discussed above, both these types of lymphomas may correspond to B-cells at a higher maturation stage. Their lower concentrations of sIg may therefore represent a maturation-associated loss of sIg. The pathway leading to sIgG positive cells may be associated with affinity maturation processes (Herzenberg et al. 1980).

A hypothetical picture of the relationship between the different lymphomas and normal B-cell maturation and differentiation as discussed above is outlined in Fig. 2.

Our findings that B-cell lymphomas can be triggered to proliferate and synthesize Ig in vitro by anti-Ig, usually in combination with TPA, represent a new approach which may help in delineating these relationships and put them on a firmer basis. It has already been shown that lymphocytic lymphomas may differentiate towards plasma cells.

Such studies may also provide important information with regard to mechanisms of B-cell triggering. Our studies so far have clearly shown that sIg of either the μ, γ, or δ type may deliver transmembrane signals giving rise to an increased influx of K^+ and in concert with other agents, especially TPA, induce proliferation and differentiation in neoplastic B-cell arrested at different stages of differentiation.

References

Black SJ, van der Loo W, Loken MR, Herzenberg LA (1978) Expression of IgD by murine lymphocytes. Loss of surface IgD indicates maturation of memory B-cells. J Exp Med 147:984–996 – Burns GF, Worman CP, Roberts BE, Raper CGL, Barker CR, Cawleys JC (1979) Terminal B cell development as seen in different human myelomas and related disorders. Clin Exp Immunol 35:180–189 Dresser DW, Parkhouse RME (1978) The effect of the parental administration of rabbit anti-(mouse)-IgD serum on the immune response of mice to sheep erythrocytes. Immunology 35:1027–1036 – Elson

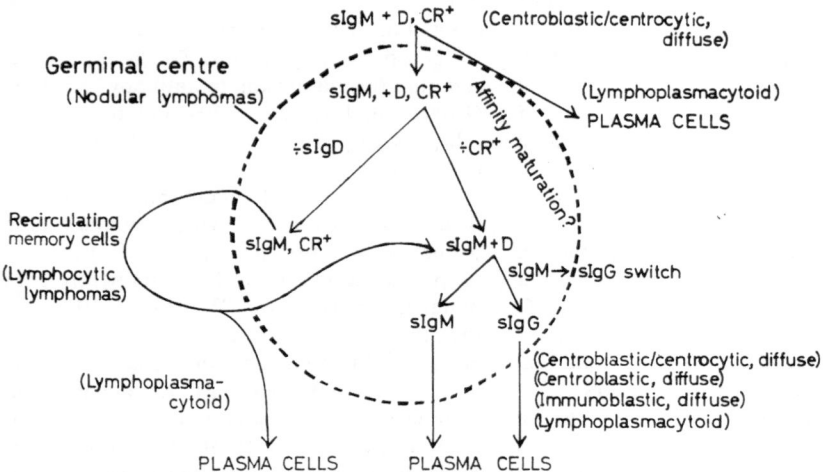

Fig. 2. Simplified and hypothetical scheme of human B-cell lymphomas in relation to normal B-cell development. The scheme suggests that plasma cell maturation may take place from different levels of B-cell differentiation. The position of different histologic types of lymphomas is indicated in brackets

CJ, Singh J, Taylor RB (1973) The effect of capping by antiimmunoglobulin antibody on the expression of cell surface immunoglobulin and on lymphocytic leukemic lymphocytes. Scand J Immunol 2:143–149 – Fialkow PJ (1976) Clonal origin of human tumors. Biochim Biophys Acta 458:283–321 – Godal T, Henriksen A, Iversen J-G, Landaas TØ, Lindmo T (1978) Altered membrane-associated functions in chronic lymphocytic leukemia cells. Int J Cancer 21:561–569 – Godal T, Lindmo T, Marton PF, Landaas TØ, Langholm R, Høie J, Abrahamsen AF (to be published) Immunological subsets in human B-cell lymphomas – Henriksen A, Godal T, Landaas TØ (1980) Mitogenic effect on human lymphocytes of insolubilized anti-immunoglobulins. I. Specificity of the stimulating agent. J Immunol 124:921–925 – Herzenberg LA, Black SJ, Tokuhisa T, Herzenberg LA (1980) Memory B cells at successive stages of differentiation. J Exp Med 151:1071–1087 – Iversen J-G (1976) Unidirectional K⁺ fluxes in rat thymocytes stimulated by concanavalin A. J Cell Physiol 89:267–276 – Klaus GGB (1979) Generation of memory cells. III. Antibody class requirements for the generation of B-memory cells by antigen-antibody complexes. Immunology 37:345–351 – Landaas TØ, Godal T, Marton PF, Kvaløy S, Langholm R, Lindmo T, Jørgensen OG, Høst H (1981) Cell-associated immunoglobulin in human non-Hodgkin lymphomas. A comparative study of surface immunoglobulin on cells in suspension and cytoplasmic immunoglobulin by immunohistochemistry. Acta path microbiol scand, sect A (in press) – Lennert K (ed) (1978) Malignant lymphomas other than Hodgkin's disease. Springer, Berlin Heidelberg New York – Levy R, Warnke R, Dorfman RF, Haimovich J (1977) The monoclonality of human B-cell lymphomas. J Exp Med 145:1014–1028 – Lindmo T, Steen HB (1977) Flow cytometric measurement of the polarization of fluorescence from intracellular fluorescein in mammalian cells. Biophys J 18:173–187 – Mason DW (1976) The requirement for C3 receptors on the precursors of 19S and 7S antibody-forming cells. J Exp Med 143:1111–1121 – Rohrer JW, Lynch RG (1979) Immunoregulation of localized and disseminated murine myeloma: Antigen-specific regulation of MOPC-315 stem cell proliferation and secretory cell differentiation. J Immunol 123:1083–1087 – Steen HB, Lindmo T (1978) Cellular and nuclear volume during the cell cycle of NHIK 3025 cells. Cell Tissue Kinet 11:69–81 – Stein H (1978) The immunologic and immunochemical basis for the Kiel classification. In: Lennert K (ed) Malignant lymphomas other than Hodgkin's disease, part 6. Springer, Berlin Heidelberg New York – Stewart CC, Ingram M (1967) A method for counting phytohemagglutinin-stimulated lymphocytes. Blood 29:628–639 – Taylor CR (1978) Immunocytochemical methods in the study of lymphoma and related conditions. J Histochem Cytochem 26:496–512 – White RG, Henderson DC, Eslami MB, Nielsen KH (1975) Localization of a protein antigen in the chicken spleen. Effect of various manipulative procedures on the morphogenesis of the germinal centre. Immunology 28:1–21 – Zan-Bar I, Strober S, Vitetta ES (1979) The relationship between surface immunoglobulin isotype and immune function of murine B lymphocytes. IV. Role of IgD-bearing cells in the propagation of immunologic memory. J Immunol 123:925–930

Haematology and Blood Transfusion Vol. 26
Modern Trends in Human Leukemia IV
Edited by Neth, Gallo, Graf, Mannweiler, Winkler
© Springer-Verlag Berlin Heidelberg 1981

Clones of Murine Functional T Cells

H. Hengartner

A. Introduction

The serologic and biochemical analysis of different classes of T cells, such as cytotoxic, helper, and suppressor T cells, has been impeded by the lack of pure populations of functional T cell lines. None of the established well characterized AKR thymoma and lymphoma T cell lines exhibit any T cell functions besides the expression of serologic T cell surface markers. To date all attempts to transform functional T cells using oncogenic viruses have failed. Although several groups reported T cell hybridomas which secrete specific and nonspecific helper or suppressor factors (Kontiainen et al. 1978; Taniguchi et al. 1979; Taussig et al. 1979), most of the described hybridomas are not very stable and have to be subcloned and selected for activity over short periods. During the past 3 years, however, several groups have succeeded in establishing and cloning functional human and mouse T cells (reviewed in Schreier et al. 1980, Immunological Reviews, Vol. 51, Ed. Möller, G., Munksgaard, Kopenhagen).

Functional T cells were expanded in vitro after in vivo immunization and kept under optimal tissue culture conditions for the appropriate T cell type. Alloreactive proliferating T cells can be kept functional by periodical restimulation using irradiated spleen cells (Fathman and Nabholz 1977), whereas the growth of cytotoxic or helper T cells after initial antigen specific stimulation, in some cases in vivo and then in vitro, is strictly dependent on the presence of T cell growth factors in the culture medium (Gillis and Smith 1977).

All attempts to establish long-term cultures of cloned or uncloned T cells appears to depend upon the following principles:

1. Expansion of the antigen-specific T cells by in vivo immunization;
2. Secondary immunization in vitro followed by the biologic assay for the appropriate T cell specificity; and
3. Maintaining the functional T cells either by periodical restimulation or by supplementing the cultures with T cell growth factor.

To prevent overgrowth by T cells which are not antigen specific, it is important to clone the cells at this point and select those clones which exhibit the biologic activity desired.

In our laboratory we have been dealing over the past 4 years with the cloning of T cells of the following types: alloreactively proliferating T cells (Fathman and Hengartner 1978, 1979; Hengartner and Fathman 1980), H-Y antigen (14) and hapten (9) specific H-2 restricted cytotoxic T cells in the mouse.

B. Alloreactive T Cells

Alloreactive T cells can be generated in an ordinary mixed lymphocyte culture where lymph node cells are stimulated by X-ray-irradiated spleen cells. Every 10 to 14 days the viable responder T cells are diluted into fresh medium and restimulated by X-ray-irradiated stimulator spleen cells. Fathman et al. (1977) described the following two long term culture systems: A/J anti-C57BL/6 (A[B6]) and A/J anti-(C57BL/6 × A/J)F₁ (A[B6A]). The bulk cultures consisted mainly of haplotype-specific proliferating T cells lacking any cytotoxic activity. After three to four restimulations, the specificity of the two systems may be analysed by stimulating 10^4 responder T cells with 10^6 X-ray-irradiated spleen cells of different haplotypes. The stimulatory effect is measured by ^{3}H-thymidine uptake during[a] 16-h period 48 or 72 h after the initiation of the cultures (Fathman et al. 1977).

The initial bulk culture A(B6) exhibited identical stimulation indexes against C57BL/6 and (C57BL/6×A/J)F$_1$ stimulator cells, and the stimulation indexes against third party stimulator cells stayed constant even after the 20th restimulation.

The bulk culture A(B6A) showed a stimulation index against (C57BL/6×A/J)F$_1$ stimulator cells which was twice as high as that against the C57BL/6 stimulator cells, suggesting a unique F$_1$ MLR determinant on the semiallogeneic stimulator cells. These proliferating T cells could be cloned in soft agar. The responder T cells were stimulated in suspension for 24 h and then seeded on soft agar in a petri dish. After 5 days colonies were picked from the agar and subsequently expanded in 0.2-ml, 2-ml, 15-ml and 45-ml cultures by restimulation with X-ray-irradiated stimulator spleen cells every 10 to 14 days. Between two restimulations the cloned alloreactive T cells undergo an activation, a proliferative, and a resting phase. The continous stimulation by allogeneic stimulator cells in vitro leads to this expansion of the alloreactive T cells.

The analysis of such cultures clearly demonstrated the existence of an F$_1$ MLR determinant expressed on semiallogeneic stimulator cells which is absent on C57BL/6 cells. The analysis of such F$_1$ alloreactive proliferating T cell clones using different recombinant F$_1$ stimulator spleen cells further demonstrated the existence of at least four different clone types with different fine specificities (Fathman and Hengartner 1979).

In the A(B6) bulk cultures we have demonstrated through cloning and subcloning the existence of a T cell clone type which can be stimulated only by C57BL/6 stimulator cells but not by the semiallogeneic (C57BL/6 ×A/J)F$_1$ stimulator cells. This suggests the expression of a unique MLR determinant on the homozygous C57BL/6 stimulator cells (Hengartner and Fathman 1980).

The alloreactive T cells can be thawed and restimulated after freezing and storage in liquid nitrogen. The chromosome number of the clones is 40 and the chromosomes do not show any obvious abnormalities.

Fathman and Weissman (1980) injected 10[7] A/J cells of one of the F$_1$ specific clones (clone A [B6A] 1-1] intraperitoneally into A/J, C57BL/6, and (C57BL/6×A/J)F$_1$ animals. After 4 weeks the F$_1$ animals exhibited enlarged lymph nodes, and the H-2 typing demonstrated the A/J origin of a large number of the lymph node cells. This clearly demonstrated the generation of a T cell lymphoma by exposing proliferating T cells to a constant stimulatory environment in the (C57BL/6 ×A/J)F$_1$ mouse.

C. Cytotoxic T Cells

The MHC-restricted cytotoxic T cells against the H-Y antigen and the hapten sp were generated in secondary mixed lymphocyte cultures 14 days after the primary immunization in vivo. Analogous to the alloreactive T cells, the cytotoxic T cells were cloned in soft agar or under conditions of limited dilution (Nabholz et al. 1980; Von Böhmer et al. 1979). In contrast to alloreactive proliferating T cells, cytotoxic T cells have to be kept in medium containing T cell growth factor. We routinely use 10% supernatant of ConA-activated (48 h) rat spleen cells in the culture medium as a source for T cell growth factor.

The growth of cloned cytotoxic T cells is strictly dependent on T cell growth factors and cells usually die within hours in regular medium. Cytotoxic T cells can not be stimulated by the specific antigens, which are X-ray-irradiated syngeneic male spleen cells or haptenated syngeneic spleen cells (Nabholz et al. 1980; Von Böhmer et al. 1979). The chromosome number of such cells is higher than 40 and occasionally even metacentric chromosomes can be demonstrated.

D. Summary

Using techniques of cloning, it became possible to generate alloreactively proliferating (Hengartner and Fathman (1980)), cytotoxic (Von Böhmer et al. 1979), and helper (Schreier and Tees 1980; Von Böhmer et al. 1979; Watson 1979) T cells. The homogeneity of functional T cells makes it possible to start to tackle problems such as the chemical nature of the T cell receptor and the organization of genes which lead to the T cell differentiation and specificity. The specific proliferation or killing observed in a complex mixture of cells after activation in a mixed lymphocyte culture can be dissected by cloning. Utilizing such clones, it might also be possible to study the phenomenon of specific activation and the still obscure phenomenon of cytolytic activity.

References

Fathman CG, Hengartner H (1978) Clones of alloreactive T cells. Nature 272:617 – Fathman CG, Hengartner H (1979) Cross-reactive mixed lymphocyte reaction determinants recognized by cloned alloreactive T cells. Proc Natl Acad Sci USA 76:5863 – Fathman CG, Nabholz M (1977) In vitro secondary mixed leucocyte reaction II. Interaction MLR determinants expressed on F_1 cells. Eur J Immunol 7:370 – Fathman CG, Weissman IL (1980) Production of alloreactive T cell lymphomas. Nature 283:404 – Gillis S, Smith KA (1977) Long term cultures of tumor specific cytotoxic T cells. Nature 268:154 – Hengartner H, Fathman CG (1980) Clones of alloreactive T cells. Immunogenetics 10:175 – T cell stimulating growth factors. Immunol Rev 51 (1980) – Kontiainen S, Simpson E, Bohrer E, Beverley PC, Herzenberg LA, Fitzpatrick WC, Vogt P, Torano A, McKenzie IFC, Feldman M (1978) T cell lines producing antigen-specific suppressor factor. Nature 274:477 – Nabholz M, Conzelmann A, Acuto O, North M, Haas W, Pohlit H, von Böhmer H, Hengartner H, Mach JP, Engers H, Johnson JP (1980) Established murine cytolytic T cell lines as tools for a somatic cell genetic analysis of T cell functions. Immunol Rev 51:125 – Schreier MH, Tees R (1980) Clonal induction of helper T cells: Conversion of specific signals into nonspecific signals. Int Arch Allergy Appl Immunol 61:227 – Schreier MH, Anderson J, Lernhardt W, Melchers F (1980) Antigen-specific T-helper cells stimulate H-2 compatible and incompatible B cell blasts polyclonally. J Exp Med 151:194 – Taniguchi M, Saito T, Tada T (1979) Antigen-specific suppressive factor produced by a transplantable I-J bearing T cell hybridoma. Nature 274:555 – Taussig MJ, Corvalàn JRF, Binns RM, Holliman A (1979) Production of H-2 related suppressor factor by a hybrid T cell line. Nature 277:305 – Von Böhmer H, Hengartner H, Nabholz M, Lernhardt W, Schreier MH, Haas W (1979) Fine specificity of a continously growing killer cell clone specific for H-Y antigen. Eur J Immunol 9:592 – Watanabe T, Kimoto M, Maruyama S, Kishimoto T, Yamamura Y (1978) Establishment of T cell hybrid cell line secreting IgE class specific suppressor factor. J Immunol 121:2113 – Watson J (1979) Continuous proliferation of murine antigen-specific helper T lymphocytes in culture. J Exp Med 150:1510

Haematology and Blood Transfusion Vol. 26
Modern Trends in Human Leukemia IV
Edited by Neth, Gallo, Graf, Mannweiler, Winkler
© Springer-Verlag Berlin Heidelberg 1981

Marker Profiles of Leukemia-Lymphoma Cell Lines

J. Minowada

During the past decade increasing number of monoclonal human leukemia-lymphoma cell lines that exhibit a relatively stable marker profile of original leukemia-lymphoma have been established. In our earlier study with 28 leukemia-lymphoma cell lines (Minowada 1978) marker profiles of these cell lines were viewed as reflecting a pattern of normal hematopoietic cell differentiation. The present study extends and modifies the attempt based on the analysis of a total of 50 leukemia lymphoma cell lines.

A. Materials and Methods

Establishment and characterization by the multiple marker analysis for each cell line have been described earlier (Greaves et al. 1978; Minowada 1978).

B. Results and Discussion

Table 1 summarizes marker profiles of a total of 50 leukemia-lymphoma cell lines (Nos. 1–50). For our convenience, these 50 cell lines are divided into three distinct groups, namely T-cell, B-cell, or non-T, non-B cell groups. The T-cell line was characterized by the presence of T-cell specific antigen, but negative for Ia-antigen, myelomonocyte antigen (MAg-I), immunoglobulins (SmIg, CyIg), and stimulating activity in "one-way" mixed leukocyte reaction. The B-cell line was characterized by the presence of immunoglobulin (monoclonal isotype on each leukemia lymphoma line), but was negative for T-cell antigen and MAg-I. The third group, i.e., the non-T, non-B cell line, is heterogeneous and characterized by the absence of both T- and B-cell markers. Figure 1 is such a scheme based on primarily the marker profiles of leukemia-lymphoma cell lines. All cell lines are thus assigned as follows: The cell lines, Nos. 1–6, are T-blast I; Nos. 7–14 are T-blast II; No. 15 is T-cell; Nos. 16–20 are pre-B-cell; Nos. 21–29 are B-blast I; Nos. 30–39 are B-blast II; Nos. 40–42 are plasma cell; Nos. 43–46 are "lymphoid precursor"; No. 47 is promyelocyte; No. 48 is myeloblast; No. 49 is "myeloid precursor"; and No. 50 is "erythroid precursor".

The attempt in this study is perhaps over simplified and in part speculative. Nevertheless, in view of similar results by others (Greaves et al. 1978; Minowada 1978; Nilsson 1978) it would provide some rational thoughts toward not only cellular origins of leukemia-lymphoma but also insight into normal hematopoietic cell differentiation.

Acknowledgments

This study was supported by USPHS grants CA-14413 and CA-17609 and contract 31-CB-74165 from the National Cancer Institute, United States.

References

Greaves MF, Janossy G, Francis G, Minowada J (1978) Membrane phenotypes of human leukemic cells and leukemic cell lines: Clinical correlates and biological implications. In: Clarkson B, Marks PA, Till JE (eds) Differentiation of normal hematopoietic cells. Cold Spring Harbor Laboratory, Cold Spring Harbor, pp 823–841 – Minowada J (1978) Markers of human leukemia-lymphoma cell lines

Table 1. Origin and marker profile of leukemia-lymphoma cell lines[a]

No. Cell line	Origin	E	EA	EAC	SmIg	CyIg	T-Ag	Ia	cALL	MAg-I	TdT	EBV	Chr	MLC-S
T-cell leukemia lymphoma lines														
1 CCRF-CEM	ALL	−	−	−	−	−	+	−	+	−	+	−	A	−
2 RPMI 8402	ALL	−	−	+	−	−	+	−	+	−	+	−	A	−
3 HPB-ALL	ALL	+	−	+	−	−	+	−	+	−	+	−	A	−
4 DND-41	ALL	+	−	+	−	−	+	−	+	−	+	−	A	−
5 HPB-MLT	ATL	+	−	+	−	−	+	−	+	−	+	−	A	−
6 HD-Mar-2	?HD	+	−	+	−	−	+	−	+	−	+	−	A	−
7 MOLT 1–4	ALL	+	−	+	−	−	+	−	−	−	+	−	A	−
8 JM	ALL	+	−	+	−	−	+	−	−	−	+	−	A	−
9 MOLT-11	ALL	+	−	+	−	−	+	−	−	−	+	−	A	−
10 P12/Ich	ALL	+	−	+	−	−	+	−	−	−	n.t.	−	A	−
11 TALL-1	ATL	+	−	−	−	−	+	−	−	−	+	−	A	−
12 MOLT-10	ALL	−	−	−	−	−	+	−	−	−	+	−	A	−
13 CCRF-HSB-2	ALL	−	−	−	−	−	+	−	−	−	−	−	A	−
14 Peer	ALL	−	−	−	−	−	+	−	−	−	−	−	A	−
15 SKW-3	CLL	+	−	−	−	−	+	−	−	−	−	−	A	−
B-cell leukemia lymphoma lines														
16 NALM-1	CML	−	−	−	−	+	−	+	+	−	+	−	A/Ph'	+
17 NALM 6–15	ALL	−	−	−	−	+	−	+	+	−	+	−	A	+
18 NALM 17,18	ALL	−	−	−	−	+	−	+	+	−	+	−	A	+
19 KOPN 1–8	ALL	−	−	−	−	+	−	+	+	−	−	−	A	+
20 HPB-Null	ALL	−	−	−	−	+	−	+	+	−	−	−	A	+
21 U-698-M	LS	−	−	−	+	−	−	+	+	−	−	−	A	+
22 EB-3	BL	−	−	−	+	+	−	+	+	−	−	+	A	+
23 Ramos	BL	−	−	−	+	+	−	+	+	−	−	−	A	+
24 DG-75	BL	−	−	−	+	+	−	+	+	−	−	−	A	+
25 Chevallier	BL	−	−	−	+	+	−	+	+	−	−	−	A	+
26 Raji	BL	−	−	+	+	+	−	+	+	−	−	+	A	+
27 HR1K	BL	−	+	−	+	+	−	+	+	−	−	+	A	+
28 Daudi	BL													
29 DND-39	BL	−	−	+	+	+	−	+	+	−	−	−	A	+
30 BALL-1	ALL	−	+	−	+	+	−	+	−	−	−	−	A	+
31 BALM 1,2	ALL	−	−	+	+	+	−	+	−	−	−	+	A	+
32 BALM 3–5	LS	−	−/+	−	+	+	−	+	−	−	−	−	A	+
33 Ogun	BL	−	−	+	+	+	−	+	−	−	−	+	A	+
34 B35M	BL	−	−	+	+	+	−	+	−	−	−	+	A	+
35 AL-1	BL	−	−	+	+	+	−	+	−	−	−	+	A	+
36 SL-1	BL	−	−	+	+	+	−	+	−	−	−	+	A	+
37 NK-9	BL	−	−	+	+	+	−	+	−	−	−	+	A	+
38 B46M	BL	−	+	−	+	+	−	+	−	−	−	+	A	+
39 BJAB	BL	−	−	+	+	+	−	+	−	−	−	−	A	+
40 RPMI 8226	MM	−	−	−	+	+	−	+	−	−	−	−	A	+
41 U-266	MM	−	−	−	+	+	−	+	−	−	−	−	A	+
42 ARH-77	MM	−	−	+	+	+	−	+	−	−	−	−	A	+
Non-T, non-B leukemia lines														
43 Reh	ALL	−	−	−	−	−	−	+	+	−	+	−	A	+
44 KM-3	ALL	−	−	−	−	−	−	+	+	−	+	−	A	+
45 NALL-1	ALL	−	−	−	−	−	−	+	+	−	+	−	A	+
46 NALM-16	ALL	−	−	−	−	−	−	+	+	−	+	−	A	+
47 HL-60	APL	−	+	+	−	−	−	−	−	+	−	−	A	+
48 ML 1–3	AML	−	+	−	−	−	−	−	−	+	−	−	A	+
49 KG-1	AML	−	+	−	−	−	−	+	−	+	−	−	A	+
50 K-562	CML	−	+	−	−	−	−	−	−	−	−	−	A/Ph'	+

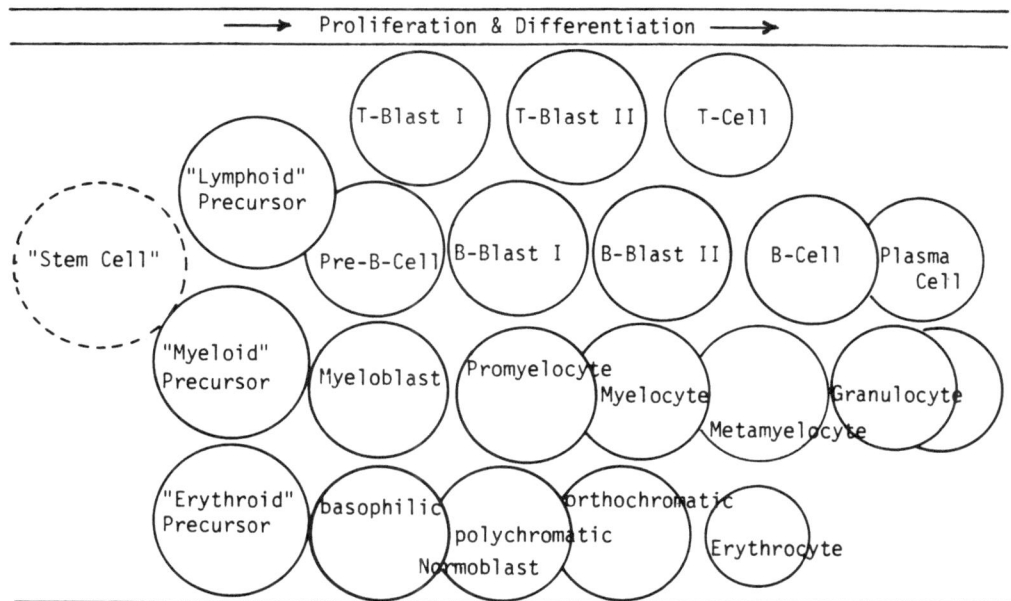

Fig. 1. Scheme for hematopoietic differentiation based on the marker profiles of 50 leukemia-lymphoma cell lines

reflect haematopoietic cell differentiation. In: Serrou B, Rosenfeld C (eds) Human lymphocyte differentiation: Its application to cancer. Elsevier/North-Holland, Amsterdam (INSERM Symposium No 8, pp 337–344) – Nilsson K (1978) Established human lymphoid cell lines as models for B-lymphocyte differentiation. In: Serrou B, Rosenfeld C (eds) Human lymphocyte differentiation: Its application to cancer. Elsevier/North-Holland, Amsterdam (INSERM Symposium No 8, pp 307–317)

◁ [a] Abbreviations used are: ALL=acute lymphoblastic leukemia; ATL=adult T-cell leukemia; ?HD=unproven Hodgkin's disease; CLL=chronic lymphocytic leukemia; CML=chronic myelocytic leukemia in blast crisis; LS=lymphosarcoma/lymphoma; BL=Burkitt's lymphoma; MM=multiple myeloma; APL=acute promyelocytic leukemia; AML=acute myeloblastic leukemia; E=sheep erythrocyte rosette; EA=rosette formed by bovine erythrocyte-IgG antibody complex; EAC=rosette formed by bovine erythrocyte-IgM antibody-complement complex; SmIg=surface membrane immunoglobulin; CyIg=cytoplasmic immunoglobulin; T-Ag=T-cell specific antigen; Ia=p28,30 glycoprotein Ia-like antigen; cALL=common ALL associated antigen; MAg-I=myelomonocyte specific antigen; TdT=terminal transferase by immunofluorescence; EBV=Epstein-Barr virus; Chr.=chromosome constitution (A=abnormal, Ph'=Philadelphia chromosome); MLC-S=stimulating activity in "one-way" mixed leukocyte culture; n.t.=not tested

Haematology and Blood Transfusion Vol. 26
Modern Trends in Human Leukemia IV
Edited by Neth, Gallo, Graf, Mannweiler, Winkler
© Springer-Verlag Berlin Heidelberg 1981

Biochemical Characterization of an Antigen Associated with Acute Lymphoblastic Leukemia and Lymphocyte Precursors

R. A. Newman, D. R. Sutherland, and M. F. Greaves

A. Introduction

Acute lymphoblastic leukemia (ALL) associated antigen (ALLA) is expressed on the surface of cells from patients with the common (or non-T, non-B) variant of ALL as well as in some cases of "undifferentiated" leukemias and chronic myeloid leukaemia (CML) in "lymphoid" blast crisis (Greaves and Janossy 1978).

This antigen has also been detected serologically on a small proportion of normal bone marrow cells (Greaves et al. 1978, 1980; Janossy et al. 1978) and is suggested to be a normal differentiation antigen of "early" hemopoietic cells which are possibly restricted to lymphoid development (Greaves and Janossy 1978; Greaves et al. 1980). Despite the lack of absolute leukemic specificity, antisera to ALLA have been useful for differential diagnosis of acute leukemia. The biochemical characteristics of this structure have been analyzed in detail using the cell line Nalm-1.

B. Results and Discussion

I. Integrity of ALLA

The ALLA, precipitated by rabbit antisera, is a single glycosylated polypeptide of approximately 100,000 daltons (gp 100) containing no intrachain disulfide linkages as judged by SDS-polyacrylamide gel electrophoresis (PAGE) under reducing and nonreducing conditions (Sutherland et al. 1978). A monoclonal anti-ALL (J-5) precipitates a similar if not identical molecule from leukemic cells (Ritz et al. 1980).

The lectin binding characteristics of gp 100 are somewhat unusual in that only 50% binds to lentil lectin, whereas 100% binds to *Ricinus communis* lectin (Fig. 1).

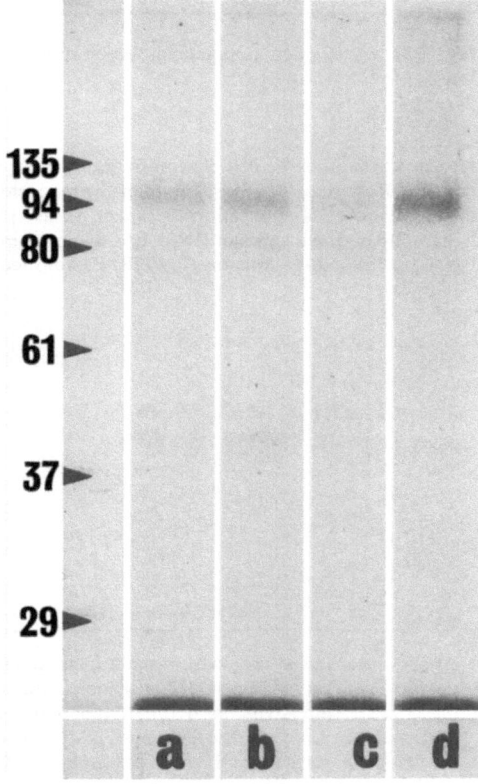

Fig. 1. SDS-PAGE of immunoprecipitates from NP-40 extracts of ^{35}S-methionine labeled Nalm-1 cells using 5 μl of rabbit anti-ALL. *a*, LcH$^+$ fraction; *b*, LcH$^-$ fraction; *c*, LcH$^-$ and RCA$^-$ fraction; *d*, RCA$^+$ fraction

Two-dimensional isoelectric focusing/SDS-PAGE of the lentil binding and lentil nonbinding forms of gp 100 over a narrow pH range gave identical homogeneous spots with a pI of 5.1–5.5. Neuraminidase treatment of both forms of gp 100 resulted in a shift of approximately 0.6 of a pH unit towards the basic end of the gel.

II. Is Carbohydrate Involved in the Antigenic Site of gp 100?

Treatment of cells with tunicamycin (20 μg/ml) and examination of immunoprecipitates from extracts on SDS-PAGE resulted in the disappearance of gp 100 with the concomitant appearance of a molecule at 75K. This was precipitable using rabbit antisera and a monoclonal anti-ALL (Ritz et al. 1980). Digestion of cell extracts with a mixture of glycosidases also gave an immunoprecipitable band of lower molecular weight. This evidence plus the heat lability of gp 100 suggests that carbohydrate, while possibly constituting up to 25% of the molecular weight, is not involved in the antigenic site.

III. Is gp 100 an Integral Membrane Protein?

As gp 100 is shed into the culture medium(s) and is also present in the sera of some leukemic patients (Kabisch et al. 1979; unpublished observations), it was of interest to establish whether or not it is an integral membrane protein.

Incubation of Nalm-1 cells with the lipophilic photoactivatable reagent, hexanoyl diiodo-N-(4-azido-2-nitrophenyl)-tyramine (Owen et al., to be published), was able to label Ia antigens but no labeling of gp 100 was evident. Charge shift electrophoresis (Helenius and Simons 1977) showed that the molecule possessed limited hydrophobicity, although this was no greater than that associated with the soluble proteins, bovine serum albumin, and lysozyme. Thus, although gp 100 possesses some hydrophobic regions, it is most likely not a true integral membrane protein. Subcellular fractionation of ^{125}I/lactoperoxidase-labeled cells, however, showed that gp 100 is strongly associated with the plasma membrane and not released into the medium as is the case with known peripheral proteins such as fibronectin (Owen et al., to be published).

IV. The gp 100 on Normal Bone Marrow Cells

Small numbers of cells in normal bone marrow react with anti-ALL (Greaves et al. 1978, 1980; Janossy et al. 1978; see also contribution by Greaves et al. in this book). Uninvolved bone marrow from three cases of children with rhabdomyosarcoma and two samples of marrow from patients in remission from leukemia were metabolically labelled with ^{35}S-methionine and immunoprecipitates of cell extracts examined by SDS-PAGE. A glycoprotein with a molecular weight of 100,000 daltons identical to that seen in leukemias and leukemic cells lines was detected. Rabbit antisera and monoclonal (J-5) antibody precipitated a similar band (Fig. 2). Peptide mapping will be required to establish

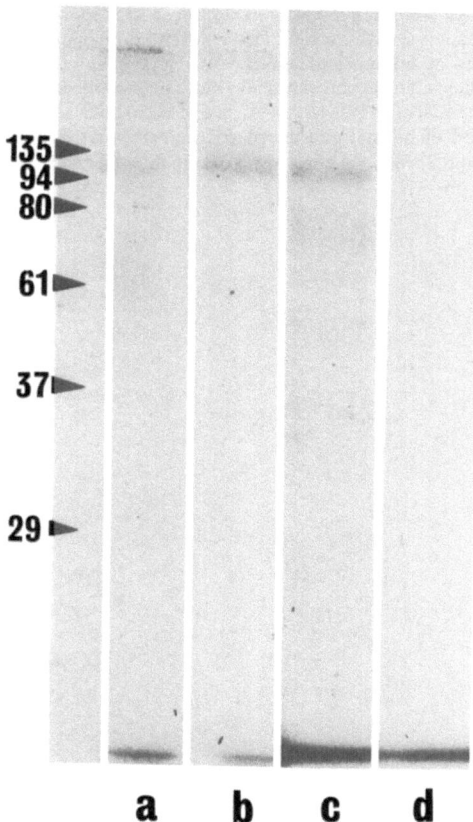

Fig. 2. SDS-PAGE of immunoprecipitates from ^{35}S-methionine labeled bone marrow cells. *a*, rhabdomyosarcoma and rabbit anti-ALL; *b*, rhabdomyosarcoma and monoclonal anti-ALL (J-5); *c*, remission marrow and rabbit anti-ALL; and *d*, remission marrow and normal rabbit serum

complete identity of gp 100 from normal marrow cells with that of leukemic cells. This data and other associated phenotypic features (see Greaves et al. pp 296–304) indicate that expression of gp 100 is likely to be a normal gene product reflecting the "target" cell for malignant transformation and/or the level of maturation arrest commonly seen in ALL.

References

Graham JM, Hynes RO, Davidson EA, Bainton DF (1975) The location of proteins labelled by the ^{125}I-lactoperoxidase system in the NIL8 hamster fibroblast. Cell 4:353–365 – Greaves MF, Janossy G (1978) Patterns of gene expression and the cellular origins of human leukaemia. Biochim Biophys Acta 516:193–230 – Greaves M, Janossy G, Francis G, Minowada J (1978) Membrane phenotypes of human leukaemic cells and leukaemic cell lines: Clinical correlates and biological implications. In: Clarkson B, Marks PA, Till JE (eds) Differentiation of normal and neoplastic hematopoietic cells. Cold Spring Harbor, New York pp 823–841 – Greaves M, Delia D, Janossy G, Rapson N, Chessells J, Woods M, Prentice G (1980) Acute lymphoblastic leukaemia associated antigen. IV. Expression on non-leukaemic 'lymphoid' cells. Leuk Res 4:15–32 – Helenius A, Simons K (1977) Charge shift electrophoresis: Simple method for distinguishing between amphiphilic and hydrophilic proteins in detergent solution. Proc Natl Acad Sci USA 74:529–532 – Janossy G, Francis GE, Capellaro D, Goldstone AH, Greaves MF (1978) Cell sorter analysis of leukaemia-associated antigens on human myeloid precursors. Nature 276:176–178 – Kabisch H, Arndt R, Becker W-M, Thiele H-G, Landbeck G (1979) Serological detection and partial characterization of the common-ALL-cell associated antigen in the serum of cALL-patients. Leuk Res 3:83–91 – Owen MJ, Knott JCA, Crumpton MJ (to be published) Labelling of lymphocyte surface antigens by the lipophilic, photoactivatable reagent, hexanoyl diiodo-N-(4-azido-2-nitrophenyl)-tyramine. Biochemistry – Ritz J, Pesando JM, McConarty JN, Lazarus H, Schlossman SF (1980) A monoclonal antibody to human acute lymphoblastic leukaemia antigen. Nature 283:583–585 – Sutherland DR, Smart J, Niaudet P, Greaves MF (1978) Acute lymphoblastic leukaemia associated antigen. II. Isolation and partial characterisation. Leuk Res 2:115–126

Haematology and Blood Transfusion Vol. 26
Modern Trends in Human Leukemia IV
Edited by Neth, Gallo, Graf, Mannweiler, Winkler
© Springer-Verlag Berlin Heidelberg 1981

Serologic Subtyping of cALL*

W.-M. Becker, W.-H. Schmiegel, H. Kabisch, R. Arndt, and H.-G. Thiele

Recently we have found that sera of patients with common ALL contain a glycoprotein reacting with antibodies directed to common ALL associated antigen (Ag cALL) (Kabisch et al. 1979). The molecular properties of the serum Ag cALL, i.e., the apparent molecular weight of 125,000 and the binding specificity to lens culinaris lectin, are in good accordance with those estimated for Ag cALL as solubilized from common ALL cells (Kabisch et al. 1978) or obtained from established leukemic cell lines (Sutherland et al. 1978). These findings indicate an in vivo shedding or secretion of this antigen.

Proceeding from the assumption that cALL cells of different patients or even single established leukemic cell lines represent distinct stages of cellular development characterized by particular patterns of cell surface structures and that shedding of Ag cALL from cALL cells may not be restricted to this antigen but may also occur with respect to other differentiation antigens, it seemed to be promising to use cell culture supernatants of such cell lines as starting material for antigen preparation and antiserum production. In comparison to intact tumor cells or membranes, secreted or shed cell material has the advantage for the purpose of immunization that the antibodies obtained will be of restricted diversity. The specificity of such antisera can be improved when before immunization the secreted or shed material is further purified and defined. Such antisera may be of value for subclassification of cALL. We here report on our preliminary results with antisera raised against distinct

glycolysated structures released into the culture medium by the established non-T, non-B cell leukemia lines Reh and Nalm (Rosenfeld et al. 1977; Minowada et al. 1977).

Purification of such structures was performed by lectin affinity chromatography on agarose immobilized (a) lens culinaris hemagglutinin (LCH), (b) ricinus communis agglutinin 60 (RCA 60), and (c) ricinus communis agglutinin 120 (RCA 120). Since purification of cell surface antigens frequently is associated with reduction of immunogenicity, the antigenic material as eluted from the lectin columns by competing sugars was incorporated into egg lecithin liposomes by use of n-octyl-glucoside following the method described by Helenius et al. (1977). After reconstitution to vesicles a significant increase of the antigenicity of Ag cALL as obtained from lectin-purified supernatants was observed in an antibody-binding inhibition assay.

Antisera were raised in rabbits by repeated injections of lectin purified antigens incorporated into liposomes (0.7–2.5 mg protein/dose). The antisera produced in this way were absorbed with AB erythrocytes, with glutardialdehyde fixed AB serum and human liver. By means of indirect immunofluorescence and by using different target cells the specificities of the three antisera were compared with that of an antiserum which had been raised by immunizing rabbits with cALL cells and which after extensive absorptions had been proved to be specific for Ag cALL (Table 1, column 1). As may be seen, antiserum 319, which was raised against LCH binding antigens derived from Nalm Cells culture supernatants, recognized membrane structures not only on Nalm cells and on cells derived from common ALL patients but also

---

* This work was supported by the Stiftung Volkswagenwerk

Table 1. Reaction of single antisera with various cell types (indirect immunofluorescence assay)[a]

Target cells	Percentage of cells reacting with different antisera			
	A-cALLS[b]	As 319[c]	As 365[d]	As 317[e]
I. ALL-derived cell lines				
REH	21	N.D.	99	89
NALM	17	55	40	30
KM-3	23	N.D.	3	6
II. Common ALL (patients)				
cALL$_{Er}$	52	51	0	42
cALL$_{Br}$	42	N.D.	31	0
cALL$_{Sc}$	72	N.D.	36	9
III. Other leukemic cells				
Acute myeloctic leukemia (AML)	0	85	0	0
Acute myelocytic-monocytic leukemia (AMML)	0	0	1	0
Acute monocytic leukemia (AMOL)	0	0	0	0
Chronic myelocytic leukemia (CML)	0	N.D.	0	0
Chronic lymphatic leukemia				
T-CLL	0	0	1	0
B-CLL	N.D.	96	12	0
T-ALL	0	0	1	5
IV. Normal cells				
Peripheral blood lymphocytes (PBL)	0	3	0	0
Bone marrow cells (BMC)	0	1	N.D.	N.D.
Tonsil lymphocytes (TOL)	0	3	11	0

[a] Second antibody: tetraethylrhodamine-isothiocyanate conjugated goat anti-rabbit globulin (Kabisch et al. 1978)

[b] Preparation of A-cALLS (Kabisch et al. 1978)

[c] Rabbit antiserum against antigen derived from Nalm cells supernatants purified by inity chromatography on LCH

[d] Rabbit antiserum against antigen derived from Reh cells supernatants purified by affinity chromatography on RCA 60

[e] Rabbit antiserum against antigen derived from Reh cells supernatants purified by inity chromatography on RCA 120

reacted with AML and B-CLL cells (Table 1, column 2).

Antiserum 365 raised to RCA 60 binding antigens derived from Reh cell supernatants revealed a different reacting pattern in that it did not react with AML but recognized a subpopulation of B-CLL as well as of tonsil lymphocytes (Table 1 column 3). When these results are compared with the selectivity of A-cALLS (Table 1, column 1), it becomes evident that antiserum 365 discriminates subtypes of Ag cALL bearing leukemic cells.

The recognition spectrum of antiserum 317 raised against RCA 120 binding antigens derived from Reh cell culture supernatants was found to be restricted to cALL cells, although its ability to discriminate cALL subtypes is evidently distinct from that of antiserum 365. Thus, antiserum 317 stained 42% of cALL cells of patient Er., whereas antiserum 365 had no labeling effect on these cells. On the other hand, antiserum 365 stained 31% and 36% of cALL cells of patients Br. and Sc., respectively. These target cells showed no (patient Br.) or only little (9%, patient Sc.) fluorescence when tested with antiserum 317.

These data confirm the assumption that antisera towards molecular-defined shed or secreted cell surface molecules with different lectin binding specificities are indeed a valuable tool for further differentiating of common ALL cells characterized by expression of Ag cALL.

References

Helenius A, Fries E, Kartenbeck J (1977) Reconstitution of semliki forest virus membrane. J Cell Biol 75:866–880 – Kabisch H, Arndt R, Thiele H-G, Winkler K, Landbeck G (1978) Partial molecular characterization of an antigenic structure associated to cells of common ALL. Clin Exp Immunol 32:399–404 – Kabisch H, Arndt R, Becker W-M, Thiele H-G, Landbeck G (1979) Serological detection and partial characterization of the common-All cell associated antigen in the serum of cALL patients. Leuk Res 3:83–91 – Minowada J, Tsubota T, Greaves MF, Walters RT (1977) A non-T, non-B human leukaemia cell line (Nalm 1): Establishment of the cells and presence of leukaemiaassociated antigens. J Natl Cancer Inst 59:83–87 – Rosenfeld C, Goutner A, Choquet C, Venuat AM, Kayibanda B, Pico JL, Greaves MF (1977) Phenotypic characterisation of a unique non-T, non-B acute lymphoblastic leukaemia cell lines. Nature 267:841–843 – Sutherland R, Smart J, Niaudet P, Greaves MF (1978) Acute lymphoblastic leukaemia associated antigen. II. Isolation and partial characterisation. Leuk Res 2:115–126

Haematology and Blood Transfusion Vol. 26
Modern Trends in Human Leukemia IV
Edited by Neth, Gallo, Graf, Mannweiler, Winkler
© Springer-Verlag Berlin Heidelberg 1981

Acute Myeloblastic Leukemia-Associated Antigens: Detection and Clinical Importance*

M. A. Baker, D. A. K. Roncari, R. N. Taub, T. Mohanakumar, and J. A. Falk

A. Abstract

Antigenic compounds from the surface of leukemic myeloblasts are shed in vitro on short-term culture. Blast cells radiolabeled by lactoperoxidase iodination release soluble compounds that react immunologically with alloantisera to leukemia-associated antigens. Partially characterized soluble antigens were used to raise heteroantisera in monkeys that are selectively reactive with leukemic myeloblasts and unreactive with nonleukemic cells. Monkey heteroantisera were used to further characterize soluble leukemia antigens. Sera from patients with acute myeloblastic leukemia inhibit the reactivity of the heteroantisera, suggesting that soluble leukemic antigen is released in vivo as well.

B. Introduction

The description of antigens on leukemic blast cells has increased our understanding of human leukemia (Greaves 1979). Heteroantisera raised in mice, rabbits, or monkeys to leukemic antigens have been useful in defining tissues of origin of leukemic cells and improving diagnostic accuracy (Baker et al. 1974, 1976, 1978, 1979). Solubilization of leukemic antigens and biochemical characterization of antigenic compounds may yield further insight into the nature of the leukemic process (Taub

* Supported by the National Cancer Institute of Canada, the Ontario Cancer Treatment and Research Foundation, The Medical Research Council of Canada, the U.S. National Cancer Institute (CA 22818 and CA 12827), and the American Cancer Society (IM 190)

et al. 1978). Biochemical studies involving extraction of leukemic cell membrane-associated antigens with proteolytic enzymes (Billing and Terasaki 1974; Metzgar et al. 1974) or hypertonic potassium chloride (Gutterman et al. 1972) have generally yielded inhomogeneous or incompletely characterized products. Assays for antigenicity have been semiquantitative and depended either on inhibition of agglutination or cytotoxicity or on the reactions to intracutaneous skin testing (Mavligit et al. 1973).

Because our preliminary observations suggested that certain membrane components may be "shed" in soluble form from blast cell surfaces (Taub et al. 1976) just as from certain normal cells (Cone et al. 1971), we have analyzed material released into the supernatant medium of cultured myeloblasts.

Partially characterized compounds from the leukemic myeloblast cell surface have been used to raise heteroantisera in monkeys that are selectively reactive with leukemic myeloblasts but are unreactive with nonleukemic cells. Sera from patients with acute leukemia inhibit reactivity of the antisera, suggesting that similar compounds are shed in vivo.

C. Methods

I. Preparation of Radiolabeled Soluble Antigen

Leukemic cells were obtained from the peripheral blood of patients with acute myeloblastic leukemia on initial presentation, with white blood cell counts greather than 50.0×10^9/l, and with greater than 99% myeloblasts on differential white count. To

1×10^8 cells in 2 ml phosphate-buffered saline (PBS; pH 7.0) were added 1.0 mC sodium iodide ^{125}I, 200 µl of lactoperoxidase (Sigma, 0.25 mg/ml), and 25 µl of 0.03% hydrogen peroxide. The cells were incubated at room temperature for 10 min; during this period 25 µl of the peroxide solution was added twice. The reaction was terminated by adding 8 ml 0.01 M cysteine and 0.01 M potassium iodide in PBS. The cells were washed thrice in Hanks balanced salt solution and placed in culture at 37°C in 5 ml minimal Eagle's medium. After 4 h the medium was discarded and the cells were washed and reincubated. The supernatant was harvested at 24 h. Cell suspensions showing less than 80% viability were not used.

II. Immunoprecipitation

To microtiter U-plate wells (Cooke Engineering Co., Alexandria, Virginia) prewashed with bovine serum albumin were added 20 µl of alloserum and 20 µl of the ^{125}I-labeled supernatant. All tests were done in triplicate. The plates were shaken and allowed to stand for 1 h at 4°C. Coprecipitation was carried out by adding 100 µl of Staphylococcal protein A (Enzyme Centre Incorporated, Boston, Mass.) to each well. The plates were shaken again, kept 15 min at 22°C, and then spun at 1800 r/min for 10 min. The supernatant liquid was gently sucked out of the wells, and the precipitates were washed three times in PBS (pH = 7.2) and transferred to cuvettes. Radioactivity was counted in a Beckmann Biogamma II gamma spectrometer.

III. Gel Filtration Chromatography

Gel filtration chromatography was conducted by applying 0.5 ml aliquots of culture supernatant on to 0.9×90 cm columns (Glenco Scientific, Inc.) of Bio-Gel A-1.5m (approximately 8% agarose, 200–400 mesh) equilibrated and eluted at 4°C with 0.01 M ammonium acetate at a hydrostatic pressure of 20 cm water.

IV. Isoelectric Focusing

Solutions for isoelectric focusing were added to 0.75 ml of 40% ampholine (pH 3.5 to 10) and applied to an LKB 8100 column at 4°C to a total volume of 110 ml with sucrose gradient solution (Abraham and Bakerman 1977).

V. LDS-Polyacrylamide Disc Gel Electrophoresis

The pooled fractions or immunoprecipitates from these fractions were boiled with 1% (weight/volume) lithium dodecyl sulfate (LDS)/0.01 M lithium phosphate buffer, pH 7.0, and then incubated further with this detergent at 37°C for 30 min. The resulting polypeptide subunits were resolved by LDS-polyacrylamide disc gel electrophoresis carried out according to Laemmli (1970) except for the substitution of LDS for sodium dodecyl sulfate in order to conduct the experiments at 4°C (Delepelaire and Chua 1979).

VI. Cells

Enriched T- or B-lymphocyte preparations were obtained either by selective rosetting of T-lymphocytes using sheep erythrocytes or by removing adherent B-lymphocytes by absorption on a flask coated with affinity-purified goat antihuman Fab. The details of T- and B-cell enrichment procedures have been published earlier (Mohanakumar et al. 1979).

VII. Preparation of Antiserum

Heterologous anti-AMLSGA serum was prepared by injecting a monkey *(M spesiosa)* intravenously and intradermally (50 µg) three times, with a period of 14 days between immunizations (Mohanakumar et al. 1974). For intradermal injections the antigen suspended in PBS pH 7.2 was mixed with an equal volume of Freund's complete adjuvant (H37Ra). The antiserum described in this report was obtained 7 days after the third inoculation with antigen.

VIII. Absorption of Antisera

Immune and the preimmune sera were heat inactivated at 56°C for 30 min and then absorbed twice for 20 min at 4°C with an equal volume of cells (pooled normal human platelets, leukocytes, bone marrow cells, or myeloblasts).

IX. Microcytotoxicity Assay

A standard Amos modification of the microtechnique described by Mittal et al. (1968) was used for unfractionated cell preparations, and the incubation time with complement was extended to 2 h when enriched B- and T-lymphocytes were used as targets. Selected nontoxic rabbit complement was used throughout.

D. Results

I. Partial Characterization of Surface Compounds

Leukemic myeloblasts radiolabeled with the lactoperoxidase iodination technique released labeled soluble compounds into supernatant media. Following 24-h incubation, cells remained >90% viable by trypan blue exclusion. Gel filtration chromatography in 8% agarose of the labeled supernatant yielded two distinct peaks, coincident in radioactivity and protein concentration. The second peak was selectively reactive by coprecipitation with antileukemic antisera obtained from patients receiving immunotherapy with leukemic myeloblasts (Taub et al. 1978).

Supernatant material derived from radiolabeled blasts and eluted in the second peak from the agarose column was applied to a DEAE cellulose column and yielded a single peak, coincident in radioactivity and protein levels. Carbohydrate content of the eluted material was estimated at 10% by weight. This material retained immunologic activity with antileukemic alloantisera as measured by coprecipitation.

II. Development of Heteroantisera

Antisera raised in monkeys to the compounds eluted from DEAE cellulose columns was tested for cytotoxic reactivity against leukemic and nonleukemic cells (Table 1). In complement-dependent cytotoxicity testing the monkey anti-AMLSGA was reactive with cells from leukemic patients but was unreactive with nonleukemic peripheral blood or bone marrow cells. Absorption of anti-AMLSGA with leukemic myeloblasts from patients with acute myeloblastic or chronic myelocytic leukemia removed all antileukemic activity. Absorption with leukemic lymphoblasts or leukemic lymphocytes removed activity against ALL or CLL cells but did not remove antimyeloblast activity. Anti-AMLSGA was unreactive with B-lymphocytes, including those of an identical twin to a patient with AML, and absorption with B-lymphocytes did not reduce antimyeloblast activity. In contrast, the rabbit anti-Ia was reactive with all nonleukemic B-lymphoytes. Antileukemic activity was not reduced by absorption of anti-AMLSGA with the enriched mononuclear fractions of nonleukemic marrow or with neutrophils from nonleukemic patients.

III. Further Characterization of Surface Compounds

The antileukemic heteroantisera were applied to the further isolation and characterization of compounds from the myeloblast cell surface. Compounds eluted from gel columns were applied to isoelectric focusing columns and fractions obtained were analyzed for reactivity by coprecipitation with the heteroantisera. A major reactive peak was obtained at pI 7.8. Analysis of the immune precipitate by LDS-PAGE yielded a homogeneous peak with molecular weight estimated between 70,000 and 80,000 daltons.

IV. Testing of Patients' Sera

Serum samples were tested for their ability to interfere with coprecipitation of soluble radio-

Table 1. Reactivity of monkey anti-AML antiserum

Serum absorbed with	Target cells					
	AML (10)[a]	CML (5)	ALL (5)	CLL (5)	T-cells (10)	B-cells (5)
Unabsorbed	+[b]	+	±	±	−	−
AML[c]	−	−	−	−	−	−
CML	−	−	−	−		
ALL	+	+	−	−		
CLL	+	+	−	−		
B-cells	+	+	±	+		

[a] Number of samples tested
[b] Plus (+) indicates all samples were reactive. Minus (−) indicates all samples were negative. Both signs (±) indicate weak positive reactions in some samples
[c] Abbreviations: AML, acute myeloblastic leukemia; CML, chronic myelocytic leukemia; ALL, acute lymphoblastic leukemia; CLL, chronic lymphocytic leukemia

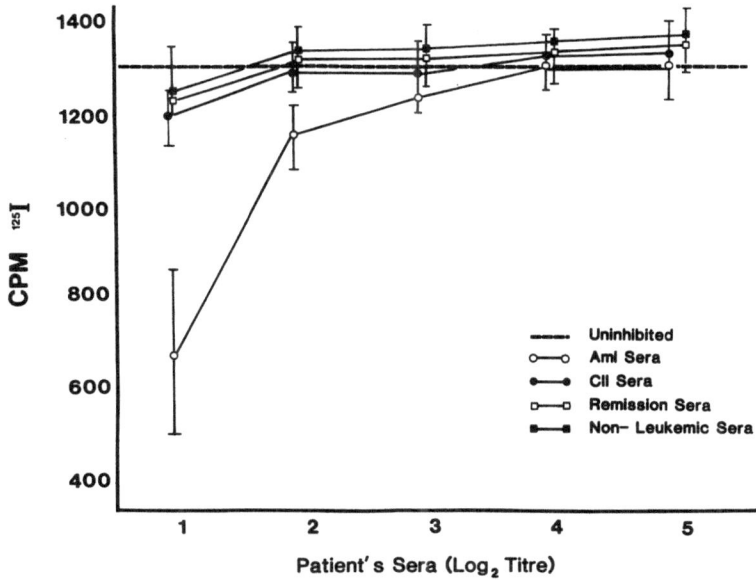

Fig. 1. Inhibition of coprecipitation by patient's sera. Sera from AML patients with high blast counts inhibit the precipitation of leukemic antigen by monkey antimyeloblast sera. Significant inhibition is obtained at the first dilution of patient's sera ($P<0.05$)

labelled leukemia antigen by antileukemic heteroantisera (Fig. 1). Sera were tested from seven patients with AML in relapse (peripheral blood blast count $>50,000/mm^3$), five patients with chronic lymphocytic leukemia (lymphocyte count $>50,000/mm^3$), five patients with AML in remission, and five patients with nonleukemic disease. Significant inhibition was seen with low dilutions of sera from patients with high myeloblast counts ($P<0.05$).

E. Discussion

The development of techniques for lactoperoxidase-catalyzed surface radioactive labeling of viable cells has provided an important tool for analysis of the composition and turnover of cell membrane components (Hubbard and Cohen 1972; Humphreys et al. 1976). An important advantage of this surface-labeling technique is that of topological as well as chemical specificity; only antigens sufficiently exposed on the membrane surface to be accessible to the action of peroxidase (Vidal et al. 1974) and consisting of substantial amounts of histidine- or tyrosine-containing protein will be heavily labeled (Hubbard and Cohen

1972). We chose to analyze material shed into the supernatant from membranes of viable cultured myeloblasts in order to circumvent the problem of contamination with HLA antigens encountered in some attempts to solublize leukemic cell membrane antigens directly. Metzgar et al. (1974) used trypsin digestion, 3 M potassium chloride extraction, or autolytic treatment to prepare soluble LAAs. Only trypsin treatment proved effective, but large amounts of HLA activity were solubilized along with LAA.

The antiserum that we have raised to this antigen is highly reactive with leukemic myeloblasts from patients with AML or CML (Ramachandar et al. 1975) and following appropriate absorption is unreactive with histocompatibility antigens, including Ia antigens, normal marrow fractions, leukemic lymphoblasts, and leukemic lymphocytes. Absorptions with normal peripheral blood cells, bone marrow cells, lymphoblasts, or CLL cells does not remove activity against myeloblasts.

Although the antiserum is selectively reactive with leukemic myeloblasts, it is not necessarily leukemia specific. The antigens recognized may be present in a cell population occurring infrequently in normal blood or marrow or may be well masked on the cell surface of nonleukemic cells (Greaves 1979). Leukemic blast cells carry oncofetal antigens (Granatek et al. 1976) or antigens characteristic of specific phases of the cell cycle (Pasternak et al. 1974), and these may be recognized by the antiserum. Selective reactivity against myeloblasts may be explained by cell surface glycoprotein changes characteristic of leukemic cells (Andersson et al. 1979; Khilanani et al. 1977; van Beek et al. 1978). Van Beek et al. (1978) have documented structural differences in fucose-containing glycopeptides in leukemic myeloblasts compared to nonleukemic leukocytes, and Andersson et al. (1979) have demonstrated surface glycoprotein patterns diagnostic of acute myeloblastic leukemia. Studies of serum and urine of patients with AML have yielded characteristic compounds resulting from alteration of normal glycoproteins (Rudman et al. 1976). Since the compounds obtained in the present study were not prepared by adding proteolytic or dissociating agents but were rather shed into the supernatant during short-term incubation, we have characterized material that is associated with the cell surface but is not likely to be an integral membrane glycoprotein; furthermore, it may represent intact native compounds rather than fragments.

We have previously described the detection of leukemic antigen in the bone marrow of patients with AML in remission (Baker et al. 1979). The increase in reactivity which occurs in marrow before relapse may allow the early use of reinduction chemotherapy. The technical difficulties inherent in studying fresh bone marrow specimens have led us to study antigen levels in serum. Further refinement of immunologic assays for detection of antigen in serum may allow trials of therapeutic intervention upon early detection of increase in tumor burden.

References

Abraham CV, Bakerman S (1977) Isolation and purification of Rh receptor component from human erythrocyte membrane by isoelectric focusing. Sci Tools 24:22–24 – Andersson LC, Gahmberg CG, Siimes MA, Teerenhoui L, Vuopio P (1979) Cell surface glycoprotein analysis: a diagnostic tool in human leukemias. Int J Cancer 23:306–311 – Baker MA, Ramachandar K, Taub RN (1974) Specificity of heteroantisera to human acute leukemia-associated antigens J Clin Invest 54:1273–1278 – Baker MA, Falk RE, Falk J, Greaves MF (1976) Detection of monocyte specific antigen on human acute leukemia cells. Br J Haematol 32:13–19 – Baker MA, Falk JA, Taub RN (1978) Immunotherapy of human acute leukemia: Antibody response to leukemia-associated antigens. Blood 52:469–480 – Baker MA, Falk JA, Carter WH, Taub RN, and the Toronto Leukemia Study Group: Early diagnosis of relapse in acute myeloblastic leukemia. N Engl J Med 301:1353–1357 – Billing R, Terasaki TI (1974) Human leukemic antigen. II. Purification. J Natl Cancer Inst 53:1639–1643 – Cone RE, Marchalonis JJ, Rolley RT (1971) Lymphocyte membrane dynamics. Metabolic release of cell surface proteins. J Exp Med 134:1373–1384 – Delepelaire P, Chua N-H (1979) Lithium dodecyl sulfate/polyacrylamide gel electrophoresis of thylakoid membranes at 4°C: Characterization of two additional chlorophyll a-protein complexes. Proc Natl Acad Sci USA 76:111–115 – Granatek CH, Hanna MG Jr, Hersh EM, Gutterman JU, Mavligit GM, Candler EL (1976) Fetal antigens in human leukemia. Cancer Res 36:3464–3470 – Greaves MF (1979) Cell surface characteristics of human leukemic cells. In: Langsben PN, Marshall RD (eds) Essays in biochemistry, vol 15. Academic Press, New York, p 78 – Gutterman JU, Mavligit G, McCredie KB, Bodey GP Sr, Freireich EJ, Hersh EM (1972) Human leukemia antigens: Partial isolation and characterization. Science 177:1114–1115 – Hubbard A, Cohen Z (1972) The Enzymatic iodination of the red cell membrane. J Cell Biol 55:390–405 – Humphreys RE, McCune JM, Chess L, Herrman HC, Malenka DJ, Mann DL, Parham P, Schlossman SF, Strominger JL (1976) Isolation and immunologic characterization of a human, B-lymphocyte-specific, cell surface antigen. J Exp Med 144:98–112 – Khilanani P, Chou T-H, Lomen PL, Kessel D (1977) Variations of levels of plasma guanosine diphosphate L-Fucose: β-D galactosyl α-2-L-Fucosyl-transferase in acute adult leukemia. Cancer Res 37:2557–2559 – Laemmli U (1970) Cleavage of structural proteins during the assembly of the head of bacteriophage T4. Nature 227:680–685 – Mavligit DM, Ambus U, Gutterman JU, Hersh EM, McBride CM (1973) Antigens solubilized from human solid tumors: Lymphocyte stimulation and cutaneous delayed hypersensitivity. Nature [New Biol] 243:183–186 – Metzgar RS, Mohanakumar T, Green RW, Miller DS, Bolgonesi DP (1974) Human leukemia antigens: Partial isolation and characterization. J Natl Cancer Inst 52:1445–1453 – Mittal KK, Mickey MR, Singal DP, Terasaki PI (1968) Serotyping for homotransplantation. XVIII. Refinement of microdroplet lymphocyte cytotoxicity test. Transplantation 6:913–927 – Mohanakumar T, Metzgar RS, Miller DS (1974) Human leukemia cell antigens: Serological characterization with xenoantisera. J Natl Cancer Inst 52:1435–1444 – Mohanakumar T, Giedlin M, DuVall C, Rhodes C, Phibbs M, Mendez G, Kaplan AM, Lee HM (1979) B-lymphocyte-specific antibodies in human renal allografts. Transplant Proc 11:397–400 – Pasternak CA, Summer MCB, Colins R (1974) Surface changes during the cell cycle. In: Padilla G, Cameron I, Zimmerman A (eds) Cell cycle control. Academic Press, New York, pp 117–124 – Ramachandar K, Baker MA, Taub RN (1975) Antibody responses to leukemia-associated antigens during immunotherapy of chronic myelocytic leukemia. Blood 46:845–854 – Rudman D, Chawla RK, Hendrickson LJ, Vogler WR, Sophianopoulos AJ (1976) Isolation of a novel glycoprotein (EDC 1) from the urine of a patient with acute myeloblastic leukemia. Cancer Res 36:1837–1846 – Taub RN, Baker MA, Roncari DA (1976) Radioimmunoassay of human myeloblastic leukemia-associated antigens. In: Proceeding of XVI International Congress of Hematology, Kyoto, Japan, 4th September 1976 – Taub RN, Roncari DAK, Baker MA (1978) Isolation and partial characterization of radioiodinated myeloblastic leukemia-associated cell surface glycoprotein antigen. Cancer Res 38:4624–4629 – van Beek WP, Smets LA, Emmelot P, Roozendaal KJ, Behrendt H (1978) Early recognition of human leukemia by cell surface glycoprotein changes. Leuk Res 2:163–171 – Vidal R, Tarone G, Perroni F, Comoglio PM (1974) A comparative study of SV40 transformed fibroblast plasma membrane proteins labelled by lactoperoxidase iodination or with trinitrobenzene sulfonate. FEBS Lett 47:107–112

Haematology and Blood Transfusion Vol. 26
Modern Trends in Human Leukemia IV
Edited by Neth, Gallo, Graf, Mannweiler, Winkler
© Springer-Verlag Berlin Heidelberg 1981

Glycophorin A as an Erythroid Marker in Normal and Malignant Hematopoiesis

L. C. Andersson, E. von Willebrand, M. Jokinen, K. K. Karhi, and C. G. Gahmberg

A. Molecular Structure of Glycophorin A

Glycophorin A (GpA), which is the major sialoglycoprotein on human red cells, is one of the best characterized mammalian integral membrane proteins (Marchesi et al. 1972; Tomita and Marchesi 1975). Its amino acid sequence is known. The protein molecule contains three distinct domains. A large hydrophilic portion, carrying the NH_2-terminal, is located on the external surface of the red cell, and the COOH-terminal is located in the cytoplasm (Bretscher 1975) and probably interacts with peripheral proteins on the inner aspect of the membrane. These two hydrophilic sequences are connected by a hydrophobic segment of 23 amino acids which must be embedded within the lipid bilayer.

An unusually large proportion (about 60%) of the GpA is made up of carbohydrates. The molecule contains 15 O-glycosidic oligosacharides with the structure of N-acetyl neuraminyl $\alpha(2-3)$-galactosyl $\beta(1-3)$ |N-acetyl neuraminyl $\alpha(2-6)$| N-acetyl galactosamine (Thomas and Winzler 1969) and one N-glycosidic oligosaccharide located at asn-26. The carbohydrate is located outside the lipid bilayer in the NH_2-terminal portion of the molecule (Fig. 1).

Glycophorin A carries the MN blood group activity of red cells (Marchesi et al. 1972; Tomita and Marchesi 1975). This is most probably due to an interaction between amino acids and O-glycosidic oligosaccharides, since either treatment with neuraminidase (Mähelä and Cantell 1958) or modifications of amino acids (Lisowska and Duk 1975) abolish the activity. GpAs from M and N cells also show different amino acid sequences in the NH_2-terminal portions (Dahr et al. 1977; Tomita and Marchesi 1975).

B. Biosynthesis of Glycophorin A

Most of our knowledge of the molecular mechanisms operating in biosynthesis of intergral membrane proteins of mammalian cells derives from studies of the glycoproteins of enveloped viruses. In these systems only a few membrane glycoproteins are made, which makes it relatively easy to follow their biosynthesis. The situation is, however, much more complex in normal cells, where a multitude of membrane proteins are simultaneously synthesized, and makes informative experiments difficult to perform.

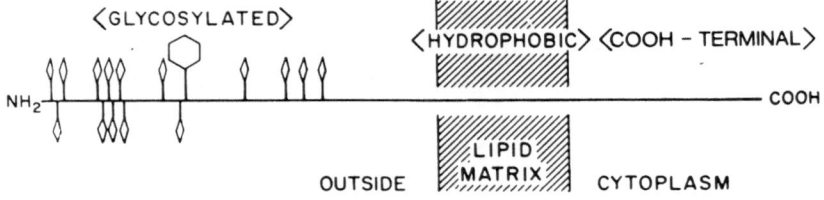

Fig. 1. Schematic drawing of glycophorin A structure. ◊ O-glycosidic chains. ⬡ N-glycosidic oligosaccharide

The detailed information available on the structure of GpA makes it an attractive candidate for biosynthetic studies. Such studies recently became possible with our finding that the human leukemia cell line K562, previously thought to be myeloid (Lozzio and Lozzio 1975), in fact shows erythroid characteristics, including the expression of GpA (Andersson et al. 1979b,c; Gahmberg et al. 1979). The reader is referred to our original reports for technical details (Gahmberg et al. 1980; Jokinen et al. 1979).

The biosynthesis of GpA in the K562 leukemia cell line was followed by pulse-chase labeling with [^{35}S] methionine. A precursor of GpA was visualized by appropriate lectin-Sepharose affinity chromatography and immune precipitation with specific anti-GpA serum (see below) and followed by polyacrylamide slab gel electrophoresis. This had an apparent molecular weight of 37,000 and contained an incompleted N-glycosidic oligosaccharide and unfinished O-glycosidic oligosaccharides. After chase for 10 min, the completed GpA with an apparent molecular weight of 39,000 was seen and it appeared at the cell surface in about 30 min. Addition of tunicamycin inhibited the N-glycosylation but not the O-glycosylation. The absence of the N-glycosidic oligosaccharide did not significantly affect the migration of the protein to the cell surface but the expression of glycophorin A was lower.

The cell-free biosynthesis of GpA was achieved by translation of glycophorin A messenger RNA which had been isolated from K562 cells in a rabbit reticulocyte system. This yielded a nonglycosylated protein with an apparent molecular weight of 19,500, which exceeded that of the glycophorin A apoprotein by about 5000. This indicates the presence of a "signal sequence" in the preprotein. When the translation was performed in the presence of microsomal membranes from dog pancreas the GpA apoprotein was both N- and O-glycosylated and the apparent molecular weight (37,000) of the synthesized protein was identical to that of the GpA precursor obtained from K562 cells.

C. Glycophorin A in Normal Hematopoiesis

To study the appearance of GpA on bone marrow cells during normal hematopoiesis we

made an antiserum to GpA. This was possible because erythrocytes from a person with the rare blood group En(a-) which lack GpA were made available (Gahmberg et al. 1976). Rabbits were immunized with isolated GpA and the antiserum was adsorbed with En(a-) red cell membranes. The specificity of the antiserum was assessed by immune precipitations from Triton X-100 lysates of normal erythrocyte membranes and bone marrow cells which were surface radiolabeled by the galactose oxidase-NaB^{3}H$_4$ method (Gahmberg and Hakomori 1973). Analysis of the precipitates by polyacrylamide gel electrophoresis (PAGE) under reducing conditions revealed that the antiserum reacted exclusively with surface molecules corresponding to the monomer (PAS2) and dimer (PAS1) of GpA (Gahmberg et al. 1978).

GpA-expressing cells in normal bone marrow were identified by the staphylococcus rosetting technique (Gahmberg et al. 1978). Suspensions of bone marrow cells were treated with antiserum followed by Staphylococcus aureus strain Cowan I, which carry protein A on their surface and therefore strongly attach to the Fc portion of IgG. The cells which bound staphylococci were identified by morphology from cytocentrifuged smears stained with May-Grünwald-Giemsa in combination with the Lephenes benzidine reaction to detect the presence of hemoglobin.

Only cells of the erythroid lineage formed rosettes with staphylococci after treatment with anti-GpA serum (Fig. 2). Weak reactivity was seen with the pronormoblasts, while the basophilic normoblasts and later stages of the erythropoiesis made strong rosettes. This indicates that the surface expression of GpA occurs slightly earlier than the onset of hemoglobin synthesis and the appearance of the ABO blood group antigens (Karhi et al. 1981) during normal red cell differentiation (Fig. 3).

D. Glycophorin A in Malignant Hematopoiesis

After our initial observations on the strong surface expression of GpA by the human leukemia cell line K562 (Andersson et al. 1979c) we have tested freshly isolated cells from leukemic patients for the presence of GpA.

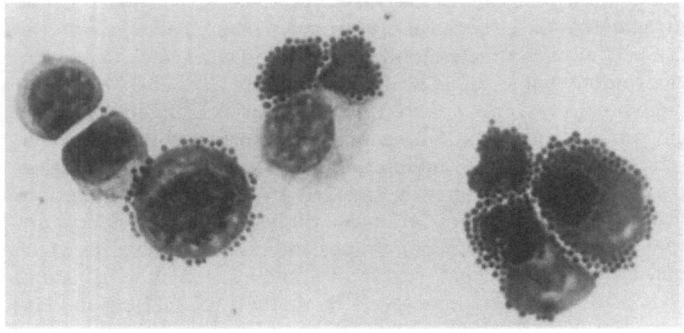

Fig. 2. Cytocentrifuged smears of bone marrow cells treated with anti-GpA serum and Staphylococcus aureus Cowan I. Benzidine-May-Grünwald-Giemsa staining

The leukemic cells were analyzed by indirect immunofluorescence using a F(ab)$_2$ preparation of the anti-GpA serum followed by a fluorescein isothiocynate-conjugated IgG preparation of sheep anti-rabbit Ig (Andersson et al. 1979a).

In 6 of 51 (12%) subsequent adult patients diagnosed as having acute myeloid or acute lymphoid leukemia we found positive staining in a large proportion (50%) of the leukemic cells. The specificity of the staining was further established by immunoprecipitation with anti-GpA serum from surface labeled leukemic cells followed by PAGE. Occassionally only the dimeric form of GpA was precipitated, while in most cases a surface protein corresponding to the monomeric form of GpA could be seen (Andersson et al. 1979a).

The GpA-expressing cells from acute leukemias were usually morphologically classified as poorly differentiated. Usually they have a basophilic, rather abundant cytoplasm lacking granulae but occasionally with azurophilic granulae and a kidney-shaped nucleus.

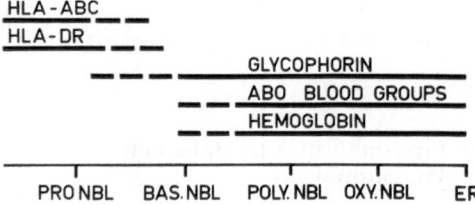

Fig. 3. Tentative sequence of appearance and disappearance of cell surface markers during erythropoiesis. *PRO NBL,* pronormoblast; *BAS.NBL,* basophilic normoblast; *POLY.NBL,* polychromatic normoblast; *OXY.NBL,* oxyphilic normoblast; *ER,* erythrocyte

Different proportions of GpA positive precursor cells can be observed during blast crisis of chronic myeloid leukemia (CML). This indicates that the arrest in maturation also involves to various degrees the erythroid lineage.

We have recently characterized the phenotype of the leukemic cells of relapsing childhood acute lymphocytic leukemia (ALL) (Andersson et al. 1980). So far we have found four cases (of a total of 30) which according to conventional surface marker analysis at initial diagnosis were classified as non-T, non-B ALL but where the majority of the leukemic blasts during relapse expressed surface GpA. In three of these the intracytoplasmic presence of fetal hemoglobin could be demonstrated in 30%–50% of the blast cells by direct staining of cold acetone fixed smears with FITC-conjugated rabbit antiserum to fetal hemoglobin. These cells, however, did not show a positive benzidine reaction, indicating low levels of hemoglobin or incomplete assembly of the hemoglobin molecule.

The phenotypic change from "lymphoid" to erythroid in relapsing childhood ALL is surprising. It is possible that in these cases the malignant transformation involves stem cells endowed with a pluripotential differentiation capacity. The anti-ALL treatment might have selected for relatively threapy-resistant clones showing early erythroid features.

These findings indicate that glycophorin A is also a useful marker of early erythroid derivation in malignant hematopoiesis. Moreover, leukemias with features of early erythroid differentiation are obviously more common than previously reported. These are, however, not identified by conventional means, since the malignant erythroid cells apparently only rarely maturate to synthesize adult hemoglobin.

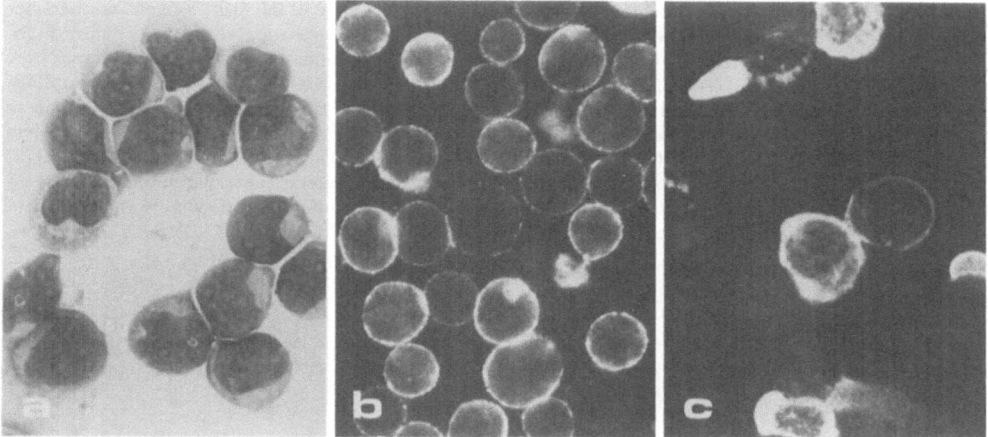

Fig. 4. a Photomicrograph of blasts from an adult patient with AML. **b** Positive membrane immunofluorescence of the same cells with a F(ab)$_2$ preparation of rabbit anti-GpA serum followed by FITC-conjugated sheep anti-rabbit IgG. **c** Direct immunofluorescence staining of acetone-fixed smears with FITC-conjugated rabbit anti-fetal hemoglobin

The recognition of leukemic cells with markers of erythroid derivation might be of clinical importance, since at least in adult acute leukemia the presence of surface GpA seems to imply poor prognosis.

Acknowledgments

We thank A. Asikainen, S. Koskinen, and L. Saraste for technical assistance. This study was supported by the Academy of Finland, the Finnish and Swedish Cancer Societies, and Finska Läkaresällskapet and was performed under a contract with the Association of Finnish Life Insurance Companies.

References

Andersson LC, Gahmberg CG, Teerenhovi L, Vuopio P (1979a) Glycophorin A as a marker of early erythroid differentiation in acute leukemia. Int J Cancer 24:717–720 – Andersson LC, Jokinen M, Gahmberg CG (1979b) Induction of erythroid differentiation in the human leukemia cell line K562. Nature 278:364 – Andersson LC, Nilsson K, Gahmberg CG (1979c) K562 – a human erythroleukemic cell line. Int J Cancer 23:143–147 – Andersson LC, Wegelius R, Borgström GH, Gahmberg CG (1980) Change in cellular phenotype from lymphoid to erythroid in a case of ALL. Scand J Haematol 24:115–121 – Bretscher MS (1975) C-terminal region of the major erythrocyte sialoglycoprotein is on the cytoplasmic side of the membrane. J Mol Biol 98:831–837 – Dahr W, Uhlenbruck G, Janssen E, Schmalisch R (1977) Different N-terminal amino acids in MN-glycoprotein from MM and NN erythrocytes. Hum Genet 35:335–340 – Gahmberg CG, Hakomori SI (1973) External labeling of cell surface galactose and galactosamine in glycolipid and glycoprotein of human erythrocytes. J Biol Chem 248:4311–4317 – Gahmberg CG, Myllylä G, Leikola A, Pirkola A, Nordling S (1976) Absence of the major sialoglycoprotein in the membrane of human En(a-) erythrocytes and increased glycosylation on band 3. J Biol Chem 251:6108–6116 – Gahmberg CG, Jokinen M, Andersson LC (1978) Expression of the major glycoprotein (glycophorin) on erythroid cells in human bone marrow. Blood 52:379–387 – Gahmberg CG, Jokinen M, Andersson LC (1979) Expression of the major red cell sialoglycoprotein, glycophorin A, in the human leukemic cell line K562. J Biol Chem 254:7442–7445 – Gahmberg CG, Jokinen M, Karhi KK, Andersson LC (1980) Effect of tunicamycin on the biosynthesis of the major human red cell sialoglycoprotein, glycophorin A, in the leukemia cell line K562. J Biol Chem 255:2169–2175 – Jokinen M, Gahmberg CG, Andersson LC (1979) Biosynthesis of the major human red cell sialoglycoprotein, glycophorin A, in a continous cell line. Nature 279:604–607 – Jokinen M, Ulmanen I, Andersson LC, Kääriäinen L, Gahmberg CG (1981) Cell-free synthesis and glycosylation of the major human red cell sialoglycoprotein, glycophorin A. Eur J Biochem (in press) – Karhi KK, Andersson LC, Vuopio P, Gahmberg CG (1981) Expression of blood group A antigens in human bone marrow cells. Blood 57:147–151 – Lisowska E. Duk M (1975)

Modification of amino-groups of human erythrocyte glycoproteins and new concept on structure basis of M and N blood-group specificity. Eur J Biochem 54:469–473 – Lozzio CB, Lozzio BB (1975) Human chronic myelogenous leukemia cell-line with positive Philadelphia chromosome. Blood 45:321–334 – Mäkelä O, Cantell K (1958) Destruction of M and N blood group receptors of human red cells by some influenza viruses. Ann Med Exp Fenn 36:366–343 – Marchesi VT, Tillack TW, Jackson RL, Segrest JP, Scott RE (1972) Chemical characterization and surface orientation of the major glycoprotein of the human erythrocyte membrane. Proc Natl Acad Sci USA 69:1445–1453 – Thomas DB, Winzler RJ (1969) Structural studies on human erythrocyte glycoproteins. J Biol Chem 244:5943–5949 – Tomita M, Marchesi VT (1975) Amino acid sequence and oligosaccharide attachment sites of human erythrocyte glycophorin. Proc Natl Acad Sci USA 73:2964–2968

Haematology and Blood Transfusion Vol. 26
Modern Trends in Human Leukemia IV
Edited by Neth, Gallo, Graf, Mannweiler, Winkler
© Springer-Verlag Berlin Heidelberg 1981

The Network Concept and Leukemia

K. Eichmann

Network regulation undoubtedly represents a major mechanism for the maintenance of steady states in the immune system. This is brought out by a large body of experimental evidence suggesting that every antigen-specific element in the immune system – antibody, soluble mediator, or lymphocyte – has its anti-idiotypic counterpart. Thus, the immune system is constructed as a series of idiotypic and anti-idiotypic compartments that regulate one another. The nature of regulation is determined by the effector functions of the antigen-specific elements in each compartment.

Since idiotypic connection is used as a major pathway for the delivery of regulatory signals, it is not surprising that idiotypic or anti-idiotypic reagents are particularly powerful means to artificially manipulate the immune system. A large body of experimental results suggests that with idiotypic and anti-idiotypic antibodies dramatic and persistant changes in immune reactivity can be induced. Furthermore, by choice of the class of antibody changes can be induced such that particular effector functions are altered, whereas others are left untouched. This is in contrast to immune manipulation by antigens and other means in which changes of the immune status are difficult to control.

What this have to do with leukemia? There are at least two ways in which the network concept could become relevant to leukemia. Firstly, one has to consider the possibility that unbalances in network control make certain lymphocytes particularly susceptible to neoplastic transformation. Examples of this appear to be certain groups of mouse myelomas, for example, those with antiphosphorylcholine specificity and T 15 idiotype. These myelomas are found in the collection of Balb/c myelomas

at a much greater frequency than would be expected if specificities were randomly distributed. The high frequency of phosphorylcholine specific myelomas is reflected in the normal lymphocyte population of Balb/c mice, and evidence is accumulating at present that this overrepresentation is due to a network unbalance. Thus, network unbalances may be cofactors in neoplastic transformation of lymphocytes.

A second area in which the network concept touches on leukemia relates to therapy. The present state of technology clearly suggests a novel strategy for specific immune therapy of leukemia: normal T cells should be recovered from patients with leukemia and restimulated in vitro with leukemic cells from the same patient. The methods for restimulation should be worked out such that a high proportion of cytotoxic T cells with specificity for idiotypic determinants on the leukemic cells arise. Such cytotoxic cells have been clearly identified by experimentation and their very special property is that they appear to be *functional in vivo*. Cytotoxic cells of all other specificities have been shown to be somehow suppressed in the in vivo situation. Thus, anti-idiotypic cytotoxicity may be the only cytotoxicity that can be exploited to kill neoplastic cells in vivo. After restimulation these cytotoxic cells should then be grown up to large quantities using TCGF technology and reinjected into the same patient.

A further relevant aspect of the network concept is that it reveals any nonspecific manipulation of the immune system to be worthless. Since the immune system is perfectly balanced through idiotypic interactions between its antigen-specific elements, only antigen-specific measures can be expected to disturb this balance in the direction of the generation of disired effector functions. Nonspecific manipulation, such as the so-called immune therapy, can at best change the absolute level of the balance with no functional consequence whatsoever.

Taken together, thinking along the lines of the network concept may open new approaches to the role of immunity in neoplastic diseases. The overall discouraging results from pervious clinical and experimental experience may have been due to our ignorance or negligence of certain basic principles in the way the immune system functions.

Reviews

Eichmann K, (1978) Adv. Immunol. 26, 195 – Jerne NK, (1974) Ann. Immunol 125 C, 373 – Jerne NK, (1976) Harvey Lect. 70, 93

Haematology and Blood Transfusion Vol. 26
Modern Trends in Human Leukemia IV
Edited by Neth, Gallo, Graf, Mannweiler, Winkler
© Springer-Verlag Berlin Heidelberg 1981

Interpretation and In Vivo Relevance of Lymphocytotoxicity Assays

E. Klein

The outcome of a short-term cell-mediated cytotoxic assay depends on the susceptibility of the target and the activation profile of the lymphocyte population. Certain cultured cell lines are highly sensitive to the lytic effect of lymphocytes of unimmunized donors, provided they have been derived from the same species; natural killing (NK) effect. This cytotoxicity seems to be independent of lymphocyte receptor-target antigen interaction but is likely due to some membrane property of the target (Ährlund et al. 1980). Specificity occurs only on the species level.

In the majority of studies which deal with characterization of the NK phenomenon one or a few lymphoblastoid cell lines are used as targets. With regard to NK sensitivity, cell lines fall into three categories, viz., those which are:

1. Sensitive in short term assays, with effector target ratios at and below 50:1. Extensive target cell damage is inflicted at low ratios which shows that the proportion of lymphocytes that can kill these targets is relatively high.
2. Sensitive only in long term assays.
3. Insensitive.

The difference between the first and second categories is probably quantitative. It seems that the lymphocyte population is heterogeneous with regard to the strength of the lytic function. Targets are characterized by a difference of the sensitivity to a lytic threshold which must be mounted by the lymphocyte. The difference between various targets is reflected in dose response experiments by the difference of the number of effector cells required to kill a certain number of targets. Increased effectivity can be achieved by manipulating the assay conditions. If a more prolonged target cell/lymphocyte interaction

is permitted to take place, the cytotoxic potential of the effector population is elevated. Interferon (IFN) production appears to play a key role in this event (Santoli and Koprowski 1979).

A. Natural Killing

"Natural killing" is an operational designation. A certain regularity appears in the human system. In short term tests T cell derived lines are more sensitive than those derived from B cells (Ono et al. 1977). Studies with the B lymphoblastoid lines showed that tumor-derived lines are more sensitive than those derived from normal cells (Jondal et al. 1978). In this connection it may be noted that the presence of EBV genome in the cell does not seem to influence NK sensitivity. EBV-negative B tumor lines and their EBV-converted sublines (derived by superinfection of the EBV-negative line with the virus) displayed no difference in sensitivity (to be published).

Experiments in mice with alternating retransplantation and explantation of tumor cells showed a change in NK sensitivity depending on whether the same target cells were harvested from the mouse or from the culture (Becker et al. 1978).

The relatively higher sensitivity of cultured cells compared to directly explanted cells (Becker et al. 1978; De Vries et al. 1975) may indicate that NK-sensitive cells are eliminated in vivo. It is conceivable that NK sensitive variants arise de novo when the population is released from the selective pressure of killer lymphocytes. Alternatively, after explantation a change of cell membrane characteristics may occur.

The majority of human blood lymphocytes with natural cytotoxic potential were found to belong to the T cell series (Kaplan and Calleweart 1978). They are heterogeneous with regard to their surface marker characteristics, however (Bakács et al. 1978). The ranking order of different subfractions derived from the nylon nonadherent lymphocyte population with regard to their "specific activity", i.e., their cytotoxic potential on a per cell basis, is as follows:

1. Non-SRBC-rosetting (which contains cells reactive with anti-T serum) subset with and without demonstrable Fc receptors;
2. SRBC-rosetting cells with relatively low avidity E receptors and concomitant expression of Fc receptors;
3. Cells with low avidity E receptors without Fc receptors;
4. Cells with high avidity E receptors and Fc receptors; and
5. Cells with high avidity E receptors without Fc receptors (Masucci et al. 1980a).

The good NK activity of nude mice without thymuses has been taken as evidence for the non-T nature of the killer cells. However, immature or precursor T cells are present in these mice and induction of differentiation by thymus implantation resulted in decrease in NK activity (Herberman and Holden 1978).

Short term exposure of lymphocytes to IFN results in a considerably enhanced NK activity (Trinchieri et al. 1978).

The non-B cells of nude mice resemble the "null" and low avidity E rosetting cell category of man in that they have a high NK activity that can be enhanced by interferon treatment. These cells may have a role in vivo, since nude mice can reject grafts of virus infected tumor cells (Minato et al. 1979).

Assays for NK and interferon activated killing (IAK) differ only operationally, in that IAK involves IFN pretreatment of the effector cells. The two systems overlap. The results with lymphocytes of individuals with high NK activity are similar to IFN-activated lymphocytes from donors which function at a lower level of natural activity. Thus different persons can be assumed to be "preactivated" at different levels. The similarities between the two systems suggest that the rules emerging from IAK experiments are likely to be valid for the NK system as well. In view of the known prompt triggering effect of interferon for

cytotoxicity, it is likely that this mechanism is important in the host response against virus infected and tumor cells.

Activation by interferon occurs before the clone of lymphocytes with antigen-specific receptors have the opportunity to enlarge. This cytotoxicity may therefore be the first active measure of the host defense by which altered cells are eliminated and virus spread is inhibited.

Interferon production is induced by viruses and by virus-carrying cells. In addition, interferon is produced during immune interactions between lymphocytes carrying specific receptors and the antigens. Thus, activation of nonselective cytotoxicity by virus-infected cells may occur through two mechanisms. The first is the effect of the virus and the second is the consequence of recognition of the altered cells and the virus by specific immunocompetent cells. The selective antigen-specific cytotoxicity appears lather, after proliferation of the clone with the specific receptor.

B. Generation of Killer Cells in Culture

The NK activity of lymphocytes gradually disappears under culture conditions (Masucci et al. 1980a). However, when lymphocytes are activated in culture by specific stimuli (e.g., in MLC), cytotoxicity is generated which affects not only targets related to the stimulus but also other cells that have no known antigenic relationship to it. In addition to alloantigens (Calleweart et al. 1978), calf serum (Zielske and Golub 1976), and some modification that occurs on the surface of cultured tumor cells (Martin-Chandon et al. 1975), EBV-transformed autologous and allogeneic lymphoid lines (Svedmyr et al. 1974) and PHA (Stejskal et al. 1973) can also trigger this type of cytotoxicity. In the allogeneic MLC system the activity was designated as "anomalous killing" (Seeley and Golub 1978). The activated lymphocyte can also affect certain targets that are NK resistant in short-term tests (Masucci et al. 1980a,b).

Since there is a quantitative correlation between generation of blastogenesis and the efficiency of the killing potential, (against K562, Molt-4, etc.) the latter can also be used as a measure of activation (Masucci et al. 1980a: Vánky et al. 1981).

The natural and the cultured activated killer (AK) cell populations show slightly different characteristics (Poros and Klein 1978). A relatively higher proportion of the AK cells adhere to nylon wool. The proportion of Fc receptor carrying killer cells in lower, and the FcR positive cells possess fewer or less avid receptors in the AK than in the NK system. T cells with high affinity E receptors are the least active both in the fresh (NK) and cultured (AK) populations.

Neither NK nor AK show the histocompatibility restriction phenomenon. The AK of a lymphocyte culture is not brought about by surviving NK cells but are triggered de novo. T cell populations depleted of the NK active subsets became cytotoxic on exposure to appropriate activating stimuli (Masucci et al. 1980); lymphocytes which have been kept in autologous plasma in vitro for several days and have lost NK activity can become cytotoxic when cultured further with K562 cells or exposed for short time to interferon (Poros and Klein 1978; Vánky and Argov 1980).

On the population level the following cytotoxicity systems can be generated in antigen-containing lymphocyte cultures:

1. Enlargement of the specific clone will result in cytotoxicity against
   (a) cells which carry the stimulating antigen and
   (b) cells which carry cross reactive antigens,
2. Transactivation will recruit lymphocytes with other specificities, and thus targets unrelated to the stimulus may be killed if the proportion of lymphocytes with receptors against their antigens is higher (Augustin et al. 1979).
3. Activated lymphocytes kill certain type of targets (cultured lines). This interaction is probably independent of antigen recognition.

Analysis of antigen-induced cytotoxic systems suggests that in any experiments the question of "specificity" on the effector level can only be asked if target cells of similar characteristics are used. As we have been proposed earlier (Martin-Chandon et al. 1975), the detection of specifically reactive cells is perhaps more meaningful at the level of the recognition step.

Awareness of these phenomena is important for interpretation of cytotoxicity experiments and to decide whether NK or AK is relevant in surveillance against virus-infected or transfor-med cells. The questions to be raised are as follows: Are lymphocytes which recognize the altered cell surfaces present in the lymphocyte population? Can these be activated by nonspecific means for cytotoxicity and can such cytotoxicity give an adequate protection? Is the viral infection or malignant transformation accompanied by changes of the plasma membrane which can interact with T lymphocytes similar to what is seen with cultured lines?

C. Killer Cells in the Blood of Acute Infectious Mononucleosis Patients

In view of the prompt triggering effect of IFN for the cytotoxic potential of lymphocytes and the wider cell panel affected by activated lymphocytes it is likely that the lytic effect of blood lymphocytes in these diseases is a consequence of activation. Infection with EBV imposes proliferation on B cells in vitro. It would be expected, therefore, that the lymphocytosis and the blasts in the blood of EBV mononucleosis are due to B cell proliferation. This is however not the case: the cells belong to the T lineage and B cells are few (Enberg et al. 1974). In fact, special measures (separation of subsets) had to be used to detect the EBV-infected B cells (Klein et al. 1975). During the acute phase when blasts are present in the blood, short term cytotoxicity of the lymphocytes is not restricted to NK sensitive targets (Svedmyr and Jondal 1975). These cells kill EBV-transformed lymphoblastoid B lines and also the ones derived from autologous lymphocytes. It is likely that in this cytotoxicity the recognition of an EBV-determined surface antigen on the target cells does not play a role but is due to the activation state of the T cells. The presence of T cell clones which recognize the EBV antigens, however, can be demonstrated later, after the acute phase subsided (Moss et al. 1978). The detection of such T cells during the acute phase would require experimental conditions in which the nonspecific effect of activated lymphocytes is eliminated. As we have shown before, the elimination of Fc receptor positive cells is not sufficient to achieve this with activated populations (Masucci et al. 1980a,b).

The autoreactive lymphocytes in the acute phase may be important for the recovery of the patient by limiting the proliferative tendency of the EBV infected B cells. However, while in the majority of IM cases the activated T cells probably have a beneficial surveillance function, in some cases they may result in autoimmune phenomena of varying severity (Purtilo et al. 1979).

D. Autotumor Reactive Cells in Patients

In the course of experiments aimed to detect tumor-specific autoreactivities of patients with solid tumors we have performed short term cytotoxicity tests with blood lymphocytes against the autologous tumor biopsy cells [autologous lymphocytotoxicity (ALC)] (Vose et al. 1977). The outcome of these experiments indicated recognition of tumor cells in 28% of the cases. In an attempt to enhance the efficiency of the cytotoxicity test the lymphocytes were pretreated with IFN prior to the assay. This measure did not alter the results in the ALC but induced cytotoxicity against allogeneic tumor biopsy cells in 50% of the cases (Vánky et al. 1980b). Without IFN treatment, 5% of the allogeneic tests with lymphocytes of tumor patients and 14% with the lymphocytes of healthy donors were positive. The results were interpreted as an IFN-induced polyclonal activation of the lymphocyte population and manifestation of cytotoxicity by those T-cells which carry receptors against the histocompatibility antigens present on the particular target.

In order to impose more efficient stimuli for activation we have attempted to generate cytotoxic cells by cultivating blood lymphocytes with autologous tumor biopsy cells or use conditions that bring about lymphocyte activation such as MLC with the patient's lymphocytes as responders (Vánky et al. 1981).

In 19 MLCs in which the patients' lymphocytes were used as responders, seven generated autologous tumor cell killers and 11/13 damaged allogeneic tumor cells (unrelated to the reactants). The effects against the allogeneic tumor cells were either due to antigenic cross reactivities between the stimulator lymphocytes and the target tumor cells and/or transactivation of alloreactive lymphocytes with other specificities.

Assuming that there was no antigenic relationship between the stimulator allolymphocytes and the autologous tumor cells, the results can be interpreted in such a way that in 40% of cases autologous tumor recognizing lymphocytes were "transstimulated" in the MLC. K562 cells were regularly killed by all MLC effectors which provided the proof that activation took place in all cultures.

Autoreactivity by specific means, i.e., in the autologous mixed cultures containing lymphocytes and tumor cells, was generated in a higher proportion of tests (12 of 19).

The most effective system to generate killer cells against autologous tumor cells was thus the autologous mixed culture. Even in those cases in which autotumor killing was not generated the lymphocytes were activated by the encounter with tumor cells because they killed the K562 cells. This indicated that recognition of the tumor cells took place in the autologous mixed cultures.

Our results with the solid tumor cells are similar to those reported by Zarling et al. (1976) and by Sharma and Odom (1979) who used freshly harvested leukemia cells. Zarling and Bach (1979) mentioned that short term IFN treatment of the lymphocytes did not induce cytotoxicity against the autologous leukemia cells. This was achieved, however, when a strong stimulus was provided by confrontation with a pool of several allogeneic lymphocytes (Zarling et al 1976) or with soluble bacterial extract (Sharma and Odom 1979). It was also shown that autologous EBV-transformed lymphoblastoid cell lines could be killed by MLC-activated lymphocytes (Seeley and Golub 1978). Killers affecting autologous leukemia cells could be induced to proliferate by exposure to TCGF (Zarling and Bach 1979).

If cytotoxic cells will be available for therapeutical administration, similar considerations which concern drug or radiotherapy may have to be raised, i.e., in addition to the antitumor effects the specifically activated lymphocyte population may damage sensitive nonmalignant cells also.

The demonstration of the occurrence of lymphocytes which recognize the autologous tumor biopsy cells indicate that immunologic recognition of the autologous tumors is a reality and further research on this line is meaningful and important. On the basis of the in vitro experiments a more convincing therapeutic effect of nonspecific immunostimulation would have been expected than has been achieved. Modification of the therapeutic strategy is perhaps still a possibility which should receive further attention.

Acknowledgments

This investigation was supported by Grant No. 5 R01 CA25250-02 awarded by the National Cancer Institute, U.S. Dept. of Health, Education, and Welfare, in part by Federal funds from the Department of Health, Education and Welfare under contract number N01 CB74144, and by the Swedish Cancer Society.

References

Ährlund-Richter L, Masucci G, Klein E (1980) Somatic hybrids between a high NK-sensitive lymphoid (YACIR) and several low sesitive sarcoma or L-cell derived mouse lines exhibit low sensitivity. Somatic Cell Genet 6:89–99 – Augustin AA, Julius MH, Casenza H (1979) Antigen-specific stimulation and transstimulation of T-cells in long term culture. Eur J Immunol 9:665–670 – Bakács T, Klein E, Yefenof E, Gergely P, Steinitz M (1978) Human blood lymphocyte fractionation with special attention to their cytotoxic potential. Z Immunitaetsforsch Immunobiol 154:121–134 – Becker S, Kiessling R, Lee N, Klein G (1978) Modulation of sensitivity to natural killer cell lysis after in vitro explantation of a mouse lymphoma. J Natl Cancer Inst 61:1495–1498 – Calleweart DM, Lighbody JJ, Kaplan J, Joroszowski J, Peterson WD, Rosemberg JC (1978) Cytotoxicity of human peripheral lymphocytes in cell mediated lympholysis, antibody dependent cell-mediated lympholysis and natural cytotoxicity assay after mixed lymphocyte cultures. J Immunol 121:81–85 – De Vries JE, Meyerung M, Van Dongren A, Rümke P (1975) The influence of different isolation procedures and the use of target cells from melanoma cell lines and short term cultures on the nonspecific cytotoxic effect of lymphocytes from healthy donors. Int J Cancer 15:391–400 – Enberg RN, Eberle BJ, Williams RC (1974) T and B cells in peripheral blood during infectious mononucleosis. J Infect Dis 130:104–111 – Herberman RB, Holden HT (1978) Natural cell-mediated immunity. Adv Cancer Res 27:305–370 – Jondal M, Spina C, Targan S (1978) Human spontaneous killer cells selective for tumour-derived target cells. Nature 72:62–64 – Kaplan J, Calleweart D (1978) Natural killer cells express human T lymphocyte antigens. J Natl Cancer Inst 60:961–964 – Klein G, Svedmyr E, Jondal M, Persson PO (1975) EBV determined nuclear antigen (EBNA)-positive cells in the peripheral blood of infectious mononucleosis patients. Int J Cancer 17:21–26 – Martin-Chandon MR, Vánky F, Carnaud C, Klein E (1975) "In vitro education" on autologous human sarcoma generates nonspecific killer cells. Int J Cancer 15:342–350 – Masucci G, Poros A, Seeley JK, Klein E (1980) In vitro generation of K562 killers in human T-lymphocyte subsets. Cell Immunol 52:247–254 – Masucci MG, Klein E, Argov S (1980a) Disappearance of the NK effect after explantation of lymphocytes and generation of similar monospecific cytotoxicity correlated to the level of blastogenesis in activated cultures. J Immunol 124:2458–2463 – Masucci MG, Masucci G, Klein E, Berthold W (1980b) Target selectivity of interferon induced human killer lymphocytes related to their Fc receptor expression. Proc Natl Acad Sci USA 77:3620–3624 – Minato N, Bloom BR, Jones C, Holland J, Reid LM (1979) Mechanism of rejection of virus persistently infected tumor cells by athymic nude mice. J Exp Med 149:1117–1133 – Moss DJ, Rickinson AB, Pope JH (1978) Long term T cell mediated immunity to Epstein Barr virus in man. I. Complete regression of virus-induced transformation in cultures of seropositive donors' lymphocytes. Int J Cancer 22:662–668 – Ono A Amos DB, Koren HS (1977) Selective cellular natural killing against human leukemic T cells and thymus. Nature 266:546–647 – Poros A, Klein E (1978) Cultivation with K562 cells leads to blastogenesis and increased cytotoxicity with changed properties of the active cells when compared to fresh lymphocytes. Cell Immunol 41:240–255 – Purtilo DT, Paquin L, DeFlorio D, Virzi F, Sakhuja R (1979) Immunodiagnosis and immunopathogenesis of the X-linked recessive lymphproliferative syndrome. Semin Hematol 16:309–343 – Santoli D, Koprowski H (1979) Mechanism of activation of human natural killer cells against tumor and virus-infected cells. Immunol Rev 44:125–162 – Sharma B, Odom LF (1979) Generation of killer lymphocytes in vitro agáinst humañ autologous leukemia cells with leukemia blasts and BCG extract. Cancer Immunol Immunotherp 7:93–98 – Seeley JK, Golub SH (1978) Studies on cytotoxicity generated in human mixed lymphocyte cultures. I. Time course and target spectrum of several distinct concomitant cytotoxic activities. J Immunol 120:1415–1422 – Stejskal V, Lindberg S, Holm G, Perlman P (1973) Differential cytotoxicity of activated lymphocytes on allogeneic and xenogeneic target cells. II. Activation by phytohemagglutinin. Cell Immunol 8:82–92 – Svedmyr EA, Deinhardt F, Klein G (1974) Sensitivity of different target cells to the killing action of peripheral lymphocytes stimulated by autologous lymphoblastoid cell lines. Int J Cancer 13:891-903 – Svedmyr E, Jondal M (1975) Cytotoxic effector cells specific for B cell lines transformed by Epstein-Barr virus are present in patients with infectious mononucleosis. Proc Nat Acad Sci USA 72:1622–1626 – Trinchieri G, Santoli D, Koprowski H (1978) Spontaneous cell-mediated cytotoxicity in humans: Role of interferon and immunoglobulins. J Immunol 120:1849–1855 – Vánky F, Argov S (1980a) Human tumor lymphocyte interaction in vitro. VII. Blastogenesis and generation of cytotoxicity against autologous tumor biopsy cells are inhibited by interferon. Int J Cancer 26:405–411 – Vánky F, Argov S, Einhorn S, Klein E (1980b) Role of alloantigens in natural killing. Allogeneic but not autologous tumor biopsy cells are sensitive for interferon induced cytotoxicity of human blood lymphocytes. J Exp Med 151:1151–1165 – Vánky F, Argov S, Klein E (1981) Tumor biopsy cells participating in systems in which cytotoxicity of lymphocytes is generated. Autologous and alloge-neic studies. Int J Cancer 27 – Vose BM, Vánky F, Klein E (1977) Lymphocyte cytotoxicity against autologous tumor biopsy cells in humans. Int J Cancer 20:512–519 – Zarling JM, Bach FH (1979) Continuous culture of T cells cytotoxic for autologous human leukemia cells. Nature 280:685–687 – Zarling JM, Raich PC, McKeough M, Bach FH (1976) Generation of cytotoxic lymphocytes in vitro against autologous human leukemia cells. Nature 262:691–693 – Zielske JV, Golub SH (1976) Fetal calf serum induced blastogenic and cytotoxic response of human lymphocytes. Cancer Res 36:3842–3846

Haematology and Blood Transfusion Vol. 26
Modern Trends in Human Leukemia IV
Edited by Neth, Gallo, Graf, Mannweiler, Winkler
© Springer-Verlag Berlin Heidelberg 1981

Acute Leukemia and Nonspecific Killer Cells

J. Milleck, P. Jantscheff, H. Thränhardt, M. Schöntube, R. Gürtler, D. Seifart, and G. Pasternak

A. Introduction

This paper is to give a contribution to two aspects of the study of leukemia: functional characterization of human leukemia cells and cellular mechanisms leading to the killing of leukemia cells. Considering that some populations of nonmatured lymphocytic and myelolytic cells are natural killer (NK) cells or effectors of the antibody-dependent cellular cytotoxicity (K cells), we have been looking for these effector cells in patients suffering from acute lymphoblastic leukemia (ALL) or acute non-lymphoblastic leukemia (ANLL). In cases with high leukemic blast counts the possibility of detection of leukemic NK or K cells may exist. Since animal experiments indicate a bone marrow origin of non-specific killer cells, we directly compared effector cell activities of mononuclear blood leukocytes (PBL) and bone marrow (BM) cells.

With regard to cellular cytotoxicity directed towards leukemia cells we previously described an antibody-dependent cellular cytotoxicity against ALL cells coated with a xenogeneic ALL antiserum (Milleck et al. 1978). In this report we want to provide some data on NK activity against human leukemia cells.

B. Patients and Methods

The ALL and half of the ANLL patients were children aged 0.5–15 years. Control groups consisted of hematologically healthy children and adults. Mononuclear PBL and BM cells were prepared by Ficoll-Visotrast centrifugation, and killer cell activities were estimated by the ^{51}chromium-release technique. Five thousand target cells in 0.1 microliter were incubated with an excess of 50 times the effector cells at 37°C for 4 h. Targets were cells of the K-562 cell line and ALL (REH) cell line (kindly provided by Dr. M. F. Greaves) for NK and mouse leukemia cells coated with antibodies for K estimation.

C. Results and Discussion

As shown in Fig. 1a, most of the ALL and ANLL patients display a very low or no NK or K cell activity, which confirms the findings of Schmidt et al. (1976). There were some patients with quite normal NK or K cell activity. This is not unexpected with patients having low leukemic blast counts in their blood. At a high ratio of blasts [percentage of blasts in PBL/BM: 90/90 (patient I.W.); 88/99 (patient T.O.); 94/n.t. (patient B.G.)] the NK or K cell activity of PBL or BM cells indicates the existence of leukemia cells with killer cell activity. Patient T.O. had a higher NK activity than K activity (Fig. 2); of patients I.W. and B.G. we tested only their K cell activity. A quite normal killer cell activity of leukemia patients was found after blood transfusion (Schmidt et al. 1978). While one patient (I.W.) was given a transfusion, the two others were not.

Some untreated leukemia patients showed a low level of NK or K cell activity in spite of the low peripheral blast counts. Since repression effect not is involved, we have to look for another explanation. It is conceivable that killer cells which have been used up in the blood or died away cannot be replaced because of the lack of supply from the leukemic bone marrow. Furthermore, it is possible that the killer cell activity of the patients involved was low for genetic reasons. This was not true for at

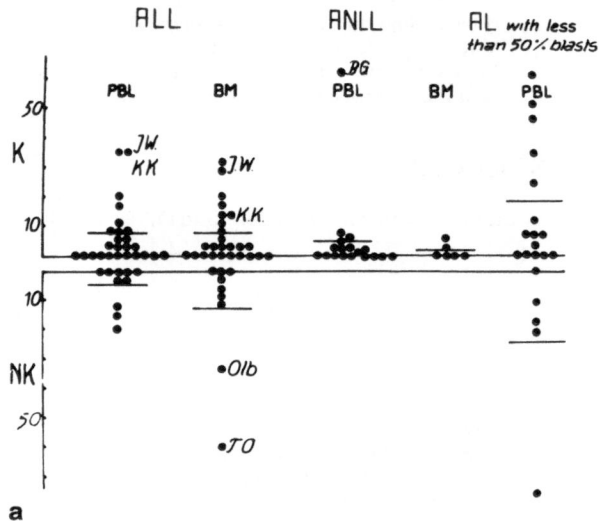

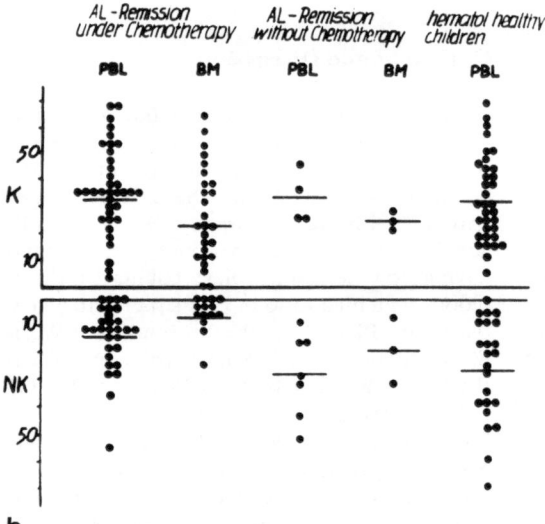

Fig. 1. NK and K cell activities (% specific ^{51}Cr-release) of mononuclear blood leukocytes, *(PBL)* or bone marrow *(BM)* cells. **a** acute non treated leukemia patients; **b** patients in a remission phase and hematologically healthy children. *ALL,* acute lymphoblastic leukemia; *ANLL,* acute nonlymphoblastic leukemia; *AL,* acute leukemia

least two patients, because their killer cell activities increased in a later remission phase.

With remission patients (Figs. 1b and 2) the K cell activity was somewhat lower compared with normal donors. Greater differences appeared in NK cell activity. The patients undergoing chemotherapy had a lower activity than remission patients without therapy or control donors. This finding suggests that chemotherapy has a stronger effect on NK cell activity than on K cell activity.

When comparing the PBL and bone marrow cells of individual hematologically healthy donors, in part coinciding killer cell activities were found, the coincidence being better on the K cell level than on the NK cell level. That PBL and BM cells stem from different sources is revealed by the proportions of E rosette forming cells: PBL: 52%±9% (64 donors) and BM cells: 19%±8% (six donors). With leukemia patients there occurred greater differences in the killer cell activity between PBL and BM cells. Differences were also observable when comparing the NK and K cell activities with each other, which indicates selective inhibition of NK or K cell receptors. But it could also be a hint to the presence of different NK and K cell populations.

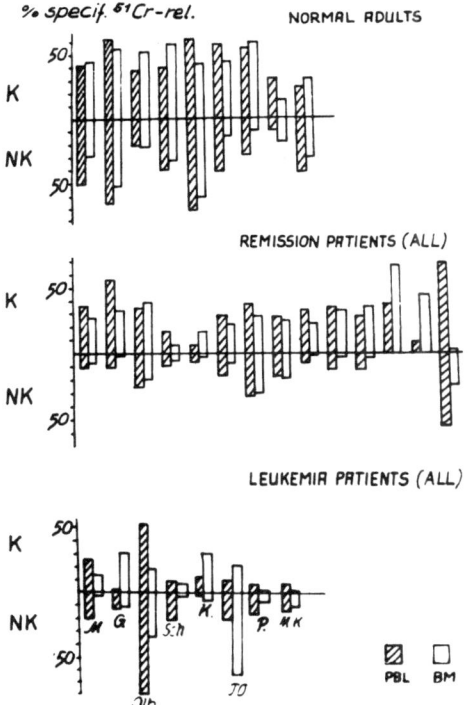

Fig. 2. Comparison of the killer cell activities between mononuclear blood leukocytes *(PBL)* and bone marrow *(BM)* cells of single acute lymphoblastic leukemia *(ALL)* patients and hematologically healthy adults

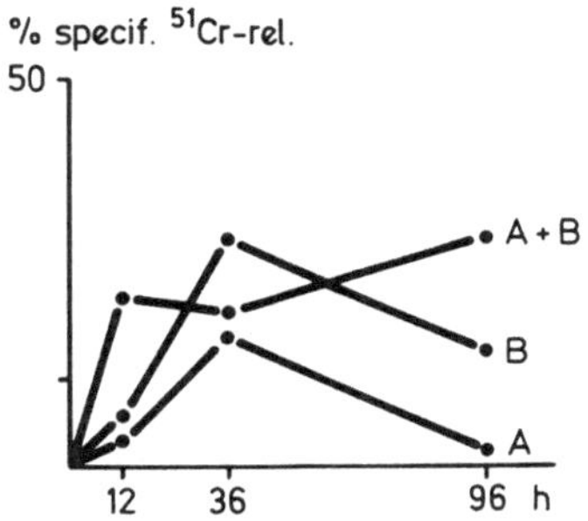

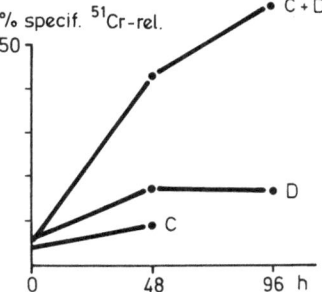

Fig. 3. Induction of NK cell activity against acute lymphoblastic leukemia *(ALL)* (REH) target cells in a mixed culture of PBL of the allogeneic donors *A* and *B*

Fig. 4. Induction of NK cell activity in a mixed culture of lymph node cells from the donors *C* and *D* (intestinal lymph node cells from tumor patients)

D. In Vitro Induction of NK Cells Against Leukemia Cells

Unlike the K cell activity against leukemia cells (Milleck et al. 1978) the NK activity is mostly low. However, immunological stimulation may give rise to NK cells destroying leukemia target cells that have not been attacked before the stimulation (Zarling et al. 1979). Figure 3 shows the induction of NK cells against the ALL (REH) cell line in a mixed culture of allogeneic PBL. Such NK cells already occurred on cultivation of the cells from the individual donors, but here the activity abated more rapidly than in the mixed culture. It is interesting to note that the NK cell induction had already occurred within a short span of time. It may be that the decrease in leukemic blasts in the peripheral blood which is sometimes observable one day after blood transfusion is attributable to similar NK cell effects. NK cells have so far been found mainly in blood, bone marrow, and spleen. Figure 4 shows that NK cells may form also in a mixed culture of lymph node cells. This shows that lymph nodes, which have so far been considered as largely inactive, harbor potential NK cells. No K cells appeared in the cocultivation of lymph node cells. This is further evidence that NK and K cells could be different cell populations.

References

Milleck J, Karsten U, Eckert R, Dörffel W, Thränhardt H, Pasternak G (1978) Antibody-dependent cellular cytotoxicity in experimental and human leukemia. In: Rainer H (ed) Immunotherapy of malignant diseases. Schattauer, Stuttgart New York, pp 323–326 – Schmidt P, Peter HH, Kalden JR, Avenarius HJ, Bodenstein H (1978) Effektorfunktion akuter Leukämiezellen in "spontanen" (SCMC) und Antikörper abhängigen zellulären Zytotoxizitätstesten (ADCC). Klin Wochenschr 56:953–962 – Zarling JM, Eskra L, Borden EC, Horoszewicz J, Carter WA (1979) Activation of human natural killer cells cytotoxic for human leukemia cells by purified interferon. J Immunol 123:63–70

Haematology and Blood Transfusion Vol. 26
Modern Trends in Human Leukemia IV
Edited by Neth, Gallo, Graf, Mannweiler, Winkler
© Springer-Verlag Berlin Heidelberg 1981

The Use of Bacteria as Markers of Leukemic Lymphocytes and for the Isolation of Natural Killer Cells

M. Teodorescu, C. Hsu, A. Bratescu, K. P. DeBoer, R. Nelson, R. Kleinman, C. M.-J. Wen, E. P. Mayer, and E. J.-M. Pang

A. Abstract

Human lymphocyte subpopulations as well as leukemic lymphocytes can be identified and enumerated in blood smears by using bacteria that bind spontaneously to lymphocytes or by using bacteria to which antibodies are chemically coupled. The mechanism of natural binding of bacteria to lymphocytes was shown to involve a lectin on the lymphocyte surface and a carbohydrate on the bacteria. Also, we found that natural killer (NK) cells can be separated by negative selection using monolayers of bacteria. A subpopulation of T cells, identified by their binding of *B. globigii,* was shown to be suppressors for NK cells.

B. Introduction

The methods used routinely to identify lymphocyte subpopulations involve the separation of lymphocytes from other blood cells followed by staining with fluorescent antibodies and/or rosette formation with erythrocytes. These procedures are all difficult to standardize and suffer from subjective interpretations. Moreover, the loss of particular subpopulations of cells and the inability to assess the cellular morphology can cause inaccuracies.

We have developed methods of identifying lymphocyte subpopulations in blood smears by using bacteria as carriers for purified antibody against cell membrane antigens or bacteria that bind spontaneously to lymphocytes (Teodorescu et al. 1977a, 1979a). Antibody-coated bacteria have been used to identify B and T cells in smears of peripheral blood and bacteria that bind spontaneously have been used to identify and enumerate B cells as well

as two B and four T cell subpopulations. Also, bacteria have been used to identify leukemic lymphocytes in cell suspensions or in blood smears (Nelson et al. 1979; Teodorescu et al. 1977b). A method has been developed to separate various lymphocyte subpopulations by bacterial adherence and functional differences among them have been demonstrated (Kleinman and Teodorescu 1978, 1979; Kleinman et al. 1980).

C. Material and Methods

I. Bacterial suspensions

Bacteria were grown and fixed as previously described (Teodorescu et al. 1979a).

II. Labeling the Lymphocytes with Bacteria in Stained Blood or Bone Marrow Smears

The procedure previously described has been followed. Briefly, heparinized blood was collected and the cells were washed. Bacteria were added in excess to small samples of blood cells, centrifuged for 6 min at 900 g to promote binding, and centrifuged twice more at 150 g for 10 min to remove the unbound bacteria. The suspension was smeared and stained with Wright's stain.

III. Separation of Lymphocyte Subpopulations by Bacterial Adherence

The procedure previously described was followed (Kleinman and Teodorescu 1978, 1979; Kleinman et al. 1980). Briefly, bacteria were coupled to glutaraldehyde-fixed gelatin layers. Monocytes were removed by glass wool adherence and the lymphocytes purified by Ficoll-hypaque gradient centrifugation. The lymphocytes were centrifuged against bacterial monolayers, and the nonadherent cells were separated from the adherent cells.

D. Results and Discussion

I. Acute Lymphocytic Leukemias

With rare exceptions, bacteria bound abundantly to lymphocytes (Fig. 1). We studied 12 patients with acute lymphocytic leukemia) (ALL) using bacteria as well as fluorescent antibodies (Hsu and Morgan 1980). Of these cases five were classified as pre-B cells based on a relatively low percentage of Ig$^+$ cells but high percentage of lymphocytes binding B melitensis, a B cell marker independent of surface Ig (Teodorescu et al. 1979b). In all five of these patients, although the percent age of Ig$^-$ Bm$^+$ cells was high, the percentage of Ig$^+$ cells was relatively low with a relatively normal $\varkappa/\lambda$ ratio (Fig. 2). This observation suggests that the cells were arrested at a stage of differentiation much earlier than that in which the surface Ig is exposed. In chronic lymphocytic leukemia (CLL) it appears that cells with undetectable surface Ig coexist with Ig-bearing cells of only one type of light chains (Nelson et al. 1979). The existence in one patient of a higher percentage of Ig$^+$ cells than cells that bound *B. melitensis* suggests that sometimes the Ig is of exogenous origin. This was also reflected by the large overlap between $\varkappa$-bearing and λ-bearing lymphocytes.

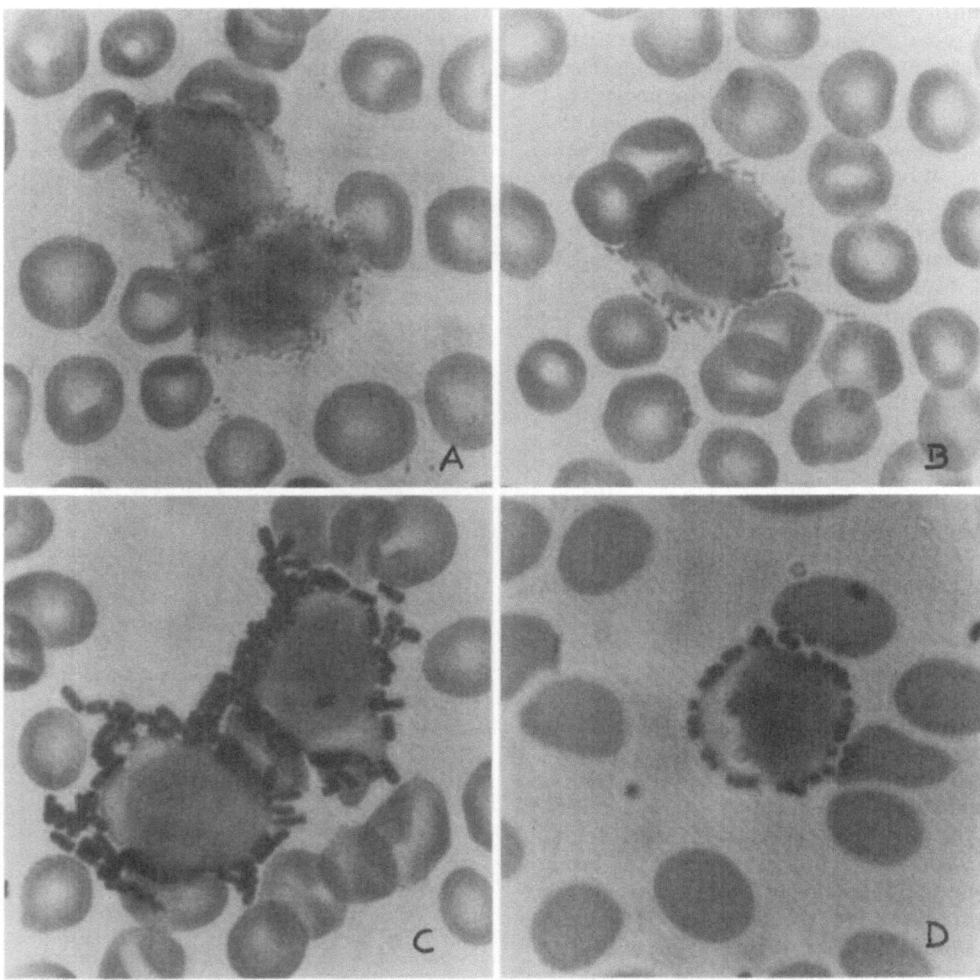

Fig. 1. Lymphocytes labeled by bacteria in blood smears of patients with leukemia. **A** *B. melitensis;* **B** *E. coli;* **C** *B. globigii* and **D** *S. aureus*

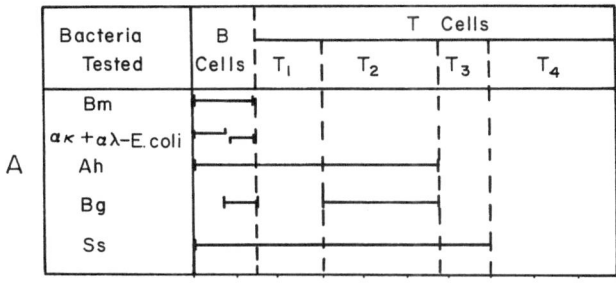

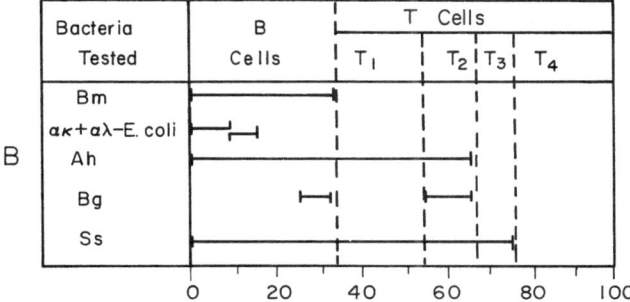

PERCENT OF LYMPHOCYTES BINDING BACTERIA

Fig. 2. The map of human lymphocyte subpopulations in blood smears of a normal donor (**A**) and a patient with ALL (**B**) Note the larger B cell population than Ig+ cell population with normal $\varkappa/\lambda$ ratio

One patient (14-month-old female) had familial chronic myelocytic leukemia (four cases diagnosed in the same family, Ph[1−]). The patient was studied here during an excerbation and found to have relatively high percentage of Bm+ lymphocytes which was much higher in the peripheral blood than in the bone marrow. At the same time the percentage Ig+ cells was normal. The coexistence of leukemic pre-B cells with CML cells was also described in 3 out of 20 cases of CML by Greaves (Greaves 1979). This observation suggests that B cells and myelocytes may have an immediate common precursor.

II. The Mechanism of Binding of Bacteria by Lymphocytes

We put forward the hypothesis that bacteria bind as the result of an interaction between a lectin on the lymphocyte surface and a carbohydrate on the bacteria (Teodorescu et al. 1979b). The following results were obtained in its support:

1. The binding of *B. melitensis* to B cells was prevented by α-methyl-D-mannoside (α-MM) but not by other sugars, suggesting that one of the lectins involved in binding is similar to Concanavalin A (Con A);

2. The binding of *B. melitensis* to B cells was prevented by pretreatment of the peripheral blood lymphocytes (PBL) with 5% α-MM, but pretreatment of bacteria had no effect;

3. An *Escherichia coli* mutant (strain 2023) which binds to B cells and part of the T cells was also agglutinated by Con A, but its parental strain was not; the binding of this mutant to B cells was also inhibited by α-MM;

4. Bacteria that bind to human lymphocytes were agglutinated at high titers by various plant lectins, while those that do not bind were agglutinated at low titers or not at all;

5. Bacteria that bind to B-cells as well as those that bind to B- and T-cells were agglutinated by Con A, *Lens culinaris* agglutinin, and *Pisum sativum* agglutinin, whose carbohydrate specificities were α-D-mannosyl- and α-D-glucosyl- residues;

6. The "receptors" on lymphocytes but not those on bacteria were sensitive to pronase, suggesting that the protein (lectin) was on the lymphocyte surface; and

7. Bacteria still bound after being heated at 121°C or being fixed with formaldehyde.

Lectin-sugar interactions have been shown to be involved in a variety of cellular interactions and recognition processes (Simpson et al. 1978). Since lymphocyte subpopulations are

357

selectively responsive to different lectins, these cells may interact among themselves or with other cells using their lectins or their carbohydrates. Thus, bacteria may recognize functional "arms" of lymphocyte subpopulations.

III. The Binding of Bacteria to CLL Lymphocytes

Both E. coli coated with anti-light chain antibody and B. melitensis bind to a substantial number of CLL lymphocytes (Nelson et al. 1979; Teodorescu et al. 1977b). Other bacteria have also been found to bind to these cells, suggesting the existence of a heterogenity within the malignant clone (Teodorescu et al. 1977b). Based on our results suggesting that lymphocytes have surface lectins, we speculated that these lectins are somehow involved in the control by other cells of malignant lymphocyte proliferation. Therefore, we put forward the hypothesis that with the progression of disease lymphocytes with less lectins are selected and grow uncontrolled.

We determined the binding of several strains of bacteria to CLL lymphocytes in blood smears of 24 patients. We found a statistically significant correlation (p=0.001) between binding indices and symptom status, i.e., the symptomatic patients had an average binding index of 35% and the asymptomatic 56.6% (Nelson et al. 1979).

Table 1. The relationship between binding indices for bacteria and survival in CLL patients[a]

Patient	Binding index	Interval between tests (months) or between the first test and death	Binding index
C.C.	70	26	55
S.F.J.	66	24	54
S.L.	60	20	53
TC	56	25	53
L.G.	46	24	46
W.J.	45	26	33
K.M.	45	25	45
F.A.	36	23	dead
K.I.	33	5	dead
B.E.	26	32	26
S.R.	11	13	dead
B.M.	7	16	dead

[a] The binding index was calculated as an average of the percentages of CLL lymphocytes that bound ten different bacteria

To demonstrate whether our observation is also relevant in predicting patient survival, we listed 12 patients in the order of binding indexes (Table 1) and followed them longitudinally. We found that the patients with low binding index also had poor survival rates, suggesting that this index may be of prognostic value.

IV. Isolation of Natural Killer Cells by Bacterial Adherence

We have previously shown that some of the lymphocyte subpopulations identified by bacterial adherence are functionally different (Kleinman and Teodorescu 1978; 1979; Kleinmann et al. 1980). Since T_4 cells do not bind any bacteria, they were readily isolated by negative selection by adsorbing on bacterial monolayers B cells, T_1, T_2, and T_3 cells. Most of the natural killer (NK) activity of the peripheral blood lymphocytes (PBL) was concentrated in the T_4 lymphocyte subpopulation (Kleinman et al. 1980). The T_4 cell population contained about 75% cells with receptors for Fc of IgG, which have been shown to be indicative of NK cells (West et al. 1977).

We investigated whether the activity of NK cells was controlled by another lymphocyte subpopulation identified by bacteria. When the ^{51}Cr release in 4-h assay was determined at increasing ratios of lymphocyte/target cells, we found that the PBL and T_4 cell curves never merge. This observation suggested that the T_4 cells were prevented from acting by another cell population. This inhibitory effect was not due to a simple dilution of NK cells, steric interference, or to a competition for targets. In fact, only when living T_2 cells were added to T_4 cells did the inhibition occur; when T_1T_3 cells were added the inhibition did not occur. Thus, T_2 cells appear to be suppressors for NK cells.

Although evidence has been accumulating that the NK activity is important in vivo in the defense against leukemic cell proliferation, the reason for the exquisite sensitivity of malignant cells to NK cells has not been demonstrated. It is worth noting that T_4 cells do not bind any of the bacteria tested (over 60 strains tested), and therefore, they are unlikely to have lectins. On the other hand, lymphoblastoid cell lines bind well and indiscriminately various bacteria. Thus, we may speculate that during malignant transformation various new lectins are exposed and attract preferentially the "lectinless" (negative replica) lymphocytes (or monocytes), resulting in killing. When we tested the binding properties of T_4 cells compared with T_2 cells, we found that the former binds exclusively to CEM lymphoblastoid cells but not to Chang hepatoma cells and that T_2 cells bound well to Chang cells but not to CEM cells.

Based on the results presented above or published elsewhere (Nelson et al. 1979) bacteria can be useful reagents for the identification and characterization of leukemic lymphocytes and of the cells that may be involved in the defense against leukemic cells. Since we have developed the necessary technology of selecting mutants of *E. coli* with various binding properties (Mayer and Teodorescu, 1980), the possibility exists of developing a large number of useful reagents that offer obvious advantages.

References

Greaves MF (1979) In: Neth R, Gallo RG, Hofschneider PH, Mannweiler K (eds) Modern trends in human leukemia III, Springer, Berlin Heidelberg New York, p 335 – Hsu CCS, Morgan ER (1980) Am J Clin Path 73:633 – Kleinman R, Teodorescu M (1978) J Immunol 120:2020 – Kleinman R, Teodorescu M (1979) Cell Immunol 48:43 – Kleinman R, DeBoer KP, Teodorescu M (1980) Clin Exp Immunol 39:510 – Mayer EP, Teodorescu M (1980) Infect Immun 29:66 – Nelson R, Bratescu A, Teodorescu M (1979) Cancer 44:1665 – Simpson DL, Thorne DR, Loh HH (1978) Life Sci 22:727 – Teodorescu M, Mayer EP, Dray S (1977a) Cell Immunol 29:353 – Teodorescu M, Mayer EP, Dray S (1977b) Cancer Res 37:1715 – Teodorescu M, Bratescu A, Mayer EP (1979a) Clin Immunol Immunopathol, 13:194 – Teodorescu M, Wen CM-J, Mayer EP (1979b) Fed Proc 38:1461 – West W, Cannon G, Kay HD, Bonnard G, Herberman R (1977) J Immunol 118:355.

Haematology and Blood Transfusion Vol. 26
Modern Trends in Human Leukemia IV
Edited by Neth, Gallo, Graf, Mannweiler, Winkler
© Springer-Verlag Berlin Heidelberg 1981

Receptor Mediated Murine Leukemogenesis: Monoclonal Antibody Induced Lymphoma Cell Growth Arrest

M. S. McGrath, L. Jerabek, E. Pillemer, R. A. Steinberg, and I. L. Weissman

A. Introduction

We have proposed a receptor-mediated leuke-mogenesis hypothesis wherein T lymphomas would be clones of T cells bearing mitogen-lin-ked surface receptors specific for the envelope determinants of the inducing MuLV (Weiss-man and Baird 1977; McGrath and Weissman 1978, 1979). We have tested a wide range of murine thymic lymphomas induced by thymo-tropic retroviruses and have shown that these cells indeed bear surface receptors highly specific for the retrovirus envelope glycopro-teins produced by these cells (McGrath et al. 1978a,b). Even closely related recombinant retroviruses bound less well than the autolo-gous retroviruses (McGrath et al. 1978b, McGrath and Weissman 1979). That these retroviruses and their interactions with T lym-phoma cell receptors might be involved in the pathogenesis of murine leukemia was sugge-sted by two kinds of experiments: First, only the leukemogenic viral isolates bound specifi-cally to lymphoma cell receptors, while non-leukemogenic but closely related viral prepa-rations bound less well or not at all (McGrath et al. 1978b, McGrath and Weissman 1979). Second, if one examined the distribution of receptor bearing cells in the thymus of a pre-leukemic AKR mouse, only T cells bearing cell surface receptors recognizing the inducing MuLV were capable of adoptive transfer of the leukemic state, whereas morphologically simi-lar cells within the same thymus were not capable of leukemic proliferation in syngeneic hosts (McGrath and Weissman 1978, 1979).

While the above described experimental results are consistent with the receptor-media-ted leukemogenesis hypothesis – and in fact were necessary postulates of the hypothesis

– they do not constitute proof of the hypothe-sis. The central postulate of the hypothesis is that continued leukemic proliferation is the result of continued antigenic stimulation of these T cell lymphomas. The purpose of this study was to design experiments aimed at testing that postulate. To do so, we raised monoclonal antibody reagents to leukemia cell surface determinants and tested the effect of these antibodies on leukemic cell proliferation in vitro as well as on specific virus binding to these cells. Several antibodies were found which inhibited lymphoma cell proliferation in vitro. Evidence is presented that this may be due to a blockade in virus binding to these cells.

B. Results

Rat monoclonal antibodies raised against the spontaneous AKR/J thymic lymphoma cell line KKT-2 were added to exponentially gro-wing KKT-2 cells in culture for 16 h, and ^{3}H-thymidine incorporation of these cells was quantitated as in Fig. 1. Antibodies recogni-zing the Thy-1 or T-80 molecules inhibited thymidine uptake by these cells, whereas anti-MuLV and antitumor-specific (43–17, 43–13) antibodies showed no effect. The inhibitory antibodies were effective at dilu-tions approaching 1:10,000 and KKT-2 growth inhibition was directly related to the level of cell surface antibody bound and the degree of interference with MuLV binding (McGrath et al. 1979, 1980a,b). Inhibitiory antibodies result in cell stasis at cell cycle phase G_1. In the initial set of experiments there was a linear fall to background in KKT-2 cell DNA synthesis, with a shift in DNA content from 4n

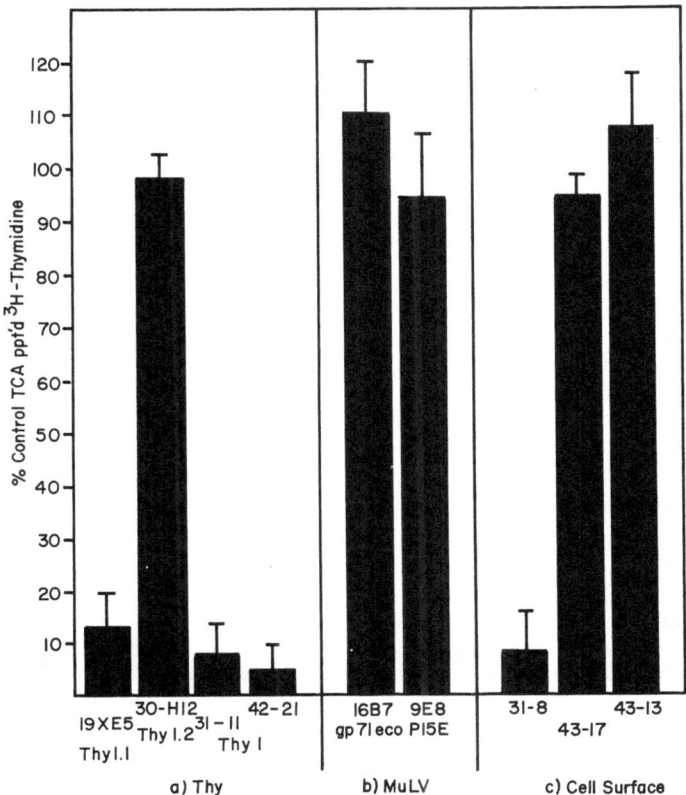

Fig. 1. Lymphoma cell growth inhibition assay. KKT-2 lymphoma cells were pelleted from subconfluent cultures and were resuspended in serum-free grwoth medium (MEM, GIBCO) for 2 h at 37°C at a density of 10^5 cells/ml. After repelleting, the cells were resuspended in cold tissue culture medium (MEM, 5% FCS) at a density of 2×10^4 cells/ml. Two and one-half milliliters (5×10^4 cells) were placed in the bottom of 25-cm^2 Corning tissue culture flasks and monoclonal antibody was added for a 1:12 final dilution. After growing for 16 h at 37°C, 0.1 ml medium containing 10 μCi [^{3}H] thymidine (NEN) was added to each culture for 2 h. Labeled cells were washed, 5% TCA precipitated, and percent growth inhibition was calculated using cells without antibody as equal to 100% growth. KKT-2 cells were tested for growth inhibition with (**a**) anti-Thy-1 (19XE5, 30-H12, 31–11, 42–21), (**b**) anti-MuLV (16B7,9E8), and (**c**) anticell surface antibodies (31-8, 43-17, 43-13). The above data represent five experiments ± standard deviations

towards 2n copies within 20 h (McGrath et al. 1979). This corresponded with a cellular size shift from large to small within 24 h culminating in noncomplement mediated cell death within 48 h (McGrath et al. 1979, 1980b).

Figure 2 shows that prebinding of KKT-2 receptors with KKT-2-SL virus protects the cell from inhibition whereas even closely related heterologous viruses do not. The level of cell surface bound antibody is not decreased by prebound KKT-2-SL virus, and preabsorption of antibody with KKT-2-SL virus does not remove inhibitory activity (McGrath et al. 1979, 1980a,b).

Prior to January 1980 antibody inhibition of KKT-2 cell growth by the inhibitory antibodies occurred rapidly in the first cell cycle following addition of the antibodies. Since that time and concomitant with a required change in tissue culture serum sources, inhibitory antibodies (42-21, 31-11, 31-8) act on KKT-2 cells only on the 2nd–4th day following addition of the antibodies. The same distribution of inhibitory and noninhibitory antibodies is seen as previously reported (McGrath et al. 1980a). The

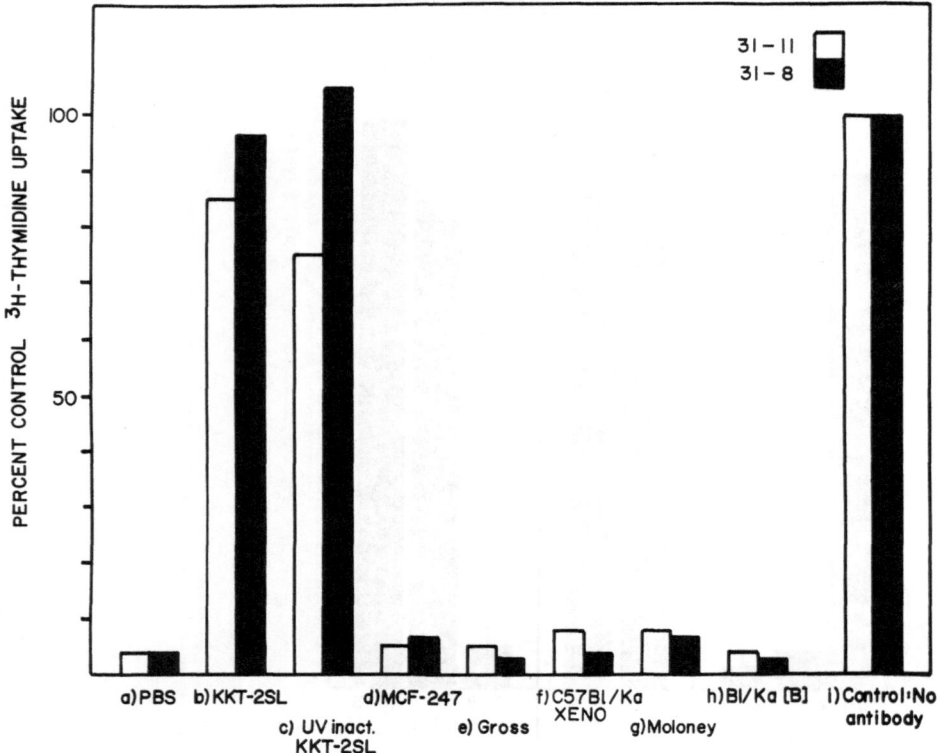

Fig. 2. The standard KKT-2 cell growth inhibition assay as outlined in Fig. 1 was carried out with 31–11 and 31–8 antibodies at a 1:250 dilution on 5×10^4 KKT-2 cells after preincubation with purified retroviruses. 0.01 a_{260} unit of Sepharose-4B-purified virus (McGrath et al. 1978c) in 0.3 ml PBS was incubated with KKT-2 cells for 60 min at room temperature prior to addition of inhibitory antibodies. This amount of virus represents a receptor saturation level as previously determined (McGrath et al. 1978b). The origin of each retrovirus population has also been previously described (McGrath et al. 1978b; McGrath and Weissman 1979). Sepharose-4B-purified KKT-2-SL virus was also UV inactivated and used to inhibit antibody-induced KKT-2 cell growth inhibition. Five milliliters of virus in PBS (1 A_{260} unit/ml) was irradiated for 145 sec at 4000 ergs/mm² prior to use (Niwa et al. 1976)

inhibitory antibodies (αThy-1 and αT80) act similarly on several other T-MuLV-induced T lymphomas. However, S49 cells are still inhibited in the first cell cycle.

Because anti-Thy-1 arrested lymphoma cell growth, we tested several mutant lymphoma cell lines for MuLV binding to determine more precisely the nature of the MuLV receptor. Table 1 shows that both Thy 1⁻ and H-2⁻ cell lines have equivalent MuLV receptor levels to those of their parental cell lines. We have not yet tested whether there is some correlation

between S49 MuLV binding, growth regulation, and level of antibody bound per cell.

Because T lymphoma cells have been shown to be susceptible to lectin, dexamethasone (Ralph 1973), and cAMP-induced (Coffino et al. 1975a) cell death, we tested several S49 mutant cell lines for susceptibility to antibody mediated growth arrest. Table 2 shows that cAMP is probably not involved in the antibody-induced growth arrest. Similarities between dexamethasone and lectin induced cell killing are currently still under investigation.

	Fluoresceinated MuLV preparations			Table 1. MuLV binding specificities: maximal percent age MuLV bound per cell[a]
	MCF-247	RadLV/VL$_3$	S49-SL	
1. KKT-2	100	68	46	
2. BL/VL$_3$	62	100	57	
3. S49 (Clone 24–32)	48	62	100	
4. S49 (Thy 1$^-$)	51	52	110	
5. L691/M.E12 (Clone E12 H-2$^-$)	250	250	N.D.	
6. L691/M (H-2$^-$)	160	160	N.D.	
7. Balb/c thymocytes	5	5	8	

[a] Maximal binding respresented by the mean fluoresceinated homologous virus bound per cell, i.e., RadLV/VL$_3$ binding to BL/VL$_3$ cells. N.D. = not done. Each entry represents the percentage of maximal fluorescence for the cell population as calculated by the following formula: % = mean fluorescence of test population/mean fluorescence of standard population × 100 where the standard population is the homologous virus-cell interaction. Fluoresceinated MuLV preparations were tested for binding specificity to four different cell populations. Binding was analyzed as described in experimental procedures and the legend to Fig. 1, and the mean fluorescence of virus bound per cell above cellular background was calculated. 100% binding was defined as virus binding to a homologous lymphoma (that is, MCF-247 to KKT-2 to RadLV/VL$_3$ to BL/VL$_3$, S49-SL to S49). The cell lines tested were: (1) spontaneous AKR/J thymic lymphoma, KKT-2; (2) RadLV-induced C57BL/Ka thymic lymphoma, BL/VL$_3$; (3) wild type spontaneous Balb/c thymic lymphoma S49, clone 24.32 (from Coffino, UCSF); (4) S49 Thy-1$^-$a mutant (Salk Institute); (5) C57/Leaden x-ray-induced T lymphoma L691, clone E12 selected for absence of H-2 (McGrath et al. 1980a and unpublished work in preparation); (6) Moloney-infected L691 producer cells, non-H-2 expressing from clone E12; and (7) normal 4-week-old Balb/c thymocytes

C. Discussion

Growth control of normal T cells and T lymphomas is extremely complex. The relationships between antigen-induced (Fathman and Weissman 1980) and growth factor induced (i.e., TCGF) (Morgan et al. 1976; Gillis et al. 1980) T cell proliferation are currently under intense investigation and the variables involved are multiple and poorly understood. As noted above, KKT-2 cells are now not inhibited in the 24 h growth assay; anti-Thy-1 antibodies no longer inhibit MuLV binding to those cells in a short-term assay. Yet this antibody does inhibit proliferation of KKT-2 cells in a 3–4 day incubation period. These findings may implicate several pathways to mitogenesis in this cell line, one of which is directly related to anti-Thy-1 and anti-T-80-induced inhibition. No experiment which we have carried out yet demonstrates the identity of the viral receptor. While αThy-1 antibodies may block T-MuLV binding and T lymphoma proliferation, the former effect must be via steric hindrance, as Thy-1 molecules need not be expressed for specific T-MuLV binding. It now becomes even more important to identify the T-MuLV receptors on T-lymphoma cells, to establish their relatedness between lymphomas, to establish whether they are products of cellular or viral genes, and to identify more precisely the viral determinants they recognize.

Table 2. Growth inhibition of S49 enzyme mutants after exposure to monoclonal antibodies[a]

S49 cell type	Treatment of cells				
	a) Control	b) Bt$_2$cAMP	c) 31–11 (1:80) Anti-Thy 1	d) 31–8 (1:80) Anti-T-80	e) PHA (10 μg/ml)
1. Wild type Clone 24.32	–	+ + + +	+ + + +	+ + + +	+ + + +
2. Protein kinase mutant	–	–	+ + + +	+ + + +	+ + + +
3. Adenylate cyclase mutant	–	+ + + +	+ + + +	+ + + +	+ + + +
4. Deathless mutant	–	+ +	+ + + +	+ + + +	+ + + +

[a] S49 cell lines were suspended at 10^5 cells per ml for 3 days in the growth inhibition assay outlined in Fig. 1. Cell growth and inhibition was quantitated by live and dead cell counting after treatment as shown above. a=control cells; b=3.3×10^{-4} M final concentration of dibutyrl cAMP (Sigma); c=1:80 final dilution of 31–11 anti-Thy-1; d=1:80 final dilution of 31–8 anti-T-80; e=10 μg/ml final concentration of phytohemagglutinin (Welcome, purified). The S49 mutant cell lines and their properties have been previously described: wild-type clone 24.32 and protein kinase mutant by Coffino et al. (1975b); adenylate cyclase mutant by Bourne et al. (1975); deathless mutant, which is arrested by cAMP but not killed, by Lemaire et al. (1977). + + + + =all cells dead; + + =cell alive; no growth; and – =no effect.

References

Bourne HR, Coffino P, Tomkins GM (1975) Selection of a variant lymphoma cell deficient in adenylate cyclase. Science 187:750 – Coffino P, Bourne H, Tomkins G (1975a) Mechanism of lymphoma cell death induced by cyclic AMP. Am J Pathol 81:199 – Coffino P, Bourne H, Tomkins G (1975b) Somatic genetic analysis of cyclic AMP action: Selection of unresponsive mutants. J Cell Physiol 85:603 – Fathman CG, Weissman IL (1980) Production of alloreactive T cell lymphomas. Nature 283:404 – Lemaire I, Coffino P (1977) Cyclic AMP induced cytolysis in S49 cells: Selection of an unresponsive "deathless" mutant. Cell 11:149 – McGrath MS, Weissman IL (1978) A receptor mediated model of viral leukemogenesis: Hypothesis and experiments. Cold Spring Harbor Symp Quant Biol – McGrath MS, Weissman IL (1979) AKR leukemogogenesis: Identification and biological significance of thymic lymphoma receptors for AKR retroviruses. Cell 17:65–75 – McGrath MS, Lieberman M, Decléve A, Kaplan HS, Weissman IL (1978a) The specificity of cell surface virus receptors on RadLV and radiation-induced thymic lymphomas. J Virol 28:819 – McGrath MS, Weissman IL, Baird S, Raschke W, Decléve A, Lieberman M, Kaplan HS (1978b) Each T-cell lymphoma induced by a particular murine leukemia virus bears surface receptors specific for that virus. Birth Defects 14:349–361 – McGrath MS, Witte O, Pincus T, Weissman IL (1978c) Retrovirus purification: Method which conserves envelope glycoprotein and maximizes infectivity. J Virol 25:923 – McGrath MS, Pillemer E, Kooistra D, Jacobs S, Jerabek L, Weissman IL (1979) T lymphoma retrovirus receptors and control of T lymphoma cell proliferation. Cold Spring Harbor Symp Quant Biol 44: – McGrath MS, Pillemer E, Weissman IL (1980a) Murine leukemogenesis: Monoclonal antibodies to T cell determinants which arrest T lymphoma cell proliferation. Nature 285:259–261 – McGrath MS, Pillemer E, Kooistra D, Weissman IL (1980b) The role of MuLV receptors on T-lymphoma cells in lymphoma cell proliferation. Cintemp Top Immunobiol 11:157 – Morgan DA, Ruscetti FW, Gallo RC (1976) Selective in vitro growth of T lymphocytes from normal human bone marrows. Science 193:1007 – Niwa O, Decleve A, Kaplan HS (1976) Conversion of restrictive mouse cells to permissiveness during sequential and mixed double infection by murine leukemia viruses. Virology 74:140–153 – Ralph P (1973) Retention of lymphocyte characteristics by myelomas and θ-lymphomas: Sensitivity to cortisol and phytohemagglutinin. J Immunol 110:1470 – Weissman IL, Baird S (1977) Oncornavirus leukemogenesis as a model for selective neoplastic transformation. In: Koprowski H (ed) Life sciences research report 7, neoplastic transformation: mechanisms and consequences. Dahlem Konferenzen, Berlin, p 135

Haematology and Blood Transfusion Vol. 26
Modern Trends in Human Leukemia IV
Edited by Neth, Gallo, Graf, Mannweiler, Winkler
© Springer-Verlag Berlin Heidelberg 1981

Effect of Bromodeoxyuridine on Endogenous Retrovirus Production in Differentiating Murine Lymphocytes

J. P. Stoye and C. Moroni

A. Introduction

Molecular hybridization studies have revealed the presence of multiple endogenous C-type viruses in germ line DNA of all mouse strains. Expression of viral information results in T-cell leukemias in AKR mice. Study of the control of these genes might be expected to provide information on both leukemogenesis and on gene regulation in eukaryotic cells. In vitro studies of virus induction have shown that bromodeoxyuridine (BrdU) incorporation into fibroblast DNA (Teich et al. 1973) leads to apparent gene derepression and the production of ecotropic and xenotropic viruses (Besmer et al. 1974).

We are interested in the control of endogenous virus expression in lymphocytes, the usual sites of C-type virus-induced diseases. As BrdU incorporation into fibroblast DNA leads to virus induction, the effect of adding BrdU to murine lymphocytes stimulated to proliferate with different mitogens was examined. Since different mitogens stimulate lymphocytes of different cell types, we could examine the effect of BrdU incorporation into different classes of lymphocytes. Surprisingly, we found that it was the target specificity of the mitogen which determined virus inducibility; only B-cells were induced by BrdU, T-cells appearing noninducible (Moroni et al. 1975; Schumann and Moroni 1976). The stimulation of cell proliferation was an absolute requirement for virus induction. In addition, it was observed that B-cell mitogens capable of promoting BrdU induction also induced low levels of xenotropic virus production (Moroni and Schumann 1975). Thus, BrdU appeared to amplify rather than to induce virus, and it remained unclear whether mitogen and BrdU

were acting synergistically or in parallel for virus induction. Two approaches to this question are described here. The first involved an examination of the dependence of induction on the stimulation of B-cell differentiation; the second, genetics.

B. Methods

Spleen cell suspensions were cultured for 3 days and assayed for reverse transcriptase and tritiated thymidine incorporation as previously described (Schumann and Moroni 1976). Antibody-secreting cells (ASC) were quantitated by the protein A coated sheep red cell plaque assay of Gronowicz et al. (1976). Xenotropic virus was assayed by the S^+L^- mink F648.1 line (Peebles 1975).

C. Results

It has been reported that terminally differentiated antibody-secreting B-cells express viral antigens (Wecker et al. 1977). Furthermore, all virus-inducing mitogens stimulate the appearance of ASC (Moroni et al., to be published). Thus it could be that ASC produce virus. However, BrdU, which amplifies virus production, inhibits the appearance of ASC. Table 1 shows the effect of BrdU on lipopolysaccharide (LPS) induction of virus in BALB/c mice, either as measured by reverse transcriptase activity or by infectious centers, and on the number of ASC. At a concentration of 5 µg/ml, which is optimal for virus induction, BrdU inhibits the appearance of ASC, without affecting the number of viable cells in LPS-stimulated cultures. These data suggested that virus induction by LPS might depend on LPS stimulation of cell differentiation, whereas

	Reverse transcriptase pmol/2×10^6 cells	Infectious centers S^+L^-foci/2×10^6 cells	ASC/2×10^6 cells
Control	0.04	0	200
LPS	0.42	2	31,800
LPS/BrdU	4.80	220	2,800

Table 1. BrdU amplification of LPS virus induction

	cpm ^{3}H-thymidine incorporated	ASC/2×10^6 cells	Reverse transcriptase pmol/2×10^6 cells	
			$-$BrdU	$+$BrdU
LPS	45,455	23,000	0.34	4.35
LPS$+\alpha$-IgM	47,147	3,600	0.24	1.37
$\dfrac{+\alpha\text{-IgM}}{\text{No}\alpha\text{-IgM}}$	1.04	0.16	0.70	0.31

Table 2. Effect of α-IgM on virus induction

virus induction by BrdU would depend on the stimulation of cell proliferation but not differentiation.

It has been shown that addition of an appropriate batch of antisera directed against mouse IgM (α-IgM) to LPS-stimulated cultures blocks the appearance of ASC without affecting cell proliferation (Anderson et al. 1974). Hence, α-IgM was added to LPS and LPS/BrdU treated cultures and reverse transcriptase measured 3 days after stimulation. Table 2 shows that virus production was reduced in both LPS and LPS/BrdU-treated cultures, but only by 30% and 69%, respectively, whereas the number of ASC was reduced by 84%. These results suggest that the stimulation of differentiation is involved in virus induction, at least in the case of LPS/BrdU. Confirmation of this point must await limiting dilution analysis to determine the effect of α-IgM on the number of cells making virus.

In a second approach to investigate B-cell differentiation we used CBA/N mice. They carry an X-chromosome linked, recessive B-cell defect (Cohen et al. 1976). Hence, we compared virus induction in age-matched (CBA/N$\times$BALB/c)F_1 males, which show the CBA/N phenotype, and females (Table 3). Virus induction with both LPS and LPS/BrdU as well as the number of ASC were much lower in males ($<25\%$) than in females. Thymidine incorporation in males was only 50% of the value in females, but we have shown that blocking DNA synthesis to 50% with hydroxyurea only results in a 50% reduction in virus induced by LPS and LPS/BrdU (data not shown). Taken together, the data with α-IgM and CBA/N mice suggest that cell differentiation is required for virus induction with both LPS and LPS/BrdU.

Since lymphocytes from a few strains of mice, e.g., 129, cannot be induced to produce infectious C-type virus, we have also taken a genetic approach to see whether genes for induction with LPS and LPS/BrdU segregate. Induction of xenotropic virus by LPS/BrdU was measured by an infectious center assay of spleen cells on mink S^+L^- cells (Table 1); induction by LPS by cocultivation of stimulated cells with mink CCL-64 cells for several

	cpm ^{3}H-thymidine incorporated	ASC/2×10^6 cells	Reverse transcriptase pmol/2×10^6 cells	
			$-$BrdU	$+$BrdU
♀	10,266	28,800	1.04	5.88
♂	5,224	4,200	0.24	0.47
♂/♀	0.51	0.15	0.23	0.08

Table 3. Induction in (CBA/N$\times$BALB/c)F_1 mice

passages (Monckton and Moroni 1980) followed by assaying for infectious xenotropic virus. BALB/c×129 crosses were kindly performed for us by Ms. Hämmerli (Tierfarm Sisseln). All BALB/c mice tested (15/15) were positive by these procedures, while all 129 mice (10/10) were negative. All (BALB/c×129)F$_1$ mice resembled BALB/c, i.e., inducibility was dominant. F$_1$ mice were backcrossed to 129 mice and tested for inducibility by LPS/BrdU; of these, 32/60 (53%) showed the BALB/c phenotype, implying that one gene controls induction by LPS/BrdU. Spleen cells from a number of the same mice were also tested for LPS induction. A perfect correlation was observed between LPS/BrdU and LPS: 17/17 LPS/BrdU positive mice were positive with LPS alone and 15/15 LPS/BrdU negative mice were noninducible with LPS. Induction with LPS and LPS/BrdU seemed, therefore, under the control of the same gene.

D. Discussion

LPS induction and BrdU "amplification" of endogenous virus production in BALB/c lymphocytes have a number of features in common. In both cases xenotropic virus is produced. Induction is controlled by the same genetic locus, probably the structural gene for BALB virus-2. The finding that BrdU increases the number of infectious centers by a factor of ten more than reverse transcriptase (Table 1) might well reflect an increased virus production per cell and hence an increased probability of detection. Both processes appear to require cell proliferation and differentiation. This suggests that murine lymphocytes release xenotropic virus at a certain stage along a normal differentiation pathway and that B-cell mitogens induce virus by stimulating the appearance of cells which produce virus. Antibody secretion itself does not appear to be required for virus production, since BrdU amplifies virus while at the same time inhibiting ASC.

Incorporation of BrdU into the DNA of three different types of cells derived from BALB/c mice has three different consequences for endogenous virus expression. In fibroblasts xenotropic and ecotropic viruses are induced, in stimulated B-cells xenotropic virus production is amplified, and in stimulated T-cells no infectious virus production occurs. The observation that α-IgM reduces the level of LPS/BrdU induction from B-cells suggests that certain differentiated functions, acquired only late in B-cell differentiation and present in fibroblasts, are required for virus induction. One class of candidates for this differentiation function are RNA-processing enzymes. The switch from surface to secreted IgM, which takes place after LPS stimulation, is thought to involve an alteration in mRNA processing (Singer et al. 1980). In a manner analogous to the failure of C-type viruses and SV40 to replicate in undifferentiated teratoma cells (Teich et al. 1977; Segal et al. 1979), the absence of the appropriate processing enzymes in T-cells might render them refractory to induction by BrdU.

References

Anderson J, Bullock WW, Melchers F (1974) Eur J Immunol 4:715 – Besmer P, Smotkin D, Haseltine W, Far H, Wilson AT, Paskin JM, Weinberg R, Baltimore D (1974) Cold Spring Harbor Symp Quant Bid 39:1103 – Cohen PL, Scher I, Mosier DE (1976) J Immunol 116:301 – Gronowicz E, Coutinho A, Melchers F (1976) Eur J Immunol 6:588 – Monckton RP, Moroni C (1980) J Gen Virol 47:59 – Moroni C, Schumann G (1975) Nature 254:60 – Moroni C, Schumann G, Robert-Guroff M, Suter ER, Martin D (1975) Proc Natl Acad Sci USA 72:535 – Moroni C, Stoye JP, DeLamarter JF, Erb P, Jay FA, Jongstra J, Martin D, Schumann G (1980) Cold Spring Harbor Symp Quant Biol 44:1205 – Peebles PT (1975) Virology 67:288 – Schumann G, Moroni C (1976) J Immunol 116:1145 – Segal S, Levine AJ, Khoury G (1979) Nature 280:335 – Singer PA, Singer HH, Williamson AR (1980) Nature 285:294 – Teich N, Lowy D, Hartley JW, Rowe WP (1973) Virology 51:163 – Teich NM, Weiss R, Martin GR, Lowy DR (1977) Cell 12:973 – Wecker E, Schimpl A, Hünig T (1977) Nature 269:598

Haematology and Blood Transfusion Vol. 26
Modern Trends in Human Leukemia IV
Edited by Neth, Gallo, Graf, Mannweiler, Winkler
© Springer-Verlag Berlin Heidelberg 1981

Modulation of Growth of Malignant Cells by Anti-Idiotypic Immunity

H. Schreiber, P. M. Flood, M. L. Kripke, and J. L. Urban

A. Introduction

One of the mechanisms capable of regulating an immune response involves the interaction of idiotypes and anti-idiotypes. In selected nontumor systems it has been shown that anti-idiotypic immunity can very specifically either suppress or stimulate immune responses (for review see Eichmann 1978). Thus, anti-idiotypic reagents may provide powerful tools for manipulating the induction or course of the host's immune responses to malignant cells.

To test this hypothesis, we have developed a tumor model in which anti-idiotypic immuni-

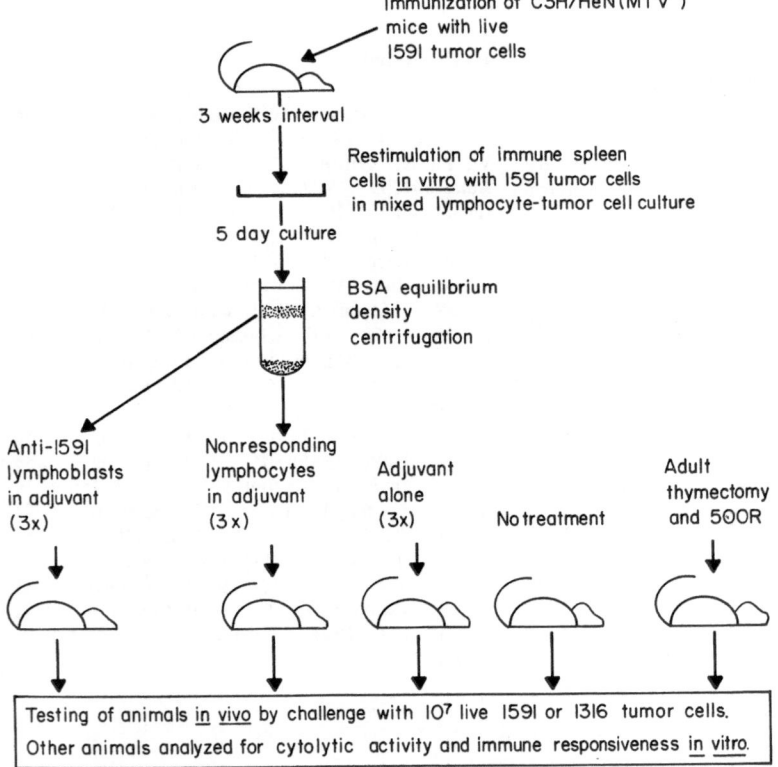

Immunization of C3H/HeN (MTV⁻)
mice with live
1591 tumor cells

3 weeks interval

Restimulation of immune spleen
cells _in vitro_ with 1591 tumor cells
in mixed lymphocyte-tumor cell culture

5 day culture

BSA equilibrium
density
centrifugation

Anti-1591
lymphoblasts
in adjuvant
(3x)

Nonresponding
lymphocytes
in adjuvant
(3x)

Adjuvant
alone
(3x)

No treatment

Adult
thymectomy
and 500R

Testing of animals _in vivo_ by challenge with 10⁷ live 1591 or 1316 tumor cells.
Other animals analyzed for cytolytic activity and immune responsiveness _in vitro._

Fig. 1. Experimental protocol used for the generation and purification of tumor-specific lymphoblasts, immunization with these cells, and subsequent testing of blast-immunized and control animals. For details see Flood et al. (1980)

ty of mice to syngeneic tumor-specific lympho-cytes can be elicited and analyzed (Flood et al. 1980). It had previously been shown that animals immunized with syngeneic purified antigen-specific lymphoblasts isolated from mixed lymphocyte cultures can produce anti-idiotypic immune responses to their own allo-antigen reactive T cells (Andersson et al. 1976, 1977; Aguet et al. 1978; Binz and Wigzell 1978). We have adapted this system to synge-neic responses against tumor antigens and we can now manipulate the immune response in such a way that tumors will grow in animals which would normally reject these tumors.

B. Materials and Methods

The fibrosarcomas 1591 and 1316 induced by ultraviolet light in C3H/HeN (MTV⁻) specific pathogen free mice were used (Kripke 1977). These tumors have non-cross-reactive tumor antigen and regularly regress upon transplantation into normal

young syngeneic C3H mice (Fisher and Kripke 1977), but grow progressively in thymectomized x-irradiated mice. The general approach for induc-tion of anti-idiotypic immunity by immunization with tumor-specific lymphocytes is shown in Fig. 1 and has previously been described in detail (Flood et al. 1980).

C. Results

We have found that immunization with tumor-specific lymphoblast induces unresponsiveness to 1591 tumor cells in vivo and in vitro (Fig. 2). Furthermore, we have found that immuniza-tion with 1591 specific lymphoblasts induced cytolytic anti-idiotypic T cells to these lympho-blasts. This was shown by an in vitro assay in which 1591 tumor-specific lymphoblasts were used as ^{51}-Cr-labeled target cells for the anti-idiotypic effector cells. Several lines of evidence suggested the specificity of the obser-ved effects. Resistance of the 1591 blast-im-

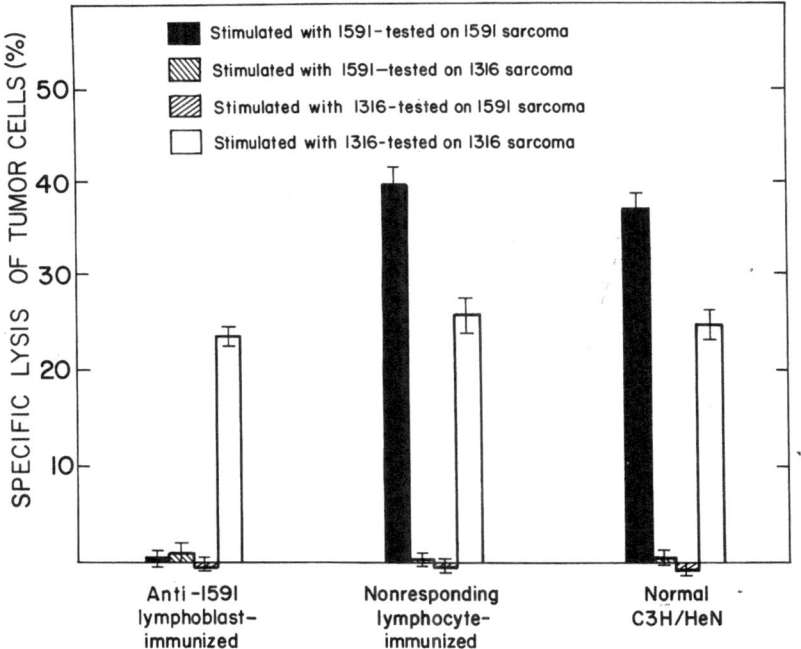

Fig. 2. Specific unresponsiveness of spleen cells from anti-1591 lymphoblast-immunized animals to 1591 tumor cells in culture. Spleen cells were stimulated in a 5 day primary mixed lymphocyte tumor cell culture with 1591 or 1316 tumor cells. The culture-generated effector cells were tested in a 3 h ^{51}Cr-release assay at a 100:1 effector to target cell ratio. Blast-immunized or control animals were tested 10 days after the third immunization

munized animals to 1316 tumor cells in vivo and responsiveness of the spleen cells from these animals in vitro were unimpaired. In agreement with this is the finding that spleen cells from the 1591 tumor-specific lymphoblast-immunized animals did not kill 1316 tumor-specific lymphoblasts. Furthermore, immunization with nonresponding lymphocytes or with lymphoblasts not having specificity for 1591 tumor cells were ineffective in inducing the observed effects.

Strong evidence indicating idiotype-specific immune reactions to tumor-specific lymphocytes came from the analysis of animals which responded to the tumor in spite of the blast immunization. These animals exhibited the same capability to specifically lyse 1591 tumor cells as control animals, yet they responded by generating 1591 specific lymphoblasts that were completely insensitive to lysis by anti-idiotypic effector cells (Table 1). This is in contrast to normal and control animals, which regularly responded by generating tumor-specific lymphocytes sensitive to the anti-idiotypic effector cells.

D. Discussion

The findings suggest that autologous idiotype-specific immunity against a tumor-specific lymphocyte clone, which is regularly present in

Table 1. Presence of a common 1591 specific idiotype on tumor-specific lymphocytes from normal and control animals which is absent in the tumor-specific lymphocytes of animals which broke idiotype-specific immune suppression

Source of target cells (anti-1591 lymphocytes)		Batch of anti-idiotypic effector cell probe (anti-anti-1591 lymphocytes)[a]	Specific lysis % of[b]	
Pretreatment	Animal no.		anti-1591 lymphoblasts	anti-1316 lymphoblasts
Normal animal	1	24-1	58	<0
	2	24-2	56	<0
	3	30-4	76	<0
	4	30-5	47	<0
	5	30-6	44	2
	6	30-7	53	<0
	7	31-1	36	<0
	8	31-2	33	N.D.
	9	35-1	44	<0
	10	35-1	50	<0
	11	35-1	56	<0
	12	35-1	54	<0
	13	35-1	44	<0
	14	35-1	43	<0
	15	44-2	56	<0
Nonresponding lymphocyte immunized animals	1	28-1	42	1
	2	28-2	54	7
	3	30-9	53	<0
	4	30-9	54	<0
Blast-immunized animals which broke suppression	1	28-1	0	1
	2	28-2	1	7
	3	30-9	1	<0
	4	30-9	0	<0

[a] Effector spleen cells were obtained from different batches of C_3H mice immunized three times with 10^7 1591-specific lymphoblasts in adjuvant

[b] Target cells were tested in a 4 h ^{51}Cr release assay using as target purified 1591-specific or 1316-specific lymphoblasts at a 250:1 effector-to-target cell ratio. These lymphoblasts were obtained after in vitro restimulation of spleen cells from normal, control, or blast-immunized tumor-responsive animals and purified by equilibrium density centrifugation

normal animals (Table 1), can be induced by the blast immunization. Thus, immunity eliminated the animals' normally predominant tumor-reactive lymphocyte clone, and these animals died of progressive tumor growth when challenged with the 1591 tumor cells, unless they were capable of breaking suppression with an idiotypically different, previously silent or undetected lymphocyte clone. The possible role of antigenic stimulation in the development of new clones (Cunningham and Pilarski 1974) is not clear in our system, but we have only observed the development of secondary 1591 specific clones in animals which have previously been blast immunized. Our experiments give strong evidence for the importance of tumor-specific lymphocytes in the primary defense of the onimmune host to malignant cells and raise the possibility that natural killer cells may not play a decisive role in the defense of C3H mice against these tumors. Interestingly, older mice or ultraviolet light irradiated young mice which are susceptible to the 1591 and 1316 tumors cannot develop 1591 specific lymphocytes in vivo or in vitro, while they do develop natural killer activity (manuscript in preparation). It will be interesting to determine whether anti-idiotypic reagents, used under defined conditions, may stimulate tumor-specific lymphocyte clones in such animals and thereby induce in these mice resistance to the malignant cells.

Acknowledgments

This research was supported by USPHS Grants R01-CA-22677 and R01-Ca 27326 to H. S and C0-75380 to M. L. K; H. S. is supported by RCDA CA-00432, P. F. by NRSA T32-AI-7090, and J. U. by T32-GMS-7281.

References

Aguet M, Andersson LC, Andersson R, Wight E, Binz H, Wigzell H (1978) J Exp Med 147:50–62 – Andersson LC, Binz H, Wigzell H (1976) Nature 264:778–780 – Andersson LC, Aguet M, Wight E, Andersson R, Binz H, Wigzell H (1977) J Exp Med 146:1124–1137 – Binz H, Wigzell H (1978) J Exp Med 147:63–76 – Cunningham AJ, Pilarski LM (1974) Eur J Immunol 4:319–326 – Eichmann K (1978) Adv Immunol 26:195 – Fisher MS, Kripke ML (1977) Proc Natl Acad Sci USA 74:1688–1692 – Flood PM, Kripke ML, Rowley DA, Schreiber H (1980) Proc Natl Acad Sci USA 77:2209 – Kripke ML (1977) Cancer Res 37:1395–1400

Haematology and Blood Transfusion Vol. 26
Modern Trends in Human Leukemia IV
Edited by Neth, Gallo, Graf, Mannweiler, Winkler
© Springer-Verlag Berlin Heidelberg 1981

Thymic Nurse Cells: Intraepithelial Thymocyte Sojourn and Its Possible Relevance for the Pathogenesis of AKR lymphomas

B. Kyewski, G. Hunsmann, R. Friedrich, U.-P. Ketelsen, and H. Wekerle

A. Introduction

Undifferentiated lymphoid precursor cells enter the thymus and differentiate there to lymphocytes clones which are diversified, both with regard to their specific antigen receptors as well as to their programmed function in the immune system. Generation of diversity and specialization of T cell subsets, both of which are fascinating examples of cell differentiation, are supposedly the result of interactions between the differentiating lymphoid cells on one side and nonlymphoid thymic stromal cells on the other. It is probable that intercellular interactions imply both communications via soluble mediators as well as direct cell-to-cell contact between the interacting cell partners. Physiologic T cell differentiation is, however, not without hazards. Within the thymus neoplastic transformation of differentiating T cells can occur, and there is evidence that this pathologic change represents an abnormal aberration of certain physiologic developmental events (McGrath and Weissman 1978).

Little is known about the exact mechanisms of physiologic and pathologic intrathymic T cell differentiation, nor do we know much about the localization of the developmental events within the organ. A quite unusual cellular phenomenon, the lymphoepithelial thymic nurse Cell (TNC) complexes, which we recently observed in dissociated rodent thymus populations, may be helpful for further understanding these problems.

TNCs are epithelial cells of enormous size which can be isolated from normal thymuses by differential trypsinization (Wekerle and Ketelsen 1980). They are specialized for incorporating large numbers of functionally intact, actively proliferating thymocytes in their cyto-plasm. The engulfed thymocytes are completely surrounded by epithelial membranes which display macromolecular specializations presumably involved in creating a special microenvironment. This finding, besides the expression of products of the H-2 subregions K,D,I-A, and I-E/C which are all believed to be centrally engaged in intercellular interactions during development and organization of the immune system, lead to a hypothesis postulating that formation of TNCs represents an intracellular differentiation cycle essentially required for intrathymic T cell maturation (Wekerle et al. 1980).

In this communication we report that TNCs from AKR/J mice are abnormal in several respects. They are of abnormally large size, containing up to 200 thymocytes. They further express retroviral products in their cytoplasms and on their membranes. And, finally, their presence in thymuses negatively correlates with the development of neoplastic thymomas in the adult AKR/J mouse.

B. Results

I. Morphologic Observations

TNCs, freshly isolated from 3-month-old AKR/J mice are abnormally large (Fig. 1). They may reach diameters exceeding 50–70 μm and contain estimated numbers of about 200 thymocytes in their cell bodies. Cytofluo-graph light scattering analyses revealed that only the TNC fractions, but not the free thymocytes, are of abnormal sizes. Ultrastructurally, the most striking observation concerns a relatively loose contact formation between engulfed thymocytes and the surrounding in-

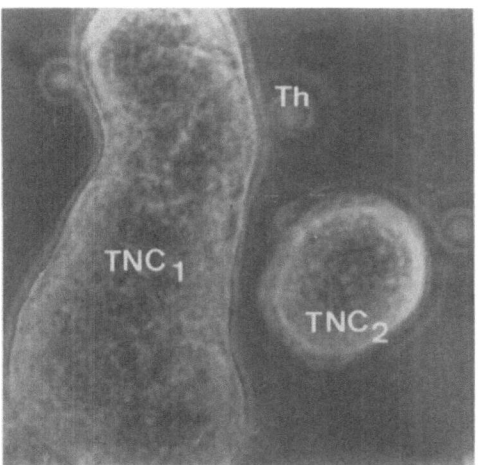

Fig. 1. Giant AKR thymic nurse cell. *Left side* Giant *TNC₁* formed by presumable one epithelial cell containing a high number of lymphoid thymocytes. *Right side, TNC₂* corresponding to normal size TNCs from nonleukemia prone mouse strains. In the background out of optical plane: free thymocytes *(Th)*

ternal epithelial membranes. The thymocytes were remarkable for their dense, ribosome-rich cytoplasms, active nuclei, and occasional mitoses (Fig. 2).

II. Occurrence of TNCs During Ontogeny

Preliminary investigations of normal mice indicate that TNCs are first dectable on day 16

of gestation. The number of demonstrable TNCs gradually increases with the growth of the organ. They can be found in thymuses at least until the age of 14 months (H. W. and G. A. Luckenbach, in preparation).

Until young adult ages the occurrence of TNCs in AKR/J mice resembles the one in normal strains. It is, however, remarkable that as soon as neoplastic conversion of thymus cells begin to occur, i.e., at the age of 6–8 months, the number of TNCs drastically declines. We never found TNCs in thymuses showing signs of neoplasia. It should furthermore be noted that in transferred thymomas we were unable to demonstrate TNC-like cell complexes.

III. Retroviral Determinants on AKR/J TNCs

The inverse relation between TNC occurrence and thymomagenesis as well as the abnormal TNC structure prompted us to search for products of C-type RNA viruses, a suspected tumorigenic agent. We applied indirect immunofluorescence using specific conventional antisera and fluorescein-labeled anti-immunoglobulin antibodies as markers. The TNCs were investigated subsequent to fixation in paraformaldehyde. We used antisera against Friend leukemia virus gp71, a glycoprotein of the viral coat. This antiserum strongly bound to the membranes of AKR/J as indicated by the bright ring shaped fluorescence (Fig. 3).

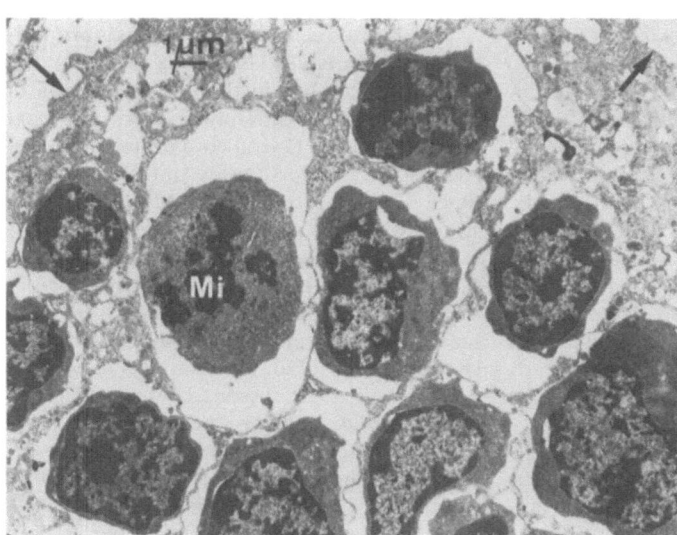

Fig. 2. Ultrastructure of AKR thymic nurse cell. Ultrathin section through TNC isolated from AKR thymus (3 months). *Arrows* mark outer TNC membrane. Note internalized thymocyte in mitosis *(Mi)*. Staining: uranyl acetate and lead citrate

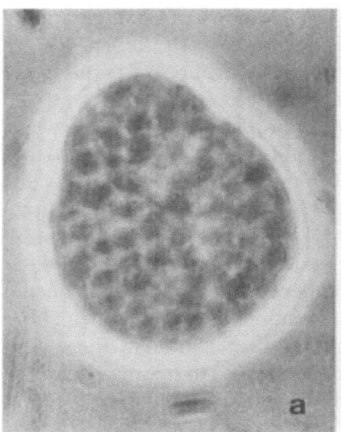
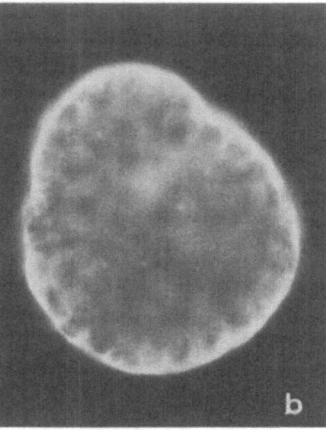

Fig. 3. Expression of retroviral gp71 on an AKR thymic nurse cell. Immunfluorescence demonstration using rabbit anti-FLV gp71 antibodies as markers and FITC-conjugated goat anti-rabbit immunoglobulin antibodies as label. TNCs were isolated from thymuses of 2-month-old AKR/J mice and fixed with 3.7% paraformaldehyde before staining. **a** Phase contrast; **b** Epifluorescence illumination.

The binding was virus specific for several reasons. First, preimmune normal serum did not stain the cells. Second, the activity could be absorbed by virus infected mouse 3T3 fibroblasts but not by unifected control cells. Third, the serum bound to transformed Friend leukemia cells but not to normal mouse lymphocytes. Except for retroviral coat gp71, AKR/J TNCs expressed Friend leukemia virus (FLV) core protein p30 determinants in their cytoplasms. This binding was also immunospecific as revealed by specificity controls similar to the ones used for gp71 determination.

Although expression of viral determinants on AKR/J cells was unequivocal, it should be noted that TNCs from mouse strains without thymoma predilection also unexpectedly expressed retroviral determinants, although to a somewhat lower degree. This was true for the other strains tested, C3H/f and C57BL/6.

To confirm the presence of RNA viruses in AKR/J TNCs, we cultured TNCs along with other thymic cell fractions and screened the culture supernatants for viral reverse transcriptase activity. We found that viral enzyme activity was demonstrable in TNC cultures from young mice, but not in cultures of single thymocytes (Fig. 4). Conversely, in preleukemic cell cultures reverse transcriptase was produced mainly in cultures of smaller cells.

C. Discussion

They key findings reported in this paper are that TNCs from young adult AKR/J mice are morphologically changed, that they are no longer demonstrable in neoplastic thymomas, and that AKR TNCs express viral products in relative high dosages.

It is known that typical pathologic changes of thymic structure precede thymomagenesis. It is well documented that starting from 4 months of age the cortical areas begin to involute, first focally and later in a generalized pattern (Arnesen 1958; Metcalf 1966; Siegler and Rich 1963).

Thus, in ontogeny of AKR mice the TNC abnormalities described here appear to be the first demonstrable changes. Since TNCs seem to be located in the thymic cortex (unpublished observations), it is probable that the preleukemic loss of TNCs in AKR thymuses is related to the cortical involution, which precedes neoplastic conversion.

Which of the cellular components is primarily changed in AKR TNCs? We demonstrated retroviral products in the epithelial parts of TNCs, using three different markers: viral coat glycoprotein gp71, viral core protein p30, and released viral reverse transcriptase. It should, however, be stressed that TNCs from mouse strains without a particular leukemia susceptibility express viral determinants as well. In fact, virus content seems to be a normal feature of thymic epithelial cells, as of virus particles have been found in EM studies of fetal (Koppenheffer et al. 1978) as well as of adult normal and AKR thymus cortical cells (DeHarven 1964). Similar to tissues of the genitourinary tract, where gp71-like determinants have been shown in copious amounts (Lerner et al. 1977), virus expression on AKR TNCs does not seem to be pathologic per se. It is

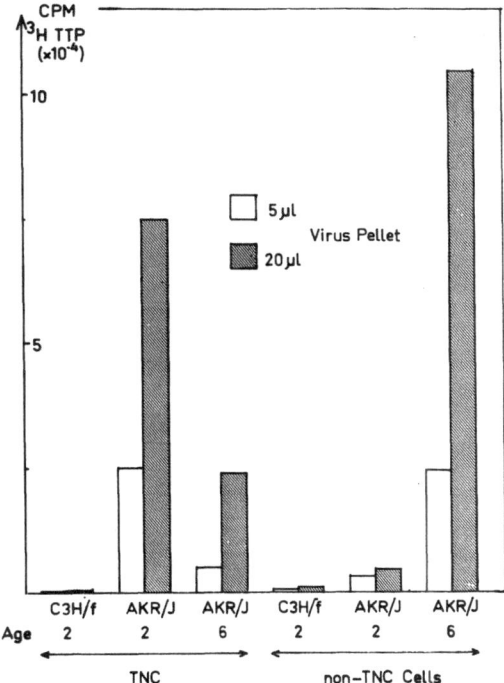

Fig. 4. Biosynthesis of reverse transcriptase in short term cultures of AKR TNC and small thymus cell populations. TNC and single thymocyte fractions of 2-month-old C3H/f and AKR/J and of preleukemic 6-month-old AKR/J mice were cultured for 4 days. Culture supernatants were harvested repeatedly and sedimentable material ("virus pellet") was assayed for reverse transcriptase activity (Novak et al. 1979)

observations on AKR thymocyte properties make such speculations quite attractive.

Weissman et al. found that few normal but a high proportion of preneoplastic and neoplastic thymocytes express receptors for retroviruses (McGrath and Weissman 1979). As has been suggested for Epstein-Barr viruses in the case of human B lymphocytes (Schwarz 1980), binding of viruses to thymic T cells in AKR thymuses is thought to trigger proliferation (McGrath and Weissman 1979). Accepting this possibility, does the AKR abnormality reside in an atypical thymocyte response pattern, and does recognition of TNC membrane-expressed viral products lead to excessive mitotic activity? Irrespective of whether this proliferation is sufficient for subsequent transformation or whether it "only" provides some of the requirements for cancerogenic cytogenetic changes to occur (Klein 1979), we believe that the study of AKR TNC components will offer an approach to reinvestigate the role of lympho-epithelial interactions, which has been a matter of debate (Haas et al. 1977; Peled and Haran-Ghera 1978; Waksal et al. 1976).

Acknowledgments

We thank Mrs. Maria Döll for her excellent technical assistence and Mrs. Rosemary Schneider for typing this manuscript. This work was supported by grants from the Deutsche Forschungsgemeinschaft.

possible, though not yet proven, that a property of the thymocytes is the basis for the changes. AKR TNCs contain enormous numbers of thymocytes, which are, as their "normal" counterparts, morphologically intact and actively proliferate within the TNCs (Wekerle and Ketelsen 1980). AKR intra-TNC thymocytes, however, often show a very loose contact between their surface membranes and the surrounding epithelial caveolar membranes. At present it is not possible to decide whether the abnormal cell numbers are due to an enhanced intra-TNC proliferation or to an increased recruitment of immigrating thymocytes.

Are the changes of AKR TNCs related to neoplastic thymocyte conversion? Lacking functional data, any consideration of this problem must be highly speculative. Yet, some

References

Arnesen K (1958) Preleukemic and early leukemic changes in the thymus of mice. Acta Pathol Microbiol Scand [A] 43:350–364 – DeHarven E (1964) Virus particles in the thymus of conventional and germfree mice. J Exp Med 120:857–868 – Haas M, Sher T, Smolinsky S (1977) Leukemogenesis in vitro induced by thymus epithelial reticulum cells transmitting murine leukemia viruses. Cancer Res 37:1800–1807 – Klein G (1979) Lymphoma development in mice and humans: Diversity of initiation is followed by convergent cytogenetic evolution. Proc Natl Acad Sci USA: 2442–2446 – Koppenheffer TL, Philips JH, Vankin GL (1978) C-type virus-lymphocyte interactions in the developing mouse thymus. Am J Anat 153:165–170 – Lerner RA, Wilson CB, DelVillano CB, McConahey PJ, Dixon FJ (1977) Endogeneous oncoviral expression in adult and fetal mice: Quantitative, histologic and physiologic studies of the major viral glycoprotein pg70. J Exp Med 143:151–166 – McGrath MS, Weissman IL (1978) A receptor-mediated model of viral leukemogenesis: Hypothesis and experiments. In: Clarkson B, Marks PA, Till JE (eds) Differentiation of normal and neoplastic hematopoietic cells. Cold Spring Harbor Laboratory, New York, pp 577–589 – McGrath MS, Weissman IL (1979), AKR leukemogenesis: Identification and biological significance of thymic lymphoma receptors for AKR retroviruses. Cell 17:65–75 – Metcalf D (1966) Histologic and transplantation studies on preleukemic thymus of the AKR mouse. J Natl Cancer Inst 37:425–442 – Novak U, Friedrich R, Mölling K (1979) Elongation of DNA complementary to 5' and of the avian sarcoma virus genome by the virion associated RNA dependent DNA polymerase. J Virol 30:438–452 – Peled A, Haran-Ghera N (1978) Lack of transformation of murine thymocytes by thymic epithelium. Nature 274:266–269 – Schwarz RS (1980) Epstein-Barr virus-oncogen or mitogen? (editorial). N Engl J Med 302:1307–1308 – Siegler R, Rich MA (1963) Unilateral histogenesis of AKR thymic lymphoma. Cancer Res 23:1774–1781 – Waksal SD, Smolinsky S, Cohen IR, Feldman M (1976) Transformation of thymocytes by thymus epithelium derived from AKR mice. Nature 263:512–514 – Wekerle H, Ketelsen U-P (1980) Thymic nurse cells – Ia-bearing epithelium involved in T-lymphocyte differentiation? Nature 283:402–404 – Wekerle H, Ketelsen U-P, Ernst M (1980) Thymic nurse cells. Lymphoepithelial cell complexes in murine thymuses: Morphological and serological characterization. J Exp Med 151:925–944

Haematology and Blood Transfusion Vol. 26
Modern Trends in Human Leukemia IV
Edited by Neth, Gallo, Graf, Mannweiler, Winkler
© Springer-Verlag Berlin Heidelberg 1981

Generation of Stable Antigen Loss Variants from Cloned Tumor Lines – An Example of Immunoadaptation During Metastasis

V. Schirrmacher and K. Bosslet

The experiments to be presented will demonstrate a new type of tumor variant which can arise with high frequency within carefully cloned tumor cell lines. As a possible mechanisms of escape from a T cell mediated antitumor immune response, the tumor cells studied reduce the expression of the tumor antigen and pass this new antigen negative phenotype on to many subsequent cell generations. These findings are interpreted as an example of adaptation of tumor cells to their microenvironment. The relevance of this finding for tumor metastasis will be discussed.

As tumor model system we chose the chemically induced DBA/2 mouse (H-2^d) lymphoma L5178Y with the two sublines Eb and ESb (Schirrmacher et al. 1979a). We previously described morphological, functional, and antigenic differences between the parental tumor line Eb and its spontaneous variant ESb which arose in 1968 and had highly increased metastatic capacity (Schirrmacher et al. 1979b, 1980). In spite of these differences the tumor lines could be shown to be closely related (Schirrmacher and Bosslet 1980). Tumor protection experiments revealed the presence of tumor-associated transplantation antigens (TATAs) on both Eb and ESb tumor cells. These TATAs were shown to be distinct and non-cross-reactive and could be detected in vitro with the help of tumor-specific syngeneic cytotoxic T lymphocytes (CTL) (Bosslet et al. 1979).

The expression of these TATAs – as tested by CTL – was investigated on tumor cells which had metastasized from a local site (s.c.) to various internal organs, such as liver, lung, or spleen. In organ selection experiments this process of tumor cell spread was repeated several times (i.e., s.c. → organ → s.c. → organ

etc.). Some of the typing results obtained with anti-Eb, anti-ESb, and anti-H-2 CTL are summarized in Table 1, others are published elsewhere (Bosslet and Schirrmacher, to be published).

While the control tumor lines were always specifically lysed, the tumor cells which had metastasized to the spleens of normal syngeneic mice could not be lysed by the antitumor CTL (see the ESb lines no. 2 and 10 and the Eb line no. 7). In contrast, tumor cells isolated under identical conditions from other internal organs (liver or lung) remained tumor antigen positive and could be specifically lysed by the respective CTL (see the ESb lines no. 3 and 11 and the Eb line no. 8). The tumor lines no 1–8 were derived from experiments performed with uncloned populations, thus allowing the interpretation of host selection of possible pre-existing antigen negative variants. The tumor lines no. 9–12 were derived, however, from a twice-cloned, antigen-positive ESb line. During spread from a s.c. site to the spleen (line no. 10) which took 10 days these tumor antigen positive cells converted to cells which could not be lysed by anti-ESb CTL. This finding was reproduced several times, not only with this line but also with another twice-cloned ESb line.

The evidence that the inability to be lysed by antitumor CTL was due to the loss of the respective tumor antigen is a follows: (1) As shown in the table, the cells could be lysed by anti H-2 CTL and were thus not generally resistant to lysis, (2) cold target competition experiments revealed that anti-ESb CTL could not bind to the spleen-derived ESb tumor lines, (3) the antigen negative variants could not induce CTL and thus did not express a new changed TATA, and (4) treatment of the cells

Table 1. Expression of tumor antigens and H-2^d antigens by various metastasizing tumor lines

No.	Name	Cloning[a]	Selection[b]	% Specific cytotoxicity with CTL[c]		
				anti-Eb	anti-ESb	anti H-2^d
1	ESb control	−	−	3	53	79
2	ESb-Met-SPL	−	s.c.-SPL, norm, 2×	3	8	85
3	ESb-Met-Liv	−	s.c.-Liv, norm, 2×	3	54	n.d.
4	ESb-Met-SPL	−	s.c.-SPL, nu/nu 2×	0	35	n.d.
5	ESb-Met-Liv	−	s.c.-Liv, nu/nu 2×	0	35	n.d.
6	Eb control	−	−	57	4	76
7	Eb-Met-SPL	−	s.c.-SPL, norm, 5×	0	0	78
8	Eb-Met-Liv	−	s.c.-Liv, norm, 3×	38	0	n.d.
9	ESb-Cl 32.2	+	−	6	78	85
10	ESb-Cl 32.2	+	s.c.-SPL, norm, 1×	0	7	56
11	ESb-Cl 32.2	+	s.c.-Lg, norm, 1×	2	42	60

[a] Cloning done by growing single cells in suspension culture in microtiterplates; ESb-Cl 32.2 is clone 32 recloned once. − =noncloned tumor cell population

[b] Selection performed in vivo by inoculation of tumor cells subcutaneously (s.c.); tumor cell containing organs (SPL=spleen, Liv=liver, Lg=lung) were removed from tumor bearing animals (10 days after inoculation of ESb or 25 days after inoculation of Eb or ESb-CL 32.2), cell suspensions prepared and, where indicated, inoculated again into normal (norm) or BALB/c nude (nu/nu) mice; this procedure was repeated several times as indicated; all cell lines were tested in the second tissue culture passage

[c] Percentage specific ^{51}Cr-release after 4 h coincubation of the indicated ^{51}Cr-labeled tumor lines with cytotoxic T lymphocytes (CTL) at an effector to target cell ratio of 40:1; n.d.=not done

with trypsin or neuraminidase did not uncover the tumor antigen.

The reduced expression or loss of tumor antigen on the clonal tumor cell variants seemed to depend on the presence of T lymphocytes in the host. Tumor lines derived from spleens of T cell deficient nude mice (Table 1, line no. 4) remained antigen positive. Also, the admixture of tumor-specific CTL with the tumor cells in a Winn-type assay led to a loss of tumor antigen on the tumor cells isolated eventually (after 4 weeks) from the s.c. site and from internal organs.

The antigen negativity of the clonal variants was a very stable type of changed phenotype: Spleen-derived antigen negative tumor variants passaged for prolonged periods in tissue culture (for more than 50 subsequent cell generations) remained antigen negative. The antigenic change thus differs from "antigenic modulation" which is usually of short duration.

It is very unlikely that the antigen negative variant derived from the twice-cloned ESb line was pre-existent, because we could not isolate such an antigen negative variant even from the original uncloned population. We also do not think that the variant arose by mutation because the changes could be reproduced with

too high a frequency and in a time period allowing for not more than 10–20 cell generations. The antigen negative variants could have arisen during a process of immunoadaptation, where T cells reacting against the TATA might have signaled to the tumor cell to repress the biosynthesis of the corresponding tumor antigen. From the stability of the antigen negativity we conclude that the variants represent gene regulatory variants.

This new type of immunoadaption observed with cloned lines of highly metastatic tumor cells could explain why these tumor cells can grow in lymphoid organs such as the spleen and also why they can survive and eventually grow even in immunized hosts. Adaptive behavior of tumor cells may not only explain a new type of immune escape mechanism. As discussed elsewhere (Schirrmacher 1980), it could have a more general biologic significance for tumor cell behavior, in particular during the complex process of metastasis.

References

Bosslet K, Schirrmacher V (to be published) Clonal tumor cell variants arising by adaptation. Proceedings of EORTC Metastasis Conference, London,

1980 – Bosslet K, Schirrmacher V, Shantz G (1979) Tumor metastase and cell-mediated immunity in a modl system in DBA/2 mice. VI. Similar specificity patterns of protective anti-tumor immunity in vivo and of cytolytic T cells in vitro. Int J Cancer 24:303–313 – Schirrmacher V (1980) Commentary. Shifts in tumor cell phenotypes induced by signals from the microenvironment. Relevance for the immunobiology of cancer metastasis. Immunobiology 157:89–98 – Schirrmacher V, Bosslet K (1980) Tumor metastases and cell-mediated immunity in a model system in DBA/2 mice. X. Immunoselection of tumor variants differing in tumor antigen expression and metastatic capacity. Int J Cancer 25:781–788 – Schirrmacher V, Shantz G, Clauer K, Komitowski D, Zimmermann H-P, Lohmann-Matthes ML (1979a) Tumor metastases and cell-mediated immunity in a model system in DBA/2 mice. I. Tumor invasiveness in vitro and metastases formation in vivo. Int J Cancer 23:233–244 – Schirrmacher V, Bosslet K, Shantz G, Clauer K, Hübsch D (1979b) Tumor metastases and cell-mediated immunity in a model system in DBA/2 mice. IV. Antigenic differences between the parental tumor line and its metastasizing variant. Int J Cancer 23:245–252 – Schirrmacher V, Cheingsong-Popov, R, Arnheiter H (1980) Hepatocyte-tumor cell interaction in vitro. I. Conditions for rosette formation and inhibition by anti-H-2 antibody. J Exp Med 151:984–989

**Virological and
Molecularbiological
Aspects**

Haematology and Blood Transfusion Vol. 26
Modern Trends in Human Leukemia IV
Edited by Neth, Gallo, Graf, Mannweiler, Winkler
© Springer-Verlag Berlin Heidelberg 1981

Transforming Genes of Retroviruses: Definition, Specificity, and Relation to Cellular DNA*

P. H. Duesberg and K. Bister

A. Abstract

The oncogenic properties of sarcoma, acute leukemia, and lymphatic leukemia viruses are interpreted in terms of their genetic structures. Highly oncogenic sarcoma and acute leukemia viruses are shown to contain transforming *onc* genes which are different from the three virion genes (*gag, pol,* and *env*) essential for replication. Biochemical and genetic approaches to define *onc* genes are discussed. The hallmark of retroviral *onc* genes is shown to be a specific RNA sequence that is unrelated to essential virion genes. On this basis five different classes of *onc* genes can be distinguished in the avian tumor virus group alone: two of these, the *onc* genes of Rous sarcoma virus (RSV) and avian myeloblastosis virus (AMV), share one design. Their coding sequence is a specific RNA section which either replaces *env* [RSV(−), AMV] or maps adjacent to the 3' end of *env* (RSV). Expression of this class of *onc* genes is mediated via subgenomic mRNAs containing sequences from the 5' end of viral RNA spliced onto the *onc* gene coding sequences. The *onc* gene product of RSV has been identified as a 60,000-dalton phosphoprotein. Three other classes of *onc* genes, namely, those of the myelocytomatosis (MC29) subgroup of viruses, avian erythroblastosis virus (AEV), and Fujinami sarcoma virus (FSV), share another design. Their coding sequences are hybrids consisting of specific as well as of *gag* or *gag* and *pol* gene-related elements. The products of these *onc* genes, translated from full size genomic RNA, are hybrid proteins carrying *gag* or *gag* and *pol* determinants in addition to specific sequences. They are phosphorylated and range in size from 75,000 to 200,000 daltons. Since viruses with totally different *onc* genes can cause the same disease (namely, RSV, FSV, AEV, and MC29 cause sarcoma and AEV, AMV, or E26 and MC29 cause erythroblastosis), it is concluded that multiple mechanisms involving multiple cellular targets exist for sarcomagenic and leukemic transformation of the avian cell. Comparisons between viral *onc* genes of the RSV-design and in particular those of the hybrid design and *onc*-related chromosomal DNA sequences of the cell suggest qualitative differences. Hence viral *onc* genes are not simply transduced cellular genes, and cellular sequences related to viral *onc* genes appear not directly relevant to cancer. It follows that viral *onc* genes are unique and more than the sum of their parts related to cellular DNA and to replicative genes of retroviruses. We speculate that *onc* genes also may plan a role indirectly in cancers caused by lymphatic leukemia viruses, although these viruses are not known to contain such genes.

B. Introduction

Retroviruses cause sarcomas, carcinomas, acute and lymphatic leukemias, or no disease in animals (Gross 1970; Beard et al. 1973; Tooze 1973; Levy 1978; Jarrett 1978; Duesberg 1980; Essex 1980). Table 1 shows schematically the pathology of representative re-

---

* With minor variations this paper has been presented at three symposia during the summer of 1980: (1) Proceedings of the Third International Feline Leukemia Meeting, St. Thomas, Virgin Islands; (2) Modern Trends in Human Leukemia IV, Wilsede, Germany; (3) 1980 International Symposium on Cancer, New York.

Table 1. Oncogenic properties of retroviruses

Viruses	Tumors in animals				Transformation in culture	
	Sarcoma	Carcinoma	Leukemia		Fibro-blast	Blood cell
			Acute	Lymphatic		
Sarcoma viruses RSV, RSV(−) FSV Mo-MuSV Ki-Ha-MuSV FeSV	+	−/+[a]	+[b]	−/+[c]	+	?
Acute leukemia class I Avian MC29 subgroup: MC29, MH2, CMII, OK10 AEV Abelson MuLV	+[d]	+[d]	+	−/+[c]	+	+
Acute leukemia class II AMV, E26	−[e]	−[e]	+	+	−	+
Lymphatic leukemia Avian leukosis and Rous-associated viruses, tdRSV, RAV(O) MuLV FeLV	−[f]	−[f]	−	+/−	−	−

[a] Liver and kidney metastases have been reported for RSV (Gross 1970; Purchase and Burmester 1972). FeSV has been shown to cause melanocarcinomas (McCullough et al. 1972; Chen et al. 1980)

[b] Observed among other nontumorous diseases with Harvey, Kirsten, and Moloney MuSV (see text) (Scher et al. 1975; Ostertag et al. 1980) and rarely with RSV (Gross 1970; Purchase and Burmester 1972)

[c] Possibly due to helper virus (Gross 1970; Purchase and Burmester 1972; Graf and Beug 1978)

[d] Not observed with Abelson virus (Rosenberg and Baltimore 1980)

[e] Some (Beard 1973; Purchase and Burmester 1972), but not all (Moscovici 1975), stocks of AMV have caused carcinomas or sarcomas, perhaps due to other helper virus components

[f] Lymphatic leukemia viruses have been described to cause sarcomas and carcinomas at low frequency and after long latent periods (Gross 1970; Purchase and Burmester 1972). However, sarcoma- or carcinoma-causing variants have not been isolated

troviruses of the avian, murine, and feline tumor virus groups. The avian, murine, and feline sarcoma viruses predominantly cause sarcomas and transform fibroblasts in culture. The Harvey (Ha), Kirsten (Ki), and Moloney (Mo) murine sarcoma viruses (MuSV) and rarely avian Rous sarcoma virus (RSV) also cause erythroid leukemia (Gross 1970; Scher et al. 1975; Ostertag et al. 1980; Duesberg 1980). This has not been observed with avian Fujinami virus (FSV) (Lee et al. 1980). Feline sarcoma virus (FeSV) in addition to sarcomas also causes melanocarcinomas (McCullough et al. 1972; Chen et al. 1981). The avian acute leukemia viruses of the MC29 subgroup and erythroblastosis virus (AEV) that transform fibroblasts [therefore termed "class I" (Duesberg 1980)] and hematopoietic cells in culture have broad oncogenic spectra including sarcomas and carcinomas in addition to acute leukemias in the animal (Beard et al. 1973; Graf and Beug 1978). However, the fibroblast-transforming murine Abelson leukemia virus has not been reported to cause sarcomas and carcinomas (Rosenberg and Baltimore 1980). By contrast the avian acute leukemia viruses AMV and E26 that do not transform fibroblasts in culture [therefore termed "class II" (Duesberg 1980)] have rather specific oncogenic spectra in the animal, where they cause myeloid and erythroid leukemias (Beard et al. 1973; Moscovici 1975; Graf and Beug 1978). The viruses listed thus far have in common that they transform quickly, within 1–2 weeks, and that transformation is an inevitable consequence of infection in susceptible animals. This implies that transforming *onc* genes are integral parts of the genomes of these viruses.

This appears not to be true for the majority of naturally occurring retroviruses, the lymphatic leukemia viruses. These are rather ubiquitous, nondefective viruses that often cause viremias but rarely and in particular not simultaneously cause leukemias (Gross 1970; Tooze 1973), as for example in chickens (Rubin et al. 1962; Weyl and Dougherty 1977), mice (Gardner et al. 1976; Levy 1978; Cloyd et al. 1980), or cats (Jarrett 1978; Essex 1980). The transformation-defective (td), *src*-deletion mutants of RSV have the same biologic (Biggs et al. 1972) and genetic properties (Wang et al. 1976) as the lymphatic leukemia viruses (Fig. 1). The RNA genome of these viruses contains a 3'terminal c-region and all three essential virion genes in the following 5' to 3' order: *gag* (for internal virion proteins or group-specific antigens), *pol* (for RNA dependent DNA *poly*merase), and *env* (for *env*elope glycoprotein). The c-region has regulatory functions in the reverse transcription of viral RNA and in the transcription of proviral DNA (Fig. 1) (Wang et al. 1975; Wang 1978; Tsichlis and Coffin 1980). The endogenous, nondefective (containing all three virion genes) retroviruses of chicken, such as RAV(0) (Tooze 1973), and of mice, such as xenotropic viruses (Levy 1978; Cloyd et al. 1980), are inherited according to Mendelian genetics. These viruses probably never cause a disease directly and appear to differ from the more pathogenic lymphatic leukemia viruses in minor genetic elements, including the c-region that influences virus expression (Tsichlis and Coffin 1980; Lung et al. 1980; Cloyd et al. 1980). Since transformation is not or is only rarely a consequence of replication by any of these viruses and only occurs after considerable latent periods, these viruses may not contain authentic *onc* genes.

In the following we will describe the definition of *onc* genes of the rapidly transforming sarcoma and acute leukemia viruses. On this basis we will then ask whether the oncogenic specificity of some and the lack of specificity by

other viruses is due to distinct *onc* genes or whether one *onc* gene can cause multiple forms of cancer. In addition, we review the question of the relationship between viral *onc* genes and cellular DNA. Finally, the question is addressed of how lymphatic leukemia viruses, which lack known *onc* genes, may cause cancer. The focus will be on avian tumor viruses, because their genetic structures are better defined than those of other viruses. This review extends two previous ones published recently (Duesberg, 1980; Bister and Duesberg 1980).

C. Definition of src, the onc Gene of RSV

The only *onc* gene of retroviruses for which nearly complete genetic and biochemical definitions are available is the *src* gene of RSV. In 1970 the *src* gene was formally distinguished from the three essential virion genes of nondefective RSV by the isolation of a mutant that was temperature-sensitive only in transformation but not in virus replication (Martin 1970) and by the isolation of nonconditional *src*-deletion mutants (Duesberg and Vogt 1970; Martin and Duesberg 1972). These transformation-defective *src* deletion mutants retain all virion genes and are physically and serologically like wild type RSV (Fig. 1) (Wang et al. 1975; Wang 1978). However the RNA of the wild type measures 10 kb (kilobases) whereas that of the tdRSV measures only 8.5 kb (Fig. 1) (Duesberg and Vogt 1970, 1973; Lai et al. 1973; Beemon et al. 1974; Wang 1978). On the basis of this difference *src* gene-specific RNA sequences were first defined by subtracting from the 10-kb RNA of RSV with the genetic structure 5' *gag-pol-env-src-c* 3' the 8.5-kb RNA of the isogenic *src* deletion mutant tdRSV with the genetic structure 5' *gag-pol-env-c* 3' (Fig. 1) (Lai et al. 1973). The 1.5 kb that set apart the wild type RSV from the *src* deletion mutant were shown to be a contiguous sequence that mapped near the 3' end of viral RNA (Wang et al. 1975).

The *src* gene was independently defined by recombination analysis in which a *src*-deletion mutant with variant virion genes (5' *gag"-pol"-env"-c* 3') was allowed to recombine with a nondefective RSV. All sarcomagenic recombinants with variant virion genes had the genetic structure 5' *gag"-pol"-env"-src-c* 3') and hence had inherited the *src* gene (Beemon et al. 1974; Wang et al. 1976; Wang 1978) (see also Fig. 1). It followed that the 1.5-kb sequence of RSV-specific RNA was necessary for transformation.

A major step towards proving that the 1.5-kb *src*-specific RNA sequence was also (almost) sufficient for transformation was ta-

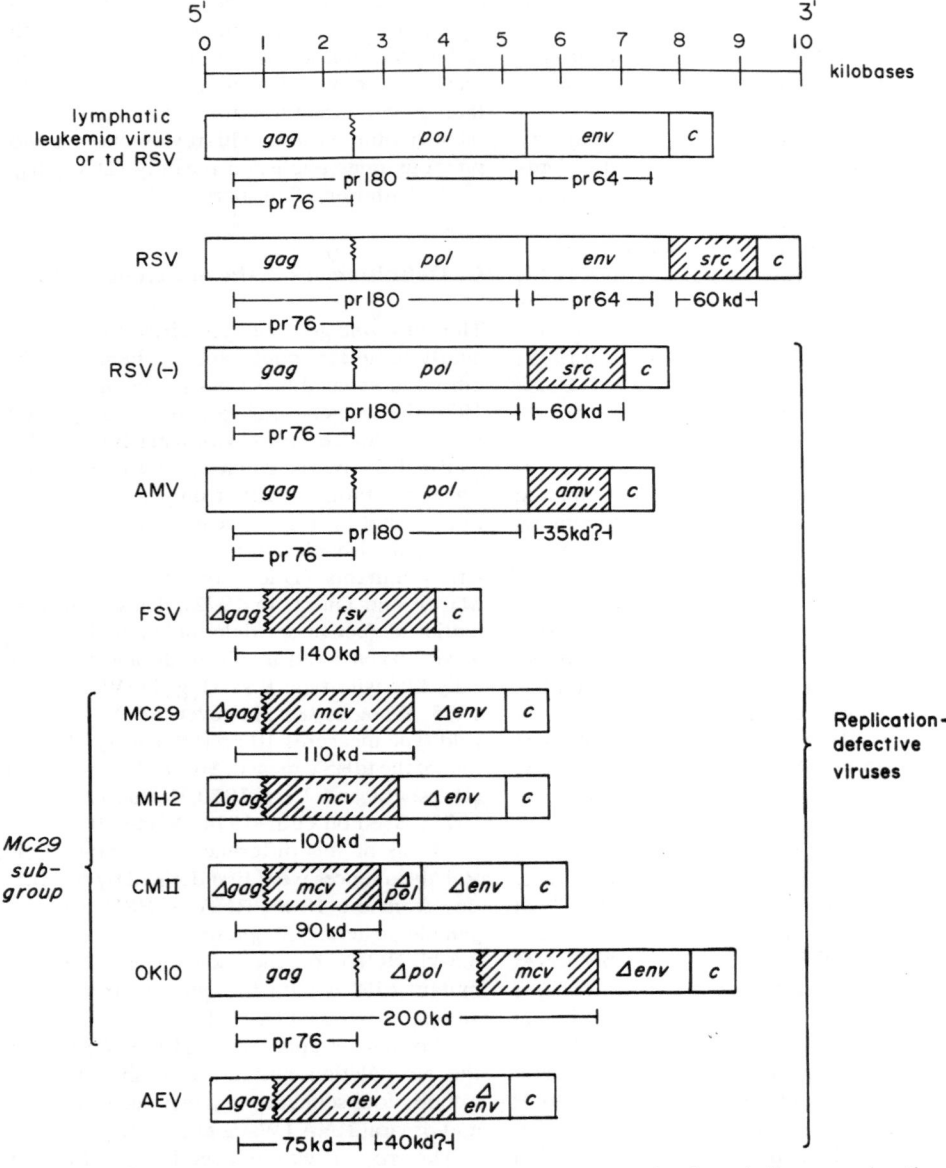

Fig. 1. Genetic structures of viruses of the avian tumor virus group. *White boxes* indicate map locations and complexities in kilobases of complete or partial (Δ) complements of the three essential virion genes *gag*, *pol* and *env* and of the noncoding *c* region at the 3′ end of viral RNAs. *Hatched boxes* indicate location and complexities of specific sequence elements which are unrelated to essential virion genes and which define five distinct RNA subgroups within the avian tumor virus group. These specific sequences represent all *(src, amv)* or part *(fsv, mcv, aev)* of the coding sequences of the five different onc genes associated with avian tumor viruses. *Undulated lines* indicate that translation crosses and *half-undulated lines* that translation may cross borders between RNA sequence elements of different genetic origin. *Lines under the boxes* symbolize the complexities in kilodaltons of the protein products encoded by the respective RNA sequences

ken when a 60-kilodalton (kd) protein product was identified in RSV-transformed cells (Brugge and Erikson 1977) that was serologically unrelated to the *gag, pol,* and *env* virion proteins. Since the genetic complexity of the 1.5-kb RSV-specific RNA sequence and of the 60-kd *src* protein are about the same, the 1.5-kb RNA must encode most or all of the protein (Fig. 1). The same *src*-specific sequence has also been identified in a *env*-deletion mutant of RSV, termed RSV($-$) (Table 1, Fig. 1) (Wang et al. 1976), and recently also in a *gag⁻, pol⁻,* and *env*-defective sarcomagenic deletion mutant of RSV (Martin et al. 1980). Transformation by the *gag⁻, pol⁻,* and *env*-defective RSV is definitive proof that the *src* gene (but not the *src*-specific RNA sequence by itself) is sufficient for transformation. Expression of the *src* gene of RSV involves a mRNA which also includes sequences derived from the 5' and 3' ends of virion RNA that are shared with *src*-deletion mutants of RSV (Mellon and Duesberg 1977). This implies that the *src*-specific sequence of RSV defined by deletion and recombination analysis does not act independently and may by itself not be sufficient for transformation.

Since the definition of the *src* gene of RSV most other acutely transforming retroviruses have been shown to contain specific sequences unrelated to essential virion genes. Such sequences appear to be the hallmark of highly oncogenic viruses, and they represent most or at least part of their *onc* genes (see below). To date the oncogenic retroviruses are the only class of viruses which have *onc* genes that are nonessential for virus replication. The only known function of these genes is their oncogenicity.

D. Identification of the Genome and Definition of the onc Genes of Replication-Defective Oncogenic Viruses

The definition of the *onc* genes of highly oncogenic viruses other than RSV is less advanced than that of *src*. This is because all highly oncogenic retroviruses, with the exception of RSV, lack essential virion genes and consequently are replication defective. The genetic phenotype of most defective sarcoma and acute leukemia viruses is: *gag⁻, pol⁻, env⁻, onc⁺* (Fig. 1) (Tooze 1973; Bister and

Vogt 1978; Graf and Beug 1978). Due to this phenotype classical deletion and recombination analysis cannot be used to define *onc* genes as was the case with *src*. An *onc* deletion of such a virus (i.e., *gag⁻, pol⁻, env⁻, onc⁻*) would obviously be undetectable by classical techniques measuring viral gene expression. Likewise the lack of secondary markers would complicate or prevent recombination analysis of *onc* genes of defective viruses.

I. Genome Identification

Defectiveness also complicates identification of the viral RNA genomes. The genome of a nondefective retrovirus is essentially identified by extracting the RNA from purified virus. Since the defective virus only replicates if complemented by a nondefective helper virus, usually a lymphatic leukemia virus, it is obtained as a complex containing defective as well as helper viral RNAs. Moreover, the two RNAs are replicated at unpredictable ratios, usually favoring the RNA of nondefective helper virus. The RNA of defective and helper virus was first separated by electrophoretic analysis of viral RNAs, which typically yields one larger RNA species measuring 8 to 9 kb and a smaller one measuring 4 to 7 kb (Maisel et al. 1973; Duesberg et al. 1977). By its absence from nondefective helper viruses, the small RNA species was shown to be necessary for transformation (Maisel et al. 1973; Duesberg et al. 1977).

Subsequent biochemical analyses directly identified the smaller RNA species, as the genome of the defective virus, which is consistent with its low complexity (Duesberg 1980; Bister and Duesberg 1980). The larger RNA species was shown to be the RNA of nondefective helper virus, whose size is invariably 8 to 9 kb as dictated by the requirement for complete *gag, pol,* and *env* genes in nondefective helper viruses (see Fig. 1 for examples).

II. Defining Transformation-Specific Nucleotide Sequences by Subtraction from the RNA of Defective Transforming Virus Sequences Shared with Nondefective Helper Viruses

Given the RNA of defective transforming virus, it can be asked whether a sequence unrelated to essential virion genes is present. Moreover in the avian system it can be asked whether this sequence is related to the genetically defined *src*. Experimentally this is accomplished by comparing the RNAs (or proviral DNAs) of defective and helper virus by various nucleic acid scopes, including hybridization of defective viral RNA with cDNA of helper viruses, comparative fingerprinting of RNase T_1-oligonucleotides, or comparison of proviral DNA fragments generated by a given restriction enzyme. By these methods two classes of sequences are distinguished in the RNAs of defective transforming viruses: helper virus related and specific sequences (Duesberg 1980). In all cases examined the specific sequences form contiguous internal map segments which are flanked by helper virus related terminal map segments (Fig. 1) (Mellon et al. 1978; Bister and Duesberg 1980; Duesberg 1980).

Although biochemical subtraction of helper virus related sequences from the RNA of a defective, transforming virus is formally analogous to deletion analysis, the subtracted (shared) RNA is not the genome of a viable deletion mutant (cf. Fig. 1). Therefore, it can only be inferred but cannot be deduced from this type of analysis that the resulting specific sequence of the defective oncogenic virus (hatched in Fig. 1) is necessary for transformation.

III. Genetic Evidence That Specific and gag-Related RNA Sequences of Avian Class I Acute Leukemia and Fujinami Sarcoma Viruses Are Necessary for Oncogenicity

Genetic evidence was used to determine whether the specific sequences of defective transforming viruses are necessary for transformation. Since due to the absence of selective markers other than *onc*, suitable recombinants have not as yet been prepared in the laboratory, different isolates of closely and distantly related avian acute leukemia viruses were used as substitutes of recombinants. The RNAs of these viral isolates were compared to each other by electrophoretic size analysis, by hybridization with cDNAs of various avian tumor viruses, and by mapping RNase T_1-resistant oligonucleotides (Duesberg et al. 1977; Bister et al. 1979; Roussel et al. 1979; Duesberg et al. 1979; Bister et al. 1980a; Bister and Duesberg 1979, 1980).

Such comparisons show that four different isolates of avian acute leukemia viruses, whose oncogenic spectra are closely related (Table 1) (Beard et al. 1973; Graf and Beug 1978), namely, MC29, MH2, CMII, and OK10, also have closely related genetic structures (Fig. 1). The hallmark of each viral RNA is an internal, helper virus unrelated sequence of about 1.5 kb (Duesberg et al. 1977, 1979; Bister et al. 1979; Bister and Duesberg 1980; Bister et al. 1980a; Roussel et al. 1979). Because the specific sequences of the four viruses are closely related and because the sequence was first identified in MC29 virus, it has been termed *mcv*. The *mcv* sequence is the structural basis for the classification of the four viruses into the MC29 subgroup of avian RNA tumor viruses (Bister et al. 1979; Bister and Duesberg 1980; Bister et al. 1980a; Duesberg 1980).

The size and the oligonucleotide composition of the *mcv* sequences appears to vary between approximately 1.5 and 2 kb in different viral strains (Fig. 1) (Duesberg et al. 1979; Bister et al. 1979; Bister et al., 1980 a). Based on oligonucleotide complexity the largest *mcv* sequence appears to be that of MC29 virus and the smallest one either that of CMII or of MH2 (Bister et al. 1980a). In MC29, CMII and MH2 the *mcv* sequence ist flanked at the 5' end by a partial (Δ) *gag* gene, termed Δgag, and in OK10 by a complete *gag* followed by a Δpol (Fig. 1). It is not clear as yet whether the Δgag sequences of MC29, MH2, and CMII have the same complexities.

At the 3' end the *mcv* sequence of MC29 and OK10 is flanked by a Δenv gene, and that of CMII, by Δpol (Fig. 1) [*env* sequences are present in MH2 RNA, but the RNA has not been analyzed sufficiently to determine whether its *mcv* sequence borders at Δenv (Fig. 1) (Duesberg and Vogt 1979)].

These comparisons of the four MC29-subgroup viral RNAs show that: (1) The 5' parts of their Δgag or *gag* sequences and most, but not all, of their *mcv* sequences are highly conserved; (2) their *env*-related sequences are related by hybridization but variable if compared at the level of shared and specific T_1-oligonucleotides (Bister et al. 1979; Duesberg et al. 1979; Bister et al., 1980a), and (3) they may have optional sequences such as the 3' half of *gag* and the Δpol at the 5' end of *mcv* in OK10 or the Δpol at the 3' end of *mcv* in CMII (Fig. 1). There are probably optional parts of the *mcv* sequence itself, because its size appears to vary in different viral strains. It would follow that most of *mcv* is an essential specific correlate and *Δgag* an essential, nonspecific (because it is shared with helper virus and other defective viruses; Fig. 1) correlate of viral oncogenicity.

These genetic analyses are confirmed and extended if one includes AEV (Bister and Duesberg 1979) and FSV (Lee et al. 1980). Each of these viruses has a genetic structure similar to the viruses of the MC29 subgroup, with a *Δgag* sequence at the 5' end and internal specific sequences, termed *aev* and *fsv* (Bister et al. 1980a), which are unrelated to essential virion genes, to *src*, to *mcv,* and to each other (Fig. 1). Thus, these viruses form an analogous series of defective transforming viruses. It follows that the internal specific sequence of each of these viruses is necessary but probably not sufficient for transformation, since oncogenicity of each of these viruses also correlates with a highly conserved *Δgag*. Hence the *onc* genes of these viruses appear to be genetic units consisting of *gag*-related and specific RNA sequences.

IV. Nonstructural, gag-Related Proteins Define Genetic Units of Helper Virus Related and Specific RNA Sequences, in Class I Avian Acute Leukemia and Fujinami Sarcoma Virus

Each of the class I avian acute leukemia viruses as well as FSV code for gag-related nonstructural phosphoproteins ranging in size from 75 to 200 kd (Fig. 1) (Bister et al. 1977; Bister et al. 1979; Hayman et al. 1979a,b; Bister and Duesberg 1980; Lee et al. 1980; Ramsay and Hayman 1980; Bister et al. 1980a). That these proteins are coded for by *gag*-related as well as specific sequences of viral RNA was deduced from in vitro translation of viral RNAs of known genetic structure (Mellon et al. 1978; Lee et al. 1980) and from peptide analyses of these proteins (Hayman et al. 1979a,b; Kitchener and Hayman 1980). This directly supports the view that the specific sequences of these viruses are not independent genetic units (Fig. 1). They function together with at least the 5' part of *gag* (or all of *gag* and part of *pol* in OK10) as one genetic unit (Fig. 1) (Mellon et al. 1978; Bister and Duesberg 1980; Lee et al. 1980; Bister et al. 1980a). To indicate that

translation crosses the border between *gag*-related or between *gag*- *Δpol*-related and specific sequence elements, these borders were drawn as undulated lines in Fig. 1, also indicating that their exact location is uncertain. Given the very similar oncogenic spectra of these viruses and assuming transforming function of these proteins, we deduce that the size differences among the 90-, 100-, 110-, and 200-kd *gag*-related proteins of CMII, MH2, MC29, and OK10 directly confirm the point made above on the basis of RNA analysis, i.e., that the *Δgag/gag-Δpol-mcv* units include optional elements (see Fig. 1).

Moreover the structure of the genetic unit coding for the 200-kd protein of OK10 which contains a complete *gag* and a *mcv* sequence which replaces only a part of *pol* (Fig. 1) is of particular interest regarding the role of *gag*-related sequences in these proteins. Based on analogy with *pol* gene expression by nondefective viruses which proceeds via a *gag-pol* precursor protein (Fig. 1), the OK10 protein could also be processed into a product that contains only *Δpol* and *mcv*. The fact that such a protein is not found in infected cells (Ramsay and Hayman 1980; our unpublished observations) suggest again that the *gag*-related portion is essential for the function of this protein. The optional nature of the *pol* sequence in OK10, already evident from its lack in other MC29 subgroup proteins, is underscored by the fact that it includes the *pol* sequences that map at the 3' end of *mcv* in CMII which are not part of the CMII protein (Fig. 1) (Bister et al. 1979, 1980a). Because the genetic units of the MC29 subgroup viruses that read *Δgag-mcv* or *gag-Δpol-mcv* share conserved 5' *gag* elements and most of *mcv* but differ in optional, internal sequences, it has been proposed that these genes and their protein products have two essential domains, one consisting of the conserved *gag*-related, the other of the conserved *mcv*-related sequences (Bister et al. 1980a).

Since the known proteins coded for by the class I acute leukemia viruses do not account for genetic information of the 3' half of the viral RNAs, it cannot be excluded that 3' terminal sequences are also necessary for transformation. Nevertheless the variability of the 3' terminal sequences, both in terms of oligonucleotide composition and in relationship to *env* and *pol* genes (Fig. 1), as well as the lack of evidence for protein products synthesized in infected cells argue that these sequences may not be translated. It was hypothesized, therefore, that these sequences may not play a direct role in transformation (Duesberg et al. 1979; Bister et al.1980a; Bister and Duesberg 1980).

In contrast, all genetic information of FSV, which has a genetic structure that is similar to that of class I acute leukemia viruses (Fig. 1), can be accounted for in terms of one known viral protein. Moreover, if one assumes that transformation requires a viral protein and that the viral RNA is translated in only one reading frame, one may argue that in the case of FSV the $\Delta gag\text{-}fsv$ sequence is not only necessary but also sufficient for transformation, since the genetic complexities of the 4.5-kb FSV RNA and of the 140-kd protein encoded by $\Delta gag\text{-}fsv$ are about the same (Fig. 1).

V. The onc Gene of Avian Myeloblastosis (AMV) and E26 Virus, Two Avian Acute Leukemia Viruses of Class II

The AMV and E26 are acute leukemia viruses which fail to transform fibroblasts and cause no sarcomas and possibly no carcinomas, signaling a unique class of onc genes (Beard et al. 1973; Moscovici 1975; Graf and Beug 1978). Until recently the analysis of AMV and related viruses has been slow, because infectious virus typically contains a large excess of nondefective helper virus. This has been changed by the discovery of defective AMV particles which are released by AMV-transformed nonproducer myeloblasts. Such particles contain a 7.5-kb viral RNA and are infectious if fused into susceptible cells together with helper virus (Duesberg et al. 1980). Consistent with the ability of AMV to produce defective virus particles, the RNA was found to contain a complete gag and pol gene, and nonproducer cells contain 76-kd gag and 180-kd gag-pol precursor proteins (Fig. 1). However there is no evidence for gag or gag and pol related nonstructural proteins in AMV-transformed cells (Duesberg et al. 1980). Between pol and a unique 3' terminal c-region AMV contains a specific amv sequence of about 1.5 kb that is unrelated to those of any other acutely transforming avian tumor virus except E26 (Fig. 1) (Duesberg et al. 1980). It appears that the genetic structure of AMV resembles closely that of RSV($-$) (Fig. 1). From this genetic structure it may be expected that the amv sequence codes possibly for a specific protein unrelated to gag and pol genes by a mRNA similar to that coding for the src protein of RSV (Mellon and Duesberg 1977). It would be expected that this protein has a transforming function. Preliminary evidence indicates that a 35-kd protein is translated in vitro from AMV RNA (Fig. 1) (Lee and Duesberg, unpublished work).

E. Two Distinct onc Gene-Designs

The onc genes described here have – as far as defined – two different designs: those with a coding sequence that is specific and unrelated to essential virion genes, for example, the src gene of RSV and possibly the onc gene of AMV, and those with a coding sequence that is a hybrid of genetic elements derived from essential virion genes and specific sequences, for example, the onc genes of MC29, AEV, and FSV. The specific sequences of the hybrid onc genes are all inserted at their 5' ends adjacent to partially deleted gag or pol genes (Fig. 1). By contrast the specific sequences of the onc genes, whose coding sequences lack genetic elements of essential virion genes, either replace env genes [RSV($-$), AMV] or are inserted between env and the c-region (RSV) (Fig. 1). For convenient reference one design is referred to as "RSV design" and the other as "MC29 design" of onc genes according to the originally identified prototypes.

The two onc gene designs also differ in their mechanism of gene expression: the hybrid onc genes, whose specific sequences replace gag or pol genetic elements, are probably translated from genomic viral RNA into gag or gag and pol related proteins like the pr76 gag or pr180 gag-pol proteins of nontransforming viruses that they replace (Fig. 1). However, there is no evidence that the hybrid gene products are subsequently processed. By contrast the src gene of RSV and probably the amv sequence of AMV, which replace env or are inserted downstream of env, are translated from subgenomic mRNAs like the env genes of nontransforming viruses (Fig. 1) (Mellon and Duesberg 1977; Hayward 1977; Duesberg et al. 1980; Lee and Duesberg, unpublished work; Gonda and Bishop, personal communication). Hence the mechanism of gene expression of the two different onc designs closely follows that of the

5' most virion gene that they partially or completely replace (Fig. 1).

To determine whether the *gag*-related elements of the hybrid *onc* genes are indeed essential for the probable transforming function of their proteins as our analyses suggest, it would be necessary to find transforming viruses in which the specific sequences of hybrid *onc* genes are not linked to *gag* or *pol* sequences. Conversely it would be interesting to know whether *src* or the *amv* sequence would have a transforming function if inserted into *gag* or *pol* genes.

It is thought that the 60-kd *src* gene product functions catalytically, probably as a phosphokinase (Erikson et al. 1980; Bishop et al. 1980), although there is evidence that kinase activity may not be the only function of the *src* gene product (Rübsamen et al. 1980; Bishop et al. 1980).

By contrast the function of the *gag*-related proteins of avian acute leukemia and Fujinami sarcoma viruses, of the Abelson MuLV, and of the feline sarcoma viruses may not be solely catalytic. Although a kinase activity again appears as a candidate for a catalytic function of these proteins, this has not been demonstrated in each of these proteins. It appears associated with the *gag*-related proteins of some strains of Abelson virus (Witte et al. 1980) and, with some uncertainty, also with the proteins of the Gardner and Snyder-Theilen strains of feline sarcoma virus (Reynolds et al. 1980) but has not been found in some avian viruses with *onc* genes of MC29 design (Bister et al. 1980b) and in the McDonough strain of feline sarcoma virus (Van de Ven et al. 1980). It is possible that these *onc* gene products have in addition to a possible catalytic function a structural function involving their *gag*-related elements. Analogous to the function of virion *gag* proteins, the *gag* portions of the nonstructural proteins of these viruses may function by binding to specific cellular and also to intracellular viral nucleic acid sequences. This specific binding may represent a regulatory function of a cellular catalytic activity or perhaps of a yet to be discovered catalytic activity of the *gag*-related proteins. This function would then correspond to one of the two domains diagnosed in the proteins of the MC29 subgroup viruses described above.

The consistent difficulties in isolating temperature-sensitive *onc* mutants of these viruses that respond fast to temperature shifts (unpublished experiments and personal communications) support the view that *onc* genes of the MC29 design may have a structural function.

F. Multiple onc Genes: Multiple Mechanisms and Multiple Targets of Transformation

Despite some insufficiencies in the definition of *onc* genes of defective viruses, it is clear that multiple, at least five different classes of specific sequences *(src, mcv, aev, fsv, and amv)* and hence probably five different *onc* genes exist in the avian tumor virus group alone. The number will increase if other viruses are analyzed and if viruses of other taxonomic groups are included. Some of these *onc* genes cause specific cancers in the animal: for example, RSV and FSV, which cause predominantly sarcomas, and AMV and E26, which cause specifically leukemias affecting myeloid or erythroid precursor cells or more primitive stem cells depending on the host [chicken or quail (Moscovici and Löliger, personal communication)]. Other *onc* genes like those of MC29 and AEV may in addition to acute leukemias cause sarcomas and carcinomas (Table 1).

The fact that different *onc* genes vary in specificity yet may cause the same cancer argues against a unique mechanism to transform a given class of differentiated cells. For example RSV, FSV, MC29, AEV, and even Kirsten MuSV (Galehouse and Duesberg 1976) all may cause sarcomas in birds and can also transform mammalian fibroblasts (not tested for FSV) (Quade 1979), although they contain totally different *onc* genes. Likewise, AEV, MC29, and E26 and AMV may cause erythroblastosis (Table 1) (Beard et al. 1973; Graf and Beug 1978), although their *onc* genes, except for those of AMV and E26 (Duesberg et al. 1980), are different. It is concluded that multiple mechanisms, involving multiple *onc* genes and *onc* gene products and presumably multiple cellular targets, exist for sarcomagenic and leukemogenic transformation. The fact that different *onc* genes cause the same cancers or that one *onc* gene may cause multiple cancers argues against the hypothesis that the transforming proteins of these viruses closely resemble specific cellular differentiation proteins and that transformation is a consequence of a competition between a specific viral transforming protein and a specific related cellular counterpart (Graf et al. 1980).

The overlap among the oncogenic spectra of different *onc* genes suggests that different *onc* genes either interact with different specific cellular targets or that *onc* genes interact with nonspecific targets. A unique target for a given form of cancer would fail to explain why different *onc* genes may cause the same disease and why in some cases one *onc* gene may cause different cancers. The nature of cellular targets for viral transformation remains to be elucidated; it is believed to include factors determining susceptibility to virus infection and replication as well as intracellular substances that interact directly with viral transforming proteins.

G. On the Relationship Between Viral onc Genes and Cellular Chromosomal Sequences

The helper virus unrelated specific sequences of acutely transforming avian, murine, and feline viruses have been shown to have closely related cellular counterparts (Scolnick et al. 1973, 1975; Tsuchida et al. 1974; Frankel and Fischinger 1976; Stehelin et al. 1976b; Spector 1978a; Frankel et al. 1979; Sheiness and Bishop 1979; Hughes et al. 1979a,b; Souza et al. 1980; Oskarsson et al. 1980). This has lent support to the hypothesis that normal cells contain viral *onc* genes and that viral *onc* genes are transduced cellular genes (Huebner and Todaro 1969; Stephenson et al. 1979; Bishop et al. 1980). If correct, this hypothesis would predict paradoxically, that normal cells contain a number of viral or cellular *onc* genes that apparently are not subject to negative selection. (At present this number is around a dozen and is going up as more *onc* genes are defined.) Thus normaly would be an admirable effort of cellular suppression of endogenous *onc* genes. Although their cellular relatives are even less well defined than most viral *onc* genes themselves, enough is known about them to deduce that viral *onc* genes are not in the cell but that some or most of their coding sequences have related counterparts in cellular DNA.

1. One example is *src* of RSV: The only form in which the specific sequence of RSV has ever been shown to have transforming function is if it is part of the viral *src* gene. As such, this sequence is expressed via a mRNA that shares 5' leader and 3' terminal *c*-region sequences with other virion genes (Mellon and Duesberg 1977). These virion sequences are not found in all veterbrates said to contain *src*-related sequences (Spector et al. 1978a) except in some strains of chicken. Moreover in chicken *src*-related and endogenous virion gene-related sequences are not located on the same restriction fragments of cellular DNA (Hughes 1979b) nor on the same chromosomes (Hughes 1979a). In addition the cellular *src*-related mRNA and DNA sequences appear not to be colinear with those of RSVs (Wang et al. 1977; Spector et al. 1978b; Hughes et al. 1979b). Hence concrete qualitative differences set apart the *src* of RSV and its relatives in normal vertebrate cells.

2. Another example of a close relationship between a viral *onc* gene and cellular alleles is the case of MuSV: Most of the helper virus unrelated 1.5-kb sequence of MuSV has a closely related, perhaps identical counterpart in the cell (Oskarsson et al. 1980; Blair et al. 1980). However, molecularly cloned "MuSV-specific" DNA from the cell or from MuSV can only transform cultured mouse fibroblasts if it is first linked with (presumably noncoding) terminal sequences from MuSV or helper MuLV. Again concrete qualitative differences exist between the *onc* gene of MuSV and related DNA sequences of the cell. Moreover transformation by these modified MuSV-related sequences from the cell is abortive, and no infectious virus is recovered. Thus transformation by this kind of DNA and by infectious virus may prove not to be the same, although they appear indistinguishable based on the fibroblast assay.

3. The transforming genes of viruses which appear to be hybrids of structural and non-structural viral genetic elements provide even more convincing evidence that viral *onc* genes and their cellular relatives are not the same thing: Although it has been shown that most but not all vertebrate cells contain sequences related to the helper virus unrelated part of MC29 and AEV, the helper virus-related elements of these viruses, in particular *gag*-related elements, do not have the same distribution and are not found in the same cells (Sheiness and Bishop 1979; Roussell et al. 1979). Hence *gag*-related sequences, thought to be an essential element of the *onc* genes of MC29 and AEV, are not part of the cellular

sequences related to those genes. Moreover, the cellular sequences related to the 3-kb AEV-specific RNA sequence have recently been shown to be distributed over a 15-kb DNA segment that includes AEV-related and AEV-unrelated sequences (J. M. Bishop, personal communication). Likewise, the cellular DNA sequence, related to the Abelson murine leukemia virus-specific RNA sequence of 3 kb (Shields et al. 1979), has been shown to be distributed over a 12-kb DNA segment that must include Abelson virus unrelated sequences (Goff et al. 1980). Hence in these cases proviral DNA and related cellular DNA sequences are not colinear. It follows that the genetic units of class I acute leukemia viruses that consist of *gag*-related and specific RNA sequences (Fig. 1) have no known counterparts in normal cells.

It is concluded that viral *onc* genes of the RSV design and in particular those of the MC29 design are different from related sequences present in the cell. The *onc* genes of the RSV design, like *src* and possibly *amv* (Fig. 1), may share most but possibly not all of their coding sequences with cellular homologs but differ from cellular relatives in essential regulatory elements. The *onc* genes of the MC29 design differ from cellular counterparts in coding (*gag* and *pol*-related sequences) as well as regulatory elements. Consequently, the cellular relatives of most viral *onc* genes are probably not present in the cell as functional *onc* genes as has been postulated (Huebner and Todaro 1969; Bishop et al. 1980) and hence are probably not directly relevant to transformation.

Instead these cellular sequences may be relevant to the archaeology of viral *onc* genes. Viral *onc* genes probably have been generated by rare transductions of cellular sequences by nondefective viruses. To generate *onc* genes of the RSV design transduction must have involved illegitimate recombination with nondefective virus. In the case of Moloney MuSV specific deletions of the parental nondefective virus also had to occur (Dina et al. 1976; Donoghue et al. 1979; Chien et al. 1979; Blair et al. 1980). Until the cellular *src*-related sequence is characterized directly, it remains unclear whether in the case of RSV the coding sequence of *src* was transduced unchanged or after alteration when RSV was generated.

Both transduction, involving again illegiti-mate recombination, as well as specific deletions of virion genes (see Fig. 1) must have been necessary to generate the *onc* genes of the MC29 design from cellular and viral genetic elements. Such events are much less likely to occur than, for example, the transduction by phage lambda of a functional galactosidase gene. It is noted that experimental evidence compatible with the transduction of cellular sequences has led to the hypothesis that viral transformation is the product of enhancing the dosage of endogenous cellular *onc* genes by homologous equivalents from exogenous viruses (Bishop et al. 1980). We submit that sequence transduction is not synonymous with the transduction of unaltered gene function which would be a necessary corollary of the gene dosage hypothesis. It would appear that viral *onc* genes are unique and more than the sum of their parts related to cellular DNA and replicative genes of retroviruses.

H. The Role of onc Genes in Carcinogenesis

Highly oncogenic viruses with *onc* genes such as those described here have only been isolated in relatively few cases from animal tumors (reviewed in Gross 1970; Tooze 1973; Duesberg 1980). By contrast leukosis and lymphatic leukemia viruses have been isolated from many viral cancers, in particular from leukemias (see above) (Gross 1970; Tooze 1973). Thus paradoxically the lymphatic leukemia viruses which lack known *onc* genes appear to be more relevant to viral carcinogenesis than retroviruses with known *onc* genes.

However, it has been argued that *onc* genes also play a role in carcinogenesis caused by lymphatic leukemia viruses (Duesberg 1980). These *onc* genes may derive from endogenous, defective retrovirus-like RNAs known to exist in some normal cells (Duesberg and Scolnick 1977; Scolnick et al. 1979) or from cellular genes acquired by processes involving illegitimate recombination and specific deletions (compare genetic structures shown in Fig. 1). The necessity for such a secondary event to occur would explain the poor correlation between the distribution of lymphatic leukemia viruses and cancers in animals (see above). The failure to find *onc* genes in most retroviral cancers may then reflect technical difficulties. These include the lack of suitable probes to detect viral RNA as the only characteristic viral structural component or nonstructural proteins as the only characteristic products of defective transforming viruses. Moreover, detection of a putative defective-transforming virus will be complicated by the fact that the ratio of defective-transforming to nondefective helper virus is low in typical stocks of defective helper virus complexes (Duesberg et al. 1977; Bister and Duesberg 1979; Duesberg et al. 1979; Lee et al. 1980). Thus, the analysis of viral *onc* genes may prove to be less academic than it appears at present – it may provide the tools and concepts necessary to understand all retroviral cancers.

Acknowledgments

We thank L. Evans, M. Nunn, and G. S. Martin for a critical review of the manuscript and D. Baltimore, J. M. Bishop, and M. Essex for communicating results prior to publication. Supported by U.S. Public Health Grant CA 11426.

References

Beard JW, Langlois AJ, Beard D (1973) Etiological strain specificities of the avian tumor virus. Bibl Haematol 39:31–44 – Beemon K, Duesberg PH, Vogt PK (1974) Evidence for crossing over between avian tumor viruses based on analysis of viral RNAs. Proc Natl Acad Sci USA 71:4254–4258 – Biggs PM, Milne BS, Graf T, Bauer H (1972) Oncogenicity of nontransforming mutants of avian sarcoma virus. J Gen Virol 18:399–403 – Bishop JM, Courtneidge SA, Levinson AD, Oppermann H, Quintrell N, Sheiness DK, Weiss SR, Varmus HE (1980) The origin and function of avian retrovirus transforming genes. Cold Spring Harbor Symp Quant Biol 44:919–930 – Bister K, Duesberg PH (1979) Structure and specific sequences of avian erythroblastosis virus RNA: Evidence for multiple classes of transforming genes among avian tumor viruses. Proc Natl Acad Sci USA 76:5023–5027 – Bister K, Duesberg PH (1980) Genetic structure of avian acute leukemia viruses. Cold Spring Harbor Symp Quant Biol 44:801–822 – Bister K, Vogt PK (1978) Genetic analysis of the defectiveness in strain MC29 avian leukosis virus. Virology 88:213–221 – Bister K, Hayman MJ, Vogt PK (1977) Defectiveness of avian myelocytomatosis virus MC29: Isolation of long-term nonproducer cultures and analysis of virus-specific polypeptide synthesis. Virology 82:431–448 – Bister K, Löliger H-C, Duesberg PH (1979) Oligoribonucleotide map and protein of

CMII: Detection of conserved and nonconserved genetic elements in avian acute leukemia viruses CMII, MC29 and MH2. J Virol 32:208–219 – Bister K, Ramsay G, Hayman MJ, Duesberg PH (1980a) OK10, an avian acute leukemia virus of the MC29 subgroup with a unique genetic structure. Proc Natl Acad Sci USA 77:7142–7146 – Bister K, Lee W-H, Duesberg PH (1980b) Phosphorylation of the nonstructural proteins encoded by three avian acute leukemia viruses and by avian Fujinami sarcoma virus. J Virol 36:617–621 – Blair DG, McClements WL, Oskarsson MK, Fischinger PJ, VandeWoude GF (1980) Biological activity of cloned Moloney sarcoma virus DNA: Terminally redundant sequences may enhance transformation efficiency. Proc Natl Acad Sci 77:3504–3508 – Brugge JS, Erikson RL (1977) Identification of a transformation-specific antigen induced by an avian sarcoma virus. Nature 269:346–348 – Chen A, Essex M, Shadduck JA, Niederkorn JY, Albert D (1981) Retravirus encoded transformation-specific polyproteins: Expression coordinated with malignant phenotype in cells from different germ layers. PNAS, in press – Chien YS, Verma IM, Duesberg PH, Davidson N (1979) Heteroduplex analysis of the RNA of clone 3 Moloney murine sarcoma virus. J Virol 32:1028–1032 – Cloyd MW, Hartley JW, Kene WP (1980) lymphomagenicty of recombinant mink cell focus – inducing murine leukemia viruses J Exp Med 151:542–552 – Dina D, Beemon K, Duesberg PH (1976) The 30S Moloney sarcoma virus RNA contains leukemia virus nucleotide sequences. Cell 9:299–309 – Donoghue BJ, Sharp PA, Weinberg RA (1979) Comparative study of different isolates of murine sarcoma virus. J Virol 32:1015–1027 – Duesberg PH (1980) Transforming genes of retroviruses. Cold Spring Harbor Symp Quant Biol 44:13–29 – Duesberg PH, Scolnick EM (1977) Murine leukemia viruses containing a ~30S RNA subunit of unknown biological activity, in addition to the 38S subunit of the viral genome. Virology 83:211–216 – Duesberg PH, Vogt PK (1970) Differences between the ribonucleic acids of transforming and nontransforming avian tumor viruses. Proc Natl Acad Sci USA 67:1673–1680 – Duesberg PH, Vogt PK (1973) RNA species obtained from clonal lines of avian sarcoma and from avian leukosis virus. Virology 54:207–219 – Duesberg PH, Vogt PK (1979) Avian acute leukemia viruses MC29 and MH2 share specific RNA sequences: Evidence for a second class of transforming genes. Proc Natl Acad Sci 76:1633–1637 – Duesberg PH, Bister K, Vogt PK (1977) The RNA of avian acute leukemia virus MC29. Proc Natl Acad Sci 74:4320–4324 – Duesberg PH, Bister K, Moscovici C (1979) Avian acute leukemia virus MC29: Conserved and variable RNA sequences and recombination with helper virus. Virology 99:121–134 – Duesberg P, Bister K, Moscovici C (1980) Genetic structure of avian myeloblastosis virus released as defective virus particle from transformed myeloblasts. Proc Natl

Acad Sci USA 77:5120–5124 – Erikson RL, Collet MS, Erikson E, Purchio AF, Brugge JS (1980) Protein phosphorylation mediated by partially purified avian sarcoma virus transforming gene product. Cold Spring Harbor Symp Quant Biol 44:907–917 – Essex M (1980) Etiology and epidemiology of leukemia and lymphoma in outbred animal species. In: Yohn DS, Lapin BA, Blakesleee JR (eds) Advances in comparative leukemia research 1979. Elsevier/North-Holland, New York, pp 432–430 – Frankel AE, Fischinger PJ (1976) Nucleotide sequences in mouse DNA and RNA specific for Moloney sarcoma virus. Proc Natl Acad Sci 73:3705–3709 – Frankel AE, Gilbert PM, Porzig KJ, Scolnick EM, Aaronson SA (1979) Nature and distribution of feline sarcoma virus nucleotide sequences. J Virol 30:821–827 – Galehouse D, Duesberg PH (1976) RNA and proteins of Kirsten sarcoma xenotropic leukemia virus complex propagated in rat and chick cells. Virology 20:970–104 – Gardner MB, Henderson BE, Estes JD, Rongey RW, Casagrande J, Pike M, Huebner RJ (1976) The epidemiology and virology of C-type virus associated hematological cancers and related diseases in wild mice. Cancer Res 36:574–581 – Goff SP, Gilboa E, Witte ON, Baltimore D (1980) Structure of the Abelson murine leukemia virus genome and the homologous cellular gene: Studies with cloned virae DVA. Cell 22:777–785 – Graf T, Beug H (1978) Avian leukemia viruses. Interaction with their target cells in vivo and in vitro. Biochim Biophys Acta 516:269–299 – Graf T, Beug H, Hayman MJ (1980) Target cell specificity of defective avian leukemia viruses: Haematopoietic target cells for a given virus type can be infected but not transformed by strains of a different type. Proc Natl Acad Sci USA 77:389–393 – Gross L (1970) Oncogenic Viruses. Pergamon, New York Oxford London Paris – Hayman MJ, Royer-Pokora B, Graf T (1979a) Defectiveness of avian erythroblastosis virus: Synthesis of a 75k gag-related protein. Virology 92:31–45 – Hayman MJ, Kitchener G, Graf T (1979b) Cells transformed by avian myelocytomatosis virus strain CMII contain a 90K gag-related protein. Virology 98:191–199 – Hayward WS (1977) The size and genetic content of viral RNAs in avian oncovirus-infected cells. J Virol 24:47–64 – Huebner RJ, Todaro GJ (1969) Oncogenes of RNA tumor viruses as determinants of cancer. Proc Natl Acad Sci USA 64:1087–1091 – Hughes SH, Payvar F, Spector D, Schimke RT, Robinson H, Payne GS, Bishop JM, Varmus HE (1979a) Heterogeneity of genetic loci in chickens: Analysis of endogenous viral and nonviral genes by cleavage of DNA with restriction endonuclease. Cell 18:347–359 – Hughes SH, Stubblefield F, Payvar F, Engel JD, Dodgson JB, Spector D, Cordell B, Schimke RT, Varmus HE (1979b) Gene localization by chromosome fractionation: Globin genes are on at least two chromosomes and three estrogen-inducible genes are on three chromosomes. Proc Natl Acad Sci USA 76:1348–1352 – Jarrett O (1978) Infectious leukemias in domestic animals. In: Neth R, Gallo RC, Hofschneider P-H, Mannweiler K (eds) Modern trends in human leukemia III. Springer, Berlin Heidelberg New York, pp 439–444 – Kitchener G, Hayman MJ (1980) Comparative tryptic peptide mapping studies suggest a role in cell transformation for gag-related proteins of avian erythroblastosis virus and avian myelomatosis virus strains CMII and MC29. Proc Natl Acad Sci USA 77:1637–1641 – Lai MMC, Duesberg PH, Horst J, Vogt PK (1973) Avian tumor virus RNA. A comparison of three sarcoma viruses and their transformation-defective derivatives by oligonucleotide fingerprinting and DNA-RNA hybridization. Proc Natl Acad Sci USA 20:2266–2270 – Lee W-H, Bister K, Pawson A, Robins T, Moscovici C, Duesberg PH (1980) Fujinami sarcoma virus: An avian RNA tumor virus with a unique transforming gene. Proc Natl Acad Sci USA 77:2018–2022 – Levy JH (1978) Xenotropic type C viruses. Curr Top Microbiol Immunol 79:111–213 – Lung ML, Hering C, Hartley JW, Rowe WP, Hopkins N (1980) Analysis of the genomes of mink cell focus-inducing murine type C viruses: A progress report. Cold Spring Harbor Symp Quant Biol 44:1269–1274 – Maisel J, Klement V, Lai MMC, Ostertag W, Duesberg PH (1973) Ribonucleic acid components of murine sarcoma and leukemia viruses. Proc Natl Acad Sci USA 70:3536–3540 – Martin GS (1970) Rous sarcoma virus: A function required for the maintenance of the transformed state. Nature 227:1021–1023 – Martin GS, Duesberg PH (1972) The a subunit in the RNA of transforming avian tumor viruses: I. Occurrence in different virus strains. II. Spontaneous loss resulting in non-transforming variants. Virology 47:494–497 – Martin GS, Lee WH, Duesberg PH (1980) Generation of non-defective Rous sarcoma virus by asymmetric recombination between deletion mutants. J Virol 36:591–594 – McCullough B, Schaller J, Shadduck JH, Yolin DS (1972) Induction of malignant melanomas associated with fibrosarcomas in cats inoculated with Gardner-feline fibrosarcoma virus. J Natl Cancer Inst 48:1893–1896 – Mellon P, Duesberg PH (1977) Subgenomic, cellular Rous sarcoma virus RNAs contain oligonucleotides from the 3′ half and the 5′ terminus of virion RNA. Nature 270:631–634 – Mellon P, Pawson A, Bister K, Martin GS, Duesberg PH (1978) Specific RNA sequences and gene products of MC29 avian acute leukemia virus. Proc Natl Acad Sci USA 75:5874–5878 – Moscovici C (1975) Leukemic transformation with avian myeloblastosis virus: Present status. Curr Top Microbiol Immunol 71:79–101 – Oskarsson MK, McClements WL, Blair DS, Maizel JV, Vande Woude GS (1980) Properties of a normal mouse cell DNA sequence (sarc) homologous to the src sequence of Moloney sarcoma virus. Science 207:1222–1224 – Ostertag W, Vehmeyer K, Fagg B, Pragnell IB, Paetz W, Le Bourse MC, Smadja-Joffe F, Klein B, Jasmin C,

Eisen H (1980) Myeloproliferate virus, a cloned murine sarcoma virus with spleen focusforming properties in adult mice. J Virol 33:573–582 – Quade K (1979) Transformation of mammalian cells by avian myelocytomatosis virus and avian erythroblastosis virus. Virology 98:461–465 – Ramsay G, Hayman MJ (1980) Analysis of cells transformed by defective leukemia virus OK10: Production of non-infectious particles and synthesis of pr76 gag and an additional 200,000 dalton protein. Virology 106:71–81 – Reynolds FW, Van de Ven WJM, Stephenson JR (1980) Feline sarcoma virus polyprotein P115 binds a host phosphoprotein in transformed cells. Nature 286:409–412 – Rosenberg N, Baltimore D (1980) Abelson virus. In: Klein G (ed) Viral oncology. Raven, New York, pp 187–203 – Roussel M, Saule S, Lagrou C, Rommens C, Beug H, Graf T, Stehelin D (1979) Three new types of viral oncogenes of cellular origin specific for haematopoietic cell transformation. Nature 281:452–455 – Rubin H, Fanshier C, Cornelius A, Hughes WF (1962) Tolerance and immunity in chickens after congenital and contact infection with avian leukosis virus. Virology 17:143–156 – Rübsamen H, Ziemiecki A, Friis RR, Bauer H (1980) The expression of pp60 src and its associated protein kinase activity in cells infected with different transformation-defective temperature-sensitive mutants of Rous sarcoma virus. Virology 102:453–457 – Scher CD, Scolnick EM, Siegler R (1975) Induction of erythroid leukemia by Harvey and Kirsten sarcoma virus. Nature 256:225–226 – Scolnick EM, Rands E, Williams D, Parks WP (1973) Studies on the nucleic acid sequences of Kirsten sarcoma virus: A model for the formation of a mammalian RNA-containing, sarcoma virus. J Virol 12:456–463 – Scolnick EM, Goldberg RJ, Siegler R (1975) A biochemical and genetic analysis of mammalian RNA-containing sarcoma viruses. Cold Spring Harbor Symp Quant Biol 39:885–895 – Scolnick EM, Vass WC, Howk RS, Duesberg PH (1979) Defective retrovirus-like 30S RNA species of rat and mouse cells are infectious if packaged by Type C helper virus. J Virol 29:964–972 – Sheiness D, Bishop JM (1979) DNA and RNA from uninfected vertebrate cells contain nucleotide sequences related to the putative transforming gene of avian myelocytomatosis virus. J Virol 31:514–521 – Shields A, Goff S, Paskind M, Otto G, Baltimore D (1979) Structure of the Abelson murine leukemia virus genome. Cell 18:955–962 – Souza LM, Strommer JN, Hillgard RL, Komaromy MC, Baluda MA (1980) Cellular sequences are present in the presumptive avian myeloblastosis virus genome. Proc Natl Acad Sci USA 77:5177–5181 – Spector DH, Varmus HE,

Bishop JM (1978a) Nucleotide sequences related to the transforming genes of avian sarcoma virus are present in DNA of uninfected vertebrates. Proc Natl Acad Sci USA 75:4102–4106 – Spector DH, Baker B, Varmus HE, Bishop JM (1978b) Characteristics of cellular RNA related to the transforming gene of avian sarcoma viruses. Cell 13:381–386 – Stehelin D, Guntaka R, Varmus HE, Bishop JM (1976a) Purification of DNA complementary to nucleotide sequences required for neoplastic transformation of fibroblasts by avian sarcoma viruses. J Mol Biol 101:349–365 – Stehelin D, Varmus HE, Bishop JM, Vogt PK (1976b) DNA related to the transforming gene(s) of avian sarcoma viruses is present in normal avian DNA. Nature 260:170–173 – Stephenson JR, Khan AS, Van de Ven WJM, Reynolds FH Jr (1979) Type C retroviruses as vectors for cloning cellular genes with probable transforming function. J Natl Cancer Inst 63:1111–1119 – Tooze J (1973) The Molecular Biology of Tumour Viruses. Cold Spring Harbor haboratory, New York – Tsichlis PN, Coffin JM (1980) Role of the c-region in relative growth rates of endogenous and exogenous avian oncoviruses. Cold Spring Harbor Symp Quant Biol 44:1123–1132 – Tsuchida N, Gilden RV, Hatanaka M (1974) Sarcoma virus-related RNA sequences in normal rat cells. Proc Natl Acad Sci USA 71:4503–4507 – Van de Ven WJM, Reynolds FH, Nalewaik RP, Stephenson JR (1980) Characterization of a 170,000 dalton polyprotein encoded by the McDonough strain of feline sarcoma virus. J Virol 35:165–175 – Wang LH (1978) The gene order of avian RNA tumor viruses derived from biochemical analyses of deletion mutants and viral recombinants. Annu Rev Microbiol 32:561–593 – Wang L-H, Duesberg PH, Beemon K, Vogt PK: Mapping RNase T_1-resistant oligonucleotides of avian tumor virus RNAs: Sarcoma specific oligonucleotides are near the poly(A) end and oligonucleotides common to sarcoma and transformation-defective viruses are at the poly(A) end. J Virol 16:1051–1070 – Wang L-H, Duesberg PH, Mellon P, Vogt PK (1976) Distribution of envelope-specific and sarcoma-specific nucleotide sequences from different parents in the RNAs of avian tumor virus recombinants. Proc Natl Acad Sci USA 73:1073–1077 – Wang SY, Hayward WS, Hanafusa H (1977) Genetic variation in the RNA transcripts of endogenous virus genes in uninfected chicken cells. J Virol 24:64–73 – Weyl KS, Dougherty RM (1977) Contact transmission of avian leukosis virus. J Natl Cancer Inst 58:1019–1025 – Witte ON, Dasgupta A, Baltimore D (1980) Abelson murine leukemia virus protein is phosphorylated in vitro to form phosphotyrosine. Nature 283:826–831

Haematology and Blood Transfusion Vol. 26
Modern Trends in Human Leukemia IV
Edited by Neth, Gallo, Graf, Mannweiler, Winkler
© Springer-Verlag Berlin Heidelberg 1981

A Cellular Protein Phosphorylated by the Avian Sarcoma Virus Transforming Gene Product

E. Erikson and R. L. Erikson

Cell transformation by ASVs is the consequence of the expression of a single viral gene, termed *src*, for sarcoma induction (Vogt 1977; Hanafusa 1977). The product of the *src* gene is a 60,000-dalton phosphoprotein termed pp60^{src} (Purchio et al. 1978). Extensively purified preparations of pp60^{src} exhibit phosphotransferase activity for various protein substrates (Erikson et al. 1979 a, b; Collett et al. 1980), implying that phosphorylation of cellular proteins may play a role in transformation. Evidence that pp60^{src} does mediate transformation via phosphorylation, however, requires the identification of a cellular protein(s) that is (are) phosphorylated directly as the result of pp60^{src} activity both in cells and in vitro and the correlation of this phosphorylation with a phenotype of transformation.

Earlier reports (Erikson et al. 1979b; Radke and Martin 1979) had described the detection of a newly phosphorylated protein in ASV-transformed chicken cells with a molecular weight of approximately 34,000 (34K) and a pI of about 7.5. In these reports no evidence was presented with regard to the possibility that this protein may be related to pp60^{src}, to its general distribution in ASV-transformed cells other than chicken, or whether it was a direct or indirect target of events initiated in cells by pp60^{src}. We describe here more direct experiments which show that this protein is a *src*-specific substrate found in normal cells and that upon transformation it is phosphorylated in ASV-infected cells of both avian and mammalian origin. The *src*-specific nature of the phosphorylation is demonstrated directly by comparative tryptic phosphopeptide analyses of this protein phosphorylated in transformed cells and in vitro.

The unphosphorylated form of 34K was purified from normal chicken embryo fibroblasts by conventional ion-exchange chromatography and tested as a substrate for pp60^{src}-specific phosphotransferase activity in vitro. Figure 1 demonstrates that 34K constituted at least 85% of the protein in the preparation and it was not detectably labeled by endogenous protein kinase activity (track 1). However, it could be phosphorylated by pp60^{src} (track 2). The *src*-specific nature of the phosphorylation is shown by the fact that anti-*src* IgG but not normal rabbit IgG (tracks 3 and 4) inhibited the phosphorylation of this protein.

However, pp60^{src} preparations are able to phosphorylate a number of proteins that may not be direct substrates of its activity in transformed cells (Erikson et al. 1979b; Collett et al. 1980), and thus the sites phosphorylated in both the protein isolated from radiolabeled transformed cells and that phosphorylated in vitro were compared by two-dimensional fingerprinting of tryptic digests. As shown in Fig. 2, there was a major and a minor phosphopeptide released by trypsin digestion of 34K prepared from transformed cells. Since the 34K preparation used for this digestion was homogeneous with respect to its migration during pH gradient gel electrophoresis (Fig. 3), the minor peptide may represent an incomplete digestion product, although there are other possible explanations for the unequal molarity consistently observed (see below). Phosphorylation of the 34K protein in vitro by pp60^{src} resulted in the phosphorylation of a peptide which comigrated with the major peptide identified in the protein from transformed cells.

Recently, it has been shown that pp60^{src} phosphorylates tyrosine residues in the immune-complex phosphotransferase reaction

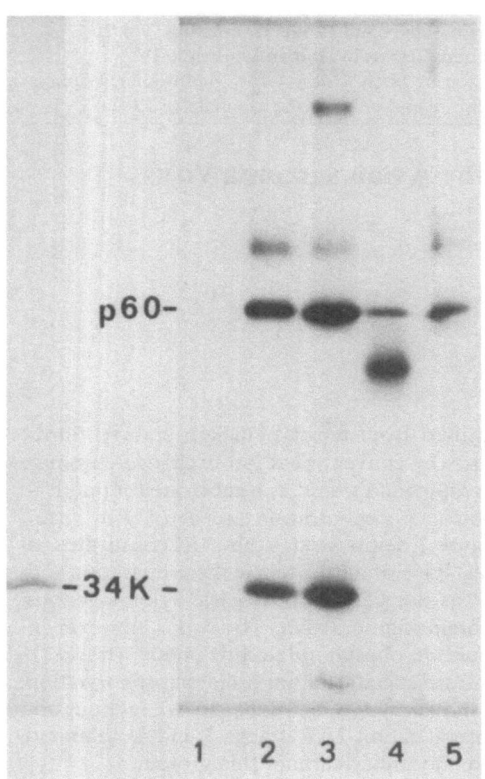

Fig. 1. In vitro phosphorylation of 34K by pp60[src]. A preparation of the 34K protein purified from normal chicken embryo fibroblasts was incubated in the protein kinase reaction mixture with pp60[src]. Reactions were carried out at 22°C for 15 min in a total volume of 35 μl as previously described (Erikson et al. 1979). Each reaction mixture contained 5 μl of partially purified pp60[src] prepared by immunoaffinity chromatography (Erikson et al. 1979), 1.5 μg bovine serum albumin, and approximately 0.5 μg 34K protein. Reactions were initiated by the addition of $MnCl_2$ and $[\gamma\text{-}^{32}P]ATP$ (400–600 Ci/mmol) to a final concentration of 2.5 mM and 1 μM, respectively. Reactions were terminated by the addition of ¼ volume of five times concentrated electrophoresis sample buffer and by heating at 95°C for 1 min. Reaction products were then analyzed by polyacrylamide gel electrophoresis and autoradiography. *Left panel* A Coomassie blue stained SDS-polyacrylamide gel after electrophoresis of the 34K preparation. *Right panel,* autoradiogram of SDS-polyacrylamide gel analysis of protein kinase reaction products: track *1,* 34K preparation alone, and with *(2)* pp60[src], *(3)* pp60[src] and normal rabbit IgG, and *(4)* pp60[src] and rabbit anti-pp60[src] IgG. Track *5* pp60[src] preparation alone. Serum containing anti-pp60[src] antibody was obtained from tumor-bearing rabbits (Brugge and Erikson 1977). The IgG fraction was obtained from the sera by ammonium sulfate precipitation. The IgGs were present in the reaction mixture at 600 μg/ml

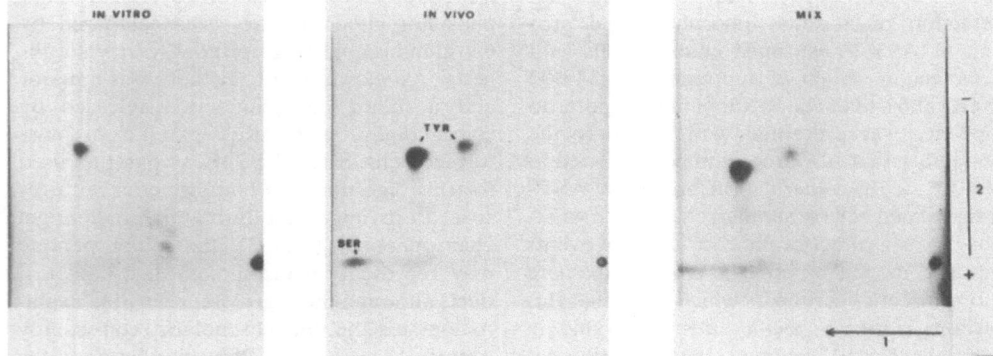

Fig. 2. Phosphopeptide analysis of 34K. Two-dimensional tryptic fingerprints of [^{32}P]-labeled 34K isolated from transformed cells *(center),* phosphorylated in vitro by pp60[src] as shown in Fig. 1, track 2 *(left),* and a mixture of the two preparations *(right).* Radiolabeled 34K was localized in preparative gels by autoradiography, excised, eluted from the gels, precipitated, and digested with trypsin. A portion of the digest was analyzed by ascending chromatography in n-propanol:s-butanol:isoamyl alcohol:pyridine:water (1:1:1:3:3) in the first dimension followed by electrophoresis at pH 3.5 [pyridine:acetic acid:water (1:10:189)] in the second dimension

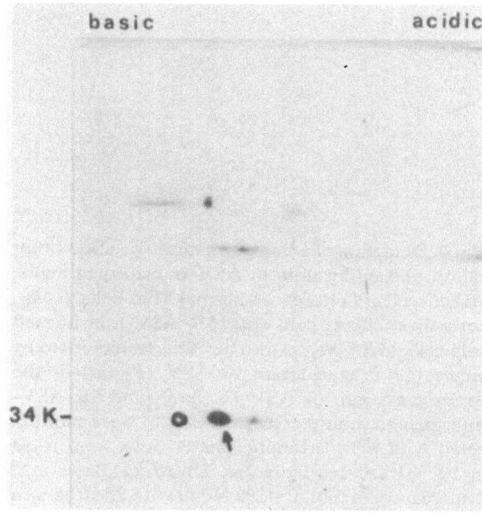

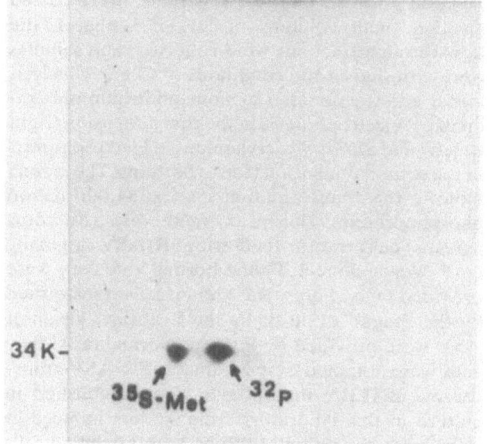

Fig. 3. Two-dimensional fractionation of 34K protein phosphorylated in vitro by pp60^src. *Upper panel* The 34K protein was phosphorylated in vitro as shown in Fig. 1, track 2. The reaction mixture was adjusted to the conditions of O'Farrell's lysis buffer (O'Farrell 1975) (9.5M urea, 5% 2-mercaptoethanol, 2% NP40, 2% ampholines) and analyzed by nonequilibrium pH gradient gel electrophoresis in the first dimension (right to left) and SDS-polyacrylamide gel electrophoresis in the second dimension (top to bottom) (O'Farrel et al. 1977). The location of Coomassie blue stained 34K is indicated by the *open circle*. The *arrow* indicates the position of [³²P]-labeled 34K. *Lower panel* Preparations of purified 34,000-dalton protein from [³⁵S]methionine-labeled normal chicken embryo fibroblasts (³⁵S-met) and [³²P]-labeled SR-ASV-transformed chicken embryo fibroblasts (³²P) were mixed and fractionated as described above

(Hunter and Sefton 1980) and in a number of protein substrates during more conventional soluble reactions as well (Collett et al. 1980). To determine whether this amino acid specificity holds for the 34K protein, phosphoamino acid analyses were carried out on 34K phosphorylated in vitro and isolated from radiolabeled transformed cells. The in vitro reaction resulted in phosphorylation of tyrosine residues exclusively, whereas the phosphoprotein from transformed cells yielded phosphotyrosine and some phosphoresine as well. In Fig. 2 the peptides labeled TYR have been shown to contain phosphotyrosine, whereas the one labeled SER contains phosphoserine (data not shown).

The 34K protein phosphorylated in vitro was also subjected to two-dimensional electrophoresis in order to gain additional information concerning the number of sites phosphorylated. The result, illustrated in Fig. 3, shows that the in vitro phosphorylation resulted in a shift in migration of the phosphate-containing polypeptide with respect to the phosphate-free polypeptide identical to that observed in vivo and indicates that each 34K molecule contains the same number of phosphate groups (probably one). Therefore, the major and minor tryptic phosphopeptides shown in Fig. 2 may be from separate 34K molecules.

The significance of such an ASV-specific phosphorylation would be clearer if it occurred in other ASV-transformed cells as well. Consequently, various mammalian cells transformed by ASV were examined for a similar phosphorylated protein and the results as shown in Fig. 4 reveal that mouse, vole, and rat cells all contained a similar phosphoprotein. Normal fibroblasts from all of these species showed either greatly reduced or undetectable levels of a phosphoprotein with a similar pI and molecular weight; two such examples are shown in Fig. 4. These 34K proteins also contain phosphotyrosine and a trace of phosphoserine (data not shown).

In this communication we have described the isolation of a protein from normal chicken embryo fibroblasts that appears to be a substrate for the phosphotransferase activity associated with pp60^src. This protein, or an analogous protein, is found to be partially phosphorylated in all ASV-transformed cells examined to date. The apparently similar nature of the protein in both avian and mammalian cells suggests that it is highly conserved. In view of

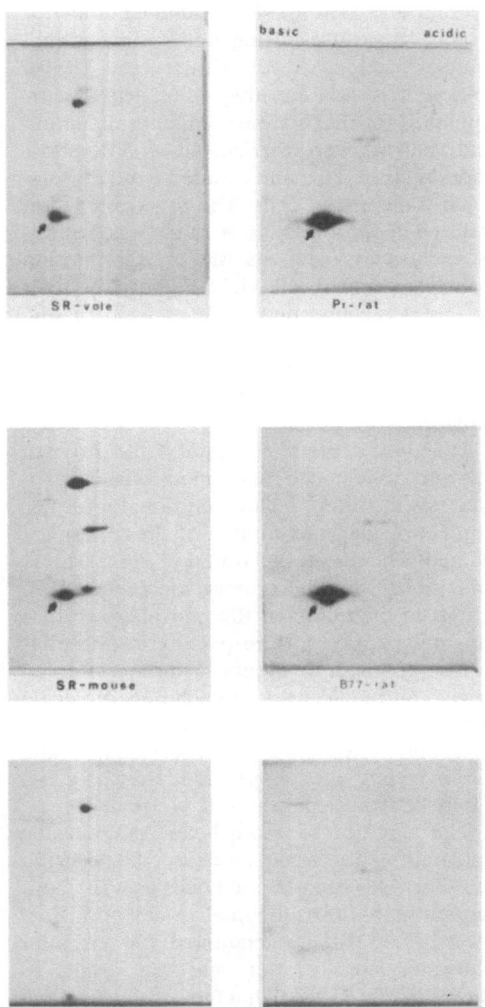

Fig. 4. Detection of a transformation-specific 34,000 dalton phosphoprotein in ASV-transformed mammalian cells. Cultures of normal vole cells *(vole)*, normal rat kidney cells *(rat)*, SR-ASV-transformed vole cells *(SR-vole)*, rat kidney cells transformed by either the Prague strain of ASV *(Pr-rat)* or the Bratislava strain of ASV *(B77-rat)* and SR-ASV-transformed mouse cells *(SR-mouse)* were radiolabeled with [^{32}P] orthophosphate. Cells were lysed in 10^{-2}M Tris-HC1 pH 7.2, 1 mM EDTA, 1 mM 2-mercaptoethanol, 0.05% NP40 with 25 strokes in a Dounce homogenizer. After clarification at 100,000 g for 30 min, the supernates were passed through small columns of DEAE-Sephacel, the flow-through fractions were collected, and samples were adjusted to the conditions of O'Farrell's lysis buffer and fractionated by nonequilibrium pH gradient gel electrophoresis in the first dimension (right to left) and SDS-polyacrylamide gel electrophoresis in the second dimension (top to bottom). The *arrows* indicate the transformation-specific 34,000 dalton phosphoprotein. European field vole (Microtus agrestis) cells transformed with SR-ASV originally by P. Vogt (clone 1-T) and normal vole cells were provided by A. Faras. Rat kidney cells transformed by the Prague strain or by the Bratislava strain of ASV were provided by P. Vogt. Normal rat kidney cells were obtained from M. Imada. SR-ASV-transformed BALB/c mouse cells were established in culture in this laboratory from tumors induced in mice by the injection of SR-ASV-transformed cells originally obtained from J. T. Parsons

the generally similar outcome of ASV transformation of fibroblasts from different species, one might expect similar targets to exist in any normal cell able to be transformed by ASV.

The pp60^{src}-specific nature of the phosphorylation is shown by the phosphorylation of 34K by pp60^{src} in vitro at a site identical to that phosphorylated in transformed cells. This result strongly suggests that 34K is a direct rather than indirect substrate of pp60^{src} in the cell. Such a result also suggests that pp60^{src} acts as a protein kinase in the transformed cell as well as in vitro and that it mediates transformation, at least in part, by phosphorylation of 34K and perhaps of other normal cell proteins. However, this conclusion does not eliminate the possibility that pp60^{src} may have other functions that influence the transformation process.

Acknowledgements

This research was supported by grants CA 21117 and CA 21326 from the National Institutes of Health and grant MV-IA from the American Cancer Society.

References

Brugge JS, Erikson RL (1977) Identification of a transformation-specific antigen induced by an avian sarcoma virus. Nature 269:346–347 – Collett MS, Purchio AF, Erikson RL (1980) Soluble protein kinase activity of purified avian sarcoma virus-transforming protein, pp60^{src}, results in the phosphorylation of tyrosine residues. Nature 285:167–169 – Erikson RL, Collett MS, Erikson E, Purchio AF (1979a) Evidence that the avian sarcoma virus transforming gene product is a cyclic AMP-independent protein kinase. Proc Natl Acad Sci USA 76:6260–6264 – Erikson RL, Collett MS, Erikson E, Purchio AF, Brugge JS (1979b) Protein phosphorylation mediated by partially purified avian sarcoma virus transforming gene product. Cold Spring Harbor Symp Quant Biol 44:907–917 – Hanafusa H (1977) Cell transformation by RNA tumor viruses. In: Fraenkel-Conrat H, Wagner RP (eds) Comprehensive virology, vol 10. Plenum, New York, pp 401–483 – Hunter T, Sefton BM (1980) Transforming gene product of Rous sarcoma virus phosphorylates tyrosine. Proc Natl Acad Sci USA 77:1311–1315 – O'Farrell PH (1975) High resolution two-dimensional electrophoresis of proteins. J Biol Chem 250:4007–4021 – O'Farrell PZ, Goodman HM, O'Farrell PH (1977) High resolution two-dimensional electrophoresis of basic as well as acidic proteins. Cell 12:1133–1141 – Purchio AF, Erikson E, Brugge JS, Erikson RL (1978) Identification of a polypeptide encoded by the avian sarcoma virus src gene. Proc Natl Acad Sci USA 75:1567–1571 – Radke K, Martin GS (1979) Transformation by Rous sarcoma virus: Effects of src gene expression on the synthesis and phosphorylation of cellular polypeptides. Proc Natl Acad Sci USA 76:5212–5216 – Vogt PK (1977) The genetics of RNA tumor viruses. In: Fraenkel-Conrat H, Wagner RP (eds) Comprehensive virology, vol 9. Plenum, New York, pp 341–455

Haematology and Blood Transfusion Vol. 26
Modern Trends in Human Leukemia IV
Edited by Neth, Gallo, Graf, Mannweiler, Winkler
© Springer-Verlag Berlin Heidelberg 1981

Correlated Loss of the Transformed Phenotype and pp60src-Associated Protein Kinase Activity

R. R. Friis, A. Ziemiecki, V. Bosch, C. B. Boschek, and H. Bauer

Summary

The decline in pp60src-associated protein kinase activity occurring after shift of Rous sarcoma virus transformation defective, mutant-infected cells was compared with changes in other parameters of transformation in an attempt to measure the relevance of the protein kinase to the overall transformed state.

Using transformation defective temperature sensitive mutants, Martin (1970) presented the first evidence that a Rous sarcoma viral gene product was continuously needed for maintainance of transformation. More recently, Ash et al. (1976) showed that a reversible return to a normal phenotype could be induced in Rous sarcoma virus transformed cells by treatment with inhibitors of protein synthesis. This was interpreted to mean that a viral gene product directly or indirectly induces the transformed state and that transformed cells, freed of this effector because of its presumably modest half-life in the cell, take on spontaneously a normal phenotype without requirement for new protein synthesis. This communication wil document a similar reversion in the transformed phenotype, induced in transformation-defective, temperature-sensitive, mutant-infected cells after a shift from the permissive to the nonpermissive temperature.

The src gene of Rous sarcoma virus apparently is entirely and uniquely responsible for inducing transformation (Wang et al. 1975). Brugge and Erikson (1977) recently demonstrated that the gene product of the src gene, called pp60src, was a phosphoprotein of 60,000 daltons which could be immunoprocipitated using tumor-bearing rabbit serum. Furthermore, a protein kinase activity capable of phosphorylating the immune precipitating IgG was detected (Collett and Erikson 1978) and is apparently associated with the pp60src. It seems also highly probable that the pp60src also acts autocatalytically to phosphorylate one site on its own molecule.

Figure 1 illustrates an experiment in which mutant (A) and wild type (B) infected cells which had been grown at 35°C (permissive) were shifted and assayed at various times after shift to 42°C (nonpermissive). A kinase reaction is shown in the first half of each polyacrylamide gel and the intensity of the IgG heavy chain serves as a measure of kinase activity. The second half of the gel presents an immunoprecipitation of in vivo orthophosphate (^{32}P)-labeled cell lysates with the pp60src band indicated. In looking at kinase activity it is clear in comparing A and B that the mutant kinase is sharply thermolabile; a loss of 5-fold in activity is measured within 30 min. This is not seen with the Schmidt-Ruppin strain wild type parent virus-infected cells which retain approximately constant kinase activity after temperature shift. As with kinase activity, ^{32}P-orthophosphate incorporated into pp60src in a pulse label at 35°C is rapidly lost in a chase at 42°C for the mutant (A), but is lost somewhat more slowly with the wild type virus-infected cells (B). Hence, the rapid loss of kinase activity seen with the mutant-infected cells upon temperature shift to 42°C correlates with a dephosphorylation occurring more rapidly than the half life of the incorporated phosphate in the cells infected by the wild type virus could account for.

Parallel studies examined the change in the rate of hexose transport shown by mutant-infected cells upon shift to the nonpermissive temperature. Within 4 h after the shift to 42°C,

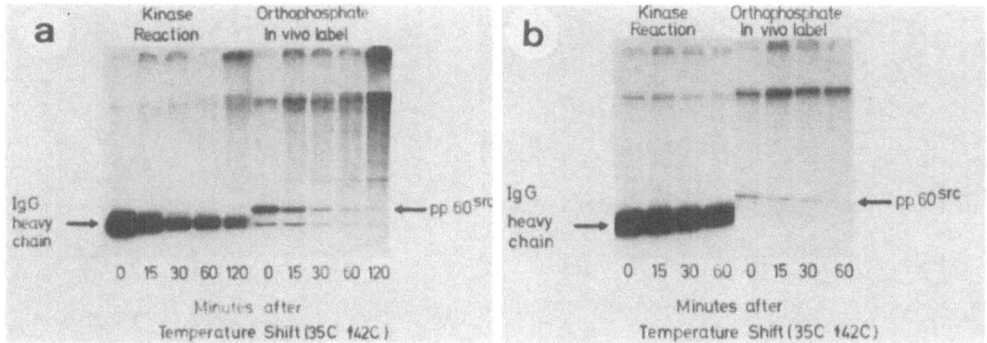

Fig. 1. Pp60^{src}-associated protein kinase activity and the half life of in vivo incorporated ^{32}P-orthophosphate are shown. The kinase reaction was performed as already described (Rübsamen et al. 1980). For the half life study, cultures were labeled for 20 min at 35°C with 1 mCI/ml of ^{32}P-orthophosphate, followed by a chase according to the times indicated at 42°C. **a** shows results obtained with NY68 (Kawai and Hanafusa 1971) infected cells, while **b** was transformed with the Schmidt Ruppin strain of Rous sarcoma virus wild type parent. *Arrows* indicate the heavy chain of IgG and pp60^{src}

cells showed a 50% reduced rate of uptake of ^{3}H-2-deoxyglucose in a 10 min incubation when compared to sister cultures maintained at 35°C.

Figure 2 illustrates the changes occurring in the organization of mutant-infected cell microfilaments concomitant with a temperature shift from 35°C to 42°C. The method used takes advantage of the high affinity binding of the fluorescent-labeled toxin, phalloidin (the generous gift of Prof. Th. Wieland, Heidelberg), to filamentous actin (Wieland and Faulstich 1978). The initial conditions (35°C) is shown in the first picture (a); all cells show few stress fibers, and several (the central cell and several to the right side) show virtually no stress fibers, with diffuse and punctate fluorescence. In pucture (b), taken just 30 min after the shift to 42°C, most cells show better outlined stress fibers and some degree of linear array in all cells. Figure 2 (c) shows notably a cell with an apparently regular punctate fluorescence and developing stress fibers array at 60 min after temperature shift. Finally, 4 h after shift to 42°C, all cells (d) display well developed stress fiber arrays.

The data presented above indicate how rapidly the change in phenotype from transformed to normal can occur. Such kinetics have been previously examined, but heretofore always using cells in the normal phenotype at 42°C shifted to 35°C in order to observe the onset of transformation (Ziemiecki and Friis, to be published). In the present study, as in the

work of Ash et al. (1976), the interesting finding is that upon loss of the *src* gene product's activity, here monitored as the associated protein kinase, the cell undergoes a rapid change to normal. Ash et al. (1976) established that this change took place without the need of new protein synthesis; their result was obtained only 12–16 h after treatment, owing to the rather long functional life of the *src* gene product under these conditions. Using mutants, in which case the loss of *src* gene function is very rapid, and without using inhibitors which might have morphological effects of their own, the same result emerged from our investigation.

Acknowledgements

We thank Prof. Dr. Th. Wieland, Heidelberg, for the gift of fluorescein isothiocyanate labeled phalloidin. This work was supported by the Sonderforschungsbereich 47 (Virologie) of the Deutsche Forschungsgemeinschaft.

References

Ash JF, Vogt PK, Singer SJ (1976) Reversion from transformed to normal phenotype by inhibition of protein synthesis in rat kidney cells infected with a temperature sensitive mutant of Rous sarcoma virus. Proc Natl Acad Sci USA 73:3603–3607
– Brugge JS, Erikson RL (1977) Identification of a transformation-specific antigen induced by avian

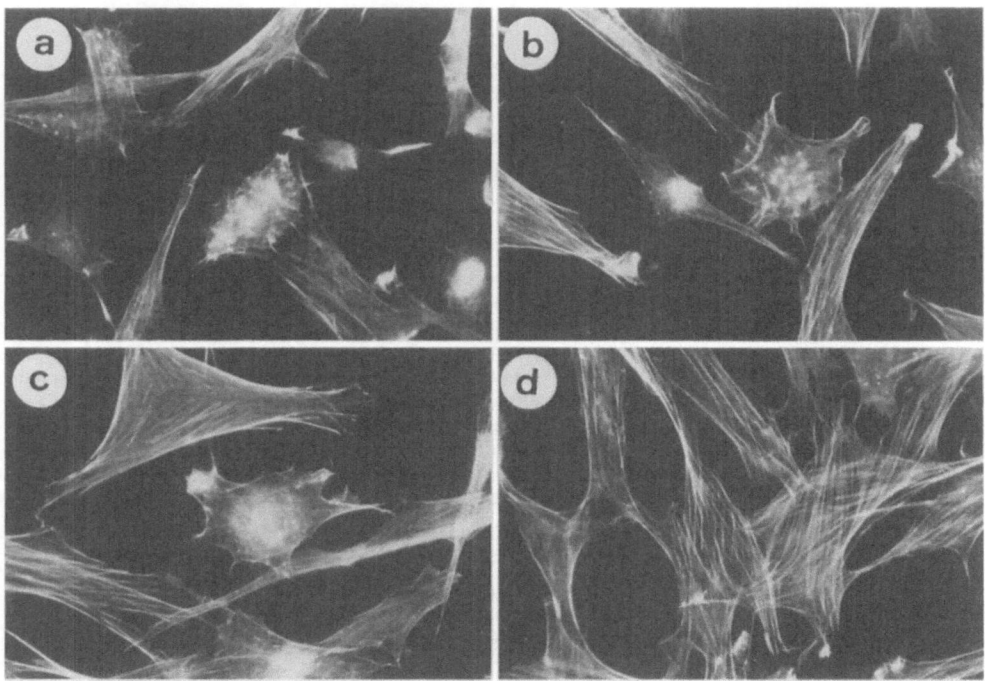

Fig. 2. Photomicrographs of NY68 infected cells fixed with 2.5% formaldehyde containing 0.2% Triton X-100 and stained with fluorescein isothiacyanate labeled phalloidin for 30 min at 25°C. Cells were prepared rapidly at the following conditions: **a** 35°C; **b** shifted to 42°C for 30 min, **c** shifted to 42°C for 60 min, and **d** shifted to 42°C for 4 h. Final magnification 592 ×

sarcoma virus. Nature 269:346–348 – Collett MS, Erikson RL (1978) Protein kinase activity associated with the avian sarcoma virus src gene product. Proc Natl Acad Sci USA 75:2021–2024 – Kawai S, Hanafusa H (1971) Effects of reciprocal changes in temperature on the transformed state of cells infected with a Rous sarcoma virus mutant. Virology 46:470–479 – Martin GS (1970) Rous sarcoma virus: A function required for the maintainance of the transformed state. Nature 227:1021–1023 – Rübsamen H, Ziemiecki A, Friis RR, Bauer H (1980) The expression of pp60src and its associated protein kinase activity in cells infected with different transformation-defective temperature-sensitive mutants of Rous sarcoma virus. Virology 102:453–457 – Wang LH, Duesberg P, Beemon K, Vogt PK (1975) Mapping RNase T$_1$-resistant oligonucleotides of avian tumor virus RNAS: Sarcoma-specific oligonucleotides are near the poly A end and oligonucleotides common to sarcoma and td-viruses are at the poly A end. J Virol 16:1051–1070 – Wieland T, Faulstich H (1978) Amatoxins, phallotoxins, phallolysin and anatmanide: The biologically active components of poisonous amanita mushrooms. Crit Rev Biochem 185–260 – Ziemiecki A, Friis RR (to be published) The role of phosphorylation of pp60src in the cycloheximide insensitive activation of the pp60src-associated kinase activity of transformation-defective temperature-sensitive mutants of Rous sarcoma virus. Virology

Haematology and Blood Transfusion Vol. 26
Modern Trends in Human Leukemia IV
Edited by Neth, Gallo, Graf, Mannweiler, Winkler
© Springer-Verlag Berlin Heidelberg 1981

The Transformation-Specific Protein pp60^{src} from an Avian Sarcoma Virus

K. Moelling, M. K. Owada, P. Donner, and T. Bunte

A. Abstract

We have detected the avian sarcoma virus (ASV) transforming protein pp60^{src} in RNA tumor virus particles and used them as a source for its isolation. The partially purified protein has a molecular weight of 60K, exhibits protein kinase activity, and is indistinguishable from its cellular counterpart. It is released from the virus by nonionic detergent. The soluble molecule easily undergoes transition to a degraded form of 50/52K. Both 60K and 50/52K forms phosphoylate themselves and reveal protein kinase activity. Embedded in the viral membrane, pp60^{src} faces the inner coat, since it is inaccessible in intact virus particles to surface iodination, antibodies, and proteases.

B. Introduction

The transforming gene product of ASV, pp60^{src}, was found in transformed cells by means of antibodies which have been prepared in tumor bearing rabbits (TBR sera) (Brugge and Erikson 1977). The heavy chain of the IgG can be phosphorylated by the enzyme, a reaction which allows one to identify the enzyme (Collett and Erikson 1978; Levinson et al. 1978). We have detected pp60^{src} in ASV virus particles (Schmidt-Ruppin strain of subgroup D, SR-D), used them as a source of the isolation of pp60^{src}, and found it associated with the viral envelope which reflects properties of the host cell membrane.

C. Results

The SR-D virus mixed with ^{35}S-methionine-labeled virus was disrupted in the presence of nonionic detergent and processed for isolation of pp60^{src} by chromatography on a DEAE cellulose and phosphocellulose column chromatography similar to previously published procedures (Moelling et al. 1978; Owada et al. 1981). Protein kinase activity was assayed by ^{32}P incorporation into casein, and furthermore ^{35}S-methionine radioactivity of the fractions was determined by acid precipitation (Fig. 1). Fractions of the phosphocellulose column (16–20) exhibited IgG phosphorylating protein kinase activity and contained ^{35}S-methionine-labeled 60K molecules (Fig. 1, bottom). The partial proteolytic cleavage pattern of the 60K band was indistinguishable from its cellular analog (not shown).

The pp60^{src} purified by this procedure was capable of phosphorylating itself in an endogenous reaction (Fig. 2, slots 1 to 4). Depending on the assay conditions it stayed intact as a 60 K molecule or underwent transition to degraded forms such as 50/52K or even 45K. Lower incubation temperatures were more favorable for conservation of the 60K form. The pp60^{src} was released from virus particles by treatment with nonionic detergent (Fig. 2). After a high-speed centrifugation insoluble material was pelleted (p) which contained 60K and 50/52K molecules, whereas the supernatant (s) revealed only the 50/52K form as tested by endogenous phosphorylation. The pelleted material was floated through a sucrose densitiy gradient for isolation of membranes according to a published procedure (Van de Ven et al. 1978). The pp60^{src} was found to be specifically associated with the viral membranes (m) where it remained in its intact 60K form (Bunte et al., J Virol, in press). The undegraded as well as the degraded forms were capable of phosphorylating IgG of TBR serum (Fig. 2).

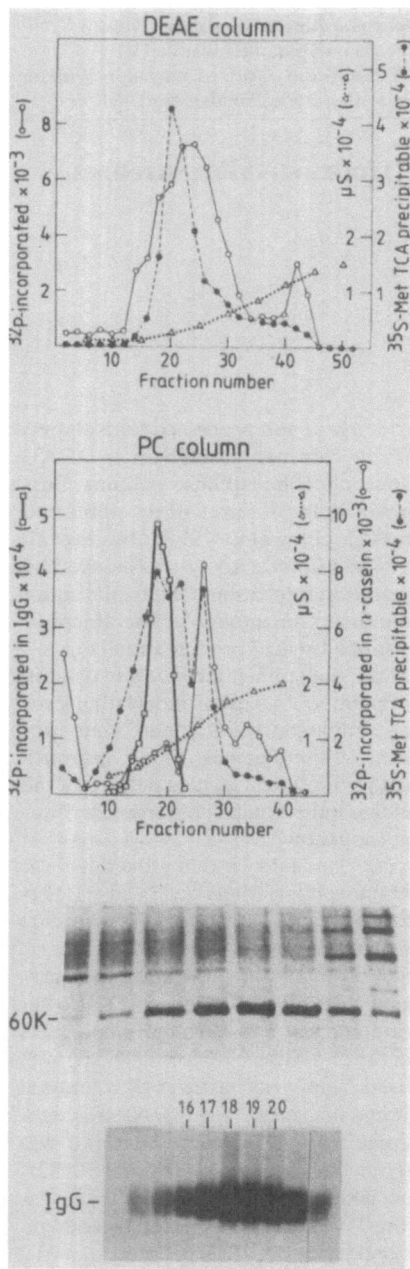

Fig. 1. Purification of ^{35}S-methionine labeled pp60[src] from SR-D virus particles by DEAE and phosphocellulose column chromatography. Fractions were tested for ^{35}S-methionine radioactivity, presence of pp60[src] by immunoprecipitation with TBR serum, and IgG phosphorylation according to published procedures (Owada and Moelling 1980)

To furhter analyze the location of pp60[src] in the viral membrane, intact and disrupted virus particles were analyzed for the accessibility of pp60[src] to antibodies, surface iodination, and protease. The results are summarized in Table 1. Intact virus did not allow binding of TBR serum as tested for by IgG phosphorylation. Furthermore, no iodination and no endogenous phosphorylation of pp60[src] or pp50/52K was achieved. Only if disruption of the virus preceded the various treatments did pp60[src] participate in these reactions. Mild proteolytic digest did not significantly affect pp60[src]. In parallel, gp85, the viral envelope glycoprotein, was analyzed and gave rise to opposite behaviors. This is in agreement with its position on the outside of the virus and indicates that pp60[src] is not located there in an analogous fashion.

D. Discussion

From these results a model was deduced (Fig. 3) which shows localization of pp60[src] inside of the virion. It is embedded in the membrane but not accessible from the outside in contrast to gp85. The 8K moeity of pp60[src], which easily breaks off, appears to be hydrophobic, since the 60K molecules can only be kept in solution in the presence of detergent, whereas the 50/52K forms do not exhibit this requirement (Donner et al., unpublished work). The hydrophobic tail may therefore be associated with the lipid bilayer. The pp60[src] sediments as a globular monomeric molecule (unpublished work) which is schematically indicated by its circular shape.

Whether pp60[src] is specifically incorporated into the virion from the cellular membrane during the budding process is unknown. Furthermore, it needs to be investigated whether pp60[src] plays a structural role in the virus particle and whether it is involved in viral transformation.

E. Materials and Methods

Protein kinase assay: 100 µl containing 0.02 M MES buffer (N-morpholino-ethane-sulfonic acid) with a pH of 6.8, 10 mM MgCl$_2$, 0.625 mg/ml of α-casein, 5 mM DTT (dithiothreitol), and 0.1 mM [γ-^{32}P]ATP (specific activity 0.5–4 Ci/mmole). Incubation was for 30 min at 30°C. Then acid precipitable radioacti-

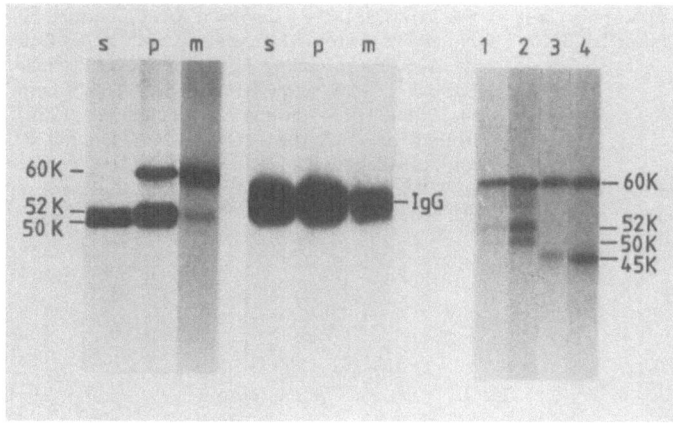

Fig. 2. SR-D virus was disrupted with (2%) NP-40, centrifuged at 45.000 rpm for 180 min at 4°C and separated into supernatant (s) and pellet (p). The pellet was used for membrane isolation (m) according to a published procedure (Van de Ven et al. 1978). Identical aliquots of s, p and m were incubated for endogenous phosphorylation and IgG phosphorylation (Owada and Moelling 1980). The purified enzyme from the phosphocellulose colum was incubated for endogenous phosphorylation under various conditions to demonstrate its proteolytic cleavage. Incubation was in *1:* 60 min, 0°C, pH 6.8; *2:* 30 min, 20°C, pH 6.8; *3.* 2 h, 0°C, pH 6.8; and *4:* 30 min, 20°C, pH 8.2

Table 1. SR-D without and with disruption (2% NP-40) was used for IgG phosphorylation, for precipitation of ³H-glucosamine radioactivity of the gp85 by antibodies, for surface iodination by means of lactoperoxidase (NEN, Radioch.), and for endogenous phosphorylation. Trypsin treatment (10 µg/ml) was for 30 min at room temperature (nt: not tested)

	Trypsin treatment	IgG-phosphorylation (cpm × 10³)	H³-glucosamine gp85 (cpm)	^{125}J-pp60^{src}	^{125}J-gp85 (cpm)	Endogenous phosphorylation		
						^{32}p-60K	^{32}P-50/52K p 19	
							(cpm)	(%)
Intact	−	52	1360	0	1064	0	0	100
Virus	+	58	603	0	532	0	0	100
Disrupted	−	512	964	169	809	77	610	100
Virus	+	564	537	146	462	72	680	2
Isolated	−	nt	nt	nt	nt	452	41	nt
Membranes	+	nt	nt	nt	nt	39	398	nt

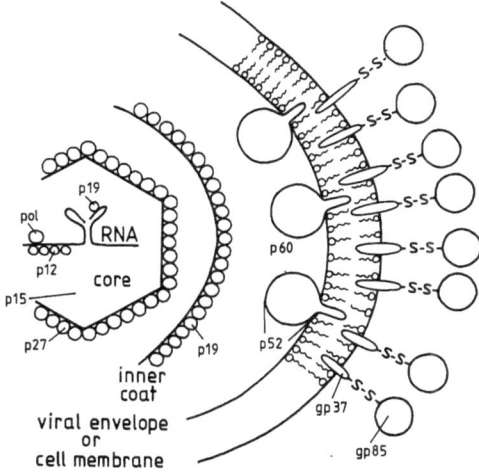

Fig. 3. Schematic presentation of the location of pp60^{src} in an avian RNA tumor virus particle. *gp,* glycoprotein

407

vity was determined. For endogenous phosphorylation casein was omitted. For pH 8.2 buffer Tris-HCl was used.

References

Brugge JS, Erikson RL (1977) Nature 269:346–348 – Collet MS, Erikson RL (1978) Proc Natl Acad Sci USA 75:2021–2024 – Levinson AD, Opperman H, Levintow L, Varmus HE, Bishop JM (1978) Cell 15:561–572 – Moelling K, Sykora KW, Dittmar KEJ, Scott A, Watson KF (1978) J Biol Chem 254:3738–3742 – Owada M, Moelling K (1980) Virology 101:157–168 – Owada KM, Donner P, Scott A, Moelling K (1981) Virology 110 – Van de Ven WJM, Vermorken AJM, Onnekink C, Bloemers HPJ, Bloemendal HJ (1978) Virology 27:595–603

Haematology and Blood Transfusion Vol. 26
Modern Trends in Human Leukemia IV
Edited by Neth, Gallo, Graf, Mannweiler, Winkler
© Springer-Verlag Berlin Heidelberg 1981

Proteolytic Processing of Avian and Simian Sarcoma and Leukemia Viral Proteins

B. Konze-Thomas and K. von der Helm

A. Introduction

Viral proteins of avian and mammalian leukemia and sarcoma viruses are synthesized in their host cells primarily as precursors. They are successively processed to smaller proteins, which then can be assembled into virus particles (Vogt et al. 1975; Arcement et al. 1976; Okasinsky and Velicer 1976; Eisenman and Vogt 1978). This processing has been found to be caused by a virus-specific proteolytic enzyme. The protease p15 is coded by the genome of leukemia/sarcoma viruses; it is part of the internal viral core, the group-specific antigen (gag) protein, and cleaves its own gag precursor (von der Helm 1977). This precursor cleavage can be demonstrated in vitro with purified p15 from AMV and gag precursor bound to an antibody (directed against gag proteins) and Staph. aureus protein A (Dittmar and Moelling 1978).

Using this system we studied whether protein precursors with gag sequences of other related or unrelated oncornaviruses could be cleaved by the avian gag protein p15.

This paper describes the cleavage of a 110 k dalton fusion protein of the replication-defective avian acute leukemia virus MC 29 (Langlois et al. 1967; Bister et al. 1977) and a gag protein precursor pr65 of Simian sarcoma virus (SSV) (Wolfe et al. 1971; Deinhardt et al. 1978) by avian p15 into discrete smaller proteins. Since protease p15 evidently cleaves off the gag sequences of the fusion protein gag-x (whereas the x sequences may represent the putative "onc"-gene sequences), we discuss how p15 could be used as a tool for mapping transformation proteins.

B. Results and Discussion

To determine the optimal conditions for cleavage of IgG-bound pr76 by the p15 protease, the immunocomplex containing ^{35}S-methionine-labeled pr76 was incubated for different periods of time and different salt concentrations in presence of p15 protease (B. Konze-Thomas and K. von der Helm, to be published). Protease p15 was isolated from virions by conventional methods (von der Helm and Konze-Thomas 1980; B. Konze-Thomas and K. von der Helm, to be published). Figure 1 shows that during 30 min of incubation in 0.15 M NaCl processing of pr76 and pr180 commenced and is completed after 6 h. In presence of higher salt concentration (i.e., 1 M NaCl) in vitro processing is already completed after 2 h of incubation. Evidence for the completion of the processing is the disappearance of the polypeptide pr32 which is an intermediate precursor to p19 (Vogt et al. 1975; von der Helm 1977). Cleavage of other non-gag-containing polypeptides (i.e., gp85) or further cleavage of the processed gag proteins (p27, etc.) has never been observed, even with very long incubation periods (not shown).

I. Cleavage of MC 29 Protein 110 k by p15

The defective avian acute leukemia virus MC 29 has among other defects a deletion of the p15 gene (Bister et al. 1977; Mellon et al. 1978). A 110 k dalton protein, the only virus-specific polypeptide synthesized in infected and transformed nonproducer cells is not processed. It is a fusion protein of an incomplete gag gene (p19 and p27) and unknown

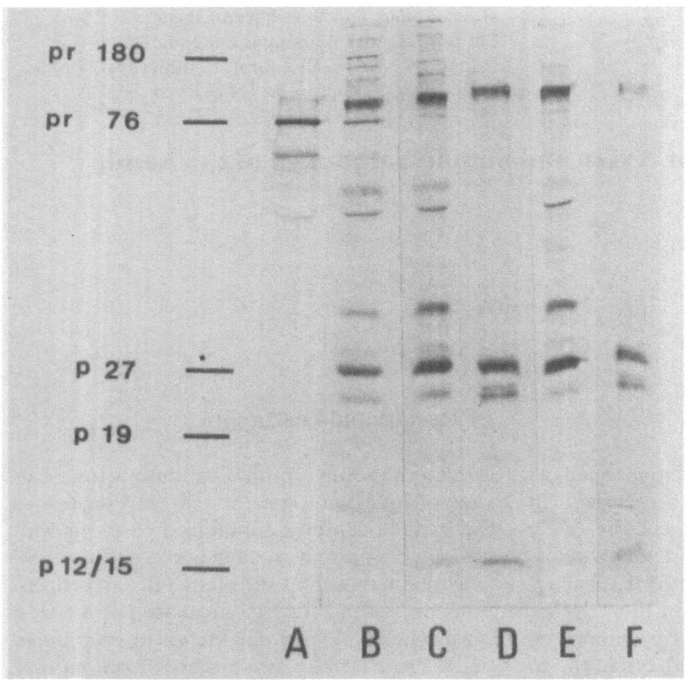

Fig. 1. In vitro cleavage of pr76 by p15. RSV-infected chicken fibroblasts were labeled for 1 h with
[35]S-methionine, lysed, and immunoprecipitated by anti-p27 serum and protein A sepharose (B.
Konze-Thomas and K. von der Helm, to be published) *(A)*, untreated control or incubated in 0.15 M NaCl at
37°C with 0.7 ug of protease p15 for ½ h *(B)*, 2 h *(C)*, 6 h *(D)* or for 2 h in 0.5 M NaCl *(E)* or 1 M NaCl *(F)*.
After incubation the samples were analysed by 12.5% SDS-PAGE and autoradiography

sequences coding for a putative transformation protein (Dittmar and Moelling 1978).

We used the p15 protease as a tool for restrictive protein cleavage in vitro and tried to cleave off the gag sequences in order to determine the size of the non-gag sequences of the 110 k dalton polypeptide. From a ^{35}S-methionine-labeled lysate of nonproducer cells, the 110 k d protein had been immunoprecipitated by a serum directed against p27 structural protein of avian leukemia/sarcoma virus (B. Konze-Thomas and K. von der Helm, 1980, to be published). After incubation of the immunocomplex with p15 the 110 k dalton protein had been cleaved into proteins of the molecular weight 75 k, 55 k, 32 k and 25/24 k dalton (Fig. 2). A comparison of these proteins by a V8 protease digestion analysis suggested that all of them derived from the 110 k dalton protein (not shown). By this analysis the 75 k d polypeptide appears to be an intermediate precursor to the 55 k d product. The 25/24 and

32 k d polypeptides react strongly with anti-gag serum, the 55 k d polypeptide, very weakly. We assume that the 24/25 k d and 32 k d polypeptides are gag-related proteins, while the 55 k d polypeptide contains no gag sequences and may represent the putative "onc" part of the fusion protein.

II. Immunoprecipitation of Intracellular SSV-Specific Proteins

Simian sarcoma virus was originally isolated from a spontaneous sarcoma of a woolly monkey (Wolfe et al. 1971). Similar to the MC 29 virus, this virus transforms cells and is replication-defective. Isolates of this virus always contain excess helper virus (SSAV) (Wolfe et al. 1971). Cells infected solely with SSV do not produce virus. We immunoprecipitated ^{35}S-methionine-labeled lysates of several SSV nonproducer or SSV (SSAV) producer cells with serum against the SSAV viral gag

410

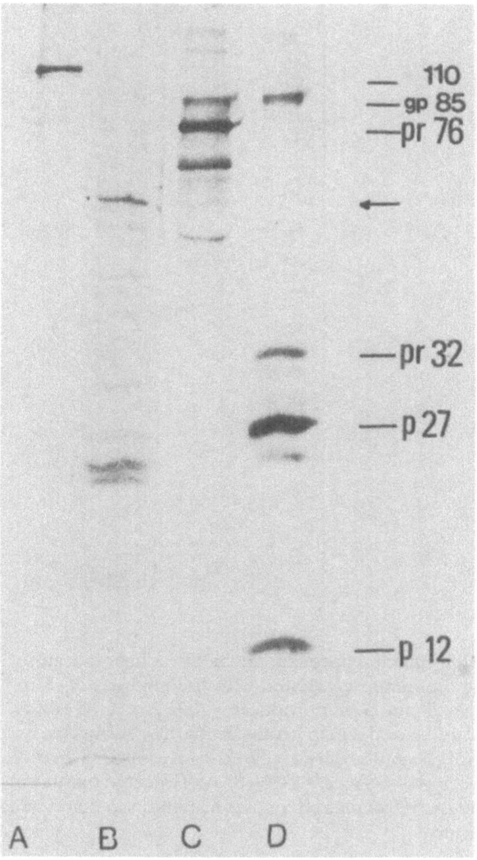
110
gp 85
pr 76
pr 32
p 27
p 12
A
B
C
D

Fig. 2. In vitro processing of the MC 29 polypeptide 110 kd. Quail cells, nonproductively infected by MC 29 (8, kindly provided by K. Bister), were radioactively labeled, immunoprecipitated *(A)* and cleaved by p15 *(B)* as in legend Fig. 1, (E). As control, ^{35}S-methionine labeled RSV infected chicken fibroblasts *(C)* were processed in vitro by p15

protein p30 (B. Konze-Thomas and K. von der Helm, to be published). Two major virus-specific polypeptides could be detected (Fig. 3a) within the different cell lines: the p30 gag protein and a polypeptide of 65 k dalton.

By a pulse chase experiment we investigated the question whether the 65 k d polypeptide is a precursor protein to p30. It can be seen from Fig. 3b that after a 6 h chase the radioactivity had been chased obviously into the p30 protein (because of the 3-h pulse labeling period some p30 appeared already in the immunoprecipitate of the pulse). We assume the 65 k d polypeptide (pr65) to be the precursor to p30.

Since the pr65 appeared in producer as well as in nonproducer cells, it might possibly be a fusion protein like the MC 29 protein containing some gag sequences plus sequences for a "transformation" protein. In order to characterize this aspect of the 65 k d polypeptide we used the protease p15 again as a tool for "mapping" cleavage.

Figure 4 shows the cleavage of the SSV protein 65 k d by protease p15 in the presence of different salt concentrations: using 0.5 M NaCl, two proteins appear, one comigrating with p30 and another polypeptide of approximately 33 k dalton that did not immunoprecipitate with anti-p30 serum at the pulse chase experiment. It is, however, possible that this 33 k d polypeptide is an intermediate precursor protein to other non-p30 gag proteins. Alternatively this protein might represent a non-gag portion of the 65 k dalton protein. During the course of this meeting evidence has been gathered by others (see Bergholz and Thiel, this volume), that this described 65 k dalton polypeptide might contain exclusively gag sequences. If so, it has to be elucidated why a polypeptide containing pure gag sequences is synthesized in a nonproducer cell.

The transforming gene product of avian sarcoma virus exhibits protein kinase activity (Brugge and Erikson 1977). There is also evidence that transformation-specific proteins of other viruses like Abelson leukemia virus (Witte et al. 1980) exhibit protein kinase activity as well. We investigated the 110 k dalton protein of MC 29 and the 65 k dalton protein of SSV (SSAV) for kinase activity by in vitro labeling with ^{32}p-ATP but could not find evidence for it (data not shown). Recently, however, evidence was presented (Bister et al., see this vol.) that the 110 dalton protein of MC 29 comprises kinase activity.

The pp60^{src} protein of avian sarcoma virus and some other virus specific transformation proteins are phosphorylated either by autocatalytic action or other kinases. We labeled RSV-, MC 29-, or SSV-infected cells for 2 h with ^{32}P-orthophosphate and immunoprecipitated the cell lysates with the respective sera. In addition, an aliquot of each immunoprecipitate had been subjected to processing by p15 protease. The results are shown in Fig. 5. The pp60^{src} (besides pr76) of RSV was phosphorylated and not cleaved by p15. From lysates of MC 29 polypeptides of 110 k, 90 k, and 75 k dalton were phosphorylated. Upon

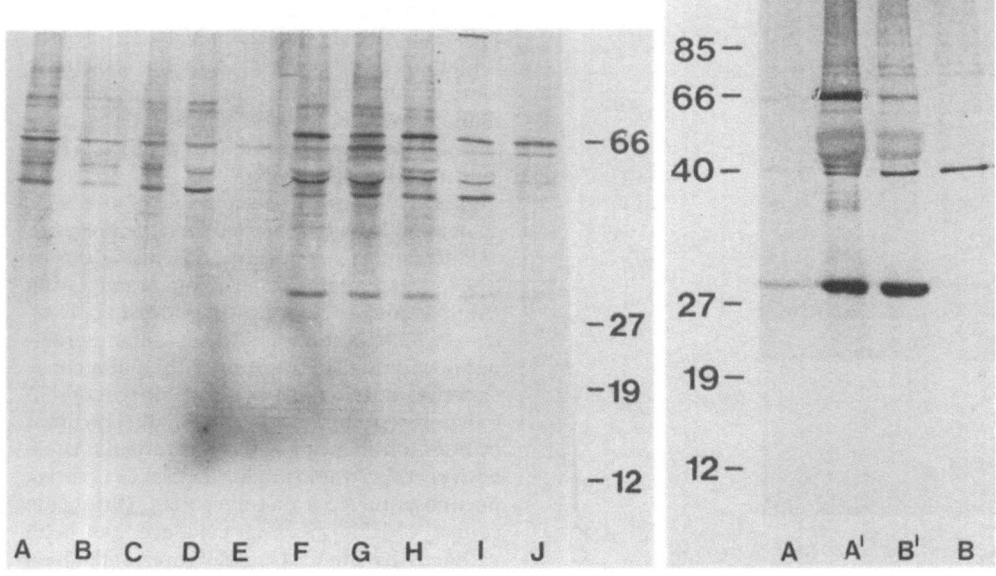

a

Fig. 3. a Immunoprecipitation of SSV specific proteins. SSV-infected producer and nonproducer marmoset (HF) cell lines were labeled for 4 h with ³⁵S-methionine, immunoprecipitated with preimmune *(A–F)* or anti-p30 serum *(F–J)*. *A* and *F*, nonproducer isolate No. 6; *B* and *G*, nonproducer isolate No. 1; *C* and *H*, producer No. 19; *D* and *I* M4-SSV, SSV(SSAV) infected and transformed producer marmoset fibroblasts; *E* and *J*, as producer No. 19, but grown in suspension culture. Samples were analysed by 12.5% SDS-PAGE and autoradiography. **b** Pulse-chase label of SSV-infected cell. M4-SSV cells [SSV(SSAV) infected marmoset fibroblasts] were pulse-labeled for 3 h with ³⁵S-methionine *(A, A″)* or chased for 6 h and immunoprecipitated *(B, B″)*. *A* and *B*, pre-immune serum; *A″ B″*, anti-p30 serum

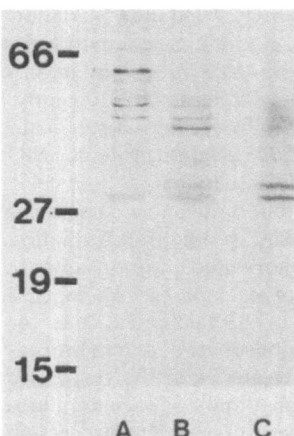

Fig. 4. Cleavage of SSV protein precursor pr65 by avian virus protein p15. M4-SSV cells were labeled and immunoprecipitated as in legend Fig. 3a *(A)* and aliquots subjected to p15-cleavage overnight in presence of 0.15 *M* NaCl *(B)* or 0.5 *M* NaCl *(C)*

addition of p15, the 75 k d polypeptide remained uncleaved, the 110 k d and 90 k d protein could be cleaved, and the radioactive label was found in two bands of about 70 and 64 k dalton and a 32 k d polypeptide (which is probably the intermediate precursor to the phosphorylated p19). However, no label could be detected in the range of 55 k dalton. We conclude that the 90, 70, and 64 k d polypeptides are intermediate precursors, that the 55 k d polypeptide is one cleavage end product which is not phosphorylated, and one of the other end products, the p32 (resp. p19), carries the phosphoryl rest.

The SSV(SSAV) 65 k dalton protein was phosphorylated. However, upon addition of p15 no significant shift of the phosphorylated 65 k d band could be detected. Further investigations now have to reveal whether this phosphorylation is implicated in an activity of a putative transformation gene product.

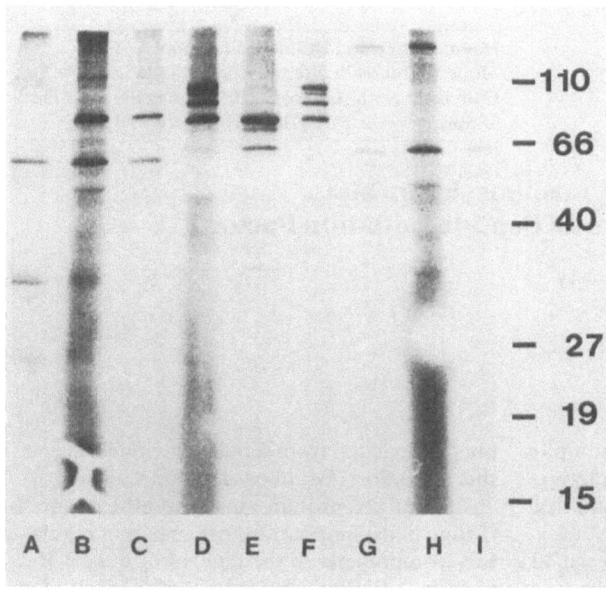

Fig. 5. Label of transformed cells in vivo by ^{32}P-orthophosphate and p15 cleavage. RSV-infected chicken fibroblasts *(A–C)*, MC 29 nonproductively infected quail cells *(D–F)*, and SSV(SSAV)-infected marmoset fibroblasts *(G–I)* were labeled with 1 uCi/ml ^{32}P-orthophosphate for 2 h, lysed, immunoprecipitated *(B, D, H)*, or subjected to an overnight incubation at 37°C in presence of p15 *(A, E, G)* or without p15-protease *(C, F, I)*. The samples were analysed by SDS-PAGE followed by autoradiography

Acknowledgments

We thank Dr. F. Deinhardt very much for his interest and support of this work. The technical assistance of Miss D. Rose is gratefully acknowledged. Preparations of AMV have been provided by Dr. J. Beard. This work was supported by the Deutsche Forschungsgemeinschaft.

References

Arcement LJ, Karshin OL, Naso RB, Jamjoom G, Arlinghaus RB (1976) Biosynthesis of Rauscher Leukemia viral proteins: Presence of p30 and envelope p15 sequences in precursor polypeptides. Virology 69:763–774 – Bister K, Hayman MJ, Vogt PK (1977) Defectiveness of avian myelocytomatosis virus MC 29: Isolation of long term non-producer cultures and analysis of viral specific polypeptide synthesis. Virology 82:431–448 – Brugge JS, Erikson RL (1977) Identification of a transformation specific antigen induced by an avian sarcoma virus. Nature 269:346–348 – Deinhardt F, Bergholz CM, Hunsmann G, Schneider J, Thiel HJ, Beug H, Schäfer W (1978) Studies of simian sarcoma and simian sarcoma associated virus. I. Analysis of viral structural proteins, and preparation and characterization of antiserum specific for viral envelope components. Z Naturforsch [C] 33:969–980 – Dittmar KJ, Moelling K (1978) Biochemical properties of p15-associated protease in avian RNA tumor virus. J Virol 28:106–118 – Eisenman RN, Vogt VM (1978) The biosynthesis of oncornavirus proteins. Biochim Biophys Acta 473:187–239 – von der Helm K (1977) Cleavage of Rous sarcoma viral polypeptide precursor into internal structural proteins in vitro involves viral protein p15. Proc Natl Acad Sci USA 74:911–915 – von der Helm K, Konze-Thomas B (1980) Avian oncornaviruses contain a virus protease (p15) which processes its own gag protein precursor and the 110 kd polypeptide of MC 29. Arch Geschwulstforsch 50:299–305 – Konze-Thomas B, von der Helm K (to be published) Processing of viral protein precursors by the avian myeloblastosis viral (AMV) protein p15 – Langlois AJ, Sankaran S, Hsiung PHL, Beard JW (1967) Massive direct conversion of chick embryo cells by strain MC 29 avian leukosis virus. J Virol 1:1082–1084 – Mellon P, Pawson A, Bister K, Martin GS, Duesberg PH (1978) Specific RNA sequences and gene products of MC 29 avian acute leukemia virus. Proc Natl Acad Sci USA 75:5874–5878 – Okasinsky GF, Velicer LF (1976) Analysis of intracellular feline leukemia virus proteins. I. Identification of a 60,000 dalton precursor of FeLV p30. J Virol 120:98–106 – Vogt VM, Eisenman R, Diggelmann H (1975) Generation of avian myeloblastosis virus structural proteins by proteolytic cleavage of a precursor polypeptide. J Mol Biol 96:471–493 – Witte ON, Dasgupta A, Baltimore D (1980) Abelson murine leukemia virus protein is phosphorylated in vitro to form phosphotyrosine. Nature 283:826–831 – Wolfe LG, Deinhardt F, Theilen GH, Rabin H, Kawakami T, Bustad LK (1971) Induction of tumors in marmoset monkeys by simian sarcoma virus, type I (Lagothrix): A preliminary report. J Natl Cancer Inst 47:1115–1120

413

Haematology and Blood Transfusion Vol. 26
Modern Trends in Human Leukemia IV
Edited by Neth, Gallo, Graf, Mannweiler, Winkler
© Springer-Verlag Berlin Heidelberg 1981

Control of Protein Synthesis. Phosphorylation and Dephosphorylation of Eukaryotic Peptide Initiation Factor 2

G. Kramer, N. Grankowski, and B. Hardesty

Differentiation, virus infection, or certain pathological conditions are examples of physiologic events that cause dramatic qualitative and quantitative changes in protein synthesis. It has been assumed and directly shown in several model systems that these changes involve a block in peptide initiation. Systems in which some of the underlying molecular mechanisms have been studied include dimethyl sulfoxide (DMSO) induced differentiation in Friend leukemia cells (FLC), iron or heme deficiency in reticulocytes or their lysates, and interferon-treated cells that are sensitive to double-stranded RNA (dsRNA). It has been shown with FLC that DMSO and other inducers of differentiation cause a rather rapid inhibition of peptide initiation that precedes the induction of hemoglobin synthesis (Bilello et al. 1979). These authors also demonstrated that inhibitors of peptide initiation, but not inhibitors of elongation, may be able to induce these cells to differentiate. Cell-free systems have been used to study the mechanism by which peptide initiation is blocked during heme deficiency and in the presence of dsRNA. It was found that the peptide initiation factor eIF-2 plays a key role in the regulation of eukaryotic protein synthesis. The activity of eIF-2 in the reaction by which Met-tRNA$_f$ is bound to 40S ribosomal subunits is controlled by phosphorylation/dephosphorylation of its smallest subunit, eIF-2α (reviewed by Kramer et al. 1980). Binding of Met-tRNA$_f$ to 40S ribosomal subunits that are dependent on eIF-2, GTP, and other initiation factor(s) is inhibited if eIF-2α has been phosphorylated by the cAMP-independent, heme-controlled reticulocyte protein kinase that is specific for this substrate (Pinphanichakarn et al. 1976). Conversely, a phosphoprotein phosphatase isolated from reticulocytes will reverse this inhibition (Grankowski et al. 1980a).

The eIF-2α protein kinase and the counteracting phosphatase thus form a pair of regulatory components in the control of eukaryotic peptide initiation. The activity of the regulatory proteins is controlled by other factors. Here we consider some aspects of the regulation of the phosphoprotein phosphatase.

A. Materials and Methods

Preparation of the following components from rabbit reticulocytes has been described in detail: eIF-2 (Odom et al. 1978), phosphatase (Grankowski et al., 1980a), and phosphatase activators (Grankowski et al. 1980b). eIF-2 was phosphorylated in its αsubunit by the heme-controlled protein kinase from reticulocytes, reisolated by chromatography on phosphocellulose, and used as substrate in the phosphatase assay as reported previously (Grankowski et al. 1980a).

B. Results and Discussion

In contrast to the highly specific protein kinase that phosphorylates eIF-2α, phosphoprotein phosphatase activity isolated from rabbit reticulocytes has been found to have a rather broad substrate range (Grankowski et al. 1980a). Proteins phosphorylated by both cAMP-independent and cAMP-dependent protein kinases are readily dephosphorylated. However, stimulation and a certain degree of substrate specificity may be imposed on phosphatase activity by specific low molecular weight, heat-stable peptides. We have purified two such peptides from reticulocytes to homogeneity (Grankowski et al. 1980b).

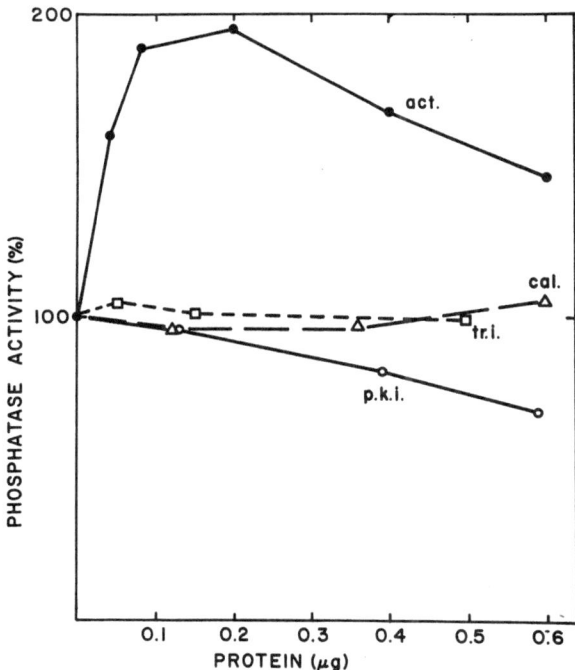

Fig. 1. Specificity of the activator that stimulates phosphatase activity for phosphorylated eIF-2α. Phosphatase (0.5 μg) was preincubated for 10 min at 37° in the absence or presence of the indicated amounts of phosphatase activator (●——●, *act.*), soybean trypsin inhibitor (□--□, *tr. i.*), calmodulin (△-△, *cal.*), or the inhibitor of cAMP-dependent protein kinases (○——○, *p.k.i.*). Then phosphatase activity was determined with [^{32}P]eIF-2α as substrate as described (Grankowski et al. 1980a)

One of them is a heat-stable, acidic, 17,400 dalton protein that specifically stimulates dephosphorylation of eIF-2α by the reticulocyte phosphatase. The results given in Fig. 1 show an increase in phosphatase activity for eIF-2α by up to 100% depending on the amount of activator added. As demonstrated in Fig. 1, no other peptide tested has been found to produce a similar effect for a few of these components (calmodulin, soybean trypsin inhibitor, and the heat-stable inhibitor of cAMP-dependent protein kinase activity, all of which are heat-stable, low molecular weight proteins with an acidic isoelectric point). This phosphatase activator does not affect dephosphorylation of phosphoproteins that have been phosphorylated by a cAMP-dependent protein kinase (Grankowski et al. 1980b). The data in Fig. 2 show that the activator increases the rate of dephosphorylation appreciably, but not the extent. The results of other experiments indicate that the activator interacts with the enzyme, not the substrate (Grankowski et al. 1980b). Thus it appears that the activator is a specific, low molecular weight peptide effector that may function in the control of phosphatase activity for eIF-2α.

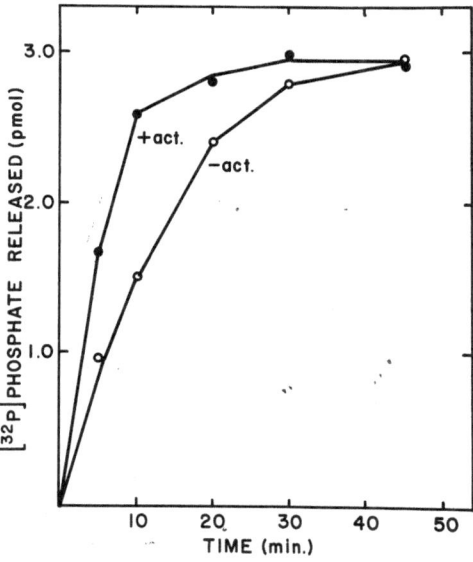

Fig. 2. Phosphatase activator increases the rate of dephosphorylation of eIF-2α. Phosphatase was preincubated in the absence or presence of the activator, then [^{32}P]eIF-2α was added and the reaction stopped at the times indicated. ●——●, *act.*, incubated in the presence of phosphatase activator

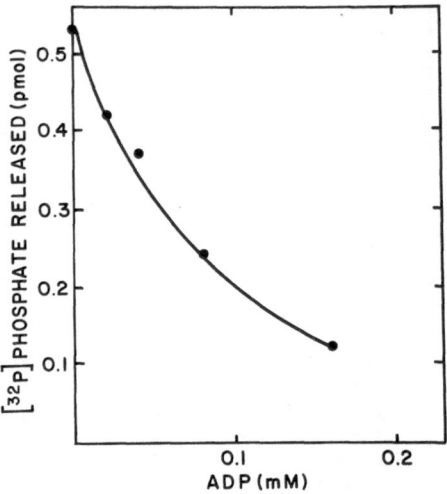

Fig. 3. Inhibition of Phosphatase Activity by ADP. ADP was included in the reaction mixture to give the concentrations shown on the abscissa. Release of [^{32}P]phosphate from eIF-2α was determined (Grankowski et al. 1980)

The results presented in Fig. 3 indicate that ADP is a potent inhibitor of eIF-2α phosphatase activity; 50% inhibition is observed with 80–100 μM. GDP has been found to be slightly less active (cf. Grankowski et al. 1980a). In vivo levels of the adenylate pool (about 2 mM) are 10-fold to 15-fold greater than the guanylate pool (Colby and Edlin 1970). The ratio of ATP to ADP appears to vary greatly and decreases under adverse nutrient conditions, thereby directly and indirectly influencing macromolecular synthetic pathways. It controls nucleoside diphosphate kinase activity affecting the conversion of GDP to GTP and thus controls protein synthesis and, especially, peptide initiation (Walton and Gill 1976). However, the direct effect of ADP on eIF-2α phosphatase activity (Fig. 3) seems to be an immediate additional way of controlling peptide initiation in situations in which the eIF-2α protein kinase is activated.

References

Bilello JA, Warnecke G, Koch G (1979) In: Neth R, Gallo RC, Hofschneider PH, Mannweiler K (eds) Modern trends in human leukemia III. Springer, Berlin Heidelberg New York, pp 303–306 – Colby C, Edlin G (1970) Biochemistry 9:917–920 – Grankowski N, Lehmusvirta D, Kramer G, Hardesty B (1980a) J Biol Chem 255:310–317 – Grankowski N, Lehmusvirta D, Stearns GB, Kramer G, Hardesty B (1980b) J Biol Chem 255:5755–5762 – Kramer G, Henderson AB, Granskowski N, Hardesty B (1980) In: Chamblis G, Craven GR, Davies J, Davis K, Kahan L, Nomura M (eds) RIBOSOMES: Structure, function, and genetics, University Park Press, Baltimore, pp 825–845 – Odom OW, Kramer G, Henderson AB, Pinphanichakarn P, Hardesty B (1978) J Biol Chem 253:1807–1813 – Pinphanichakarn P, Kramer G, Hardesty B (1976) Biochem Biophys Res Commun 73:625–631 – Walton GM, Gill GN (1976) Biochim Biophys Acta 447:11–19

Haematology and Blood Transfusion Vol. 26
Modern Trends in Human Leukemia IV
Edited by Neth, Gallo, Graf, Mannweiler, Winkler
© Springer-Verlag Berlin Heidelberg 1981

Characterization of the Hematopoietic Target Cells of Defective Avian Leukemia Viruses by Velocity Sedimentation and Density Gradient Centrifugation Analyses

T. Graf, B. Royer-Pokora, E. Korzeniewska, S. Grieser, and H. Beug

A. Introduction

As in man, several distinct types of leukemia occur in animals, e.g., lymphoid, myeloid, and erythroid leukemia. In the three best examined animal systems, i.e., chickens, mice, and cats, these neoplasms are caused in the majority by the infection or activation of C-type retroviruses. Two main categories of leukemia viruses can be distinguished: (1) replication competent viruses which have a long period of latency and cause predominatly lymphatic leukemia and (2) replication-defective viruses (DLV), which cause various types of acute leukemia within a short period of latency and are capable of inducing an in vitro transformation in both hematopoietic and nonhematopoietic tissues (Hanafusa 1977; Graf and Beug 1978).

In the avian system a large number of nondefective viruses causing lymphoid leukosis have been isolated, the prototype of which is represented by the Rous associated viruses (RAV). These viruses lack a detectable oncogene and are nontransforming in vitro. Therefore, new techniques had to be developed to study their mechanism of transformation, as is discussed by Hayward et al. elsewhere in this volume.

About 30 to 50 isolates of DLVs from chickens have been described over the past 50 years (for review see Graf and Beug 1978). Because of their ability to transform in vitro, the comparatively few surviving strains have been intensively investigated during recent years. As shown in Table 1, the eight DLV strains studied in more detail can be subdivided into three categories according to the types of neoplasms they predominantly induce and the types of transforming sequences (oncogenes) they harbor (Roussel et al. 1979). These

oncogenes differ from the *src* gene of Rous sarcoma virus (Stéhelin and Graf 1978).

As described previously the hematopoietic cells transformed by the above DLV strains (Table 1) can be grouped into the same three categories according to the phenotype of differentiation they express: AEV-type viruses induce transformed cells with the phenotype of erythroblasts, MC29-type viruses give rise to transformed cells resembling macrophages, and AMV-type strains induce myeloblast-like transformed cells (Beug et al. 1979).

The hematopoietic target cells of these viruses have been partially characterized using a number of functional (adherence, phagocytosis) and antigenic markers (differentiation-specific cell surface antigens). By these means they were shown to correspond to immature erythroid cells for AEV and to immature myeloid cells for MC29 and AMV (Graf et al. 1976a,b; Graf et al. 1981).

The present study was undertaken to characterize the hematopoietic target cells of DLVs according to physical parameters, that is, sedimentation velocity at unit gravity (providing a measure of their relative size) and centrifugation in density gradients using Percoll (to determine their relative buoyant density). Included is a comparison of the DLV target cells to the normal granulocyte/macrophage colony-forming cells (CFU-C) which develop together with the DLV-transformed cells under our conditions of culturing.

B. Materials and Methods

I. Viruses

The origin and properties of the DLV strains used (AEV-ES4, MC29, and AMV BAI-A) have been described elsewhere (Graf et al. 1980b).

Table 1. Oncogenic potential of avian leukemia viruses in vitro and in vivo

Virus	Strain	Type of neoplasms predominantly induced	Type of hematopoietic cell transformed in vitro and in vivo[a]	Transforming sequences[b]
RAV		Lymphoid leukosis, osteopetrosis, erythroblastosis[c]	B-lymphoblast (only in vivo)	–
AEV	R ES4	Erythroblastosis, sarcomas, carcinomas?[d]	Erythroblast	*erb*
MC29	MC29 CMII OK10 MH2	Myelocytomatosis, sarcomas carcinomas[d]	Macrophage	*mac*
AMV	BAI/A E26	Myeloblastosis, carcinomas?[d]	Myeloblast	*myb*

[a] Beug and Graf 1978; Beug et al. 1979
[b] Roussel et al. 1979; Bister and Duesberg 1980
[c] Neoplasms induced within a relatively long period of latency (several months to years)
[d] Neoplasms induced within weeks after infection

II. Target Cell Assay

This assay, which was shown to give a reliable (although possibly minimum) estimate of the proportion of DLV target cells in a given test tissue, has been described elsewhere (Graf et al. 1981). Briefly, bone marrow cells were prepared from 1–3-week-old white leghorn chicks of the Spafas flock. Different dilutions of bone marrow cell preparations or of fractions thereof were infected with an excess of virus, mixed with methylcellulose (Methocel)-containing medium and seeded in 35 mm dishes containing a macrophage feeder layer. Colonies were evaluated 8–12 days after infection.

III. Velocity Sedimentation at Unit Gravity

The method used was essentially that described by Miller and Phillips (1969). The apparatus used consisted of a cylindrical chamber (diameter 11 cm, height 8 cm) with a conical base. Turbulence occuring upon filling or emptying of the chamber was reduced by a stainless steel flow deflector. All operations were carried out at 4°C. The chamber was loaded first with 100 ml of 7.2 phosphate buffered saline (PBS) containing 5% serum and then with a linear gradient prepared from 400 ml 15% serum mixture in PBS and 400 ml of 24.5% serum mixture in PBS. The serum mixture consisted of 60% fetal calf serum, 35% calf serum, and 5% chicken serum. In this gradient the cells retained full viability during the experimental period, which was 12 h for each run. The chamber was then loaded with 2×10^8 cells

in 30 ml PBS containing 3% fetal calf serum. After the run, 14 fractions were collected at a rate of 25 ml/min. The first and last 50 ml were discarded. Cells from each fraction were counted, sedimented for 5 min at $800 \times g$, and resuspended in 2 ml target cell assay medium (Graf et al. 1981); aliquots corresponding to 6 parts for AEV, 1 part for MC29, and 3 parts for AMV were infected with undiluted stocks of the corresponding viruses as described for the target cell assay. In fractions with high cell numbers cells were diluted before testing. Each cell aliquot was adjusted to a volume of 1 ml before infection.

IV. Density Centrifugation

The method used was basically that described by Pertoft and Laurent (1977). A stock solution of Percoll (Pharmacia, Uppsala, Sweden) was first mixed at a ratio of 10:1 with $10 \times$ PBS and then diluted with growth medium to yield a final density of 1.080 g/cm³. Then, 2×10^7 bone marrow cells in 5 ml growth medium were layered on top of 30 ml Percoll suspension and centrifuged in the rotor R30 of Beckman Instruments at 19,000 rpm for 30 min at 4°C (no brakes). Cells were fractioned from the top of the gradient with a bent Pasteur pipette into 15 fractions per tube and aliquots separated for counting and for determination of density using a refractometer. After adding 5 ml of growth medium to each fraction, cells were sedimented at $800 \times g$ for 5 min, resuspended in 2 ml of target cell assay medium, and handled as described above for the sedimentation velocity studies.

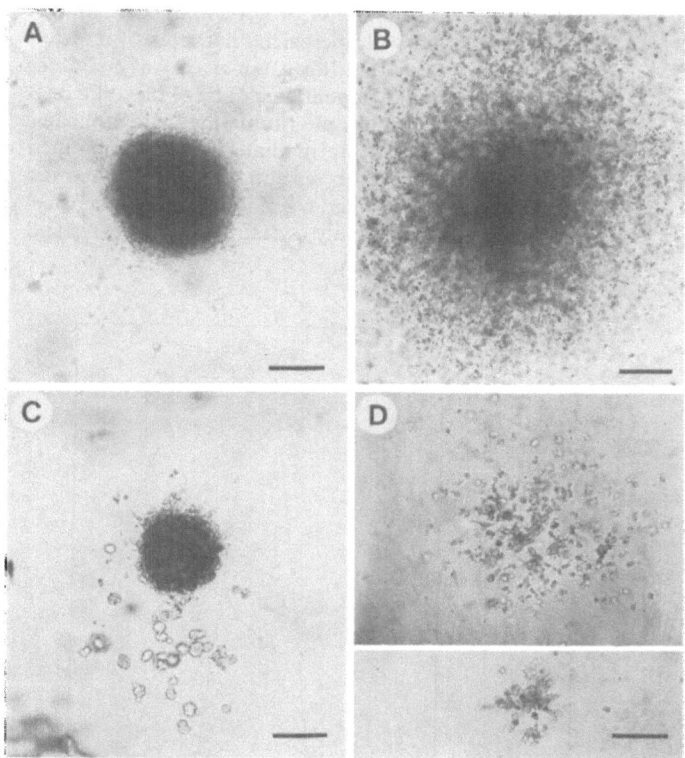

Fig. 1. Colonies of bone marrow cells transformed by AEV **(A)**; MC29 **(B)** and AMV **(C)** viruses photographed 9–12 days after infection. **D** Normal macrophage/granulocyte colonies (CFU-C) photographed 10 days after seeding bone marrow cells in Methocel-containing medium. *Bars* in **A, C,** and **D** 100 μm and in **B** 250 μm

C. Results

Colonies of bone marrow cells transformed by the three prototype DLV strains, i.e., by AEV, MC29 and AMV, are shown in Fig. 1 in comparison to a CFU-C colony. The morphology of each type of colony is characteristic for the type of infecting virus. Furthermore, cells of the DLV-induced colonies can be isolated and grown in tissue culture for up to about 30–40 generations, whereas cells isolated from CFU-C colonies cannot be grown to a significant extent. The characterization of the transformed cells thus isolated has been reported previously (Beug et al. 1979).

In order to characterize DLV target cells and CFU-C on the basis of size, normal bone marrow cells from 2-week-old chicks were subjected to sedimentation through a serum gradient at unit gravity. After sedimentation, fractions were collected and aliquots thereof tested for their content of transformable DLV target cells as well as of CFU-C cells using a newly developed target cell assay (Graf et al.

1981). The results of a typical separation experiment are shown in Fig. 2 A and B. As can be seen, colony forming target cells of all three DLVs exhibited a modal sedimentation velocity of about 5 mm/h. In several experiments the AEV target cells appeared to be slightly smaller than those of MC29 and AMV, and the distribution of AMV target cells was broader than that of MC29. In contrast, the CFU-C cells sedimented significantly more slowly, with a modal distribution of about 4.3 mm/h. Results obtained in several independent experiments are in agreement with the data shown except that in some experiments the distribution of MC29 target cells was broader than that of AMV target cells.

Next, attempts were made to separate DLV target cells on the basis of their density, using gradients containing Percoll. The results obtained after separating normal bone marrow cells on a Percoll gradient and infecting aliquots of each fraction with the three DLV virus strains are shown in Fig. 3. As can be seen, again it was not possible to obtain a clear separation of the

419

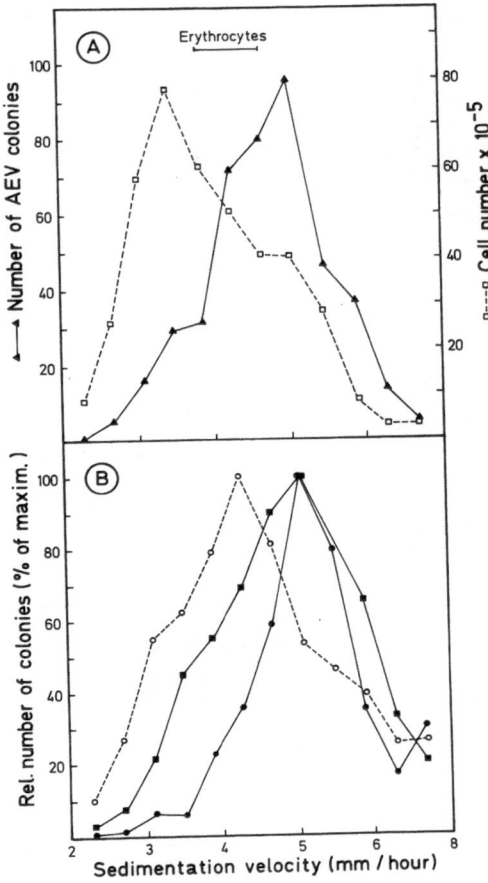

Fig. 2. Unit gravity sedimentation of chick bone marrow cells. Values shown in **A** and **B** were obtained in the same experiments using bone marrow cells of a 9-day-old chick. Maximum number of colonies per dish obtained in **B** corresponded to 442 for MC 29 (●——●), 405 for AMV (■——■), and for CFU-C (●---●)

determine whether or not colony formation is inhibited with increasing numbers of infected cells. Fraction I (lowest density) was characterized by the appearance of large blastlike cells together with some (immature) macrophages. Fraction II (intermediate density) contained mainly reticulocytes and some myelocytes and granulocytes, and fraction III (highest density) almost exclusively contained erythrocytes and

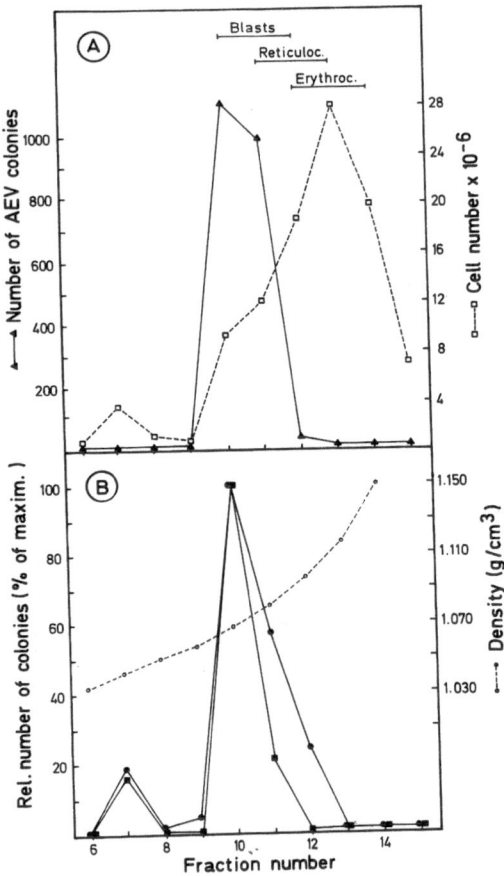

Fig. 3. Percoll density gradient centrifugation of chick bone marrow cells. Values shown in **A** and **B** were obtained in the same experiment using a pool of bone marrow cells from two 7-day-old chicks. Fractions number 1 to 5 were ommitted from the drawing since they contained negligible amounts of cells and target cells. Maximum number of colonies per dish obtained in **B** were 1900 for MC29 (●---●) and 510 for AMV (■——■). The values shown for AEV, MC29, and AMV correspond to 1/2, 1/15, and 1/5 of the total number of cells in each fraction, respectively

DLV target cells nor of the CFU-C cells. However, as reproducibly seen in several experiments, there was a fraction of MC29 target cells which appeared to be of higher density than those of AMV. Since this difference might be due to the presence of cells sedimenting at high density which inhibit the colony formation of AMV target cells, as is indeed suggested by mixing experiments (data not shown), we pooled cells from three defined regions of the Percoll gradient. By this procedure a sufficient number of cells could be obtained to perform a dilution series and to

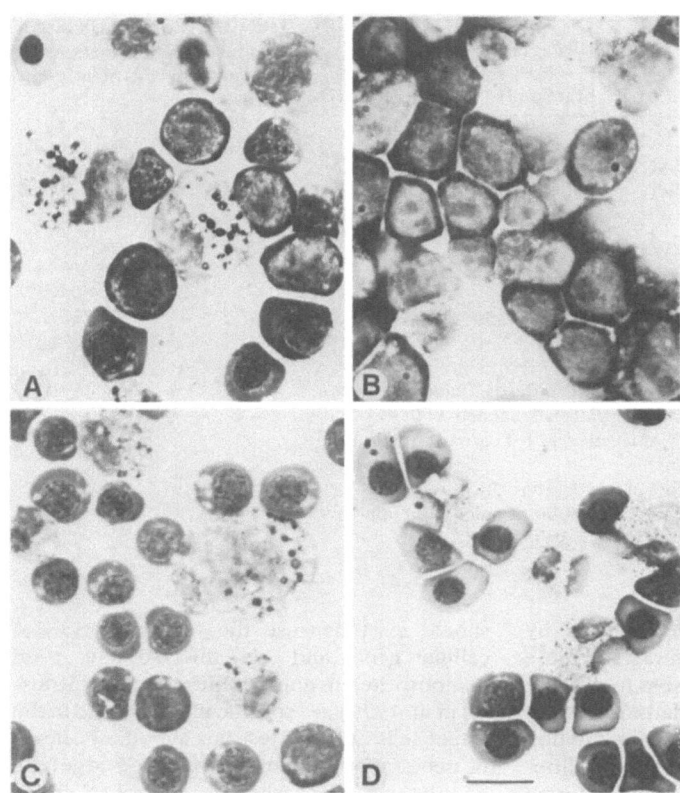

Fig. 4. Smears of bone marrow cells obtained from fractions of different density of a gradient containing Percoll. **A** Cells before centrifugation, **B** Cells from fraction I; **C** Cells from fraction II; **D** Cells from fraction III (see methods).Smears were stained with an eosine-methylene blue stain (Diff-Quik, Harleco, Herstal, Belgium). *Bar:* 10 μm

mature eosinophilic granulocytes (Fig. 4). As shown by the results in Table 2, the dense fractions II and III contained few or no target cells of AMV and AEV. In contrast, fraction II and to a lesser extent fraction III still contained MC29 target cells. Within the normal range of standard deviation, the dose-response curve obtained was in all cases linear. This indicates that the differences in the density distribution of the various types of target cells seen were not (or not only) caused by inhibitory cells.

D. Discussion

Our results show that in general target cells for all three DLV types are most abundant in those fractions which consist mainly of blast-like, immature bone marrow cells. They are similar to each other with respect to both size and density. In comparison to erythrocytes, granulocytes, and CFU-C cells they are relatively large. They are also much lighter than erythrocytes and granulocytes. Together with results

described elsewhere (Graf et al. 1976a,b; Gazzolo et al. 1979; Graf et al. 1981) these results suggest that DLV target cells are rather immature but already committed to the erythroid or myeloid lineages. They are also in accord with the notion supported by earlier work (Graf et al. 1978, 1981) that DLVs upon transformation block the differentiation of their target cells.

Our finding that a fraction of the MC29 target cells differs from those of AEV and AMV with respect to density is in accord with results described elsewhere which show that about half of the MC29 target cells in bone marrow are phagocytic and adherent, suggesting that these MC29 target cells are more mature than those of AMV, which do not express such functional markers (Graf et al. 1981).

Our data concerning the relationship between normal macrophage/granulocyte colony forming cells (CFU-C) and the target cells of MC29 and AMV are still very incomplete but suggest that they are not identical. This is also

Expt. No.	Infecting virus	Proportion of target cells[a]		
		Fraction I	Fraction II	Fraction III
1[b]	AEV	17 ± 3.5	6 ± 5	1
	MC29	3470 ± 832	2600 ± 915	353 ± 47
	AMV	1167 ± 290	356 ± 32	52 ± 8
2[b]	AEV	12.8 ± 3.9	4.3 ± 1.5	NT[d]
	MC29	1058 ± 316	1321 ± 22	NT
	AMV	370 ± 26	150 ± 14	NT
3[c]	MC29	7100 ± 415	950 ± 350	355 ± 106
	AMV	5000 ± 1300	42 ± 10	5

Table 2. Distribution of target cells for DLVs in fractions of bone marrow cells of different density

[a] Number of transformed colonies per 10^6 infected cells (average values- ± standard deviation from 4 to 6 assay dishes seeded with twofold dilutions of cells). Average density of fraction I: 1.05 g/cm³; fraction II: 1.09 g/cm³; fraction III: 1.13 g/cm³.
[b] Cells tested were from bone marrow of 2-week-old chicks
[c] Cells tested were from the nonadherent fraction of chick bone marrow cultures maintained in growth medium for 7 days
[d] NT = Not tested

in agreement with conclusions reached by Gazzolo et al. (1979). In contrast to these authors, however, we were unable to observe a rapidly sedimenting subpopulation of AMV target cells in our unit gravity sedimentation studies. This could be due to technical differences in both the unit gravity sedimentation and target cell assay techniques employed by the two laboratories.

An important question concerning the target cell specificity of DLVs is whether or not these viruses specifically infect and replicate in their target cells only. Recent studies performed on this question showed that this is clearly not the case. AEV is capable of infecting normal bone marrow macrophages without inducing any detectable transformation, while it replicates in them to almost the same titer as found in target cells. Similarly, MC29 and AMV are capable of replicating in ts34 AEV-transformed nonproducer erythroblasts without affecting their capacity to differentiate after shift to the nonpermissive temperature (Graf et al. 1980). On the basis of these observations and our earlier work (for review, see Beug and Graf 1978) we have proposed that the observed restriction of DLV-transforming capacity to specific cell types in the bone marrow may operate at the posttranslational level (Beug and Graf 1978; Graf et al. 1978; Graf et al. 1979). In addition, we have proposed that cellular proteins homologous to the transforming proteins of DLVs (which

should exist because the respective normal cellular genes and their mRNAs have been demonstrated in normal chicken cells by Roussel et al. 1979) are specifically expressed in the target cells only. To test this hypothesis, it will be necessary to characterize purified target cell populations. The techniques described in this paper could be useful as a first step in such a purification.

References

Beug H, v. Kirchbach A, Döderlein G, Conscience JF, Graf T (1979) Chicken hematopoietic cells transformed by seven strains of defective avian leukemia viruses display three distinct phenotypes of differentiation. Cell 18:375–390 – Bister K, Duesberg PH (1980) Classification and structure of avian acute leukemia viruses. Cold Spring Harbor Symp Quant Biol 44:801–822 – Gazzolo L, Moscovici C, Moscovici MG, Samarut J (1979) Response of hemopoietic cells to avian acute leukemia viruses: effects on the differentiation of the target cells. Cell 16:627–638 – Graf T, Beug H (1978) Avian leukemia viruses: interaction with their target cells in vivo and in vitro. Biochim Biophys Acta 516:269–299 – Graf T, Royer-Pokora B, Beug H (1976a) In vitro transformation of specific target cells by avian leukemia viruses. In: Baltimore D, Huang A, Fox F (eds) ICN-UCLA Symposia on molecular and cellular biology, Vol V. Academic Press, New York, pp 321–338 – Graf T, Royer-Pokora B, Beug H (1976b) Target cells for transformation with avian leukosis viruses. In: Neth R, Gallo

RC, Mannweiler K, Moloney W (eds) In: Modern trends in human leukemia II. Lehmann, Munich pp 169–176 – Graf T, Ade N, Beug H (1978) Temperature-sensitive mutant of avian erythroblastosis virus suggests a block of differentiation as mechanism of leukaemogenesis. Nature 257:496–501 – Graf T, v. Kirchbach A, Beug H (1979) Mechanism of target cell specificity by defective avian leukemia viruses: a hypothesis. Neth R, Gallo RC, Hofschneider PH, Mannweiler K (eds) In: Modern trends in human leukemia III. Springer, Berlin Heidelberg New York, pp 429–438 – Graf T, Beug H, Hayman MJ (1980) Target cell specificity of defective avian leukemia viruses: hematopoietic target cells for a given virus type can be infected but not transformed by strains of a different type. Proc Natl Acad Sci USA 77:389–393 – Graf T, v. Kirchbach A, Beug H (1981) Characterization of the hematopoietic target cells of AEV, MC29 and AMV avian leuke-mia viruses. Exp Cell Res 131:331–343 – Hanafusa H (1977) Cell transformation by RNA tumor viruses. In: Wagner RR, Fraenkel-Conrat H (eds) Comprehensive virology vol 10, Viral gene expression and integration. Plenum, New York, pp 401–483 – Miller RG, Phillips RH (1969) Separation of cells by velocity sedimentation. J Cell Physiol 73:191–202 – Pertoft H, Laurent TC (1977) Isopycnic separation of cells and organelles by centrifugation in modified silica gradients. In: Catsimpolas N (ed) Methods of cell separation. Plenum, New York, pp 25–65 – Roussel M, Saule S, Lagrou C, Rommens C, Beug H, Graf T, Stéhelin, D (1979) Defective avian leukemia viruses: three new types of viral oncogenes of cellular origin specific for haematopietic cell transformation. Nature 281:452–455 – Stéhelin D, Graf T (1978) Avian myelocytomatosis and erythroblastosis viruses lack the transforming gene src of avian sarcoma viruses Cell 13:745–750

Haematology and Blood Transfusion Vol. 26
Modern Trends in Human Leukemia IV
Edited by Neth, Gallo, Graf, Mannweiler, Winkler
© Springer-Verlag Berlin Heidelberg 1981

PRCII, a Representative of a New Class of Avian Sarcoma Viruses

P. K. Vogt, J. C. Neil, C. Moscovici, and M. L. Breitman

A. Abstract

The Poultry Research Center Virus II (PRC
II) is a replication-defective avian sarcoma
virus with envelope determinants of the A and
B subgroups. In nonproducing cells transformed by PRCII the products of the replicative
genes *gag*, *pol*, and *env* are not demonstrable,
but a single polyprotein of Mr 105,000 (p105)
can be detected. P105 contains peptides of the
gag proteins p19 and p27 plus transformation-
specific sequences. It does not contain peptides
of gPr95^{env} of Pr180$^{gag-pol}$ (with the possible
exception of one *pol* peptide). The transformation-specific sequences of p105 are distinct
form those of p100 of avian carcinoma virus
MH2, of p110 coded for by avian myelocyto-
ma virus MC29, and of p75 or p40 of avian
erythroblastosis virus AEV. They also show no
resemblance to p60^{src} of Rous sarcoma virus.
P105 is phosphorylated on a tyrosine residue
and has an associated phosphokinase activity.
P105 appears to be capable of autophosphorylation and of phosphorylating homologous
immunoglobulin.

B. Introduction

Until recently all avian sarcoma viruses were
thought to have fundamentally the same genetic structure. The investigated strains, chiefly
Rous sarcoma virus (RSV) and its relatives,
contain an about 1.8-kilobase (kb) insertion at
the juncture of the *env* gene and the C region
(Duesberg and Vogt 1970; Wang et al. 1975).
This transformation-specific insertion, termed
src, was found to be of cellular origin and to
code for a protein kinase of Mr 60,000 with
preference for tyrosine as a phosphoacceptor

(Stehelin et al. 1976; Spector et al. 1978;
Brugge and Erikson 1977; Collett and Erikson
1978; Levinson et al. 1978; Hunter and Sefton
1980). In contrast to RSV, avian acute leukemia viruses code for polyproteins that are
derived from a gene in which *gag* sequences at
the 5' terminal part of the genome are fused to
transformation-specific, cell-derived sequences in the middle of the genome. The cell-derived sequences form a substitution for replicative information of the *gag*, *pol*, and *env* genes
(Bister et al. 1977; Hu et al. 1979; Lai et al.
1979; Sheiness and Bishop 1979; Roussel et
al. 1979; Sheiness et al. 1980). As a consequence of this missing information, the acute
avian leukemia viruses are replication defective (Ishizaki and Shimizu 1970; Graf 1975;
Bister and Vogt 1978; Hu and Vogt 1979).
A genome organization similar to that of avian
acute leukemia viruses has also been found in
Abelson and radiation leukemia virus of mice
and in feline sarcoma virus (Witte et al. 1978;
Manteuil-Brutlag et al. 1980; Barbacid et al.
1980; Sherr et al. 1980; Van de Ven et al.
1980).

Recently a new class of avian sarcoma
viruses has been described which lack *src* and
have a genetic structure related to the avian
acute leukemia viruses (Breitman et al. 1981;
Hanafusa et al. 1980; Kawai et al. 1980; Lee et
al. 1980; Neil et al. 1981). The viruses
belonging to this group are Fujinami sarcoma
virus (FSV), Y73, which is a recent field
isolate, and PRCII. Even though these viruses
have transformation-specific sequences which
are different from the *src* of RSV, their
transformation-specific proteins bear some
intriguing functional resemblance to p60^{src}.
This functional similarity suggests possible
common elements in the mechanism of trans-

formation by RSV and the new avian sarcoma viruses. The present paper will briefly summarize our studies on PRCII as an eample of the new class of avian sarcoma viruses (Breitman et al. 1981; Neil et al. 1981).

C. Results

PRCII was isolated from a spontaneous mesenterial sarcoma in a chicken and was shown to cuase sarcomas which could be distinguished histologically from the growths induced by RSV (Carr and Campbell 1958). The virus belongs to envelope subgroups A and B (Payne and Biggs 1966; Duff and Vogt 1969). PRCII causes only sarcomas in chikkens, and compared to RSV, it is a less virulent agent: Of 50 chickens inoculated with about 10^4 focus-forming units of virus, only 13 came down with tumors within an observation time of 4 weeks. In chick embryo fibroblast cultures PRCII induced foci of predominantly fusiform transformed cells; but no transformation was seen in cultures of hematopoietic cells derived from chicken bone marrow or chicken embryo yolk sac. Infectious center tests showed that while a focus of PRCII-transformed cells could be induced by a single particle, a focus which also released infectious progeny was the result of double infection with transforming virus and nontransforming helper virus. PRCII-transformed cells which failed to release infectious virus have been isolated. Such nonproducer lines also failed to produce noninfectious virions, an indication that the replication defects in PRCII extend into the *gag* gene (Bister et al. 1977; Bister and Vogt 1978; Hu et al. 1978; Hu and Vogt 1979). Superinfection of these nonproducing cells with avian leukosis helper viruses led to the rescue of infectious PRCII.

In order to search for virus-specific products in PRCII-transformed cells, virus producing and nonproducing transformed fibroblasts were labeled with [^{35}S]methionine (50 to 20 µCi/ml) and tested in immunoprecipitation using a variety of antisera. The precipitates were resolved by polyacrylamide gel electrophoresis and analyzed by autoradiography (Fig. 1). Rabbit sera prepared against whole virions of the Prague strain of RSV and sera against the structural *gag* protein of avian leukosis viruses precipitated from PRCII-transformed cell lysates a virus-specific protein

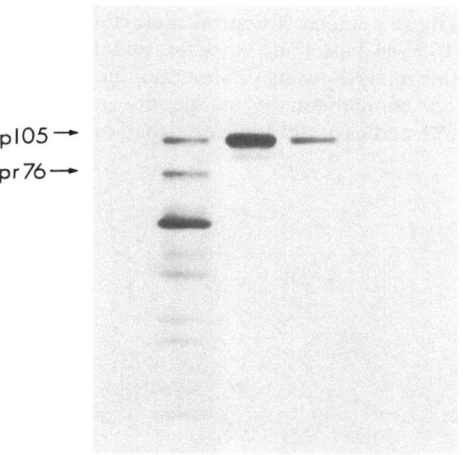

Fig. 1. Immunoprecipitation of virus-specific proteins in PRCII-transformed producing and nonproducing cell clones. Cells were labeled with [^{35}S]methionine and proteins resolved on a 6%–18% SDS-polyacrylamide slab gel (Breitman et al. 1981). Cell lysates and precipitating sera were: PRCII-transformed producing cells with (a) normal rabbit serum, (b) anti-whole virus serum; and PRCII-transformed nonproducing clone with (c) anti-whole virus serum, (d) anti-p27 serum, (e) RSV tumor-bearing rabbit serum preabsorbed with disrupted whole virus, and (f) antiglycoprotein serum

of about Mr 105,000 (p105). In nonproducer cells this was the only virus-specific product that could be identified. P105 was not found in cells infected by nontransforming PRCII-associated helper virus. Lysates of PRCII nonproducer cells did not react with sera directed against the group-specific determinants of the virion surface glycoprotein and against the virion polymerase. There also was no immunologic cross reaction between p105 and a broadly reacting rabbit anti-p60^{src} serum nor did such a serum precipitate another protein from PRCII-transformed cell lysates. Therefore, we conclude that PRCII does not code for a functional *env* or *pol* gene product and that although PRCII is a pure sarcoma virus, it does not produce a transformation-specific protein that cross reacts in immunoprecipitation with antisera against p60^{src} of RSV. The p105 does, however, contain *gag*-related sequences. But since gag codes for a protein of only Mr 76,000, p105 must contain additional non-*gag* sequences, provided its *gag* portion is not reiterated.

A more detailed structural characterization of p105 was based on two-dimensional tryptic peptide analysis, using [35S]methionine as a label. A comparison of the peptide maps of Pr76^{gag} and of p105 indicated that some but

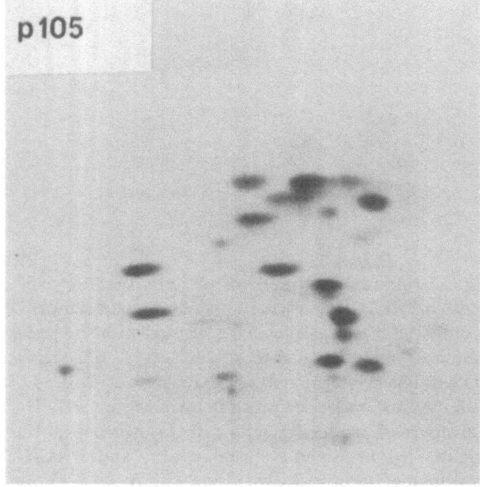

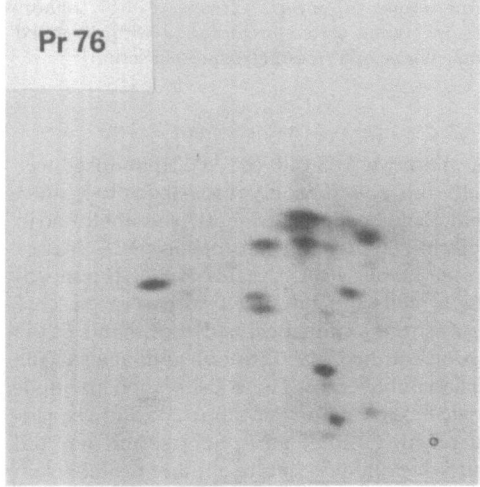

Fig. 2. Tryptic peptide maps of PRCII p105 and of Pr76 of PRCII-AV. [35S]methionine-labeled proteins were separated by PAGE and located by autoradiography. The bands were excised and the proteins eluted and oxidized with performic acid and digested with TPCK-trypsin. The resultant peptides were separated by TLC electrophoresis (pyridine:acetic acid, pH 4.5) at 600 V for 100 min and by chromatography for 4 h in n-butanol:acetic acid:pyridine:water (75:15:60:60)

not all of the *gag* peptides were present in p105 and that p105 contained additional peptides not seen in Pr76^{gag} (Fig. 2). Petide maps of the individual *gag* proteins p19, p27, and p15 were also obtained. The fourth *gag* protein, p12, does not contain useful [35S]methionine peptides. These maps of three individual *gag* proteins showed that all of the p19 and p27 but none of the p15 peptides were present in p105. Identification of the common peptides was confirmed by appropriate mixing experiments. These results lead to the conclusion that p105 contains the 5′ portion of the *gag* gene encompassing p19 and p27 but lacks the 3′ of *gag* with p15. No statement can be made concerning the presence or absence of p12 sequences in p105. However, we found a rabbit antiserum prepared against p27 which did not react with p105, although it precipitated p27. Therefore, not all of the determinants of p27 appear to be present in p105. If the order of the *gag* proteins is N-p19-p27-p12-p15-C (Shealy et al. 1980), then p105 may lack p12 and p15 together with a portion from the carboxyterminus of p27. The *gag*-related part of p105 can then account for roughly half of the p105 molecule. In order to test for the possiblity that the remainder of p105 contains partial, immunologically nonreactive sequences derived from the *pol* or *env* genes, tryptic peptide maps of gPr95^{env} and of Pr180$^{gag-pol}$ of the PRCII helper virus were prepared. There was no overlap between any of the gPr95^{env} peptides and those of p105. Of the *pol* peptides in Pr180, one comigrated with a peptide of p105, and this observation was confirmed in a mixing experiment. However, considering the relative complexity of the Pr180 map, this overlap may be fortuitous and requires further examination. We conclude that p105 does not contain significant portions of the helper virus *env* or *pol* genes.

Two-dimensional tryptic maps were also obtained of the transformation-specific proteins of (p110), of carcinoma virus MH2 (p100), of avian erythroblastosis virus AEV strain ES-4 (p75 and p40), and of the p60^{src} protein from several genetically distinct lines of the Schmidt-Ruppin strain of RSV as well as of the endogenous p60^{src} of chicken cells. The p60^{src} proteins, the AEV p40, and the non-*gag* portions of AEV p75, MC29 p110, and MH2 p100 did not contain peptides coinciding with any of p105. We conclude that PRCII contains new transformation-specific sequences not found in RSV or in avian acute leukemia viruses AEV, MC29, or MH2.

Cells transformed by PRCII were labeled with [^{32}P]orthophosphate (1 mCi/ml) and followed by analysis by immunoprecipitation with anti-virion sera. Electrophoresis and autoradiography indicated that p105 was heavily phosphorylated. This degree of phosphorylation was greater than could be accounted for by the presence of the phosphorylated *gag* protein p19 in p105. The most abundant phosphoamino acid in p105 was tyrosine. These observations suggest that p105 is phosphorylated in its non-*gag* portion, probably at one or several tyrosine residues. In order to test for phosphokinase activity associated with p105, immunoprecipitates were incubated with [^{32}P]ATP according to published procedures before immunoprecipitation, electrophoresis, and autoradiography. Under these conditions both p105 and the heavy chain of IgG were phosphorylated. We suggest that p105 is a phosphoprotein with associated kinase activity capable of autophosphorylation and of phosphorylating homologous IgG.

D. Discussion

PRCII is a representative of a new class of avian sarcoma viruses that lack *src,* have a genetic structure similar to avian acute leukemia viruses, and code for a transformation-specific *gag*-related polyprotein. Other members of this class are FSV and avian sarcoma virus Y73 (Hanafusa et al. 1980; Kawai et al. 1980; Lee et al. 1980). FSV and Y73 have been shown to contain a small (26 S) RNA genome. Our preliminary data suggest that the genome of PRCII has also a size of about 26 S. PRCII and FSV habe some common transformation-specific sequences as detected by nucleic acid hybridization (Shibuya et al. 1980), and the proposal has been made to refer to these sequences as *fps* (*FSV, PRCII* Sarcoma) (J. Coffin et al. to be published). Y73 appears to have no appreciable sequence relationship in its transformation-specific information to either PRCII, FSV, or RSV (Shibuya et al. 1980; M. Yoshida et al. 1980, personal communications). The transformation-specific sequences of FSV have also been found to be related to those of the Snyder-Theilen and Gardner-Arnstein strains of feline sarcoma virus (Shibuya et al. 1980; Barbacid

et al. 1981). Since the latter sequences have been detected in normal feline cells where they code for a cellular protein homologue (Barbacid et al. 1981) one can expect *fps* to be also cell derived. The transformation-specific polyproteins of FSV, Y73, PRCII, and feline sarcoma virus are all phosphorylated and show phosphokinase activity. The predominant phosphoacceptor for these polyproteins is tyrosine (Hanafusa et al. 1980; Kawai et al. 1980; Neil et al.1981; Barbacid et al. 1980). For PRCII and the Snyder-Theilen strain of feline sarcoma virus it has also been shown that phosphotyrosine levels in transformed cells are substantially increased over normal cells (Barbacid et al. 1980; K. Beemon 1980, personal communication). Phosphorylation and kinase activity are also characteristic of p60^{src}, and cells transformed by RSV contain elevated levels of phosphotyrosine (Collett and Erikson 1978; Levinson et al. 1978; Hunter and Sefton 1980). These parallels suggest that even though sarcoma viruses may carry different transforming genes, the mechanisms of viral sarcomagenesis could share common elements in protein function and cellular targets.

Acknowledgment

Supported by U.S. Public Health Service Research Grants No. CA 13213 and 19725 awarded by the National Cancer Institute.

References

Barbacid M, Beemon K, Devare SG (1980) Proc Natl Acad Sci USA 77:5158–5162 – Barbacid M, Lauver AV, Devare SG (1980) J Virol 33:196–207 – Barbacid M, Breitmann ML, Lauver AV, Long LK, Vogt PK (1981) Virology 110:411–419 – Bister K, Hayman MJ, Vogt PK (1977) Virology 82:431–448 – Bister K, Vogt PK (1978) Virology 88:213–221 – Breitman ML, Neil JC, Moscovici C, Vogt PK (1981) Virology 108:1–12 – Brugge JS, Erikson RL (1977) Nature 269:346–348 – Carr JG, Campbell JG (1958) Brit J Cancer 12:631–635 – Collett MS, Erikson RL (1978) Proc Natl Acad Sci USA 75:2021–2024 – Duesberg PH, Vogt PK (1970) Proc Natl Acad Sci USA 67:1673–1680 – Duff R, Vogt PK (1969) Virology 39:18–30 – Graf T (1975) Z Naturforsch 30:847–849 – Hanafusa T, Wang L-H, Anderson SM, Karess RE, Hayward W, Hanafusa H (1980) Proc Natl Acad Sci USA

77:3009–3013 – Hu SSF, Moscovici C, Vogt PK (1978) Virology 89:162–178 – Hu SSF, Vogt PK (1979) Virology 92:278–284 – Ishizaki R, Shimizu T (1970) Cancer Res 30:2827–2831 – Hunter T, Sefton BM (1980) Proc Natl Acad Sci USA 77:1311–1315 – Kawai S, Yoshida M, Segawa K, Sugiyama H, Ishizaki R, Toyoshima K (1980) Proc Natl Acad Sci USA 77:6199–6203 – Lai MMC, Hu SSF, Vogt PK (1979) Virology 97:366–377 – Lee WH, Bister K, Pawson A, Robins T, Moscovici C, Duesberg PH (1980) Proc Natl Acad Sci USA 77:2018–2022 – Levinson AD, Oppermann H, Levintow L, Varmus HE, Bishop JM (1978) Cell 15:561–572 – Manteuil-Brutlag S, Liu SI, Kaplan HS (1980) Cell 19:643–652 – Neil JC, Breitman ML, Vogt PK (1981) Virology 108:98–110 – Payne LN, Biggs PM (1966) Virology 29:190–198 – Roussel M, Saule S, Lagrou C, Rommens C, Beug H, Graf T, Stehelin D (1979) Nature 281:452–455 – Shealy DJ, Mosser AG, Rueckert RR (1980) J Virol 34:431–437 – Sheiness D, Bishop JM (1979) J Virol 31:514–521 – Sheiness D, Bister K, Moscovici C, Fanshier L, Gonda T, Bishop JM (1980) J Virol 33:962–968 – Sherr CJ, Fedele LA, Oskarsson M, Maizel J, Vande Woude G (1980) J Virol 34:200–212 – Shibuya M, Hanafusa T, Hanafusa H, Stephenson JR (1980) 77:6536–6540 – Spector D, Varmus HE, Bishop JM (1978) Proc Natl Acad Sci USA 75:4102–4106 – Stehelin D, Varmus HE, Bishop JM, Vogt PK (1976) Nature 260:170–173 – Van de Ven WJM, Khan AS, Reynolds FH jr, Mason KT, Stephenson JR (1980) J Virol 33:1034–1045 – Wang L-H, Duesberg PH, Beemon K, Vogt PK (1975) J Virol 16:1051–1070 – Witte ON, Rosenberg N, Paskind M, Shields A, Baltimore D (1978) Proc Natl Acad Sci USA 75:2488–2492

Haematology and Blood Transfusion Vol. 26
Modern Trends in Human Leukemia IV
Edited by Neth, Gallo, Graf, Mannweiler, Winkler
© Springer-Verlag Berlin Heidelberg 1981

Identification of the Avian Myeloblastosis Virus Genome

L. M. Souza, D. G. Bergmann, and M. A. Baluda

In addition to neoplasias caused in chickens by helper viruses of the avian myeloblastosis virus (AMV) complex, acute myeloblastic leukemia is induced by a defective leukemogenic component. To identify the leukemogenic viral genome the unintegrated and integrated viral DNA intermediates were chracterized. Linear viral DNA isolated from the cytoplasm of helper virus (MAV-1 or MAV-2) infected chicken embryonic fibroblasts (CEF) has a mass of 5.3 million daltons (md) (Bergmann et al. 1980). The linear MAV-1 and MAV-2 DNAs can be distinguished from one another by cleavage with the restriction endonuclease Hind III, because MAV-1 DNA contains one more Hind III recognition site than does MAV-2. Linear viral DNA isolated from the cytoplasm of CEF infected with standard AMV (AMV-S) which contains the defective leukemogenic component showed a minor molecular species of 4.9 md in addition to the major species of 5.3 md. Eco RI or Hind III digestion of the linear viral DNA from AMV-S-infected CEF generates specific fragments in addition to those unique for MAV-1 or MAV-2 viral DNA (Bergmann et al. 1980). A Hind III digest of AMV-S linear viral DNA also indicates that more than 90% of the AMV-S virus complex is MAV-1 like, while the remainder represents both the leukemogenic and MAV-2-like viruses (Souza et al. 1980).

The arrangement of endogenous proviral DNA in the chicken genome was determined prior to AMV infection. Infections were carried out both in vitro and in vivo using viral stocks of AMV-S, AMV-B, or AMV-C. (Souza and Baluda, to be published; Souza et al., to be published a). AMV-B contains only viruse of subgroup B, whereas AMV-S contains both subgroup A and B viruses. AMV-C originated from a clone of nonproducer myeoloblasts superinfected with tdB77 subgroup C. Peripheral blood leukemic myeloblasts induced by AMV contained two specific restriction enzyme fragments, an Eco RI 2.2 md and a Hind III 2.6 md, in addition to the endogenous proviral pattern. These two fragments were also detected in the appropriate digest of AMV-S linear viral DNA. DNA from 16 clones of leukemic myeloblasts isolated from AMV-converted yolk sac cell cultures contained the Eco RI 2.2 md and Hind III 2.6 md fragments, regardless of the endogenous complement or the pseudotype of AMV used for conversion. In addition, 2 of the 16 leukemic myeloblast clones contained the two leukemia-specific fragments in the absence of any detectable helper provirus (1). (Souza and Baluda, to be published; Souza et al., to be published a).

Juncture fragments between cellular and proviral sequences could be detected in the leukemic myeloblast clones, but were generally not seen in peripheral blood leukemic myeloblasts. The number of differently sized juncture fragments detected in the leukemic myeloblast clones indicated that the DNA intermediates of the AMV complex can integrate at multiple sites in host DNA (Souza et al., to be published a)

Recombinant DNA clones were constructed by inserting 16–20-kilobase fragments of Eco RI partially digested leukemic myeloblast DNA into phage λ Charon 4a (Soza et al. 1980, to be published b). Clones containing proviral sequences were identified by hybridization with ^{125}I-AMV-S RNA. Restriction enzyme analysis of one clone, λ11A1-1, showed that the proviral DNA is flanked by cellular sequences on either side, contains both the Eco

RI 2.2 md and Hind III 2.6 md leukemia specific fragments, and has a mass of approximately 4.9 md (Souza et al. 1980). This molecular mass is the same as that of an unintegrated linear viral DNA found in CEF infected by AMV-S but not in CEF infected by MAV-1 or MAV-2. Therefore, this provirus could represent the AMV genome responsible for acute myeloblastic leukemia. Another λ-chicken hybrid clone, λ10A2-1, contained 85% of a MAV-1-like genome starting from the 5' end with respect to viral RNA. Comparison of the AMV genome from λ11A1-1 with the MAV-1-like genome from λ10A2-1 by restriction endonuclease mapping (Fig. 1) and

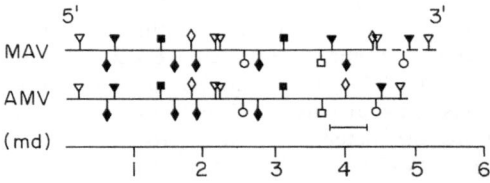

Fig. 1. Restriction enzyme maps of the presumptive AMV and MAV-1-like genomes. Restriction endonuclease sites are localized for the proviral DNA of the presumptive AMV provirus in λ-hybrid 11Al-1 and the partial MAV-1-like provirus in λ-hybrid 10A2-1. The *dashed line* in the MAV map indicates that part of the MAV-1-like genome not present in the λ10A2-1 hybrid. The location of the 3' terminal enzyme sites in MAV-1 were determined with linear viral DNA. Enzyme sites: (∇) Hind III, (◇) Eco RI, (○) Xba I, (□) Kpn I, (◆) Bam HI, (■) Bgl II, and (▼) Xho I. The *bar* under the AMV map represents the region of cellular substitution

heteroduplex analysis indicated both genomes are homologous over 3.6 md from the 5' terminus and lack homology on the 3' side of the single Kpn I site in each genome (Souza et al., to be published a,b). R-loop analyses carried out with the λ-recombinant containing the AMV genome and 35S AMV-S RNA revealed two types of R-loops (Souza et al., to be published b). The first type showed the RNA hybridized over the entire length of the presumptive AMV genome, while the second type showed the RNA hybridzed for approximately 5700 bases from the 5' end of the provirus, displaced by a DNA-DNA duplex for the next 900 bases, and hybridized again for the remaining 700 bases to the 3' terminus.

The first type is interpreted to represent an R-loop of AMV RNA and the second type, and R-loop of MAV RNA to the AMV genome in which a contiguous 900 base substitution exists.

Southern blots of Eco RI digested DNA from various strains of uninfected chickens were hybridized with either ^{125}I-labeled RAV-0, MAV-2, or AMV-S RNA. In addition to the Eco RI fragments containing endogenous proviral sequences detected by the MAV-2 or RAV-0 probe, two AMV-S-specific fragments of 3.7 and 1.5 md were detected by the AMV-S probe (Souza and Baluda 1978). ^{32}P-DNA probes prepared from the 3' region of the AMV DNA genome were hybridized to Eco RI DNA blots prepared from various strains of uninfected chickens (Souza et al. to be published b). The ^{32}P-AMV probes detected the same cellular sequences, i.e., the same Eco RI fragments that were detected with ^{125}I-AMV-S RNA. AMV-specific sequences could also be detected in uninfected Peking duck Eco RI DNA blots using the ^{32}P-labeled AMV probes. Ducks do not contain endogenous proviral DNA homologous to the known avian retroviruses. A ^{32}P-labeled probe made from a similar region of the MAV-1-like provirus contained only homology to endogenous proviral sequences in chicken DNAs and no homology to the Peking duck DNA (Souza et al., to be published b). These hybridization studies have demonstrated that the AMV genome contains a cellular substitution. The physical mapping studies place this substitution in the region of the genome normally occupied by the envelope gene. Thus, this cellular substitution in AMV may be responsible for its leukemogenic potential and its defectiveness.

AMV differs from avian defective transforming viruses such as MC-29, AEV, and MH2 in the following: (1) AMV is only slightly smaller than its natural helper(s), (2) the substitution if contains is half the size of the substitution contained in the other defective viruses, (3) the substitution in AMV appears to only have replaced the env gene, whereas the substitutions in the other defective viruses have replaced part of gag, pol, and env, and (4) AMV does not make an unprocessed transforming protein containing part of gag (Silva and Baluda, to be published). However, the AMV genome resembles physically that of Bryan RSV, a defective avian sarcoma virus.

References

Bergmann DG, Souza LM, Baluda MA (1980) Characterization of the avian myeloblastosis associated virus DNA intermediates. J Virol 34:366–372 – Silva RF, Baluda MA (to be published) Avian myeloblastosis virus proteins in leukemic chicken myeloblasts. J Virol – Souza LM, Baluda MA (1978) Qualitative studies of the endogenous provirus in the chicken genome. In: Stevens J, Todaro GJ, Fox CF (eds) ICN-UCLA Symposium on Molecular and Cell Biology. Academic Press, New York, pp 217–229 – Souza LM, Baluda MA (to be published) Identification of the avian myeloblastosis virus genome. I. Identification of restriction endonuclease fragments associated with acute myeloblastic leukemia. J Virol – Souza LM, Komaromy MC, Baluda MA (1980) Identification of a proviral genome associated with avian myeloblastic leukemia. Proc Natl Acad Sci USA 77:3004–3008 – Souza LM, Briskin MJ, Hillyard RL, Baluda MA (to be published a) Identification of the avian myeloblastosis virus genome. II. Restriction endonuclease analysis of DNA from λ-proviral recombinants and leukemic myeloblast clones. J Virol – Souza LM, Strommer JN, Hillyard RL, Komaromy MC, Baluda MA (to be published b) Cellular sequences are present in the presumptive avian myeloblastosis virus genome. Proc Natl Acad Sci USA

Haematology and Blood Transfusion Vol. 26
Modern Trends in Human Leukemia IV
Edited by Neth, Gallo, Graf, Mannweiler, Winkler
© Springer-Verlag Berlin Heidelberg 1981

Genetics of Leukemogenesis by Avian Leukosis Viruses

J. M. Coffin, P. N. Tsichlis, and H. L. Robinson

A. Introduction

Oncoviruses of chickens can be classified into one of three groups, depending on their effects on cells in culture and their pathogenicity and lifestyle in the chicken (Fig. 1). The most intensely studied but rarest of these viruses are the transforming acute leukemia and sarcoma viruses. These viruses cause rapid disease in animals and transform appropriate target cells in culture, properties attributable to an extra gene in place of (or, in the case of nondefective Rous sarcoma virus, in addition to) the three replicative genes. These *onc* genes are most likely normal genes of the host cell taken under the control of the very efficient sequences that the virus uses for its own expression and therefore expressed at 100- to 1000-fold higher levels than in the uninfected cell (Spector et al. 1978; Stehelin et al. to be published). Since these transforming viruses are very

rapidly pathogenic and are transmitted horizontally very poorly, it is improbable that they exist as infectious agents of epidemiological significance. Rather, they probably arise at low frequency by some recombinational process between leukosis virus and host cell information and, if not given a good home in the laboratory, would die out quickly.

The second group of viruses is the more common natural agent of neoplastic disease in many species, for example lymphoid leukosis in the chicken. They do not transform cells in culture and induce disease only after a long latent period. Their genomes do not appear to contain any information in addition to that required for virus replication. There are three types of virus which behave this way: field isolates of lymphoid leukosis virus (LLV); Rous-associated viruses (RAV), which have been isolated as helpers for defective sarcoma viruses; and transformation-defective *(td)* de-

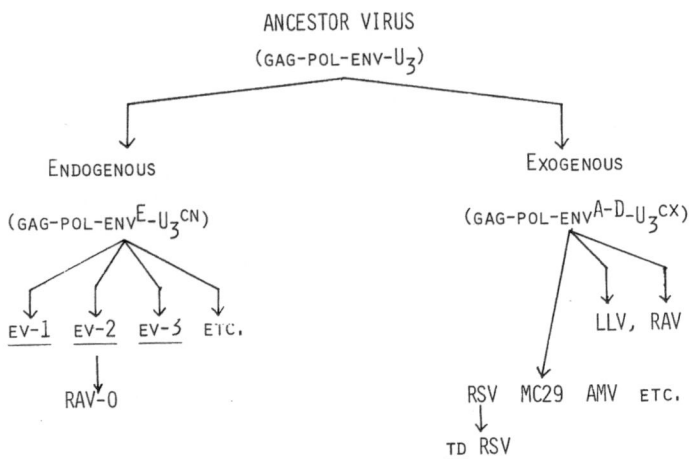

Fig. 1. Relationships among avian tumor virus groups. The hypothetical pattern shown is consistent with the relationships inferred from experiments as in Fig. 2. *RAV*, Rous-associated virus; *LLV*, lymphoid leukosis virus; and *EV-1, etc*, distinct loci of endogenous proviruses of chickens

letion mutants of nondefective sarcoma viruses (Biggs et al. 1973; Vogt 1971). All three types have very similar genome structure.

The third group of avian oncovirus are the endogenous viruses which reside primarily as integrated proviruses in the chromosomal DNA of chickens (for review, see Robinson 1978) and are inherited as though they were usual cellular genes. The endogenous proviruses of chickens have been typed by integration site and phenotype of expression into numerous distinct loci, termed *ev-1, 2,* etc. (Astrin 1978). The endogenous viruses, when expressed as infectious agents, differ from the former two groups (the exogenous viruses) in several interesting ways: they are nonpathogenic in chickens, even when viremia is present (Motta et al. 1975); they replicate somewhat more poorly in cell culture (Linial and Neiman 1976; Robinson 1976); and they have a distinct host range (subgroup E) (Vogt and Friis 1971). They are, however, very closely related to the exogenous nontransforming viruses with a nearly identical genome structure (Coffin et al. 1978b; Neiman et al. 1977).

In this report, we will describe some experiments in which we exploit the biological differences between endogenous and exogenous viruses of chickens to obtain information regarding the roles of various portions of the exogenous virus genome in pathogenicity, particularly in lymphoid leukosis.

B. Results and Discussion

I. Relationship of Endogenous and Exogenous Virus Genomes

There are numerous field and laboratory strains of avian tumor viruses and there are numerous distinct endogenous viral loci. Thus a detailed survey of nucleic acid sequences of genomes of many members of the two groups should allow us to determine in general terms the historical relationships between them, for example, whether the different endogenous viruses are independently derived from germ line integration of an exogenous virus or represent a distinct lineage of viruses derived only from another endogenous virus. To obtain such information, we have subjected the genomes of various endogenous and exogenous viruses to T_1 oligonucleotide mapping (Coffin et al. 1978b), a method sensitive to one

base change per 600 nucleotides. Figure 2 shows a selection of different endogenous and exogenous avian tumor virus genomes by comparison with the genome of RAV-0 (a prototype endogenous virus). Note that the absence of a marker oligonucleotide could be due to as little as a single base change or as much as a deletion or a substitution of completely unrelated information. It can be seen that the endogenous viruses are distinguishable from one another by the presence or absence of specific markers. However, no two of these genomes differ from one another by more than 1%. By contrast, all the exogenous viruses examined differ substantially from one another and from the endogenous viruses, with distinctive markers in many places in the genome. We conclude that these viruses represent two distinct but closely related lineages, a conclusion which is consistent with the relationship scheme for the viruses shown in Fig. 1.

II. Role of the U_3 Region in Growth

Although specific point markers distinguishing endogenous from exogenous viruses are distributed all over the genome, the greatest divergence is in the U_3 region near the 3' end of the genome (Coffin et al. 1978b; Neiman et al. 1977; Wang et al. 1977). We have termed the exogenous allele of this region *cx* and the endogenous type *cn* (Tsichlis and Coffin 1980). Major regions of inhomology were also found in a region to the left of U_3 and in the S (subgroup-coding) region of *env* (Coffin et al. 1978b).

To assess the roles of the various regions in growth and pathogenicity of the viruses, we prepared a series of recombinants between RAV-0 and either Pr-B (a nondefective transforming virus) or its *td* derivative. Recombinants were selected for their ability to infect turkey (T/BD) cells due to the env^E gene of RAV-0 and for transformation and/or rapid growth from the Pr-B parent. Selection for transformation and rapid growth led to selection of *src,* a region immediately to its left, and a short region in *gag.* Selection for rapid growth only was accompanied in all cases by selection of only the U_3^{cx} region of Pr-B. The isolation of one particularly useful recombinant is shown in the top portion of Fig. 3. On initial screening one recombinant "clone" (MRE-1) was found to be a mixture of

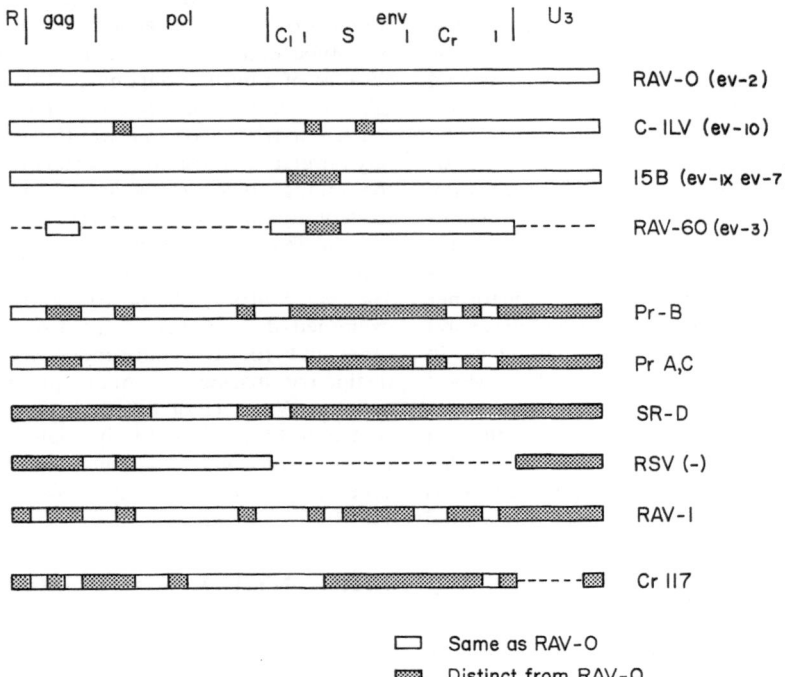

Fig. 2. Genomes of endogenous and exogenous avian tumor viruses. The genomes are displayed as oligonucleotide maps by comparison with that of RAV-0 (Coffin et al. 1978b). Regions identical to RAV-0 (by the presence of an identical oligonucleotide) are shown as an *open box,* regions which differ by a *shaded box,* and undetermined or deleted regions by a *dashed line.* The *top four lines* show RAV-0 and the products of other *ev* loci [ev-3 is defective, and the map shown was inferred from RAV-60 recombinants (Coffin et al. 1978a)]. The *remaining lines* show exogenous viruses. *Pr-B, Pr-C,* and *SR-D* are nondefective transforming virus. *RAV-1 and 2* are lab strains of nontransforming viruses, and *Cr-117* is a new field isolate of LLV

recombinants, all of which were $env^E - U_3^{cx}$, but which were heterogenous in other portions of the genome. Recloning of this virus by focus formation led to the selection of a virus (TRE-14) which contained all the regions found to accompany transformation. When recloned by infection of QT6 cells (Moscovici et al. 1977), a virus, NTRE-7, was isolated which was entirely derived from RAV-0 except for the 200 to 300 nucleotide U_3^{cx} region.

The repeated selection of the U_3^{cx} allele suggested that was responsible for the difference in the growth rate between endogenous and exogenous viruses. NTRE-7 allowed us to test this hypothesis, since it was congenic with RAV-0 except in U_3. We therefore compared the growth of this virus with RAV-0 and with various RAV-60s, a similar set of

recombinants between exogenous and endogenous viruses (Hanafusa et al. 1970; Hayward and Hanafusa 1975), which have various contributions from the exogenous parent in several parts of the genome (Fig. 3, bottom). Parallel cultures of chicken (C/0) cells were infected at various multiplicities of infection and challenged 4 days later with RSV (RAV-60). The extent to which focus formation by the challenge virus was reduced provided a measure of the relative amount of virus replication. As shown in Fig. 4, RAV-0 and the endogenous viruses tested (open symbols) had a virtually identical growth rate, whereas NTRE-7 and the various RAV-60s (closed symbols) had a growth rate 30-fold higher than all the endogenous viruses. Since the only consistent feature distinguishing these recom-

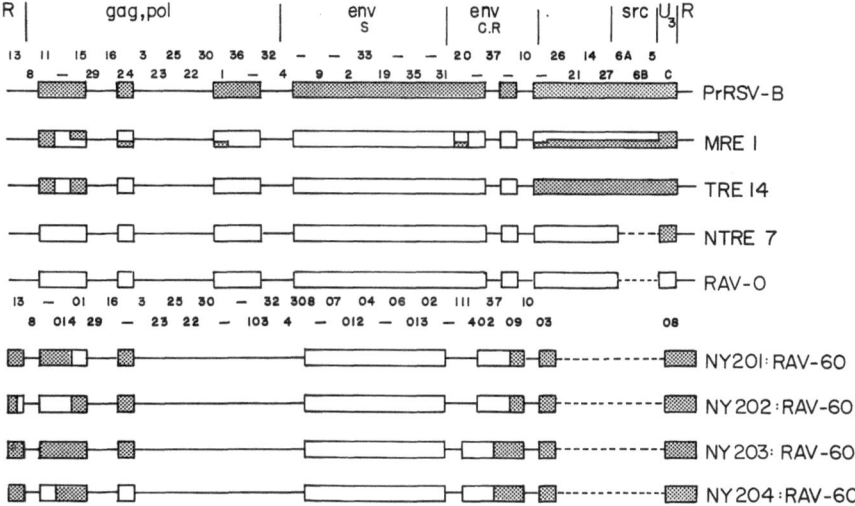

Fig. 3. Recombinants between exogenous and endogenous viruses. The *top section* shows a cross between Pr-B *(shaded bars)* and RAV-0 *(open bars)* leading to a mixture of recombinants, designated *MRE-1,* which was subcloned to select a transforming *(TRE-14)* and a nontransforming virus *(NTRE-7). Solid* lines indicate regions indistinguishable in the two parents, *dashed lines* the *src* deletion in RAV-0 and NTRE-7. The *lower panel* shows 4 RAV-60 strains originally isolated by Hanafusa et al. (1970). Again, regions derived from the endogenous parent are shown by *open boxes* and from the exogenous by *shaded boxes*

binants from the endogenous viruses was the U_3^{cx} allele, we conclude that this small region of the genome is the major determinant responsible for the more rapid growth of exogenous viruses.

The nucleotide sequence of the U_3^{cx} region of several different avian tumor virus strains has been determined (Schwartz and Gilbert, personal communication; Czernilofsky et al., to be published; Yamamoto and Pastan 1980), as has that of one U_3^{cn} region (Hishinuma et al., personal communication), and it is improbable that a protein is encoded by this region. However, this region is reduplicated at the left end of the provirus during DNA synthesis (Hsu et al. 1978; Shank et al. 1978). Since the RNA transcript of the provirus (i.e., the genome) does not contain a copy of the left U_3 region, it is likely that U_3 contains a promoter for virus RNA synthesis and that the distinction between the two U_3 alleles is in the efficiency of the promoters they contain.

III. Role of the U_3 Region in Leukemogenesis

The structure of the integrated provirus suggests a possible mechanism for carcinogenesis

without a specific "transforming" gene. If the left U_3 region carries an efficient promoter, then there must also be one on the right of the provirus where the same combination of sequences is found. Since integration of the provirus into chromosomal DNA is more or less random (Hughes et al. 1978; Sabran et al. 1979), an occasional infected cell might have a provirus integrated to the left of a potentially "transforming" gene. Efficient promotion of transcription of such a region could induce the expression of this gene to oncogenic levels. Compelling evidence for this sort of mechanism has been provided by Hayward et al. (see this book) and by Payne et al. (personal communication).

In its simplest form this model would predict that the nonpathogenicity of endogenous viruses is a consequence of an inefficient U_3 promoter sequence. Again, NTRE-7 and the various RAV-60s allowed us to test this hypothesis directly. A full account of the methods used for this experiment can be found in Robinson et al. (to be published). In brief, susceptible chicks were injected with equal amounts of RAV-1, RAV-0, NTRE-7, or the RAV-60s. Figure 5 shows the level of viremia

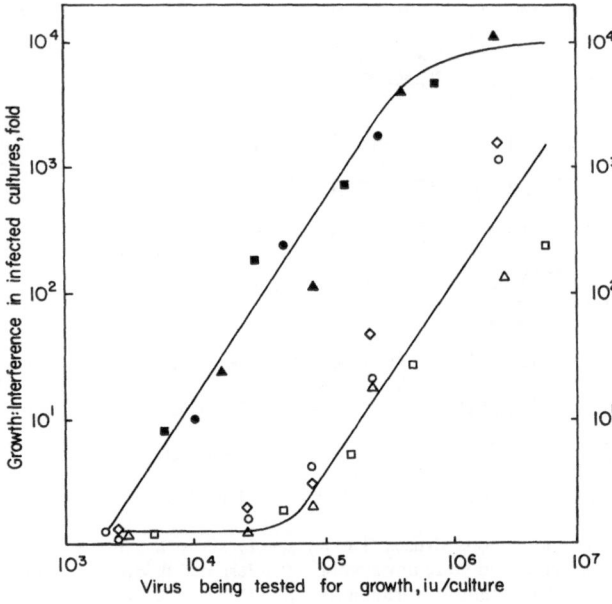

Fig. 4. Relative growth rates of various viruses. C/0 gro+ chicken embryo-fibroblasts (Robinson et al., to be published) were infected at various multiplicities with either the endogenous viruses RAV-0 (○), C-ILV (◇), 15B×K16 ILV (△), 15B E-virus (□), or the recombinant viruses NTRE-7 (●), NY 201 (▲), and NY 203 (■) RAV-60. Four days after infection the cultures were superinfected with B-RSV (RAV-60) and foci were counted 5–7 days later. The extent of interference was determined by dividing the titer of the challenge virus in uninfected control cultures by the titer in the various infected cultures

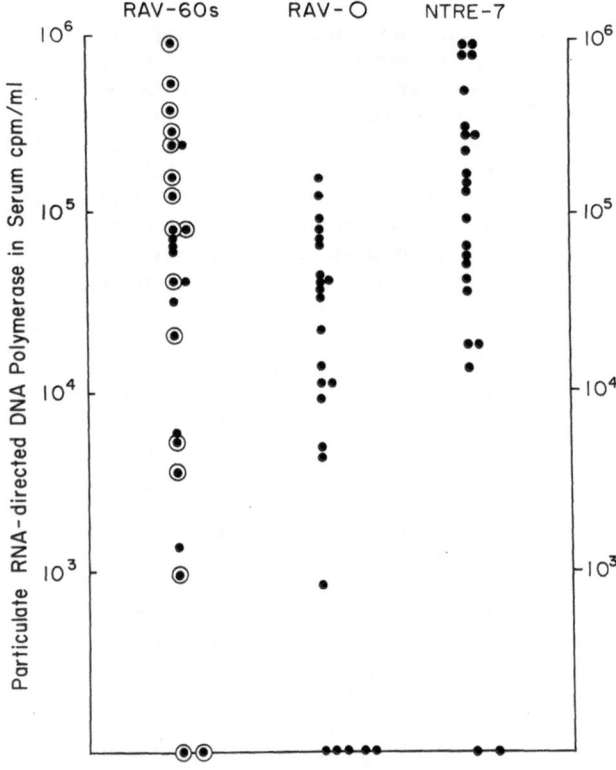

Fig. 5. Growth of NTRE-7, RAV-0, and RAV-60 in birds. Each *point* shows the level of serum viremia in C/0 chickens 1 month after infection with 10^6 infectious units of each virus as measured by particulate reverse transcriptase in serum. *Circled points* show birds which were later diagnosed as having lymphoid leukosis

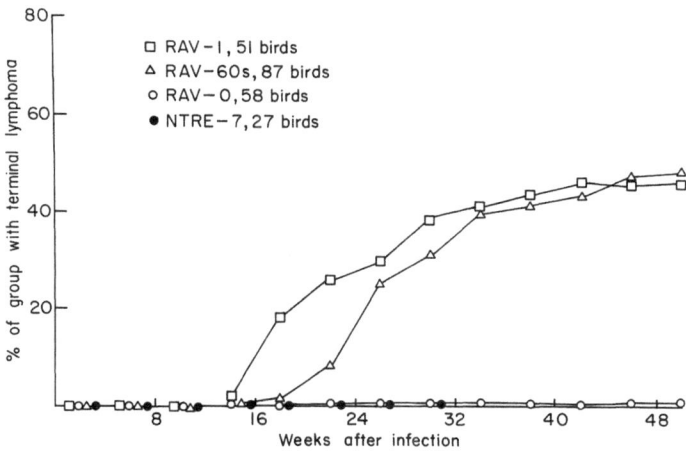

Fig. 6. Pathogenicity of NTRE-7, RAV-0, and RAV-60s. The figure shows cumulative disease incidence in the same birds as in Fig. 5 as a function of time after injection with 10^6 infectous units of *RAV-1* ($\square$), RAV-0 (O), NTRE-7 ($\bullet$) and pooled data for the four RAV-60s shown in Fig. 3 ($\triangle$). All diagnoses were histologically confirmed. A small additional incidence of other neoplasms in the RAV-60 and RAV-1 groups is not included. Data taken in part from Robinson et al. (to be published)

in the latter three groups at 1 month of age. Although there was substantial variation from bird to bird, the growth of the viruses in vivo seemed to mimic that in cell culture, with RAV-0 growing to a median value about 10-fold less than NTRE-7 or the RAV-60s.

Figure 6 shows the incidence of leukosis in all the birds tested. The incidence and latent period for the RAV-60 strains were not significantly different from the RAV-1. Thus, the subgroup E host range does not contribute to the nonpathogenicity of endogenous viruses. Similar results were found by Crittenden et al. (1980). As previously reported (Motta et al. 1975), RAV-0 was nonleukemogenic. Although the test of NTRE-7 is not yet complete, the results to date are quite surprising. In the first 34 weeks, there has been no disease whatever, compared with 40% in the RAV-60 infected birds. While we cannot yet conclude that NTRE-7 is completely nonpathogenic, it may well be so, and it is at least significantly slower than the RAV-60s. We must also point out that although td sarcoma viruses have been reported to be leukemogenic (Biggs et al. 1973; Halpern and Hanafusa, personal communication), td Pr-B has not yet been tested.

In any case, this result clearly separates growth rate from leukemogenicity, since RAV-60s and NTRE-7 show identical growth both in vitro and in vivo. This result is inconsistent with the simplest predictions of the downstream promotion model as well as models which invoke pathogenic side effects of the virus gene products. We have additional

recombinants available for testing which should provide us with a suggestion of which region of the genome is responsible for these differences. A comparison of the structures of NTRE-7 and the RAV-60s gives a hint of where to look (Fig. 3). The only exogenous virus region besides U_3 consistently inherited by these viruses is immediately to the left of U_3. This region is at present undefined. There are a number of reasons why such a sequence might have a role in pathogenicity, the most interesting of which is the regulation of downstream promotion by either the sequence itself or its product.

We believe that the nonpathogenicity of the endogenous viruses is an important adaptive feature to their quiescent lifestyle, for which it is quite important that they not harm the host. Experiments such as we have presented here should be useful in identifying and characterizing the regions of the virus genomes relevant to this adaptation and also in exploiting the differences in these regions in different viruses to probe the molecular mechanisms of viral leukemogenesis.

Acknowledgements

We thank M. Champion and L. Lieberman for expert technical assistance. This work was supported by grants CA17659, CA24530, and CA23086 from the National Cancer Institute. J. Coffin was a recipient of a Faculty Research Award from the American Cancer Society, and P. Tsichlis was a postdoctoral fellow of the National Cancer Institute.

References

Astrin S (1978) Endogenous viral genes of white leghorn chickens: A common site of residence as well as sites associated with specific phenotypes of viral gene expression. Proc Natl Acad Sci USA 75:5941–5945 – Biggs P, Milne B, Graf T, Bauer H (1973) Oncogenicity of non-transforming mutants of avian sarcoma viruses. J Gen Virol 18:399–403 – Coffin JM, Champion MA, Chabot F (1978a) Genome structure of avian RNA tumor viruses: Relationships between exogenous and endogenous viruses. In: Barlati C, deGiuli-Morghen C (eds) Avian RNA tumor viruses. Piccin, Padua, pp 68–87 – Coffin J, Champion M, Chabot F (1978b) Nucleotide sequence relationships between the genomes of an endogenous and an exogenous avian tumor virus. J Virol 28:972–991 – Crittenden LB, Hayward WS, Hanafusa H, Fadley AM (1980) Induction of neoplasms by subgroup E recombinants of exogenous and endogenous avian retroviruses (Rous-associated virus type 60). J Virol 33:915–919 – Czernilofsky A, Delorbe W, Swanstrom R, Varmus H, Bishop JM (to be published) The nucleotide sequence of "C" an untranslated but conserved domain in the genome of avian sarcoma virus. Nucleic Acids Res – Hanafusa T, Hanafusa H, Miyamoto T (1970) Recovery of a new virus from apparently normal cells by infection with avian tumor viruses. Proc Natl Acad Sci USA 67:1797–1803 – Hayward WS, Hanafusa H (1975) Recombination between endogenous and exogenous RNA tumor virus genes as analyzed by nucleic acid hybridization. J Virol 15:1367–1377 – Hsu J, Sabran J, Mark G, Guntaka R, Taylor J (1978) Analysis of unintegrated avian RNA tumor virus double-stranded DNA intermediates. J Virol 29:819–818 – Hughes S, Vogt PR, Shank PR, Spector PH, Kung HJ, Breitman ML, Bishop JM, Varmus HE (1978) Proviruses of avian sarcoma viruses are terminally redundant, coextensive with unintegrated linear DNA, and integrated at many sites in rat cell DNA. Cell 15:1397–1410 – Linial M, Neiman PE (1976) Infection of chick cells by subgroup E virus. Virology 73:508–520 – Moscovici C, Moscovici MG, Jimenez H, Lai MMG, Hayman MJ, Vogt PK (1977) Continuous tissue culture cell lines derived from chemically induced tumors of Japanese quail. Cell 11:95–103 – Motta J, Crittenden L, Purchase H, Stone H, Okazaki W, Witter R (1975) Low oncogenic potential of avian endogenous RNA tumor virus infection or expression. J Natl Cancer Inst 55:685–689 – Neiman PE, Das S, MacDonnel D, McMillan-Helsel C (1977) Organization of shared and unshared sequences in the genomes of chicken endogenous and sarcoma viruses. Cell 11:321–329 – Robinson HL (1976) Intracellular restriction on the growth of induced subgroup E avian type C viruses in chicken cells. J Virol 18:856–866 – Robinson H (1978) Inheritance and expression of chicken genes which are related to avian-sarcoma viruses. Curr Top Microbiol Immunol 83:1–36 – Robinson HL, Pearson MN, Desimone DW, Tsichlis PN, Coffin JM (to be published) Subgroup E avian leukosis virus associated disease in chickens. Cold Spring Harbor Symp Quant Biol 44 – Sabran J, Hsu T, Yeater C, Kaji A, Mason W, Taylor J (1979) Analysis of integrated avian RNA tumor virus DNA in transformed chicken, duck, and quail fibroblasts. J Virol 29:170–178 – Shank PR, Hughes S, Kung HJ, Majors JE, Quintrell N, Guntaka RV, Bishop JM, Varmus HE (1978) Mapping unintegrated forms of avian sarcoma virus DNA: Both termini of linear DNA bear a 300 nucleotide sequence present once or twice in two species of circular DNA. Cell 15:1383–1395 – Spector DH, Smith K, Padgett T, McCombe P, Roulland-Dussoix D, Moscovici C, Varmus HE, Bishop JM (1978) Uninfected avian cells contain RNA unrelated to the transforming gene of avian sarcoma viruses. Cell 13:371–379 – Stehelin D, Varmus HE, Bishop JM, Vogt PK (1976) DNA related to the transforming gene(s) of avian sarcoma virus is present in normal avian DNA. Nature 260:170–172 – Stehelin D, Soule S, Roussel M, Sergeant A, Lagrou C, Rommens C, Raes MB (to be published) Three new types of viral oncogenes in defective avian leukemia viruses. Cold Spring Harbor Symp Quant Biol 44 – Tsichlis PN, Coffin JM (1980) Recombinants between endogenous and exogenous avian tumor viruses: Role of the C region and other portions of the genome in the control of replication and transformation. J Virol 33:238–249 – Vogt PK (1971) Spontanous segregation of nontransforming viruses from cloned sarcoma viruses. Virology 46:939–946 – Vogt PK, Friis RR (1971) An avian leukosis virus related to RSV(0): Properties and evidence for helper activity. Virology 34:223–234 – Wang SY, Hayward WS, Hanafusa H (1977) Genetic variation in the RNA transcripts of endogenous virus genes in uninfected chicken cells. J Virol 24:64–73 – Yamamoto T, Jay G, Pastan I (1980) Unusual features in the nucleotide sequence of a cDNA clone derived from the common region of avian sarcoma virus messenger RNA. Proc Natl Acad Sci USA 77:176–180

Haematology and Blood Transfusion Vol. 26
Modern Trends in Human Leukemia IV
Edited by Neth, Gallo, Graf, Mannweiler, Winkler
© Springer-Verlag Berlin Heidelberg 1981

Avian Lymphoid Leukosis is Correlated with the Appearance of Discrete New RNAs Containing Viral and Cellular Genetic Information

W. S. Hayward, B. G. Neel, J. Fang, H. L. Robinson, and S. M. Astrin

Lymphoid leukosis (LL) is a B-cell lymphoma of birds which is caused by a class of RNA tumor viruses called avian leukosis viruses (ALVs). These viruses also occasionally cause other neoplasms such as sarcomas and nephroblastomas. ALVs induce tumors in infected animals only after a latent period of 4–12 months and do not transform cells at detectable frequency in tissue culture (Hanafusa 1977). Despite intensive efforts, no transforming gene has been identified in these viruses. This suggests that the mechanism involved in neoplastic transformation by ALV is fundamentally different from that of the avian acute transforming viruses (sarcoma viruses and acute leukemia viruses). The acute viruses induce tumor formation within about 2 weeks, transform appropriate target cells in tissue culture, and code for transforming proteins (Bister et al. 1979; Erikson 1980; Graf und Beug 1978; Hanafusa 1977; Hanafusa et al. 1980; Hayman et al. 1979; Lee et al. 1980).

We have analyzed the virus-related RNA and DNA from more than 20 ALV-induced tumors. The data suggest that integration of the provirus of ALV induces increased expression of one or more normal cellular genes by providing a strong upstream promoter. We propose that enhanced expression of these cellular genes causes neoplastic transformation.

A. Results

I. Incidence of Tumor Induction

ALV ($\sim 10^7$ I.U./bird) was injected intravenously into 2–7-day-old chicks. Four virus strains were used: RAV-1, RAV-2, td103, and td107A. The latter two viruses are deletion mutants of RSV, lacking most or all of the *src* gene (Halpern et al. 1979; Kawai et al. 1977). No strain-specific differences were observed in the experiments described below.

Lymphomas were first detected at 4 months, and by 6 months (when all surviving birds were sacrificed) approximately 40% of the birds had developed visible tumors. The most commonly involved tissues were bursa, liver, kidney, and spleen. Of 23 tumors used for RNA analyses, 22 were diagnosed as lymphomas and one (#16L) was a fibrosarcoma in the liver. We also analyzed a continuous cell line, RP9, derived from a RAV-2-induced lymphoma (kindly provided by W. Okazaki).

II. Virus-Related RNAs in Tumor Cells

Tumor cell RNAs were analyzed by a modification (Brian Seed, personal communication) of the Northern transfer technique (Alwine et al. 1977). Virus-related RNA was identified by hybridization to ^{32}P-labeled "strong stop" DNA (cDNA$_{ss}$), which corresponds to the 5' 101 nucleotides of the viral RNA (Haseltine et al. 1977).

The normal 35S and 21S RNAs of ALV (Hayward 1977; Weiss et al. 1977) were present in many, though not all, of the lymphomas analyzed. In addition, 19 out of 22 lymphomas (from 14 of 17 birds) contained new RNA species not found in uninfected cells or in nontransformed infected cells. These tumor-specific RNAs fell into three size classes of 2.5, 2.9, and 5.45 kb (designated classes I–III, respectively; examples are shown in Fig. 1, top). Other new RNAs were detected in some samples (e.g., RP9 and 19K), but these RNAs were not found in more than one tumor. In all cases where more than one tumor from the same animal were examined (e.g., 7L, 7K, 10B, 10L, 11B, 11L, 9B, 9K) the same new tumor-specific RNA was found in each tumor, suggesting that metastases were derived from the same initial clonal event.

RNAs of classes I and II were not detectable with cDNA$_{rep}$, a probe representing the entire viral genome (Fig. 1, bottom). Thus these RNAs contain little, if any, viral information other than the 5′ sequences and presumably contain cellular sequences. The absence of viral sequences (other than 5′) in these RNAs was confirmed by both liquid and Northern gel hybridization using probes specific for different regions of the viral genome (data not shown). RNA of class III could be detected with cDNA$_{rep}$, but the intensity of the bands suggested that only a small portion of the information in these RNAs (not enough to

account for their size) could be virus-specific. Analyses with other probes indicated that class III RNAs contain some gag-specific information, but no pol- or env-specific sequences.

RNA from several tumors was analyzed by liquid hybridization to determine the relative abundance of the virus-related RNAs. Three of the tumors selected (7K, 23L, and 9B) contained low or undetectable amounts of 35S and 21S RNAs in the Northern analysis. In each of these tumors the level of RNA detected with cDNA$_{ss}$ was at least 20-fold higher than that detected with cDNA$_{rep}$ (Table 1). The ss-containing RNA, presumably representing the new tumor-specific RNAs, was present at levels ranging from 100–1300 copies per cell. In other tumors the contribution of tumor-specific RNAs was obscured by the high levels of 35S and 21S RNAs.

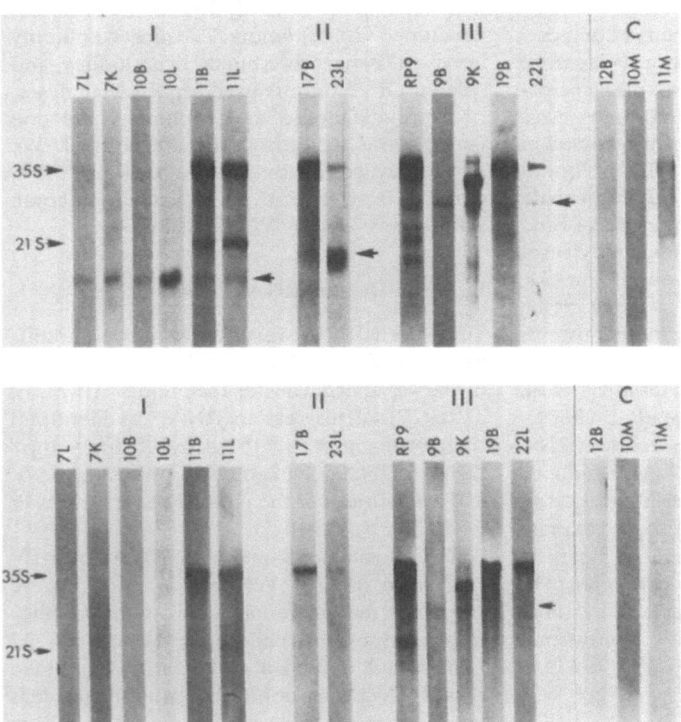

Fig. 1. Virus-related RNAs in lymphoma cells. Poly (A)-containing RNA from normal and tumor tissues were analyzed by the Northern gel transfer technique (Alwine et al. 1977). *Top panels,* RNAs detected with a probe (cDNA$_{ss}$) representing the 5′ 101 nucleotides of RAV-2. *Bottom panels,* RNAs detected with a probe (cDNA$_{rep}$) representing the entire RAV-2 genome. Sample designations indicate the animal number and the tissue involved: L, liver, K, kidney, B, bursa, M, muscle. Control RNAs *(C)* were from a normal bursa from an uninfected bird *(12B)* or from nonneoplastic tissues of infected birds *(10M, 11M)*. Tumor-specific RNAs of classes I, II, and III are indicated by arrows

Table 1. Viral and transformation-specific RNAs in tumor tissues

Tissue	RNA size (kb)[a]	RNA (copies/cell)[c]					
		s.s.	rep	src	erb	myb	fps
12B (uninfected)	–	<1	<1	3	2	3	1
31L (uninfected)	–	<1	<1	2	4	1	1
7K (lymphoma)	2.5[b]	100	2	4	6	5	1
11B (lymphoma)	8.4, 3.3, 2.5[b]	2500	2000	3	2	4	2
23L (lymphoma)	8.4, 2.9[b]	100	5	5	2	3	1
9B (lymphoma)	5.45[b]	1300	1000	5	4	2	1
22L (lymphoma)	8.4, 5.45[b], 3.3, 2.5	300	300	4	N.D.[d]	5	2
RP 9 (cell line)	8.4, 7.2[b], 5.45[b], 4.0[b], 3.3, 2.9[b]	4000	1500	3	3	40	1
16L (sarcoma)	8.4, 6.7[b], 3.3	2000	1500	4	5	2	300

[a] Sizes were estimated by Northern gel analysis of glyoxalated RNA (see Fig. 1) using RAV-2 35S and chicken 27S and 18S RNAs as markers. [b] New RNA species not present in normal ALV-infected cells
[c] RNA concentrations were determined by liquid hybridization as described previously (Hayward 1977). cDNA probes used were: "strong-stop" (s.s.), corresponding to the 5′ 101 nucleotides of RAV-2 RNA; "rep," containing a relatively uniform distribution of all RAV-2 sequences; unique (presumably transformation-specific) sequences of RSV *(src)*, AEV *(erb)*, AMV *(myb)*, and Fujinami sarcoma virus *(fps)*
[d] Not determined

III. Expression of Cellular Transformation-Specific Sequences

Normal cells contain genes closely related to (and probably progenitors of) the putative transforming genes of the acute avian viruses (Chen, to be published; Erikson 1980; Hanafusa et al. 1977; Sheiness and Bishop 1979; Stehelin et al. 1976; to be published; Wang et al. 1979). To test whether these cellular genes are encoded in the new tumor-specific RNAs, we prepared probes corresponding to the unique sequences of RSV (termed *src*), AEV *(erb)*, AMV *(myb)*, and Fujinami sarcoma virus *(fps)*. None of the lymphoma tissues contained elevated levels of these RNA sequences (Table 1). However, the lymphoma-derived cell line, RP9, contained a higher level of *myb*-specific RNA (40 copies/cell vs 1–3 copies in control tissues). This RNA comigrated with a 4.0 kb RNA detected with cDNA$_{ss}$, but we do not yet know whether the ss and *myb* sequences are covalently linked.

An elevated level of *fps*-specific RNA was found in tumor 16L (the only fibrosarcoma found in our ALV-infected birds). Preliminary evidence indicates that this tumor was induced by a defective virus related to, but not identical to, Fujinami sarcoma virus. The origin of the virus in the fibrosarcoma is unknown, but one possibility is that it was derived by recombination between the infecting ALV and endogenous *fps*-specific sequences. We can find no evidence for participation of a defective transforming virus in any of the lymphomas examined.

IV. Restriction Analysis of Tumor DNAs

Tumor cell DNA was digested with the restriction endonuclease Eco R-1, size fractionated on agarose gels, and transferred to nitrocellulose paper by the technique of Southern (1975). Virus-specific restriction fragments were detected by hybridization with cDNA$_{ss}$. This combination of enzyme and probe identifies two fragments for each integrated provirus: an internal fragment from the left end and a virus-cell junction fragment from the right end.

Figure 2 compares the restriction patterns of DNA from normal and neoplastic tissues from three different birds. Restriction fragments from endogenous proviruses were detected in both normal (left panels) and tumor DNAs. The most frequent were the 8.4 and 18-kb fragments of ev-1, which were present in all birds used (Astrin 1978). In each case, however, new tumor-specific restriction fragments (indicated by arrows) were present in lympho-

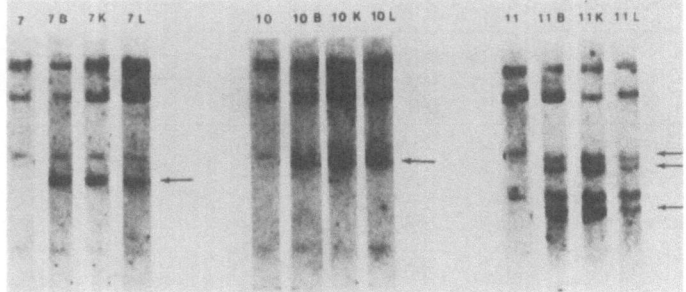

Fig. 2. Restriction analysis of DNAs from metastatic tumors. DNA was isolated from lymphomas of bursa *(B)*, kidney *(K)*, and liver *(L)* and from nonneoplastic muscle tissue *(M)* from three different birds. DNAs were digested with Eco R-1 and analyzed by the gel transfer technique of Southern (1975). Restriction fragments encoding 5' sequences of ALV were identified by hybridization to ^{32}p-cDNA$_{ss}$. Tumor-specific junction fragments are indicated by *arrows*

ma DNAs. These fragments contain both viral and cellular sequences ("junction fragments") as they are not detected with cDNA$_{rep}$ (data not shown). The fact that distinct junction fragments could be detected argues strongly that all or most of the cells in each tumor are derived from a single infected cell. (Distinct junction fragments are not detected in randomly infected cell populations, since integration occurs at many different sites.) All tumors from a single bird contained the same tumor-specific junction fragments (Fig. 2); thus metastatic tumors are clonally derived. Similar observations have been reported by others (Neiman et al. 1980; G. Payne, J. M. Bishop and H. Varmus, personal communication; H.-J. Kung, personal communication).

The integrated proviruses in tumors from birds 7 and 10 are apparently defective, since these DNAs lack the 2.6-kb internal fragment (which would be below the tumor-specific bands indicated by arrows). This is consistent with the absence of 35S and 21S viral RNAs in these tumors (Fig. 1).

New tumor-specific junction fragments were found in all tumors analyzed (21 birds). Four size classes of junction fragments, designated class A (3.8 kb), B (3.2 kb), C (3.0 kb), and D (3.5 kb), were found to be common to more than one tumor (Fig. 3). All tumors tested contained one of these new junction fragments. These data are consistent with the interpretation that each tumor contains viral information at one of four common sites, but further analyses of the flanking cellular sequence are needed before any final conclusions can be drawn.

The presence of a specific junction fragment correlated with the presence of a specific new tumor-specific RNA in eight of the ten birds in which both RNA and DNA were analyzed. (The exceptions were birds 7 and 19). In general, class A DNA correlated with class I RNA, class B, with class II, and class C with class III.

B. Discussion

From these data we conclude that expression of viral genes is not required for maintenance of neoplasia, since many tumors (at least 30%) lack complete proviruses and do not express the normal viral 35S and 21S mRNAs. The data suggest that lymphoma induction occurs only when the provirus integrates at one of a limited number of sites on the host cell chromosome. The provirus could induce the expression of an adjacent cellular gene, analogous to the endogenous transformation-related genes, by read-off from the strong viral promoter. We call this the "promoter insertion" model of leukemogenesis.

The promoter for viral RNA synthesis is located at both the left and right ends of the provirus, within the "3'" region of the terminal repeat (Dhar et al. 1980; Sutcliffe et al. 1980; Yamamoto et al. 1980), (see Fig. 4). Read-off from the right end promoter of a normal provirus (Fig. 4, top) would generate an RNA transcript containing viral 5' sequences plus adjacent cellular sequences. Alternatively, read-off could occur from the left end promoter of a permuted (Fig. 4, bottom) or defective

442

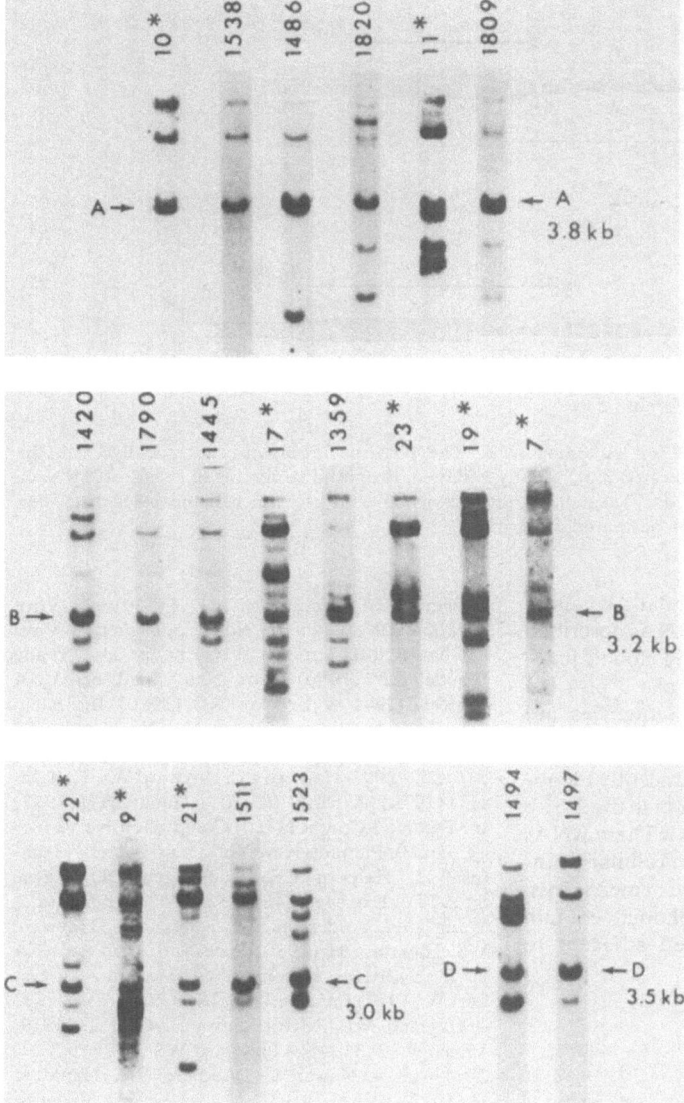

Fig. 3. Restriction analysis of DNAs from ALV-induced lymphomas. Lymphoma DNAs from 21 birds were analyzed as in Fig. 2. Junction fragments common to more than one tumor fell into four size classes *(A–D)* as indicated by *arrows*

(not shown) provirus, generating a transcript containing viral 5′, (possibly) gag, and cellular information. The latter mechanism would explain the presence of gag-specific sequences in class III RNA.

The major assumption of the promoter insertion model is that cell transformation is caused by the elevated expression of a normal cellular gene. If this model is correct, it seems likely that oncogenesis by other, nonviral agents could occur by similar mechanisms. Expression of one of these cellular genes could be altered by mutation or structural rearrangements induced by external agents such as radiation or chemical carcinogens rather than by insertion of the viral promoter. While we

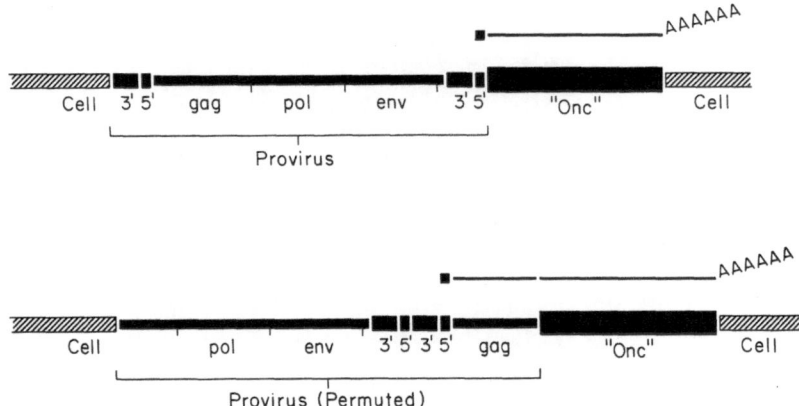

Fig. 4. Promoter insertion model for leukemogenesis. The provirus is shown schematically, with the terminally repeated sequences (indicated 3'5') greatly enlarged. Proposed structures of "read-off" RNAs, containing both viral and cellular ("onc") sequences, are shown above the provirus structures (see text). *Top,* normal integrated provirus. *Bottom,* permuted provirus

have not yet identified the cellular sequences encoded in the tumor-specific RNAs described above, studies in progress using cloned junction-fragment DNAs should make it possible to determine whether these sequences are involved in nonviral cancers.

Note added in proof: We have recently identified the cellular sequences present in the 2.5 kb and 2.9 kb tumor-specific RNAs. These RNAs are transcribed from c-*myc*, the cellular counterpart of the transforming gene of mc2a virus. Nearly all ALV-induced lymphomas contain proviral information integrated adjacent to c-*myc*.

Acknowledgments

We thank N. Goldberg for excellent technical assistance; J. Benedetto for typing the manuscript; T. Hanafusa, H. Hanafusa, and L.-H. Wang for providing some of the birds used in this study; W. Okazaki for providing the lymphoma cell line; and J. Walberg for performing histologic analyses. This work was supported by Public Health Service Grants CA16668 (W.S.H.), CA23086 (H.L.R.), and CA06927 (S.M.A.) from the National Cancer Institute.

References

Alwine JC, Kemp DJ, Stark GR (1977) Proc Natl Acad Sci USA 74:5350–5354 – Astrin SM (1978) Proc Natl Acad Sci USA 75:5941–5945 – Bister K, Löliger HC, Duesberg PH (1979) J Virol 32:208–219 – Chen JH (to be published) J Virol – Dhar R, McClements WL, Enquist LW, Vande Woude GF (1980) Proc Natl Acad Sci USA 77:3937–3941 – Erikson RL (1980) In: Klein G (ed) Viral Oncology. Raven, New York, pp 39–53 – Graf T, Beug H (1978) Biochim Biophys Acta 516:269–299 – Halpern CC, Hayward WS, Hanafusa H (1979) J Virol 29:91–101 – Hanafusa H (1977) In: Fraenkel-Conrat H (ed) Comprehensive Virology, Vol 10. Plenum, New York, p 401–483 – Hanafusa H, Halpern CC, Buchhagen DL, Kawai S (1977) J Exp Med 146:1735–1747 – Hanafusa T, Wang L-H, Anderson SM, Karess RE, Hayward WS, Hanafusa H (1980) Proc Natl Acad Sci USA 77:3009–3013 – Haseltine WA, Maxam AM, Gilbert W (1977) Proc Natl Acad Sci USA 74:989–993 – Hayman MJ, Royer-Pokora B, Graf T (1979) Virology 92:31–45 – Hayward WS (1977) J Virol 24:47–63 – Kawai S, Duesberg PH, Hanafusa H (1977) J Virol 24:910–914 – Lee WH, Bister K, Pawson A, Robins T, Moscovici C, Duesberg PH (1980) Proc Natl Acad Sci USA 77:2018–2022 – Neiman P, Payne LN, Weiss RA (1980) J Virol 34:178–186 – Sheiness D, Bishop JM (1979) J Virol 31:514–521 – Southern EM (1975) J Mol Biol 98:503–517 – Stehelin D, Varmus HE, Bishop JM, Vogt PK (1976) Nature 260:170–173 – Stehelin D, Saule S, Roussel M, Lagrou C, Rommens C (to be published) Cold Spring Harbor Symp Quant Biol 44 – Sutcliffe JG, Shinnick TM, Verma IM, Lerner RA (1980) Proc Natl Acad Sci USA 77:3302–3306 – Wang LH, Moscovici C, Karess RE, Hanafusa H (1979) J Virol 32:546–556 – Weiss SR, Varmus HE, Bishop JM (1977) Cell 12:983–992 – Yamamoto T, Jay G, Pastan I (1980) Proc Natl Acad Sci USA 77:176–180

444

Haematology and Blood Transfusion Vol. 26
Modern Trends in Human Leukemia IV
Edited by Neth, Gallo, Graf, Mannweiler, Winkler
© Springer-Verlag Berlin Heidelberg 1981

The Molecular Basis of Avian Retrovirus-Induced Leukemogenesis

H. J. Kung, Y. K. Fung, L. C. Crittenden, A. Fadly, and S. K. Dube

A. Introduction

There is overwhelming evidence that infection by retroviruses can lead to transformation of the infected cell and to tumor development in the target organ of the host. However, the mechanism by which virus-induced oncogenic transformation occurs is not clearly understood. The viral tumorigenesis involves several steps, including infection by the virus, integration of provirus, transformation of the target cells, tumor development, and in some cases metastasis. In an attempt to gain insight into the molecular mechanism of this process, we have studied the avian leukosis virus [(ALV) e.g., RAV-1] induced lymphoid leukosis (LL) by following the fate of proviral DNA of infecting virus through preleukosis, leukosis, and metastasis stages. The results of these studies presented below have indicated that there are multiple sites in the cellular genome of the target tissue where the proviral DNA of infecting virus can integrate, that there may be a few preferred sites at which integration can lead to tumor formation, that deletions and other structural alterations in the proviral DNA may facilitate tumorigenesis, that origin of LL tumors is clonal, and finally that metastasis arise by migration of a primary clone to the secondary site.

B. Experimental Approach

I. Source of DNA

Sixteen newborn chickens from an inbred line $15I_5 \times 7_2$ of Regional Poultry Research Laboratory, East Lansing, Michigan, United States were used for these experiments and each was infected with 10^5 clone-purified RAV-1 viruses. Bursal specimens at 4 and 8 weeks post infection were obtained by biopsy. Around 16–20 weeks after infection chickens showed signs of leukosis. Bursal tumors could be felt by palpation and were surgically removed. Visual inspection of dissected chickens showed that in several cases tumors had metastasized, and distinct-looking foci from liver and spleen were excised. DNA from all specimens was extracted (Huges et al. 1978) and analyzed by the Southern technique (Southern 1975).

II. Hybridization Reagents

$cDNA_{rep}$: 32p-labeled DNA probe complementary to RAV-1 RNA and representative of the entire genome was synthesized using reverse transcriptase (RT) and calf thymus DNA primer (Hughes et al. 1978; Taylor et al. 1976). $cDNA_{3'}$: A probe complementary to the 3' terminus of RAV-1 RNA and specific for RAV-1 (Neiman et al. 1977; Coffin et al. 1978) was synthesized using RT and oligo dT_{12-18} primer (Tal et al. 1977). $cDNA_{5'}$: This probe was synthesized using an endogenous reaction (Friedrich et al. 1977) and the 101-nucleotide-long "strong-stop" fragment (Haseltine et al. 1976) was purified by polyacrylamide gel electrophoresis (Friedrich et al. 1977). DNA_{gag}: This probe was prepared by nick translation (Rigby et al. 1977) of a gag containing EcoRI-SacI segment of the cloned proviral DNA (Fig. 1a).

III. Identification of Exogeneous Provirus

We have used restriction endonucleases SacI or EcoRI and viral probes capable of distinguishing between endogenous and RAV-1-speci-

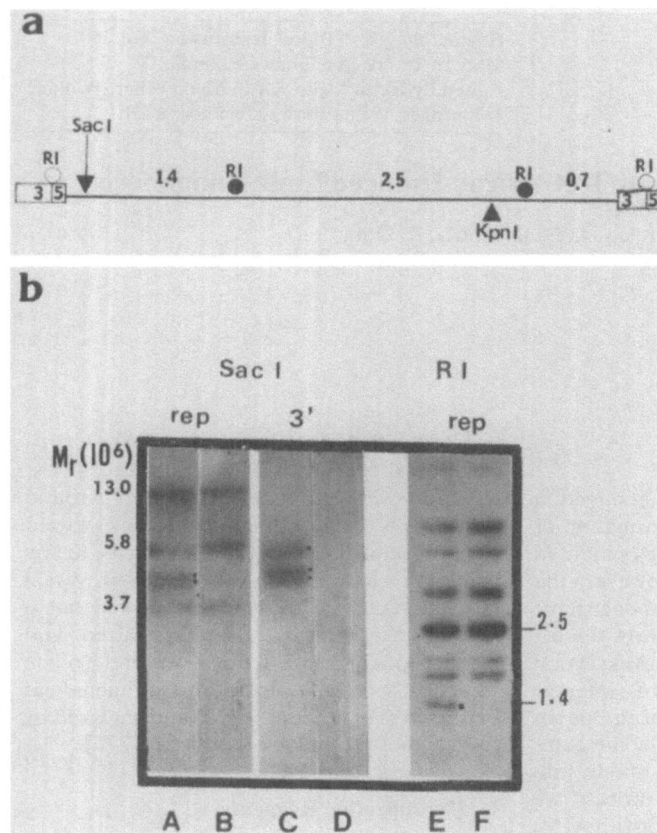

Fig. 1. The restriction-enzyme cleavage maps of RAV-1 DNA and the identification of tumor-specific (TS) proviral DNA. **a** The cleavage maps of restriction enzymes EcoRI, SacI, and KpnI. *Open triangles* indicate EcoRI sites not present in the ev sequences. The *boxed 35* represents the large terminal repeat (LTR), which is located at both termini of the viral DNA and carries the 3' and 5' terminal sequences of the RNA genome. **b** Restriction enzyme digestion analysis of proviral DNA. The DNA samples were extracted from bursa tumor #1 *(lane A and C)*, from the nontumorous thymus *(lane B and D)* of the same bird, and from the in vitro RAV-1-infected *(lane E)* or uninfected *(lane F)* chicken embryo fibroblasts of line $15I_5 \times 7_2$. They were digested with SacI or EcoRI, analyzed on 0.8% agarose gel and by Southern blotting hybridizations with cDNA$_{rep}$ or cDNA$_3$

fic sequences. The rationale of the method is outlined below.

The $15I_5 \times 7_2$ has three ev loci (Astrin 1978) which are readily revealed as three bands of molecular weight 13 md (ev-6), 5.8 md (ev-1), and 3.7 md (ev-2) upon cleavage of genomic DNA with SacI and hybridization with cDNA-$_{rep}$. In the example shown in Fig. 1b both nontumor and tumor tissue DNA display these three bands (lane A,B). However, tumor DNA has two additional bands. Since they are present only in tumor DNA, we refer to them as tumor-specific or TS bands. Their exogenous origin was established by hybridization with cDNA$_{3'}$ (lane C,D), since the 3' terminal region of the RAV-1 genome does not share homology with any endogenous virus sequence (Neiman et al. 1977; Coffin et al. 1978). The specificity of this probe is demonstrated by the complete absence of ev-related fragments in lane D. The tumor DNA shows three distinct bands; two of these are identical to TS bands

detected by cDNA$_{rep}$, and the third was presumably obscured by ev-1 in the cDNA$_{rep}$ hybridization.

Since SacI has a single site in proviral DNA, the fragment size is determined not only by the location of this site in viral genome but also by the nearest enzyme cleavage site in the flanking cellular sequence. Therefore, SacI can provide information concerning the integration site of proviral DNA. On the other hand, there are several cleavage sites for EcoRI in the viral genome allowing for the probing of internal structural arrangement of proviral DNA (Fig. 1a). In addition, the ev sequences lack the two outer sites (indicated by open circles) which are present in the exogenous proviral DNA. Consequently, either the 1.4-md or 0.7-md fragment can be used to demonstrate the integration of infecting virus. As shown in lane E and F, the 1.4-md fragment is present in infected but not in uninfected cells.

C. Results

I. Preleukosis

Analysis of SacI-cleaved DNA from bursal specimens obtained at 4 weeks post infection showed a complete absence of TS bands (Fig. 2a). This was not due to inefficient infection of target tissue because the RAV-1 specific 1.4-md EcoRI fragment could be clearly identified at this stage in the inoculated (I) samples (Fig. 2b). Since the TS bands contain viral-cell junction sequences, their absence indicates that proviral DNA integrates in multiple sites in cellular genome. The data in Fig. 2b also provide an estimate of the extent of infection in the target organ at this early stage; based on the relative intensities of the RAV-1 (1.4-md fragment) and ev fragments, at least 25% of the bursal tissue had been infected at the 4 week stage. The analysis of bursal DNA from specimens 8 weeks after infection gave similar results (data not shown) except that the extent of infection was greater.

II. Leukosis

In contrast, SacI-cleaved tumor DNAs from all 16 chickens showed new bands. The results are summarized in Table 1 and gel patterns of representative tumor samples are shown in Fig. 3. In some instances (e.g., 3, 4, and 5 in Fig. 3a) the TS bands were very faint as detected by $cDNA_{rep}$. However, they could be readily detected using a highly specific $cDNA_{3'}$ probe (Fig. 3b). These data taken together with the observation in the preceding section indicating multiplicity of integration sites suggest that only a small population of the infected cells develops into a tumor and the origin of tumor, therefore, must be clonal.

The results also show a size variation of TS bands in different tumors suggesting that integration in a number of sites can lead to the development of a tumor. However, the other equally plausible but not mutually exclusive possibility is that deletion within the proviral DNA contributes to size variation. This possibility was examined using a DNA_{gag} probe for hybridization (Fig. 3c). Most striking are the results of tumor DNAs 2 and 5 where DNA_{gag} failed to detect any TS bands, although these bands were readily detectable by $cDNA_{3'}$. This immediately suggests that gag sequences in the proviral DNA of these tumors have been deleted.

Further evidence for the deletion of gag

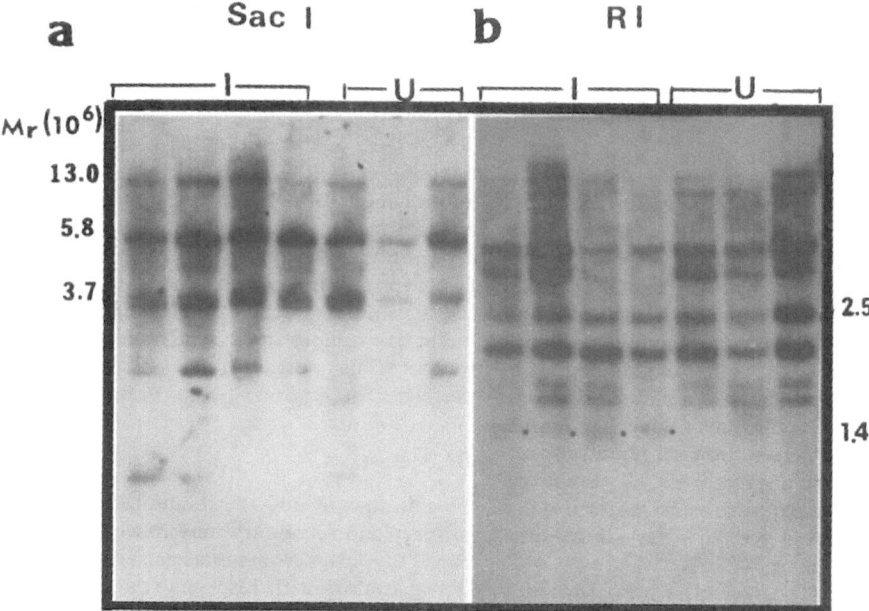

Fig. 2. The structure of proviral DNA in bursa tissues at the preleukosis stage. The DNA samples extracted from the bursae of the uninoculated *(U)* or inoculated *(I)* animals at 4 weeks post inoculation were digested with SacI or EcoRI and analyzed by hybridization with $cDNA_{rep}$

Table 1

Sample	Tissue	TS fragment[a] (SacI/3′)	Right end[b] cell-viral junction (EcoRI/5′)	Deletion and insertion, etc.
1	Bursa	5.8, 4.5, 4.3	1.1, 0.9	−
2	Bursa	8.0, 4.7	ND[c]	−
3	Bursa	8.0	2.3	RI–1.4 (−)[d], gag (Δ)[e]
4	Bursa	5.2, 4.5	1.7	RI–1.4 (−)
5	Bursa	5.3, 4.5, 2.9	2.8, 1.7	RI–1.4 (−), gag (Δ)
6	Bursa	5.8, 5.5	1.7	−
7	Bursa	5.8, 4.8, 4.5 3.0	1.7, 1.58	RI–1.4 (−)
8	Bursa	6.0	0.8	−
9	Bursa	9.0, 5.3	2.1	−
10	Bursa	2.5	2.3, 2.0	RI–1.4 (−)
11	Bursa	8.0, 7.8, 7.5	0.6	−
	Liver	8.0	2.3, 2.0	RI–1.4 (−)
12	Bursa	8.0, 4.0	1.43	RI–1.4 (−)
13	Bursa	5.0	ND	RI–1.4 (−), gag (Δ)
14	Bursa	4.5, 1.2	1.7	−
15	Bursa	8.0, 4.8, 4.2	2.8, 2.6	RI–1.4 (−), Insertion[f]
16	Bursa	−	0.6	RI–1.4 (−)

[a] TS fragment is defined as the SacI fragment which can be detected only in the tumor tissue and is hybridizable to cDNA$_{3'}$. Molecular weight in 10^6 daltons
[b] Right-end cell-viral junction fragment is defined as the EcoRI fragment which hybridizes only to cDNA$_{5'}$ but not to cDNA$_{rep}$
[c] ND = Not determined
[d] EcoRI viral specific 1.4×10^6 fragment is absent
[e] gag gene is deleted
[f] Insertion of a stretch of cellular sequence ca. 2.4×10^6 at the left end, which replaces the gag gene

sequences from these DNAs was provided by an experiment in which EcoRI-cleaved tumor DNA was hybridized with a cDNA$_{5'}$ probe (Fig. 3d). As shown in Fig. 1a, cDNA$_{5'}$ can detect the right end viral-cell junction fragment and the 1.4-md gag-containing fragment. Indeed, in tumor DNAs 2, 3, and 5 (Fig. 3d), the 1.4-md fragment is completely missing. A survey of all 16 chickens (Table 1) demonstrates that deletions in the viral genome occur rather frequently in tumor DNA. Some of these deletions are quite extensive; for instance, tumor DNA 5 contains very little viral sequence other than the LTR.

Hybridization with cDNA$_{5'}$ also provides a more reliable information concerning the right end integration site of proviral DNA, since the results are not influenced by extensive deletions in the viral genome. The size heterogeneity of the end fragments (indicated by dots in Fig. 3d; also see Table 1) clearly argues for a multiplicity of integration sites. However, it is noteworthy that some fragment sizes are more prevalent than others, i.e., 1.7 md in five tumors and 2.3 md in another three tumors. This suggests that there may be preferred integration sites for tumorigenesis.

III. Metastasis

To gain insight into the relationship between primary and secondary tumors we have compared the DNA from metastasized tissues and bursal tumors with respect to proviral DNA sequences. The results (Fig. 4a) show striking similarity in KpnI-derived TS band patterns from liver and bursa, suggesting that primary and secondary tumors share the same clonal

448

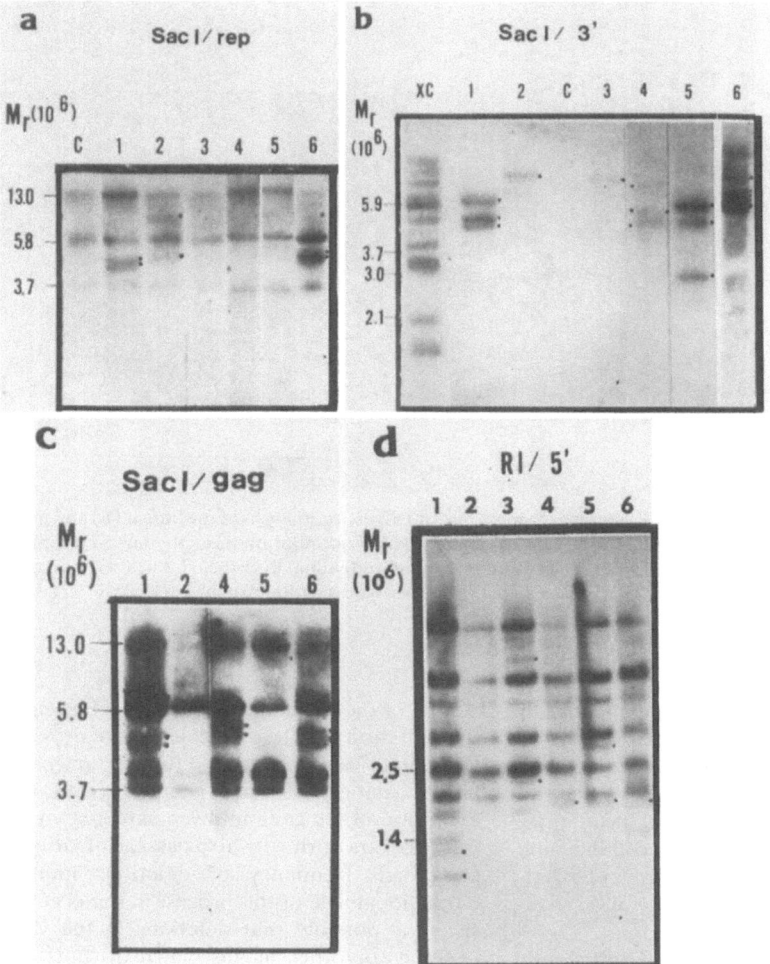

Fig. 3. The structure of proviral DNA in bursa tumor. The DNA samples isolated from the bursal tumors developed in animals Nos. 1 to 6 were digested with SacI or EcoRI and analyzed as described in legend to Fig. 1. The hybridization probes employed are cDNA$_{rep}$ **a)**, cDNA$_{3'}$ **(b)**, DNA$_{gag}$ **(c)**, and cDNA$_{5'}$ **(d)**. *Lane C* in either **a** or **b** shows SacI digested thymus DNA isolated from animal No. 2, which was included as a control sample for nontumorous tissue. XC represents EcoRI-cleaved high-molecular-weight DNA from Rous sarcoma virus transformed XC cells, which serves as a molecular size marker

origin. Furthermore, Fig. 4b shows that different liver foci (L1 to L4) from another chicken have identical band patterns which indicates that individual foci derive from a single clonal population. The figure also shows that liver foci have a single SacI-TS band while in bursa there were at least three closely spaced TS bands (Fig. 4b). This suggests that only one of the original multiple tumor clones in bursa was selected for secondary spread.

D. Discussion

As a first step toward characterization of the oncogenes, we have employed EcoRI digestion of tumor DNA in conjunction with cDNA$_{5'}$ hybridization to specifically identify the right end cell-viral junction (i.e., integration sites) of ALV proviruses. Among 16 tumors analyzed, at least ten different size classes could be identified. However, a few size

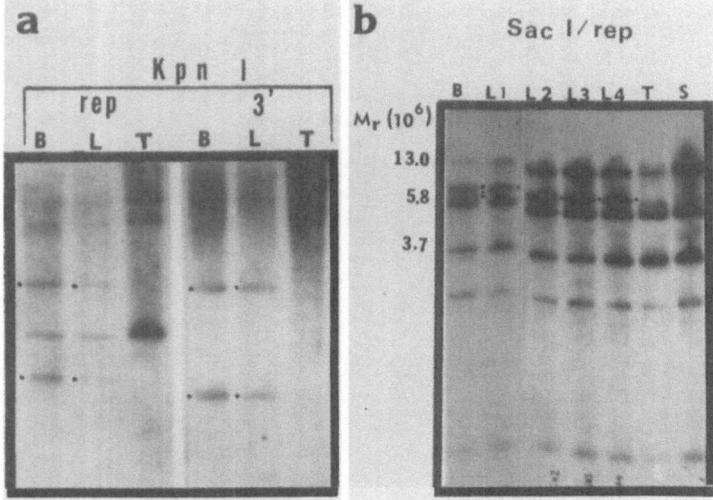

Fig. 4. The structure of proviral DNA in metastic tumors. **a** KpnI digestion analysis of the bursal *(B)* and liver *(L)* tumor DNA of animal No. 8. Included as control is the DNA from nontumorous thymus *(T)*. **b** SacI digestion analysis of the DNA isolated from the bursa *(B)* and four individual liver foci *(L1* to *L4)* of animal No. 12. Nontumorous thymus DNA *(T)* is used as a control. The hybridization probe is cDNA$_{rep}$

classes, e.g., 1.7 md and 2.3 md, appeared to be more prevalent than others. If size variation truly reflects the sequence diversity of the integration sites, our data suggest that all tumors are not the consequence of the integration of provirus into a unique cellular site. Similar conclusions have been drawn by Neiman et al. (1980) from their study of ALV-induced tumors.

Although our sampling is not sufficiently large to give a reliable estimate of the total number of integration sites in the entire genome, the observation that cell-viral junction fragments of identical sizes are present in many tumors does indicate a certain degree of specificity of integration of proviral DNA. Our data, therefore, are consistent with the view that there are a limited number of gene(s) which, upon activation by provirus, could trigger the transformation process. Whether this gene(s) is involved directly in the initiation of transformation·process (in a manner similar to the src gene product) or indirectly in the induction of a transforming protein awaits further characterization. To further understand the nature of the downstream sequence, we have recently obtained a clone-purified SacI-TS sequence from two of the tumors, and experiments are underway to characterize their structures.

One of the striking features in our finding is the detection of extensive deletions of proviral DNA in at least 35% of the tumors analyzed. Since deletion of viral genome (with the exception of src gene in avian sarcoma virus) rarely occurs during in vitro passage of viruses, such high frequency of deletions implies a functional role of this process in tumorgenesis. It is possible that deletions in the viral genome (or other means which disrupts the transcriptional program of viral RNA) facilitate the downstream promotion by the right LTR. This possibility is particularly attractive in view of the fact that the two LTRs flanking the viral genome are strong promotors for RNA transcription (Tsichlis and Coffin 1980) and the left end LTR directs the synthesis of viral genomic and messenger RNA (Weiss et al. 1977). Although the functional state of the right LTR remains to be determined, a not unlikely possibility is that it is normally masked by the ongoing RNA synthesis which starts at the left LTR and extends into the 5' sequence of the right LTR (Yamamoto et al. 1980). However, a disruption of the transcriptional program affected by deletions in the proviral DNA may expose the right LTR, facilitate the RNA polymerase binding, allow efficient transcription of the downstream cellular sequence, and activate gene(s) involved in onco-genesis. The detection of novel mRNA species (W. Hayward, see this volume; G. Payne and H. E. Varmus, personal communication) carrying the viral promotor joined with cellular sequences lends further support to this notion.

The deletion of viral sequence may also play a role in the selective growth of the tumor clones. The first sign of lymphocyte transformation after avian leukosis virus inoculation is the appearance of enlarged follicles in the Bursa of Fabricius at 8 weeks of age (Cooper et al. 1968). These enlarged follicles, identified only at the microscopic level, are believed to be the descendents of a single transformed cell and the precursors to the terminal tumors. They number 10 to 100 per infected bursa (Neiman et al. 1979); the terminal tumor follicles, however, are much fewer (i.e., only one or two). This observation led to the suggestion that some of the transformed clones regressed and only a small fraction acquired the ability to develop into tumor. We would like to speculate that deletion of viral genome which stops the synthesis and expression of the viral antigens (especially exogenous virus specific *env* product) on the cell surface would render the cell less immunogenic and furnish it with the ability to cope with the host immunity. Since in this study, due to the reagents and methods employed, most of the deletions are mapped near the gag region, it is likely that more extensive analysis would reveal deletions in other regions as well.

Irrespective of the implication of deletion of provirus in the tumorigenic process, it is evident from our data that the presence of a complete provirus and, hence, virus production is not required at the terminal stage of the tumor. This finding lends further support to the hypothesis that the oncogene(s) involved in the maintenance of cells in the transformed and tumorous state is (are) of cellular rather than of viral origin.

The characteristic proviral DNA structure of each tumor as revealed by SacI digestion provides strong evidence that LL tumors are clonal growth and that primary and secondary tumors share common clonal origin. Furthermore, the metastic tumor consists of a subpopulation of the primary tumor. The factors which dictate the metastatic potential of the primary tumor cells are currently unclear, though deletion of the provirus of the tumor cell may enhance such potential, since we found that the provirus in almost all the metastatic tumors carries extensive deletions.

Acknowledgments

This research was supported in part by a grant from the National Cancer Institute (CA 24798-01) to H.J.K. S.K.D. is a Leukemia Society of America Scholar. We thank Ms. Sue Uselton for excellent technical assistance in the preparation of the manuscript.

References

Astrin S (1978) Proc Natl Acad Sci USA 75:5941–5945 – Coffin JC, Champion M, Chabot F (1978) J Virol 28:972–991 – Cooper MD, Payne LN, Dent PB, Burmester BR, Good RA (1968) 373–389 – Friedrich R, Kung HJ, Baker B, Varmus HE, Goodman HM, Bishop JM (1977) Virology :198–215 – Haseltine WA, Kleid DG, Panet A, Rothenberg E, Baltimore D (1976) J Mol Biol 106:109–131 – Hughes SH, Shank PR, Spector DH, Kung HJ, Bishop JM, Varmus HE, Vogt PK, Breitman ML (1978) Cell 15:1397–1410 – Neiman PE, Das S, McMillin-Helsel C (1977) Cell 11:321–329 – Neiman PE, Payne LN, Jordan L, Weiss RA (1979) In: Viruses in naturally occuring cancer, vol 7. Cold Spring Harbor Laboratory. New York – Neiman P, Payne LN, Weiss RA (1980) J Virol 34:178–186 – Rigby PWJ, Dieckmann M, Rhodes C, Berg P (1977) J Mol Biol 113:237–251 – Southern EM (1975) J Mol Biol 98:503–517 – Tal J, Kung H-J, Varmus HE, Bishop JM (1977) Virology 79:183–197 – Taylor JM, Illmensee RI, Tausal LR, Summers J (1976) In: Baltimore D, Huang AS, Fox CF (eds) Animal Virology. Academic, New York, pp 161–173 – Tsichlis P, Coffin J (1980) J Virol 33:238–249 – Weiss SR, Varmus HE, Bishop JM (1977) Cell 12:983 – Yamamoto T, Jay G, Pastan I (1980) Proc Natl Acad Sci USA 77:176–180

Haematology and Blood Transfusion Vol. 26
Modern Trends in Human Leukemia IV
Edited by Neth, Gallo, Graf, Mannweiler, Winkler
© Springer-Verlag Berlin Heidelberg 1981

Studies of the Association of Leukemogenic and Oncogenic Properties in Avian Leukemia Viruses

H.-C. Löliger, D. von dem Hagen, and W. Hartmann

A. Introduction

The transmission of avian leukosis virus (ALV) in chickens doesn't cause only leukosis, but also nonleucocytic neoplasias (Carr 1960; Graf and Berg 1978; Löliger 1964). After inoculation with avian myeloblastosis virus (AMV), kidney tumors (nephroblastomas) and osteopetrosis or osteosarcomas distinctly different to leukemia may develope in the infected, susceptible chickens. The nephroblastomas, which might be compared with the Wilm's tumor in man, are mostly consisting of different neoplastic cellformations, such as cystoma, adenoma, endothelioma, hemangioma and fibrocytic neoplasias. It is not known that other avian tumor viruses, which don't belong to the ALV group, such as the Marek's disease herpes virus (MDHV), reveal a similar tumor spectrum.

Investigations to separate and characterize the non leucocytic tumor factors (Ogura et al. 1974; Smith and Moscovici 1969) might suggest that this factor of the AMLV is not identical with the leucocytic factor but belongs to the same ALV subgroup antigens A and B. In order to determine the susceptibility of chicken lines having different homozygous cell type properties – c/A, c/B, c/AB, c/O – for AMLV, we investigated the development of leucocytic and nonleucocytic neoplasias in the individual chicken lines to clarify the following:

1. Influence of the chicken lines on incidence and type of the leucocytic and the nonleucocytic neoplasias;
2. Identification of the leucotic and non leucocytic tumor inducing factors in the standard AMLV by differential susceptibility of host cells to ALV subgroups; and

3. Comparison of the tumor development in chicken following experimental infection with AMLV and MDHV.

B. Material and Methods

I. Chicken Lines

The following lines were used: Leghorn line R with sublines celltype c/0, c/A and c/AB;
2. Leghorn line M with sublines celltype c/0 and c/AB;
3. Leghorn line G with subline celltype c/B;
4. Line UM of dysgammaglobulinemic chicken, celltype c/0; and
5. SPAFAS line, free from endogenous ALV, celltype c/0.

The homozygoty of celltype properties were tested by challenge with RSV BH-RAV-1 and BH-RAV-2 (14).

II. Virus Strains

Standard avian myeloblastosis virus (AMV) – strain BAI-A – were obtained by Dr. Bauer, Giessen; – also used was MDHV, strain Celle. Chickens were infected by the intraperitoneal route within 48 h after hatching with the plasma of birds with acute AMV leukemia or the whole blood of birds with acute Marek's disease. The observation extended over 140 days in the first trial and 112 days in the second.

III. Clinical and Pathomorphological Observations

Blood smears and hematocrit were taken from the chicks at the 11th, 15th and 21st day after infection and from moribund chicken before killing. Autopsies were performed on all dead chickens. Touching smears of bone marrow and histologic preparation from bone marrow, liver, bursa, and kidney were done.

C. Results and Discussion

Leukemia and nephroblastomas developed after infection with standard AMV in chickens of all the tested lines homozygous for celltype c/0, c/A, and c/B, but not for cell type c/AB. MDHV induced only lymphoid cell reticulosis, but no leukosis, nephroblastomas, or osteosarcomas within 20 weeks (Table 1).

Pretumorous lesions in the kidney by proliferation of capillary endothel and retothelial cells in the nephron can already be observed in 3-week-old chicks. Gross lesions with clinical symptoms and death by nephroblastoma occur at the earliest at 56 days and mostly between 70 and 112 days after infection. In general leucocytic lesions are not present in chickens older than 50 days (Fig. 1).

Table 1. Incidence of leukemia, nephroblastoma (incl. ovarycystoma), and osteosarcoma in chickens of various lines and different cell susceptibility for the ALV subgroup viruses after experimental inoculation with standard AMV at 1 day age. Observation time: 112 and 140 days

chicken			leukemia complex %			Nephrobl. %	Osteosarc.[a] %	Total %
Line	Cell type	n	Anemia	Erythrobl.	Stemc.-1.			
R	C/0	59	0	0	57.6	35.6	0	93.2
R	C/A	58	0	0	22.4	48.3	1.7	70.7
R	C/AB	46	0	0	0	0	0	0
M	C/0	51	0	0	68.6	25.5	7.8	94.1
M	C/AB	84	0	0	0	0	0	0
G	C/B	58	0	0	8.6	32.8	0	41.4
UM	C/0	146	4.8	0	89.7	4.8	22.6	99.3
SPAFAS	C/0	18	11.1	44.4	11.1	33.3	16.7	100.0

[a] Osteosarcoma occurs together with leukosis or nephroblastoma

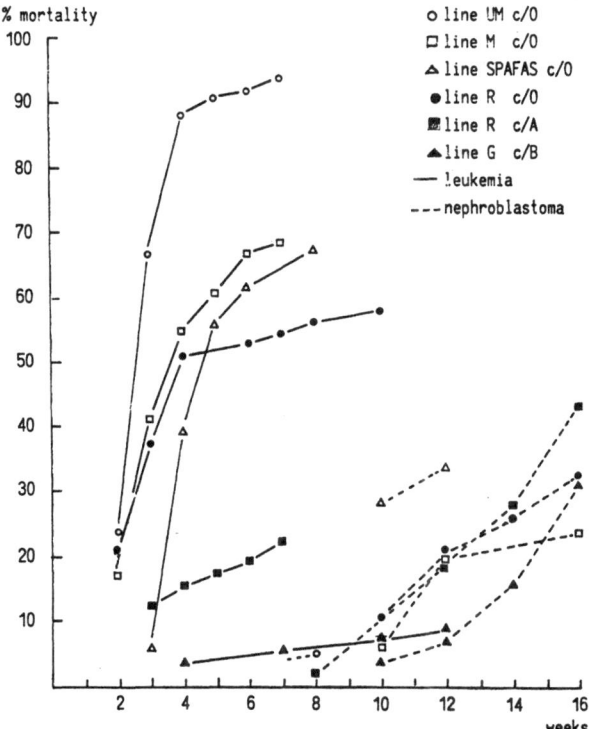

Fig. 1. Development of leukemia and leucocytic neoplasias (nephroblastoma) in chicken of different lines after infection with standard AMV

Osteopetrosis and osteosarcomas occur most often in chicken of lines M, UM, and SPAFAS. Osteosarcomas were observed in young chicken with acute stem cell leukemia as well as in older pullets with nephroblastomas (Table 1).

The frequency of clinic-evident nephroblastomas increases at low frequency of acute leukemia among the young chickens. AMV-infected susceptible chicks, which survive the acute leukemia stage, sicken mostly at a high percentage for nephroblastomas (Fig. 1).

In susceptible chickens of lines R, M, and G the acute stage of AMV infection is evident from agranulocytic stem cell leukemia at 2 to 5 weeks after infection. Among the dysgammaglobulinemic chicken of line UM the first stage observed within 12–15 days was an aplastic anemia with medullar fibrosis which was followed by the stem cell leukemia stage. In the SPAFAS chicken at first an erythroblastosis occurs, followed by stem cell leukemia and later by chronic nephroblastomas (Table 1).

These results indicate that leukemic lesions, nephroblastomas of mixed cell type, and osteosarcomas are caused only by the RNA avian leukosis viruses. Within AMLV both subgroup antigens A and B comprise leukemogenic and nonleucocytic tumor properties. The target cell of these seems to be the pluripotential retothelial cell of mesenchymal origin in the young chicks.

The kind of evident lesions, i.e., leukemia or nonleucocytic tumors, depends on the pathogenicity or amount of the infective agent and on the genetical susceptibility of the retothelial target cells. The more intensive the early hemoblastic disorders (aplastic or leukemic) in the host, the lower is the chance of development of nonleucocytic tumors, especial the late nephroblastomas, by neoplastic transformation of other cells with AMV-infected retothelial cells.

Basing on these etiologic relationships between leukemias, nephroblastomas and osteopetrosis or osteosarcomas in chickens it might be allowed to inaugurate, speculatively, similar etiologic relationships between the leukemias. Wilm's kidney tumors and osteosarcoma in man, especially in young man. This comparative speculation is the mind of our contribution about the association of leucemogenic and oncogenic properties in avian leukemia viruses.

References

Carr JG (1960) Kidney carcinomas of the fowl induced by the MH$_2$ reticulo-endothelioma virus. Br J Cancer 14:77–82 – Graf T, Beug H (1978) Avian leukemia viruses; interaction with their target cells in vivo and in vitro. Biochem Biophys Acta 516:269–299 – Löliger HC (1964) Atypische Veränderungen in den Nieren von Hühnern nach experimenteller Infektion mit einem übertragbaren Leukosestamm. Dt Tierärztl. Wschr 68:517–521 – Ogura H, Gelderblom H, Bauer H (1974) Isolation of avian nephroblastoma virus from avian myeloblastosis virus by the infectious DNA technique. Intervirology 4:69–76 – Smith RE, Moscovici C (1969) The oncogenic effects of nontransforming viruses from avian Myeloblastosis virus. Cancer Res 29:1356–1366

Haematology and Blood Transfusion Vol. 26
Modern Trends in Human Leukemia IV
Edited by Neth, Gallo, Graf, Mannweiler, Winkler
© Springer-Verlag Berlin Heidelberg 1981

Genetic Approaches Toward Elucidating the Mechanisms of Type-C Virus-Induced Leukemia

S. A. Aaronson, M. Barbacid, C. Y. Dunn, and E. P. Reddy

A. Introduction

Type-C RNA viruses may be horizontally transmitted as infectious cancer-inducing viruses or vertically transmitted from one generation to the next, often in an unexpressed form, within the host genome (for review see Aaronson and Stephenson 1976). To date the translational products of three leukemia viral genes have been identified (Baltimore 1975). The *gag* gene product is a polyprotein precursor that undergoes cleavage to form the major nonglycosylated viral structural proteins, which for mammalian type-C viruses are p30, p15, p12, and p10. It has been possible to determine that the information within the murine viral *gag* gene is arranged 5'-p15-p12-p30-p10-3' (Barbacid et al. 1976). The products of the *pol* and *env* genes are, respectively, the viral reverse transcriptase and a precursor protein containing the major envelope glycoproteins, gp70 and p15E. Evidence primarily from the avian system indicates that the type-C viral genes are ordered 5'-*gag-pol-env*-3' (for review see Wang et al. 1976).

The lack of an in vitro transformation assay for type-C helper leukemia viruses has so far impaired efforts to elucidate the mechanisms by which these viruses cause tumor development in the animal. Thus, it is not known whether there exists a discrete viral gene that codes for a product that transforms a specific target cell population or whether the malignant potential of these viruses is exerted through a more indirect mechanism. The present report reviews biologic approaches currently underway within our laboratory to elucidate the mechanisms by which murine type-C viruses induce leukemia.

B. Results

I. Lymphoid Cell Targets for Transformation by Rauscher and Moloney MuLV Strains

In an effort to study target cells for leukemia induction by murine leukemia virus (MuLV), we analyzed the kinetics of tumor formation and the histopathology of tumors induced by clonal strains of two oncogenic replication-competent mouse type-C viruses, Rauscher and Moloney MuLV. The susceptibility of newborn NIH/Swiss mice to tumor induction by each virus was comparable. Gross enlargement of spleen and lymph nodes occurred as early as 10–11 weeks following inoculation of 5×10^4 XC pfu of either virus. As few as 5×10^2 XC pfu of each virus were capable of causing 50% mortality within 23 weeks. With Rauscher MuLV affected organs invariably included the spleen and (less frequently) liver and peripheral or visceral lymph nodes. Thymic involvement was not detected in 50 tumor-bearing animals examined. In contrast, Moloney MuLV caused gross evidence of tumor involvement of the thymus in the majority of animals. Other lymphoid organs were also affected at high frequency. Histopathologic analysis of tumors revealed no obvious differences in the morphology of the neoplastic lymphoid cells.

II. Distribution of T and B Cell Markers Associated with MuLV-Induced Tumors

As seen in Table 1, Moloney MuLV induced tumors and lymphoma cell lines exhibited Thy. 1 antigen in the absence of detectable Fc or C3 receptors, indicating their T cell origin. Rauscher MuLV primary tumors and lymphoma

Table 1. T and B lymphoid markers on cell membranes of cultured Rauscher MuLV and Moloney MuLV-induced lymphoma cell lines[a]

Lymphoma cell line	% Positive cells		
	Thy.1 antigen	Fc receptor	C'3 receptor
Rauscher MuLV induced			
6E	<1	95	<2
13-2-6	<1	89	<2
13-1	<1	94	<2
Moloney MuLV induced			
19-1-2	>99	<1	<2
19-1-5	>99	<1	<2
P1798	>99	<1	<2
L691 (spontaneous)	>99	<1	<2
129J (X-ray)	>99	<1	<2
Normal spleen	45	47	42

[a] The assays for Thy. 1 antigen and Fc and C'3 receptors were performed as described previously (Reddy et al. 1980). In the Fc receptor assay, SRBC alone did not yield rosettes. In the C'3 receptor assay, SRBC alone or SRBC coated with SRBC antibody did not give rosettes

cell lines of the same mouse strain, however, invariably exhibited Fc receptors in the absence of Thy.1 antigen, suggesting that these tumors were of the B lymphoid lineage. The pattern of immunoglobulin synthesis by individual Rauscher MuLV tumor cell lines was determined by both biosynthetic and radioimmunologic techniques. Rauscher MuLV lymphoma lines generally expressed immunoglobulin heavy (μ) chain in the absence of detectable light (●——● or λ) chains. These findings established that the target of neoplastic transformation in response to Rauscher MuLV is an immature cell within the B lymphoid lineage (Burrows et al. 1979; Siden et al. 1979).

III. Generation of Recombinants Between Oncogenic and Nononcogenic Mouse Type-C Viruses in Tissue Culture

An important approach toward defining viral genes required for transformation might result from the generation of recombinants between oncogenic and nononcogenic type-C viruses or between oncogenic viruses with different targets for transformation. We initially set out to obtain recombinants between a prototype ts mutant of the oncogenic Rauscher strain of MuLV (Stephenson and Aaronson 1973) and the endogenous xenotropic BALB:virus-2. Use of these viruses permitted the design of

a protocol for recombinant virus isolation based upon specific virus growth requirements (Aaronson and Barbacid 1980). By assay at 39°C on NIH/3T3 cells, the replication of the ts mutant and xenotropic parental viruses, respectively, was effectively blocked. However, recombinants possessing Rauscher MuLV envelope functions and BALB:virus-2 sequences in genes affected by the ts lesions might be expected to grow efficiently in mouse cells at the nonpermissive temperature.

To generate potential recombinant viruses, we utilized a wild mouse embryo cell line, WM-C, which was permissive for replication of certain mouse xenotropic viruses. WM-C cells were first chronically infected with BALB:virus-2 and then superinfected with the Rauscher MuLV ts mutant at the permissive temperature (31°C). The mutant utilized, ts 25, represented a class known to accumulate noncleaved *gag* gene precursors at the nonpermissive temperature, 39°C (Stephenson et al. 1975). To control for mutant leakiness or reversion, WM-C cells were infected with the mutant alone and passaged under identical conditions. After 4 weeks, virus released from each culture was tested for infectivity for NIH/3T3 cells at the restrictive temperature. Only if the infectivity of the virus at 39°C was significantly enhanced by passage of the mutant through WM-C cells replicating the xenotropic virus were individual virus clones selected by the microtiter procedure for further analysis.

IV. Immunologic Identification of Recombinant Viruses

Type-specific antigenic determinants have been readily demonstrated in the p15 and p12 *gag* gene coded proteins as well as in the reverse transcriptase and envelope glycoprotein (gp70) of mouse leukemia viruses (for review see Stephenson et al. 1977). Furthermore, using appropriate antisera, type-specific determinants have also been demonstrated even in the more broadly immunoreactive proteins such as p30 (Boiocchi and Nowinski 1978) and p10 (M. Barbacid and S. A. Aaronson, unpublished observations).

We submitted clonal viruses isolated according to the above protocol to immunologic analysis. The origin of the viral sequences of each recombinant virus was determined by the ability of its respective gene products to compete in corresponding Rauscher MuLV or BALB:virus-2 homologous radioimmunoassays. The results, summarized in Figure 1, indicate the generation of individual recombinants that contained different amounts of genetic information of each parent. In some cases, as with rec 25e–8, recombination appeared to involve more than one cross-over.

V. Oncogenicity of Recombinants Between Rauscher MuLV and Balb:Virus-2

We have investigated the biologic properties of some of the recombinant viruses so far generated. Their infectivity in tissue culture for NIH/3T3 cells was found to be similar (data not shown). However we observed striking differences in their ability to infect and replicate in newborn NIH/Swiss mice. As shown in Table 1, the Rauscher MuLV parental virus induced readily detectable levels of MuLV p30 in serum within 5 months with as few as 10 XC pfu inoculated. Rec 25b–14 showed almost comparable infectivity. In contrast, recombinants, including rec 25c–3, rec 25d–22, and rec 25e–8, were markedly less able to induce sustained virus replication in vivo. It should be noted that these viruses each contain substantially more genetic information of the xenotropic parental virus than did rec 25b–14. The ability of a given virus to chronically replicate in vivo was highly predictive of subsequent tumor formation. As shown in Table 2, both Rauscher MuLV and rec 25b–14 induced tumors by 10 months with as few as 10^2 XC pfu inoculated, whereas each of the other recombi-

GENETIC MAPPING OF *IN VITRO* GENERATED RECOMBINANTS
BETWEEN RAUSCHER-MuLV ts 25 AND BALB:VIRUS 2

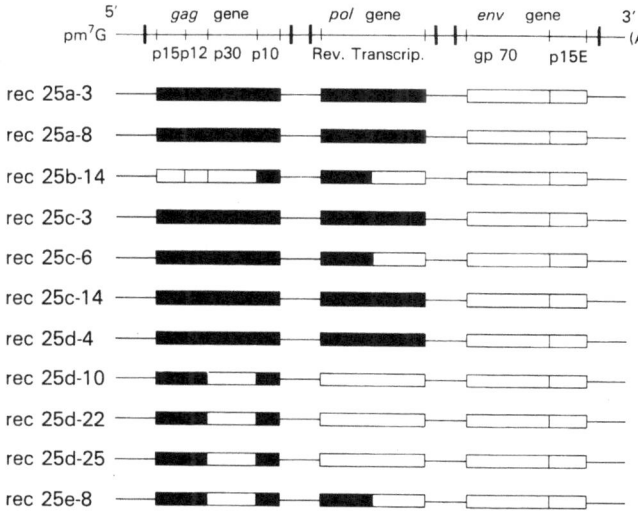

Fig. 1. Proteins exhibiting parental Rauscher-MuLV (☐) or BALB:virus-2 (▰) antigenic determinants are indicated. Where intracistronic crossing-overs are depicted, the relative localization and extent of Rauscher-MuLv and BALB:virus-2 derived genetic information have been arbitrarily assigned

457

Table 2. In vivo growth and oncogenicity of recombinants between Rauscher MuLV and BALB:virus-2

Virus	In vivo infectivity[a] MuLV p30 in serum at 5 months[b]				Tumorigenicity Tumor at 10 months[b]		
	XC pfu inoculated				XC pfu inoculated		
	10^4	10^3	10^2	10^1	10^4	10^3	10^2
Rauscher MuLV	10/10	10/10	10/10	7/10	9/10	7/7	3/7
rec 25b-14	10/10	10/10	9/10	1/10	5/9	5/7	1/8
rec 25c-3	0/10	ND	ND	ND	0/9	ND	ND
rec 25d-22	7/10	0/10	ND	ND	0/10	ND	ND
rec 25e-8	0/10	ND	ND	ND	0/10	ND	ND

[a] NIH/Swiss mice were injected at birth with 0.2 ml of the appropriate virus dilution
[b] Animals positive/total animals inoculated

nant viruses tested was at least 100-fold less tumorigenic.

C. Discussion

The present studies demonstrate that the target cells for transformation by two clonal mouse leukemia virus strains, Rauscher and Moloney MuLV, contain markers that differentiate them readily within the lymphoid cell lineage. Our finding that Moloney MuLV caused tumors in NIH/Swiss mice containing T but not B cell markers (Reddy et al. 1980) confirms previous studies indicating that T cells are the in vivo target for transformation by this virus (Moloney 1960). Rauscher MuLV tumors of the same strain, tested either directly or as cell lines established in culture, invariably contained markers of B lymphoid cells. This in combination with their lack of Thy. 1 antigen, a well established marker of T lymphoid cells, provides the first demonstration of a B cell target for neoplastic transformation by a replication-competent MuLV (Reddy et al. 1980).

Among the most important biologic questions pertaining to replication-competent type-C viruses concerns the mechanism by which they cause neoplasia. Recombinants generated and characterized in this report should be useful in determining what regions of the viral genome are essential for oncogenicity. Our preliminary data indicate that recombinant viruses, which have a similar capacity to infect and replicate in mouse cells in tissue culture, show striking differences in their abilities to replicate and induce tumors in the animal. In collaborative studies with P. Arnstein (National Cancer Institute), it has been possible to show that each recombinant virus was capable of inducing tumors in (Nu/Nu) mice on an NIH/Swiss genetic background. Under the same conditions only the parental Rauscher MuLV and rec 25b–14 produced tumors in (Nu+/Nu) heterozygous mice. These results indicate that the ability of the host to mount an immune response plays an important role in the ability of recombinant viruses to replicate in the mouse. Further studies will be necessary to dissect other host genetic factors that may also influence the expression of the viruses in vivo. Nonetheless, our studies to date argue for the importance of active virus replication in order for mouse type-C viruses to induce disease in their host.

Leukemia viruses might be postulated to induce transformation as a result of their site of integration or due to their coding for a specific transforming gene product from an already identified structural gene or an as yet unidentified transforming gene. Accumulating evidence indicates that there is no specificity with respect to the site of virus integration. This conclusion is derived both from analysis of the arrangement of added viral information in the cellular genome of individual virus-induced leukemias (Canaani and Aaronson 1979; Steffen and Weinberg 1978) and by DNA sequence analysis of cellular junctions of individual molecularly cloned integrated DNA proviruses (McClements et al. 1980; Shimotohno et al. 1980). Recently, Hayward (this volume) has obtained evidence that at least some cellular messages found in leukemia virus transformants contain information of the viral large terminal redundancy (LTR) in the absence of detectable information derived from the rest of the viral genome. This has led to the hypothesis that a viral promoter in the LTR may be responsible for transformation by causing derepression of a cellular gene by means of "downstream" promotion. If this hypothesis were correct, the transformation of different target cells by Rauscher and Moloney MuLV would have to be explained on the basis of differences in susceptibility of target cells for virus infection.

The possibility that the leukemia virus mediates its transforming action on the host by means of one or more of its gene products must also be considered. To date, there is no direct evidence that the leukemia virus contains a discrete transforming gene that codes for a nonviral structural transforming gene product. However, continued genetic analysis will be necessary to completely exclude this possibility. It has been postulated that viral structural products, specifically the *env* gene product, gp70, may directly (McGrath and Weissman 1979) or indirectly (Lee and Ihle 1979) cause chronic blastogenesis of lymphoid cells. This chronic antigenic stimulation of cell division has been postulated to result in the eventual selection of a spontaneously transformed clone. Our findings argue that blastogenesis in response to different leukemia viruses would have to be very specific if this mechanism were to explain the reproducibly distinct lymphoid cell targets for transformation by different leukemia viruses. Studies are presently underway to generate recombinants between Rauscher and Moloney MuLV. Such recombinants may make it possible to map the region within the viral genome responsible for transformation of specific lymphoid cell populations and shed further light on the mechanisms by which these viruses induce malignancy.

References

Aaronson SA, Barbacid M (1980) Viral genes involved in leukemogenesis. I. Generation of recombinants between oncogenic and nononcogenic mouse type-C viruses in tissue culture. J Exp Med 151:467–480 – Aaronson SA, Stephenson JR (1976) Endogenous type-C RNA viruses of mammalian cells. Biochim Biophys Acta 458:323–354 – Baltimore D (1975) Tumor Viruses: 1974. Cold Spring Harbor Symp Quant Biol 39:1187–1200 – Barbacid M, Stephenson JR, Aaronson SA (1976) The gag gene of mammalian type-C RNA tumor viruses. Nature 262:554–559 – Boiocchi M, Nowinski RC (1978) Polymorphism in the major core protein (p30) of murine leukemia viruses as identified by mouse antisera. Virology 84:530–535 – Burrows P, LeJeune M, Kearney JF (1979) Evidence that pre-B cells synthesize μheavy chains but no light chains. Nature 280:838–841 – Canaani E, Aaronson SA (1979) Restriction enzyme analysis of mouse cellular type-C viral DNA: emergence of new viral sequences in spontaneous AKR/J lymphomas. Proc Natl Acad Sci USA 76:1677–1681 – Lee JC, Ihle JN (1979) Mechanisms of C-type viral leukemogenesis. I. Correlation of in vitro lymphocyte blastogenesis to viremia and leukemia. J Immunol 123:2351–2358 – McClements WL, Enquist LW, Oskarsson M, Sullivan M, Vande Woude GF (1980) Frequent site-specific deletion of coliphage λ murine sarcoma virus recombinants and its use in the identification of a retrovirus integration site. J Virol 35:488–497 – McGrath MS, Weissman IL (1979) AKR leukemogenesis: identification and biological significance of thymic lymphoma receptors for AKR retroviruses. Cell 17:65–75 – Moloney JB (1960) Biological studies on a lymphoid leukemia virus extracted from sarcoma 37. I. Origin and introductory investigations. J Nat Cancer Inst 24:933–951 – Reddy EP, Dunn CY, Aaronson SA (1980) Different lymphoid cell targets for transformation by replication-competent Moloney and Rauscher mouse leukemia viruses. Cell 19:663–669 – Shimotohno K, Mizutani S, Temin HM (1980) Sequence of retrovirus provins resembles that of bacterial transposable elements. Nature 285:550–554 – Siden EJ, Baltimore D, Clark D, Rosenberg NE (1979) Immunoglobulin synthesis by lymphoid cells transformed in vitro by Abelson murine leukemia virus. Cell 16:389–396 – Steffen D, Weinberg RA (1978) The integrated genome of murine leukemia virus. Cell 15:1003–1010 – Stephenson JR, Aaronson SA (1973) Characterization of temperature-sensitive mutants of murine leukemia virus. Virology 54:53–59 – Stephenson JR, Tronick SR, Aaronson SA (1975) Murine leukemia virus mutants with temperature-sensitive defects in precursor polypeptide cleavage. Cell 6:543–548 – Stephenson JR, Barbacid M, Tronick SR, Hino S, Aaronson SA (1977) Proteins of type-C RNA tumor viruses. In: Gallo R (ed) Cancer research: Cell biology, molecular biology and tumor virology. CRC, Cleveland, pp 37–50 – Wang L, Galehouse D, Mellon P, Duesberg P, Mason WS, Vogt PK (1976) Mapping oligonucleotides of Rous sarcoma virus RNA that segregate with polymerase and group-specific antigen markers in recombinants. Proc Natl Acad Sci USA 73:3952–3956

Haematology and Blood Transfusion Vol. 26
Modern Trends in Human Leukemia IV
Edited by Neth, Gallo, Graf, Mannweiler, Winkler
© Springer-Verlag Berlin Heidelberg 1981

The Long Terminal Repeat of Moloney Sarcoma Provirus Enhances Transformation

D. G. Blair, M. Oskarsson, W. L. McClements, and G. F. Vande Woude

A. Introduction

Transforming retroviruses are generally thought to arise from a recombination between nontransforming viruses and sequences of cellular origin. Until recently, it has not been possible to test whether the acquired cell sequences *(onc)*[1] of transforming retroviruses act in concert with the conserved retrovirus sequences to establish transformation or whether the *onc* sequences alone are sufficient to cause transformation. For example, if retrovirus sequences are not essential, a finite number of naturally occurring malignancies would be expected to be caused by expression of *C-onc* sequences. Alternatively, if a region(s) of the retrovirus genome is (are) required for expression of the malignant phenotype, then the properties of this viral sequence may reveal how a normal cell sequence is modified to activate its transformation potential. We have cloned from normal mouse cell genomic DNA a sequence, *C-mos* that is homologous to the Moloney sarcoma virus (MSV) acquired *V-mos* sequence (Oskarsson et al. 1980). This cloned fragment and cloned integrated MSV proviral DNA have provided a direct means for addressing these questions and for testing the transforming activity of various combinations between the *V-mos, C-mos,* and MSV sequences derived from Moloney murine leukemia virus (M-MuLV).

The biologic activity of both in vitro synthesized and molecularly cloned MSV proviral DNA has been demonstrated (Oskarsson et al. 1980; Andersson et al. 1979; Vande Woude et al., to be published; Canaani et al. 1979; Aaronson et al., to be published; Blair et al. 1980). These studies showed that subgenomic DNA fragments of MSV could transform cells in a direct DNA transfection assay and that the entire MSV genome was not essential for efficient transformation. Here we review evidence (Oskarsson et al. 1980; Vande Woude et al., to be published; Blair et al. 1980) demonstrating that the long terminal repeat (LTR) of the MSV retrovirus enhances cell transformation by an internal MSV fragment containing *V-mos.* Furthermore we show that a single LTR placed covalently 5' to *C-mos* activates the transforming potential of the otherwise inactive *C-mos.*

The LTR sequences of MSV are direct repeats of 588 base pairs (bp) in length which bracket the MSV provirus (Vande Woude et al. 1979, to be published; Dhar et al. 1980; McClements et al., to be published b). The LTR is derived from the 5' and 3' ends of the genomic viral RNA during proviral DNA synthesis and for MSV are conserved from the parental M-MuLV (Dhar et al. 1980; Shoemaker et al., to be published). The nucleotide sequence of the MSV LTR reveals putative transcription control sequences (Dhar et al. 1980) and bears several striking parallels to the prokaryotic insertion sequence (IS) elements (Dhar et al. 1980; McClements et al., to be published a,b).

---

[1] *Onc* is a general term for all cellular sequences with malignant transforming potential. These are designated *C-onc* when part of the cell genome and *V-onc* in the retrovirus genome. Mos has been adopted as the name for the acquired sequence in MSV. Thus *mos* is a member of the set of *onc* sequences present in mice. This nomenclature supersedes utilization of *src* and *sarc* for viral and cellular transforming sequences

B. Results

I. LTR Enhances Transformation by V-mos

Figure 1 shows physical maps of integrated HT1 MSV provirus cloned in phage λ(λHT1) (Vande Woude, to be published, 1979) together with clones of subgenomic portions of the provirus cloned in pBR322. The biologic activity of the complete provirus in the DNA transfection assay is compared to the activities of the cloned subgenomic fragments (Table 1) (Blair et al. 1980). A cloned internal MSV fragment, pHT10, containing approximately 800 bp of M-MuLV derived sequences and 1200 bp of *V-mos,* transforms NIH 3T3 cells with a specific infectivity ∼10,000-fold lower than the intact HT1 MSV DNA (λHT1). Two clones of external MSV fragments, pHT15 and pHT13, containing respectively the 5' or 3' LTR, lack *V-mos* and are inactive in this assay. When sequences in pHT13 are added to the

MSV sequences in pHT10, reconstructing the 3' end of HT1 MSV provirus as in pHT21 and pHT22, the efficiency of transformation is enhanced 1000-fold over pHT10 (Table 1) (Oskarsson et al. 1980; Blair et al. 1980). Also shown in Table 1 is clone pHT25 which contains the entire 5' portion of HT1 MSV through *V-mos* and transforms with the same efficiency as pHT21 and pHT22. The only sequence in common among these three subclones, besides the MSV sequences in pHT10, is the LTR.

II. Cotransfection-Transformation by V-mos plus LTR

We have used deletion mutants of the hybrid λMSV phages to further demonstrate that transformation enhancement is due to the LTR. When either λHT1 or λml [a hybrid phage containing the integrated provirus of the ml strain of MSV (Vande Woude et al. 1979, to

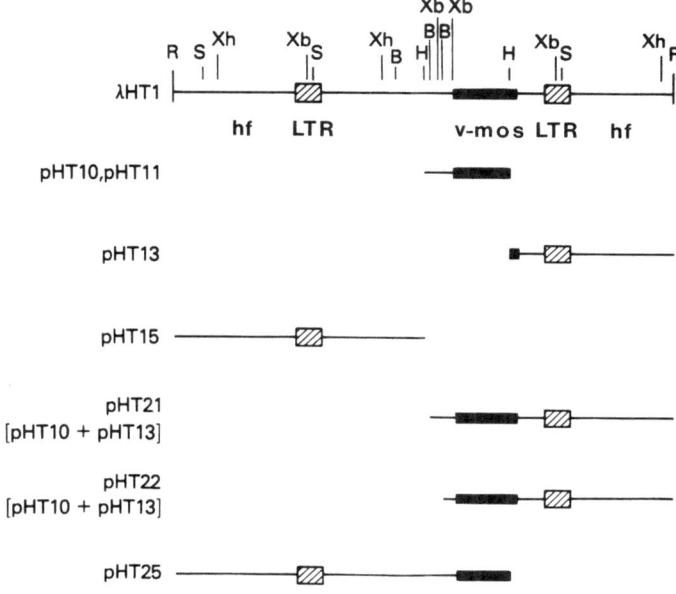

Fig. 1. Physical maps of HT1 MSV and subclones. The simplified map of the integrated provirus is shown indicating the *V-mos (heavy line),* LTR *(cross hatch),* and hf *(host flank)* sequences. Pertinent restriction endonuclease sites are shown: *R, Eco* RI; *Xb,Xba* I; *S, Sac* I; *B, Bg1* II; *Xh, Xho* I; *H, Hind* III. The specific portions of λHT1 subcloned in pBR322 are indicated. Plasmids pHT10 and pHT11 are identical, independently derived clones of the 2.1 kb *Hind* III *V-mos* fragment of λHT1. Plasmids pHT15 and pHT13 were generated by *Hind* III digestion of the purified *Eco* RI insert of λHT1 and cloned into the *Hind* III and *Eco* RI sites of pBR322. Partial *Hind* III digestion of the same *Eco* R1 fragment allowed construction of pHT25. Plasmids pHT21 and pHT22 were made in vitro by cloning the *Bg1* II-*Hind* III MSV fragment of pHT10 into pHT13. All subclones have been characterized by restriction mapping

Table 1. Transforming activity of cloned MSV fragments

Fragment Tested[a]	ffu/pmole[b]
λHT1	37,000
pHT10	7
pHT15	ND
pHT13	ND
pHT21	6,900
pHT22	8,100
pHT25	7,800

[a] DNA was transfected onto NIH 3T3 cells as previously described (Andersson et al. 1979; Blair et al. 1980; Graham and van der Eb 1973; Lowy et al. 1977)
[b] Focus-forming units (ffu) per picomole. ND = no foci were detected. Data from Blair et al. (1980)

Table 2. MSV LTR enhancement of transformation by *V-mos*

Plasmid	ffu/pmole
pHT10[a]	7
pm1sp	ND
pHT1sp	ND
pm1sp + pHT10	2,100
pHT1sp + pHT10	850
pBR322 + pHT10	ND

[a] The concentration of each plasmid was 0.25 µg/ml applied to each plate containing 3×10^5 NIH 3T3 cells/dish using the Ca^{++} precipitation procedure (Graham and van der Eb 1973; Lowy et al. 1977). ND = no foci were detected

be published)] is propagated in *E.coli* a specific deletion in the inserted fragment is readily detected in a percentage of the phage progeny (Vande Woude et al., to be published; McClements et al., to be published b). The inserts of these deletion mutants retain one LTR and the bracketing host sequences, while one LTR and the unique MSV sequences are lost. The generation and physical characterization of these has been described in detail elsewhere (Vande Woulde et al., to be published; McClements et al., to be published b). The retained sequences have been cloned in pBR322 and designated "pmlsp" and "pHT1sp" (Fig. 2B); they are compared to the λTH1 and λml maps in Fig. 2A (Vande Woude et al. 1979, to be published).

We have shown that pmlsp enhances transformation by the *V-mos* sequences in pHT10 when a mixture of both is transfected onto NIH 3T3 cells (Blair et al. 1980; McClements et al. 1980, to be published a). In experiments summarized in Table 2 neither pmlsp nor pHT1sp produces foci of transformation. However, when either is cotransfected with pHT10, the number of foci produced is between 100- and 300-fold higher than pHT10 alone. No stimulatory effect is observed when the vector, pBR322, is cotransfected with pHT10. The only MSV sequences in common between pHT1sp and pmlsp is the single LTR (Vande Woude et al., to be published; McClements et al., to be published b). These data suggest that the LTR is responsible for enhancement of transformation.

III. The Effect of MSV Sequences of Transformation by C-mos

We have cloned and characterized the C-mos sequences from normal Balb/c mouse genomic DNA and have shown that C-mos is inactive in the transfection-transformation assay (Oskarsson et al. 1980; McClements et al., to be published a). Moreover, when pHT13 sequences are linked 3' to *C-mos,* this new clone (λLS$_1$) is still inactive. This data, from Oskarsson, et al. (1980), is shown in Table 3. Recall that in the analogous procedure linking pHT13 sequences 3' to *V-mos* enhanced transformation ∼1000-fold (cf. pHT21 and pHT22, Table 2 to λLS$_1$, Table 3). From these results, we have proposed that the M-MuLV sequences immediately 5' to *V-mos* in pHT10 contribute to its transforming activity. To test this hypothesis a hybrid, λLS$_2$, was constructed by covalently linking 5' MSV sequences from λml to *C-mos.* This hybrid is structurally equivalent to the 5' end of mlMSV thru *V-mos* (Fig. 2, 0–4.2-kb map units) and analogous to the pHT25 subclone of HT1 MSV (Table 2) (Blair et al. 1980). Like the latter, λLS$_2$ transforms NIH 3T3 cells efficiently (Table 3). This result demonstrated that the *C-mos* sequences can transform cells if the normal Balb/c sequences 5' to *C-mos* are replaced with MSV sequences of M-MuLV origin (Oskarsson et al. 1980). These M-MuLV-derived sequences include the LTR and portions of the *gag, pol,* and *env* genes (Vande Woude et al., to be published; Sherr et al. 1980). This result

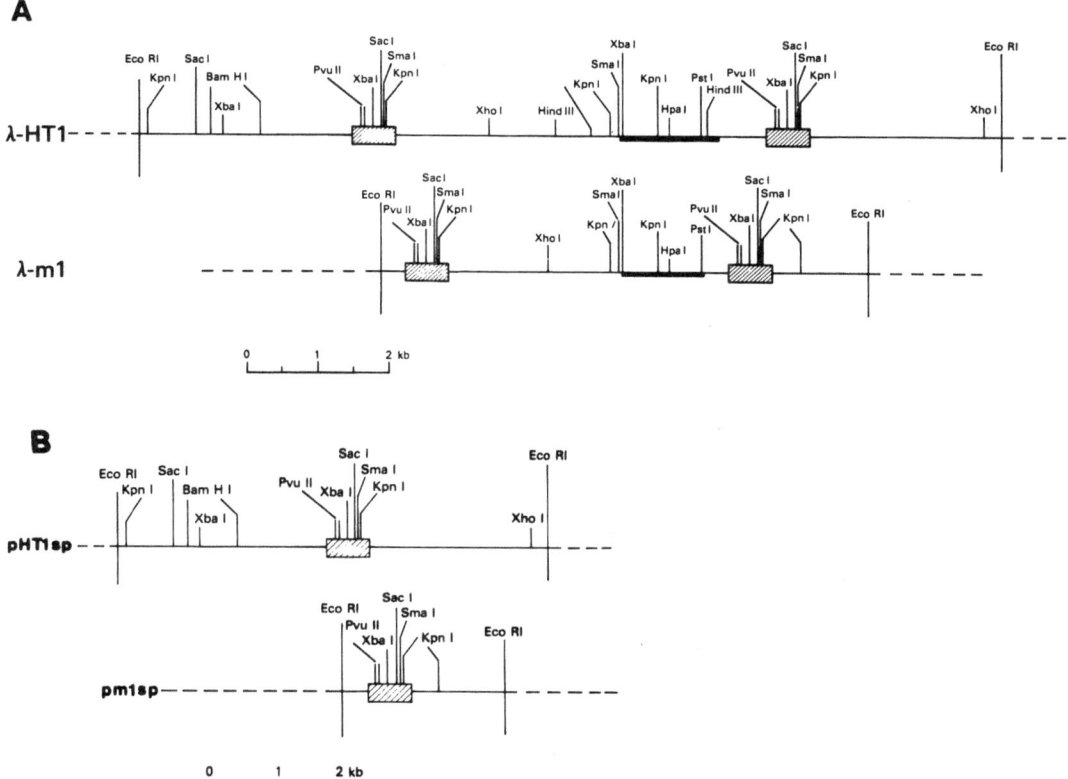

Fig. 2. Physical maps of cloned integrated MSV and their deletion mutants. **A** The maps show some of the restriction endonuclease sites in the inserted Eco R1 DNA fragments of λHT1 and λml (Vande Woude et al. 1979, to be published; McClements et al., to be published b). Additional *Pst 1*, *Bg 1* II and *PvuII* sites in MSV and mink flanking sequences are not shown. The *solid horizontal lines* represent insert DNA, the *heavy lines* represent *V-mos*, the *crossed-hatched rectangles* are the long terminal repeats (LTR), and the *dashed lines* represent the prokaryotic vector sequences. **B** The deleted inserts pHT1sp and pm1sp were subcloned in pBR322. The characters and symbols are the same as in A above

taken with the pHT10 result suggests a contribution of the *env* gene sequences that immediately preceed *V-mos* in pHT10 or *C-mos* in λLS$_2$ to the activation of the transforming potential (Oskarsson et al. 1980; McClements et al. 1980). We have proposed that an *env* gene splice acceptor site could facilitate activation of *V-mos* expression by an upstream promoter, perhaps the one in the LTR (Dhar et al. 1980). To test whether *env* sequences are absolutely required for *C-mos* expression, we covalently linked the mlMSV LTR to cellular sequences ∼600 bp from the 5' end of *C-mos* generating the hybrid pTS$_1$ (Table 3). This hybrid transformed with an efficiency equiva-

lent to that of a subgenomic fragment of MSV such as pHT25, pHT22, or pHT21 but aside from the LTR lacked all other M-MuLV-derived sequences.

C. Discussion

We have demonstrated that the normal cell sequence *C-mos* does not transform cells in the DNA transfection assay (Table 3) (Oskarsson et al. 1980). In contrast, as part of the viral genome *V-mos* does transform. Using recombinant DNA techniques, we have identified portions of the viral genome that are essential

Table 3. Transformation activity of C-mos

Clone designation	Schematic of fragment tested[a]	DNA ng	Foci (No.)	Activity (ffu/ pmole)
λM$_{C-mos}$		570	0	ND[b]
		1000	0	ND
	R B$_2$ H B$_2$ R	3200	0	ND
pMS$_1$		420	0	ND
		2100	0	ND
λLS$_1$(pHT13 + λM$_{C-mos}$[c])		90	0	ND
		810	0	ND
	H	1350	1	4
		1800	1	3
λLS$_2$(λml + pMS$_1$)		141	78	2600
		30	13	2400
	R B$_1$	15	12	4000
pTS$_1$(pm1sp + pMS$_1$)		100	136	5900
		50	36	3300
	R Sb	25	17	3000

[a] To approximate scale ..... indicates normal mink sequences flanking the integrated proviral DNA; ○○○ = the 588-bp-long terminal repeat sequences (LTR) of the provirus (Dhar et al. 1980); ***** = MSV sequences of M-MuLV origin (Vande Woude et al., to be published; × × × × V-mos sequences (Vande Woude et al., to be published); ----- = normal Balb/c sequences flanking C-mos; ●●●● = C-mos sequences. The approximate location of restriction endonuclease sites used in the construction of λLS$_1$, λLS$_2$ and pTS$_1$ are indicated; R = Eco R1; H = Hind III; B$_1$ = Bg1 I; B$_2$ = Bg1 II; and S = Sma I. Sb indicates that Ba1 31 exonuclease digested pMS$_1$ (∿600 bp 5' to C-mos) was ligated to the Sma I site in the MSV LTR to generate the plasmid pTS$_1$

[b] ND = no foci detected

[c] See schematic of pHT13 in Fig. 1 and its biologic activity given in Table 1. λLS$_1$ was generated by joining pHT13 sequences to the 3' end of C-mos at their common Hind III site. λLS$_2$ was generated from λml MSV by joining the entire 5' MSV portion of ml MSV at the Bg1 I site in V-mos to the 3' portion of C-mos at its Bg1 I site. pTS$_1$ was generated by blunt-end ligation of a Ba1 31 digested pMS$_1$ to the Sma I site of the MSV LTR

for activating the transforming potential of C-mos.

In experiments with subgenomic portions of the MSV provirus we demonstrated that an MSV fragment containing an LTR placed covalently either 3' or 5' to V-mos enhanced transformation. Also, simply cotransfecting a plasmid containing V-mos sequences with a second plasmid containing a single LTR enhanced transformation. Clearly, the enhancement of transformation could be associated with one or several biologic functions of the LTR. It could be that in this assay the LTR is providing a maintainance function (e.g., an origin of replication) or an integration function by facilitating a stable association of mos with the genome of the transfected cell. However, the LTR possesses putative transcription con-

trol elements (Dhar et al. 1980), and it is likely that at least one of its transformation enhancement activities is due to the promotion of mos transcription. We have shown that the MSV LTR has several structural and at least one functional feature in common with bacterial IS elements (Blair et al. 1980; Dhar et al. 1980; McClements et al., to be published a,b). It is well known that IS elements are involved in the transposition (and integration) of DNA sequences, and some IS elements are believed to contain transcriptional control signals that affect expression of adjacent genes (see review in Bukhari et al. 1977). The LTR may be acting in a manner analogous to IS elements.

Our results with λLS$_2$ in which the cellular sequences preceeding C-mos were replaced by M-MuLV-derived MSV sequences suggested that in addition to the LTR, MSV sequences immediatly preceeding *V-mos* are required for transformation (McClements et al. 1980). However, the data do not rule out the possibility that the mere removal of these cellular sequences allows transformation by *C-mos*. There may be controlling cellular sequences preceeding *C-mos* that block its expression. The activation of *C-mos* in clone pTS$_1$ is consistent with this interpretation if (1) the LTR sequences override the cellular control elements or (2) the putative controlling cellular sequences are more than approximately 600 bp before *C-mos*. The latter possibility suggests that removing normal cell sequences 5' to *C-mos* should activate its malignant potential in the transfection assay. Indeed, this is consistent with the model proposed by Cooper et al. (1980) to explain the transforming activity of normal cellular DNA after shearing.

Because the LTR is directly repeated at both ends of the provirus it could be expected to allow transcription to occur from the 3' LTR into the cell genome. Thus, random integration of retroviruses into multiple sites in the host cell genome (see Weinberg 1980 for review) could result in the activation of normally quiescent cell genes. For example, 17 out of 19 tumors isolated from birds infected with avian leukosis virus show evidence for activation of expression of normal cell sequences by LTR sequences (Hayward et al. this volume). The loss of almost all of the retrovirus genome in some of the tumors, except for a residual LTR, could mean that LTR-promoted expression of normal cell sequences is responsible for the disease. Certainly in this case all other avian leukosis viral genes can be excluded. We have shown with pTS$_1$ (Table 3) that a single LTR which is linked 5' to *C-mos* activates transformation. This in vitro construction is analogous to a retrovirus integrating 5' (upstream) to a normal cell sequence (e.g., *C-mos*) in vivo, whereby the 3' LTR could activate expression of this sequence and cause transformation. This may be a useful model for other (nonviral) forms of transformation. Normal cellular sequences with functional properties of an LTR (e.g., an eukaryotic IS element) could become juxtaposed to quiescent cellular genes with transformation potential as a result of either chemically induced, radiation induced, or simply spontaneous genomic arrangements.

References

Aaronson S, Canaani E, Robbins K, Andersson P, Tronick S (to be published) Cellular origin of the transforming gene of Moloney murine sarcoma virus. Cold Spring Harbor Symp Quant Biol 44 – Andersson P, Goldfarb MP, Weinberg (1979) A defined subgenomic fragment of in vitro synthesized Moloney sarcoma virus DNA can induce cell transformation upon transfection. Cell 16:63–75 – Blair DG, McClements W, Oskarrson M, Fischinger P, Vande Woude GF (1980) The biological activity of cloned Moloney sarcoma virus DNA: terminally redundant sequences may enhance transformation efficiency. Proc Natl Acad Sci USA 77:3504–3508 – Bukhari AI, Shapiro JA, Adhya SL (eds) (1977) DNA insertion elements, plasmids and episomes. Cold Spring Harbor Laboratory, New York – Canaani E, Robbins KC, Aaronson SA (1979) The transforming gene of Moloney murine sarcoma virus. Nature 282:378–383 – Cooper GM, Okenquist S, Silverman L (1980) Transforming activity of DNA of chemically transformed and normal cells. Nature 284:418–421 – Dhar R, McClements W, Enquist LW, Vande Woude GF Nucleotide sequences of integrated Moloney sarcoma virus Long Terminal Repeats and their host and viral junctions. Proc Natl Acad Sci USA 77:3937–3941 – Graham FL, van der Eb AJ (1973) A new technique for the assay of infectivity of human adenovirus 5 DNA. Virology 52:456–467 – Lowy DR, Rands E, Scolnick EM (1977) Helper independent transformation by unintegrated Harvey sarcoma virus DNA. J Virol 26:291–298 – McClements WL, Blair DG, Oskarsson M, Vande Woude GF (1980) Two regions of the Moloney leukemia virus genome are required for efficient transformation by src/sarc. In: Fields B, Jaenisch R, Fox C (eds) Animal virus genetics ICN-UCLA symposia on molecular and cellular biology. Academic Press, New York – McClements WL, Dhar R, Blair DG, Enquist LW, Oskarsson M, Vande Woude GF (to be published a) The terminal repeats of integrated Moloney sarcoma provirus are like bacterial insertion sequence (IS) elements. Cold Spring Harbor Symp Quant Biol 45 – McClements WL, Enquist LW, Oskarsson M, Sullivan M, Vande Woude GF (to be published b) Frequent site-specific deletion of coliphage λmurine sarcoma virus recombinants and its use in the identification of a retrovirus integration site. J Virol 35 – Oskarsson M, McClements WL, Blair DG, Maizel JV, Vande Woude GF (1980) Properties of a normal mouse cell DNA sequence (sarc) homologous to the src sequence of Moloney sarcoma virus. Science 207:1222–1224 – Sherr CJ, Fedele LA, Oskarsson M, Maizel J, Vande Woude GF (1980) Molecular cloning of Snyder-Theilen feline leukemia and sarcoma viruses: comparative studies of feline sarcoma virus with its natural helper and Moloney sarcoma virus. J Virol 24:200–212

– Shoemaker C, Goff S, Gilboa E, Paskind M, Mitra SW, Baltimore D (to be published) Structure of a cloned circular Moloney murine leukemia virus DNA molecule containing an inverted segment: implications for retrovirus integration. Proc Natl Acad Sci USA 77 – Vande Woude GF, Oskarsson M, Enquist LW, Nomura S, Sullivan M, Fischinger PJ (1979) Cloning of integrated Moloney sarcoma virus proviral DNA sequences in bacteriophage λ. Proc Natl Acad Sci USA 76:4464–4468 – Vande Woude GF, Oskarsson M, McClements WL, Enquist LW, Blair DG, Fischinger PJ, Maizel J, Sullivan M (to be published) Characterization of integrated Moloney sarcoma proviruses and flanking host sequences cloned in bacteriophage λ. Cold Spring Harbor Symp Quant Biol 44 – Weinberg RA (1980) Integrated genomes of animal viruses. Ann Rev Biochem 49:197–226

Haematology and Blood Transfusion Vol. 26
Modern Trends in Human Leukemia IV
Edited by Neth, Gallo, Graf, Mannweiler, Winkler
© Springer-Verlag Berlin Heidelberg 1981

Ontogeny of Abelson Murine Leukemia Virus Target Cells

G. L. Waneck and N. Rosenberg

A. Introduction

Abelson murine leukemia virus (A-MuLV) is a replication defective retrovirus that induces a thymus-independent lymphoma after a short, 3–5 week latent period (Abelson and Rabstein 1970). The virus is unique among murine retroviruses in its ability to transform lymphoid cells in vitro (Rosenberg and Baltimore 1976; Rosenberg et al. 1975). The lack of thymic involvement in the disease (Abelson and Rabstein 1970; Siegler et al. 1972) and the susceptibility of athymic nu/nu mice to the virus (Raschke et al. 1975) coupled with an inability to detect T lymphocyte markers on the tumor cells (Sklar et al. 1975) has suggested that this lymphoma is made up of malignant cells related to B lymphocytes. The ability to detect immunoglobulin (Ig) in some tumors further supports the involvement of cells of the B lymphocyte lineage in this malignancy (Potter et al. 1973; Prekumar et al. 1975).

A significant percentage of clonally derived in vitro transformants isolated from adult bone marrow also express Ig (Boss et al. 1979; Pratt and Strominger 1977; Rosenberg and Witte 1980; Siden et al. 1979). Like the in vivo derived tumor cells, these isolates lack phenotypic markers characteristic of mature T or B lymphocytes (Boss et al. 1979; Silverstone et al. 1978). A very large number of the isolates express terminal deoxynucleotidyl transferase (TdT) (Rosenberg and Witte 1980; Silverstone et al. 1978), an enzyme associated with many T lymphocytes and probably with immature B lymphocytes (Chang 1971; Kung et al. 1975; Silverstone et al. 1978).

The studies of the phenotypic markers expressed by A-MuLV-transformed cells suggest that they may be analogous to a normal cell present early in the B lymphocyte lineage. While this type of study may serve as a useful guide to predicting the nature of the cell(s) susceptible to A-MuLV, no conclusive evidence of a correlation between the phenotype of the transformed cell and the phenotype of the target cell(s) has been presented.

Direct examination of A-MuLV target cells is difficult because of the heterogeneity of hematopoietic cell preparations and the low frequency of these cells in the population. The observation that bone marrow contains the highest number of A-MuLV susceptible cells among adult hematopoietic tissues (Rosenberg and Baltimore 1976; unpublished work) is consistent with the hypothesis that A-MuLV transforms fairly undifferentiated cells. The ability to eliminate more than 90% of A-MuLV target cells from bone marrow with a monoclonal antibody that reacts with normal pre-B lymphocyte colony forming cells (Shinefeld et al. 1980; Kincade, and Sato, personal communication) also supports this notion.

Recently, we have examined the appearance of A-MuLV target cells during ontogeny by determining the frequency of these cells in fetal liver at various times of gestation. These experiments demonstrate that cells susceptible to A-MuLV-induced transformation arise within a defined 24 h period between day 12 and day 13 of gestation and increase in number until birth. Study of Ig and TdT expression in clonally derived lines arising from livers at different times during gestation demonstrates that the frequency of cell lines expressing these markers varies depending upon the gestation time. Because of the consistent frequency of expression of these markers in adult bone marrow derived cell lines, the variations observed with the cell lines of fetal origin may

467

indicate a shifting of target cell populations during ontogeny.

B. Results

I. Presence of A-MuLV Target Cells in Fetal liver

Fetal livers from embryos at various stages of gestation were examined for the frequency of cells susceptible to A-MuLV-induced transformation using the quantitative agar assay (Rosenberg and Baltimore 1976). Consistent with previous results (Rosenberg and Baltimore 1976; Rosenberg et al. 1975), infection of late gestation livers resulted in high numbers of transformants (Fig. 1). The maximum number of foci was found in 18–19 day fetal livers where the frequency was about twice that

observed in adult bone marrow. Examination of earlier gestation livers revealed a gradual decrease in the number of transformants, with only 1.3 foci/ 10^6 nucleated white blood cells being observed at day 13. No foci were observed when livers from day 11 and day 12 of gestation were examined. After birth the number of foci observed after infection of liver cells had declined drastically and cells susceptible to A-MuLV could be detected in bone marrow (Fig. 1).

II. Lack of Toxicity in Fetal Liver Preparations

The failure to detect A-MuLV transformants in early fetal liver and the low frequency of foci in 13–14 day fetal liver could result from either a lack of target cells or from the presence of toxic factors or cells that suppress the expression of potential transformants. To distinguish

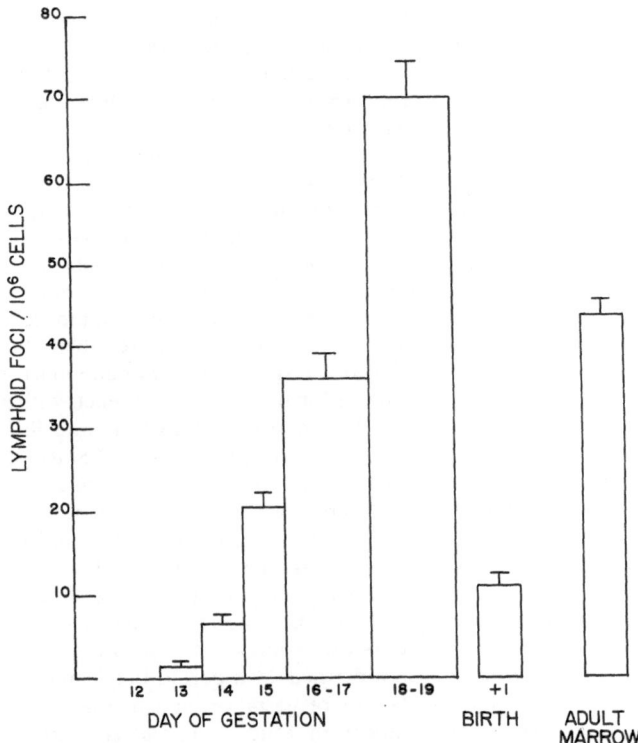

Fig. 1. Ontogeny of A-MuLV target cells. Fetal livers at various points in gestation were removed from embryos, dissociated, and infected with A-MuLV P160 (Rosenberg and Witte 1980). Gestation times were determined by vaginal plug with the morning of detection being considered day 0 of gestation. Bone marrow from 6–10-week-old adult mice was also examined. Foci were measured using the agar transformation assay. The results of 2–4 experiments have been pooled. The *error bars* indicate the standard error of the mean number of foci/well

468

between these two possibilities, fetal liver cells from gestation times when the number of transformants observed was low were infected and plated either alone or after dilution with an equal number of adult bone marrow cells (Table 1). The mixed cultures contained the same total number of cells as each of the cultures in which the two types were plated alone. Thus, the expected number of foci in the mixed plating was calculated by halving the sum of the foci observed when the two types of cells were plated separately. In all cases, the expected and observed frequency of transformants coincided closely (Table 1).

III. Phenotypic Markers Expressed by Fetal Liver Clones

Clones of A-MuLV-transformed cells were removed from agar with a pasteur pipette and either examined morphologically after Wright-Giemsa staining or adapted to grow as continuous cell lines. Study of over 50 colonies from various times of gestation revealed that all of these clones were composed of lymphoid cells characterized by a large nucleus with one or more nucleoli and a scant cytoplasm that lacked granules. No morphologic features distinguishing these clones from clones isolated from adult bone marrow were noted.

The expression of Ig and TdT was examined by SDS polyacrylamide gel analysis of ^{35}S-methionine-labeled immunoprecipitates. These two lymphocyte markers are expressed by a large number of A-MuLV transformants derived from adult bone marrow. For example, one survey of 22 such clonally derived isolates revealed that 68% of them were μ positive and 91% expressed TdT (Rosenberg and Witte 1980).

Nearly all the cells lines derived from foci of transformed neonatal bone marrow or liver cells expressed both Ig in the form of μ chain and TdT (Table 2). When a large number of late fetal liver-derived cell lines were examined, about the same frequency of μ positive clones was observed but TdT synthesis was not detected in any of the cell lines. A reversed pattern of TdT and μ expression was observed when foci from early fetal liver were examined. In this case, only 14% of the isolates expressed μ while 64% synthesized TdT (Table 2).

C. Discussion

Cells susceptible to A-MuLV-induced transformation appear in fetal liver within a defined, less than 24 h period between day 12 and day 13 of gestation. The inability to detect transformants in earlier fetal liver is due to a lack of detectable numbers of target cells and not the result of inhibitory cells or factors in these tissues.

Sensitive immunofluorescent staining techniques have detected Ig-positive cells in fetal liver at days 11–12 of gestation (Raff et al. 1976). However, precursors of functional mitogen- responsive B lymphocytes are first detected at day 13 of gestation (Melchers 1977). The kineties of appearance of this lymphocyte precursor cell parallels the appearance of A-MuLV target cells. The coincident appearance of cells with these two properties

Day of Gestation	Foci/ 10^6 Cells			
	Plated separately		Plated together	
	Liver	Adult marrow	Observed	Expected
12	<0.5	44	21	22
13	3.0	28	20	16
14	13	32	24	23
15	21	54	36	37
newborn	22	32	28	27

Table 1. Detection of A-MuLV transformants in liver and bone marrow mixtures[a]

[a] Liver and bone marrow cells were infected with virus separately or as 1:1 mixtures and then plated. The total cell number in both cases was the same. Transformation was examined using the agar assay. The expected number of foci was derived by halving the sum of the foci observed when each cell type was plated alone

Source of clones	No. clones tested	% Clones positive for marker	
		μ	TdT
Neonatal liver	4	100	100
Neonatal marrow	3	67	100
17–19 d fetal liver	16	75	<6
13–14 d fetal liver	14	14	64

Table 2. Expression of μ and TdT by A-MuLV-transformed cells[a]

[a] Cultures of cells were examined within 3–4 weeks after removal from agar. Expression of μ and TdT was detected by SDS polyacrylamide gel analysis of ^{35}S-methionine-labeled immunoprecipitates as previously described (Rosenberg and Witte 1980; Witte and Baltimore 1978). The goat anti-Moloney virus, polyspecific rabbit antimouse Ig and the rabbit anti-TdT sera used in these studies have been previously described (Rosenberg and Witte 1980; Silverstone et al. 1980; Witte and Baltimore 1978; Witte et al. 1978)

does not mean that the mitogen-responsive precursors and A-MuLV target cells are identical. However, the appearance of the mitogen-responsive precursor cells may signal the onset of active lymphopoiesis in the fetal liver, even though a few Ig-positive cells are present prior to day 13.

Results obtained with adult bone marrow indicate that actively cycling cells are most susceptible to A-MuLV-induced transformation (unpublished work). Thus, the time at which target cells appear in fetal liver could reflect both the appearance of appropriate lymphocytes and the entry of significant numbers of these cells into the cell cycle.

The frequency of clones expressing μ and TdT varies depending upon the age of gestation of the fetus. This variation is probably significant because the frequency of expression of the markers is quite constant among the large numbers (>75) of cell lines isolated from adult bone marrow. In addition, clones from neonatal animals are similar to the clones from adult tissue with respect to frequency of μ and TdT positive cells. Thus, changes in the frequencies of μ and TdT expression among fetal liver-derived cell lines probably reflect changes in the predominant target cell population during ontogeny. This shift may result from the different proportions of certain types of lymphoid precursors existing in rapidly cycling states at different times during gestation.

Acknowledgments

This work was supported by Public Health Service Grant CA-24220 and Program Project grant CA-24530 from the National Cancer Institute. N.R. is a recipient of an American Cancer Society Research Scholar Award (Massachusetts Division).

References

Abelson HI, Rabstein LS (1970) Lymphosarcoma: Virus-induced thymic-independent disease in mice. Cancer Res 30:3313–2222 – Boss M, Greaves M, Teich N (1979) Abelson virus transformed haemopoietic cell lines with pre-B cell characteristics. Nature 278:551–553 – Chang LMS (1971) Development of terminal deoxynucetidyl transferase activity in embryonic calf thymus gland. Biochem Biophs Res Commun 44:124–131 – Kung PC, Silverstone AE, McCaffrey RP, Baltimore D (1975) Murine terminal deoxynucleotidyl transferase: Cellular distribution and response to cortisone. J Exp Med 141:855–865 – Melchers F (1977) Blymphocyte development in fetal liver II. Frequencies of precursor B cells during gestation. Eur J Immunol 482–486 – Potter M, Sklar MD, Rose WP (1973) Rapid viral induction of plasmacytomas in pristane-primed BALB/c mice. Science 182:592–594 – Pratt DM, Strominger J Parkaman R, Kaplan D, Schwaber J, Rosenberg N, Scher CD (1977) Abelson virus – transformed lymphocytes: Null cells that modulate H-2. Cell 12:683–690 – Prekumar E, Potter M, Singer PA, Sklar MD (1975) Synthesis, surface deposition, and secretion of immunoglobulins by Abelson virus – Transformed lymphosarcoma cell lines. Cell 6:149–159 – Raff MC, Megson M, Owen JJT, Cooper MD (1976) Early production of intracellular IgM by B-lymphocyte precursors in mouse. Nature 259:224–226 – Raschke WC, Ralph P, Watson J, Sklar M, Coon H (1975) Brief communication: Oncogenic transformation of murine lymphoid cells by in vitra infection with Abelson leukemia virus. J Natl Cancer Inst 54:1249–1253 – Rosenberg N, Baltimore DA (1976) Quantitative assay for transformation of bone marrow cells by

Abelson murine leukemia virus. J Exp Med 143:1453–1463 – Rosenberg N, Witte ON (1980) Abelson murine leukemia virus mutants with alterations in A. MuLV specific P120 molecule. J Virol 3:340–348 – Rosenberg N, Baltimore DR, Scher CD (1975) In vitro transformation of lymphoid cells by Abelson murine leukemia virus. Proc Natl Acad Sci USA 72:1932–1936 – Shinefeld L, Sato V, Rosenberg N (1980) Monoclonal rat antimouse brain antibody detects Abelson murine leukemia virus target cells in mouse bone marrow. Cell 20:11–18 – Siden ET, Baltimore D, Clark D, Rosenberg N (1979) Immunoglobulin synthesis by lymphoid cells transformed in vitro by Abelson murine leukemia virus. Cell 16:389–396 – Siegler R, Fajdel S, Lane E (1972) Pothogenesis of Abelson-virus-induced murine leukemia. J Natl Cancer Inst 48:189–218 – Silverstone A. E, Rosenberg N, Sato VL, Scheid MP, Boyse EA, Baltimore D (1978) Correlating terminal deoxynuckotidyl transferase and cell surface makers in the pathway of lymphocyte ontogeny. In: Clarkson B, Till JE, Marks PA (eds) Cold Spring Harbor conferences on cell proliferation, vol 5. Cold Springs Harbor Press, Cold Spring Harbor, pp 432–452 – Silverstone AE, Sun L, Witte ON, Baltimore D (1980) Biosynthesis of murine terminal deoxynucleotidyl transferase. J Biol Chem 255:791–796 – Sklar MD, Shevach EM, Green I, Potter M (1975) Transplantation and preliminary characterization of lymphocyte surface markers of Abelson virus-induced lymphomas. Nature 253:550–552 – Witte ON, Baltimore D (1978) Relationship of retrovirus polyprotein cleavages to viron maturation studied with temperature – Sensitive murine leukemia virus mutants. J Virol 26:750–761 – Witte OM, Rosenberg N, Paskind M, Shields A, Baltimore D (1978) Identification of an Abelson murine leukemia virus-Encoded protein presnets in transformed fibroblasts and lymphoid cells. Proc Natl Acad Sci USA 75:2488–2492

Haematology and Blood Transfusion Vol. 26
Modern Trends in Human Leukemia IV
Edited by Neth, Gallo, Graf, Mannweiler, Winkler
© Springer-Verlag Berlin Heidelberg 1981

Structural and Functional Studies of the Friend Spleen Focus-Forming Virus: Structural Relationship of SFFV to Dualtropic Viruses and Molecular Cloning of a Biologically Active Subgenomic Fragment of SFFV DNA

L. H. Evans, P. H. Duesberg, D. L. Linemeyer, S. K. Ruscetti, and E. M. Scolnick

A. Introduction

The Friend virus induces an acute erythro-proliferative disease in adult mice characterized by splenomegaly and pronounced erythroblastosis. In early stages of the disease, discrete splenic foci of proliferating erythroid cells are apparent, and thus the virus has been termed the spleen focus-forming virus (SFFV) (Axelrad and Steeves 1964). As is the case with nearly all retroviruses which cause acute proliferative diseases, SFFV is defective in replication and is associated in a complex with a helper virus, termed the Friend murine leukemia virus (F-MuLV), which provides replicative functions (Dawson et al. 1968; Rawson and Parr 1970; Steeves et al. 1971; Troxler et al. 1977c). Several substrains of SFFV have been derived from the original isolate, some of which have pathologic properties distinguishable from others (Troxler et al. 1980). The present report deals with the structure and function of a polycythemia-inducing strain of SFFV originally obtained by Lilly and Steeves (SFFV$_{LS}$) (Lilly and Steeves 1973). We describe structural analyses which indicate that SFFV$_{LS}$ is a deletion mutant of a dualtropic Friend mink cell focus-inducing virus. In addition, we describe the derivation of molecularly cloned SFFV$_{LS}$ as well as a subgenomic fragment of this clone, both of which contain the information necessary to encode all pathogenic properties of the intact virus.

B. "Specific" Sequences of SFFV: Characterization and Location in the SFFV Genome

I. Specific Sequences Defined by Hybridization Studies

In all known replication-defective retroviruses which induce acute proliferative diseases, two classes of RNA sequences have been identified. One class is closely related to RNA sequences of associated helper viruses, and a second class is unrelated to helper virus RNA and, therefore, specific to the defective retrovirus genome (Duesberg 1980). The specific sequences very likely correspond to the genes encoding the pathogenic functions of these viruses. Hybridization analyses of SFFV, using specific cDNA probes prepared from SFFV-F-MuLV complexes, have also identified sequences closely related to F-MuLV as well as F-MuLV-unrelated sequences (Bernstein et al. 1977; Mak et al. 1978; Pragnell et al 1978; Troxler et al. 1977a,b). In contrast to the initial findings of others studying different isolates of SFFV, our analyses indicated that the specific sequences of SFFV$_{LS}$ exhibited homology to the RNAs of helper-independent dualtropic (infecting murine and nonmurine cells) and xenotropic (infecting preferentially nonmurine cells) viruses. Subsequent work by us (Troxler et al. 1980) and others (Bernstein et al 1979) identified dualtropic sequences in all SFFV isolates tested. It is likely that the earlier discrepancies were the result of xenotropic or dualtropic sequences present in helper virus RNA preparations used for the construction of SFFV-specific probes.

II. Identification and Location of Specific Sequences in SFFV RNA by RNase T₁-oligonucleotide Fingerprinting Analyses

In the hybridization analyses discussed above, the SFFV genome had not been examined directly. Rather, SFFV RNA from nonproducer cells (Troxler et al. 1977c) or mixtures of SFFV and F-MuLV RNAs were utilized (Berstein et al. 1977; Mak et al. 1978; Pragnell et al. 1978). Thus, the location of specific and F-MuLV-related sequences in SFFV RNA had not been determined. Our approach to the structural analysis of Friend virus RNA components has been to identify the large RNase T₁-resistant fragments (T₁-oligonucleotides) of each RNA and to determine the order of the oligonucleotides along the RNA relative to the 3' poly A terminus (Wang et al. 1975; Coffin and Billeter 1976). A direct comparison of the oligonucleotide maps in many cases will identify related and specific sequences of the RNAs.

The SFFV genome was identified as a 50S virion RNA consisting of monomers of approximately 6–7 kilobases (kb) by rescue of the SFFV component from nonproductively infected cells (Evans et al. 1979). This size is considerably smaller than the RNA monomers of F-MuLV (9 kb); thus, SFFV RNA could be isolated free of helper virus RNA sequences on the basis of size. The comparison of SFFV RNA to F-MuLV RNA by T₁-oligonucleotide fingerprinting was complicated by the existence of numerous minor sequence differences between related sequences of the two RNAs. Although SFFV RNA was 85%–90% homologous to F-MuLV by hybridization, only 8 of 24 SFFV oligonucleotides were found in F-MuLV RNA. This problem was circumvented by the identification of T₁-oligonucleotides in SFFV RNA-F-MuLV cDNA hybrids. Briefly, ^{32}P-labeled RNA was hybridized to F-MuLV cDNA, and the reaction mixture was digested with RNase to remove unhybridized RNA. The hybrid was then isolated, denatured, and fingerprinted to identify oligonucleotides from homologous sequences. This procedure identified 21 of the 24 SFFV T₁-oligonucleotides as F-MuLV related. The three specific SFFV oligonucleotides defined a region on the SFFV genome extending from approximately 2 to 2.5 kb from the 3' terminus of SFFV. A comparison of the three specific SFFV oligonucleotides with oligonucleotides of dualtropic viruses indicated that they were sequence elements of dualtropic *env* genes (Evans et al. 1979, 1980). Thus, SFFV is comprised entirely of sequences closely related to a combination of different helper virus RNAs. SFFV is fundamentally different from other retroviruses which induce rapid proliferative disease in that SFFV does not contain specific sequences unrelated to helper virus RNA.

C. Structural relationship of SFFV to F-MuLV and to Dualtropic Viruses

I. Structure of the Dualtropic Friend Mink Cell Focus-Inducing Virus

Dualtropic viruses are generated by recombination of ecotropic (murine host range) MuLVs with *env* gene sequences of uncertain origin (Faller and Hopkins 1978; Rommelaere et al. 1978; Shih et al. 1978). Since SFFV was shown above to be comprised of sequences related to F-MuLV and dualtropic envelope sequences, it is plausible that a dualtropic variant of F-MuLV may contain all SFFV sequences. To test this possibility, we have compared the structure of a dualtropic variant of F-MuLV, termed the Friend mink cell focus-inducing virus (F-MCF) (Troxler 1978), to F-MuLV and subsequently to SFFV (see below). A direct comparison of the oligonucleotide fingerprints of F-MuLV and F-MCF indicated that approximately 75% of their oligonucleotides were shared and about 25% of the oligonucleotides in each virus were unique. A comparison of the oligonucleotide maps of F-MuLV and F-MCF indicated that the two viruses were virtually indentical in all regions except for a region located about 1.5 to 3.3 kb on the oligonucleotide maps corresponding to the viral envelope gene. Within this region no oligonucleotides were shared. Such a relationship is typical of many dualtropic viruses with respect to their ecotropic parents (Faller and Hopkins 1978; Rommelaere et al. 1978; Shih et al. 1978) and is shown schematically in Fig. 1.

II. Structural Relationship of SFFV to F-MCF

Initial hybridization results of SFFV RNA with F-MCF cDNA indicated that virtually all SFFV RNA is closely related to the F-MCF genome; however, only 14 of 24 SFFV oligo-

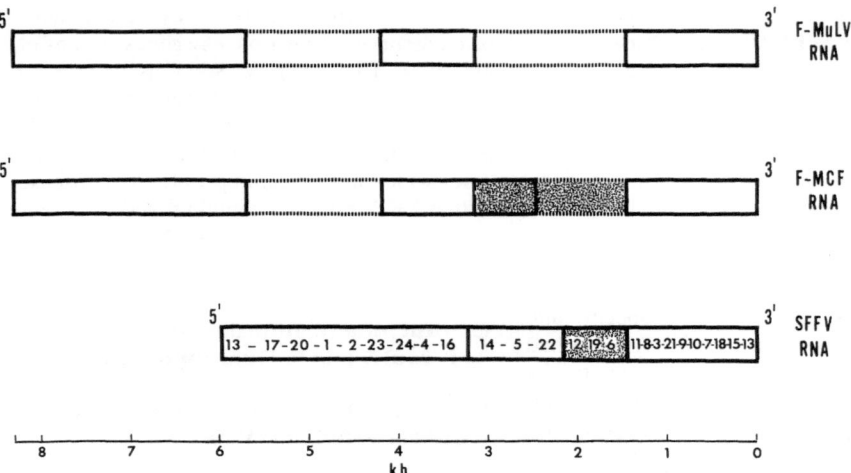

Fig. 1. Structural relationships of F-MuLV, F-MCF, and SFFV RNAs. RNA sequences of each viral genome which are shared with ecotropic F-MuLV RNA are *unshaded*. RNA sequences shared with F-MCF RNA but not with F-MuLV RNA are *shaded*. Sequences shared with SFFV RNA are bordered by *solid lines* and those not shared with SFFV RNA are bordered by *dashed lines*. The positions of RNase T_1-resistant oligonucleotides (designated by Nos. 1 through 24) are shown for SFFV RNA

nucleotides have identical counterparts in F-MCF. To determine the F-MCF-related oligonucleotides in SFFV, the oligonucleotides present in an SFFV RNA-F-MCF cDNA hybrid were identified. It was found that all SFFV oligonucleotides were hybridized; thus, our prediction that all SFFV sequences may be contained in a single replication-competent retrovirus was confirmed.

Since F-MCF does not cause an acute disease, but contains all sequences of SFFV, including those responsible for Friend disease, it would appear that the pathogenicity of SFFV is the result of a particular configuration of F-MCF-related sequences. It is; therefore, important to determine what structural features distinguish F-MCF sequences from F-MCF-related sequences in SFFV. To determine which T_1-oligonucleotides correspond to SFFV-related sequences in F-MCF, the oligonucleotides in a hybrid of F-MCF RNA with molecularly cloned SFFV DNA (Linemeyer et al. 1980; also see below) were determined. This analysis indicated that the structure of SFFV$_{LS}$ corresponds to an F-MCF which has deleted two large contiguous sequences (Fig. 1): one region which extends from 1.5 to 2.5 kb from the 3' end in F-MCF and corresponds to about one-half of the dualtropic sequences and a second region extending from approxi-

mately 4.2 to 5.8 kb which would include most of the polymerase gene and probably a portion of the *gag* gene which encodes the major virion core proteins.

D. Molecular Cloning of SFFV-Specific DNA

The structural analyses described above imply that the SFFV genome may encode defective *gag* gene and *env* gene products. Both defective *gag* proteins (Ruscetti et al. 1980; Bernstein et al. 1977; Barbacid et al. 1978) and defective *env* proteins (Dresler et al. 1979; Ruscetti et al. 1979) have been described in SFFV-infected cells. *Gag* gene related proteins have been detected in cells infected with only certain strains of SFFV, and these proteins vary considerably in size and in their antigenic properties. In contrast, cells infected with any strain of SFFV always express an *env* gene related protein of 52,000–55,000 daltons which contains antigenic determinants of dualtropic viral envelope glycoproteins. No evidence exists to determine directly whether either protein is involved in the SFFV erythroid disease. Thus, we have taken a molecular approach to study the genetics of the erythroproliferation induced by this virus.

474

I. Molecular Cloning of Complete SFFV Proviral DNA

The SFFV proviral DNA has been recently molecularly cloned in the plasmid vector pBR322 (Linemeyer et al. 1980). Briefly, a culture of normal rat kidney fibroblasts was infected with a helper viral pseudotype of $SFFV_{LS}$. The unintegrated viral DNA was extracted by the Hirt procedure (Hirt 1967), electrophoresed through a 1% agarose gel, and the fractions enriched for the linear form III and closed circular form I SFFV-specific DNA molecules were collected and pooled. An analysis of the 6.3 kilobase pair (kbp) unintegrated linear SFFV DNA was performed using single and double restriction endonuclease digestions to develop the physical map of restriction enzyme recognition sites shown in Fig. 2A. The map was oriented 5' to 3' according to the viral genomic RNA by hybridizing enzyme digestion fragments to a ^{32}P-labeled cDNA prepared from the 3' end of F-MuLV RNA, which shares homology to the 3' end of SFFV RNA (Evans et al. 1979).

A single Hind III digestion site was found to be located 2.6 kbp from the 3' end of the linear molecule (Fig. 2A). The closed circular form I SFFV DNA was then linearized by cleavage at this single Hind III site, and SFFV-specific DNA molecules were cloned in Escherichia coli with the plasmid vector pBR322 using the unique Hind III site as described (Linemeyer et al. 1980). The clones of SFFV proviral DNA generated by this protocol were, thus, circularly permuted about the Hind III site with respect to the in vivo linear DNA. After growth of the bacterial clones and extraction of the recombinant plasmid SFFV DNA, physical restriction enzyme maps of the cloned SFFV DNAs were determined. The map of one clone (clone 4–1a3) is shown in Fig. 2B. This molecule is only 5.7 kbp in size and lacks 0.6 kbp of DNA and one Kpn I restriction enzyme site found in the in vivo linear DNA. This variation can be accounted for by the absence of one copy of the terminally redundant sequences which contain the Kpn I recognition site and which have been previously reported for murine and avian retroviruses (Gilboa et al. 1979; Hager et al. 1979; Hsu et al. 1978). To demonstrate the completeness of this 5.7 kbp clone of DNA, we showed that it was able to hybridize to all the T_1-oligonucleotides of SFFV genomic RNA (Evans et al. 1980), thus indicating that it contains at least one copy of all the sequences present in the SFFV genome.

II. Molecular Cloning of a Subgenomic Fragment of SFFV Proviral DNA

Using the 5.7-kbp clone of SFFV DNA we have now molecularly cloned a subgenomic fragment of SFFV DNA, again using the plasmid vector pBR322. We accomplished this by cleaving the recombinant circular pBR322-SFFV-cloned DNA with Pst I and inserting the resulting DNA fragments into fresh pBR322 molecules which were linearized by digestion at the unique Pst I site. The resulting SFFV DNA fragment pBR322 molecules were cloned in E. coli and identified as containing SFFV sequences by hybridization to a ^{32}P-labeled cDNA which has homology to SFFV. The plasmid DNA of various clones was then isolated and restriction endonuclease digestion products were analyzed. One clone was found to contain, along with an extra Pst I to Hind III

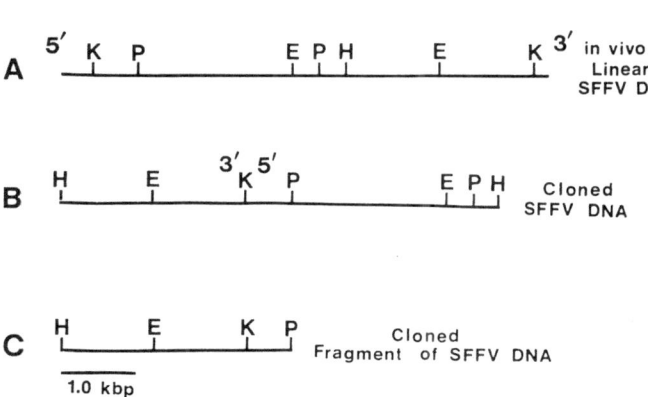

Fig. 2. Schematic map of restriction endonuclease recognition sites located on SFFV DNA. The relative positions of the recognition sites for the enzymes EcoRI (E), Hind III (H), Kpn I (K), and Pst I (P) are shown on (A) unintegrated linear SFFV proviral DNA, (B) molecularly cloned complete SFFV DNA, and (C) molecularly cloned subgenomic fragment of SFFV DNA. The areas homologous to the 3' and 5' ends of the SFFV genomic RNA are also shown

475

fragment of pBR322 DNA, a 3.0-kbp SFFV-specific DNA fragment (Fig. 2C) with restriction enzyme sites analogous to the lefthand *Hind* III to *Pst* I portion of the cloned SFFV DNA shown in Fig. 2B. This fragment of SFFV DNA should, therefore, contain 2.0 kbp of information analogous to the 3' end of the SFFV viral genome, one copy of the 0.6 kbp terminally redundant sequences, and 0.4 kbp of information analogous to the 5' end of the viral genome.

To further substantiate the portion of the SFFV proviral genome cloned, we hybridized the cloned fragment DNA to ^{32}P-labeled SFFV genomic RNA and fingerprinted the T_1-oligonucleotides which formed hybrids. Fifteen out of 24 large SFFV T_1-oligonucleotides were found to hybridize, and these oligonucleotides correspond to a contiguous segment of the SFFV T_1-oligonucleotide map which extends from the 3' end to approximately 3 kb (oligonucleotides No. 5 to No. 15 including the terminally redundant oligonucleotide No. 13, see Fig. 1). It is especially important to note that these oligonucleotides include Nos. 6, 19, and 12, which are unrelated to F-MuLV, but have identical counterparts in dualtropic MuLVs (Evans et al. 1979, 1980; Rommelaerre et al. 1978; Shih et al. 1978). Thus, these results indicate that the cloned subgenomic fragment of SFFV DNA represents the 3' half of the SFFV RNA genome and the terminally redundant sequences of the proviral DNA and contains very little of the 5' *gag* gene sequences.

E. Biologic Activity of Cloned DNA

To determine whether the cloned SFFV proviral DNA had biologic activity, NIH 3T3 fibroblasts were transfected with recombinant pBR322-SFFV DNA which had been digested with *Hind* III to linearize the plasmid molecule and to release the SFFV DNA from the vector. Since SFFV does not transform fibroblasts, it was necessary to assay for the biologic activity of the cloned DNA in the mouse. Since SFFV is also replication defective, a replication-competent helper virus must be used to rescue the SFFV sequences and allow infection of the adult mice used for the assay. Therefore, it is essential that the helper virus used does not cause a erythroid disease in adult mice.

It is possible to rescue the transfected SFFV sequences from the transfected fibroblasts by superinfecting these cells with competent helper viruses, but we have found that this rescue is accomplished more efficiently by a cotransfection protocol. In this procedure the fibroblasts are transfected with both molecularly cloned infectious helper viral DNA and cloned SFFV DNA after the two DNAs are precipitated together using CaCl$_2$ as described (Linemeyer et al. 1980). After the cotransfected cells begin to produce virus, measured by release of reverse transcriptase (1 to 3 weeks), the cell-free supernatant of these cultures is injected intravenously into adult NIH Swiss mice. The mice are then observed for the characteristics of the SFFV-induced disease from 2 to 4 weeks after injection. The results obtained from such cotransfection studies are shown in Table 1. Cotransfections using the complete 5.7-kbp cloned SFFV DNA and either cloned F-MuLV helper virus DNA (Oliff et al. 1980) or cloned Moloney MuLV (Mo-MuLV) helper virus DNA (Wei et al., unpublished work) yield virus preparations which induce splenomegaly, polycythemia, and splenic foci in the adult mice. These disease characteristics are identical to those induced by actual virus preparations of SFFV$_{LS}$. Importantly, transfections of either helper virus DNA alone produce viruses which do not induce the characteristics of SFFV-induced disease (see Table 1).

Nearly identical results are produced when the 3.0 kbp *Hind* III to *Pst* I fragment of SFFV DNA is used in the cotransfections instead of the 5.7 kbp DNA (Table 1). These results indicate that this 3' subgenomic fragment of SFFV proviral DNA contains the information responsible for the induction of the erythroproliferative disease.

F. Protein Expression of Cells Transfected with Cloned SFFV DNA

We were interested in whether the subgenomic fragment of SFFV DNA, which contained the 3' *env* gene related sequences, encoded the information necessary to express the *env* gene related gp52 SFFV protein. Cells from a culture of NIH 3T3 fibroblasts cotransfected with Mo-MuLV DNA and the SFFV DNA fragment were cloned. Twenty-three single cell

Table 1. Biologic properties of virus produced from cells transfected with cloned SFFV DNA released from the plasmid by *Hind* III digestion[a]

Exp. No.	Transfection of *Hind* III-digested cloned SFFV DNA	Rescue of SFFV activity by cotransfection with DNA	Days after mouse injection	Spleen wt[b] (g)	Hemato-[b] crit	Splenic foci production
I	5.7-kbp clone	F-MuLV clone 57	15	0.71, 0.95	46	+
			28	2.2, 4.9	62,69	
	None	F-MuLV clone 57	48	0.20, 0.31	47	−
	5.7-kbp clone	Mo-MuLV clone 1387	15	0.23, 2.2	50	+
			28	2.0, 5.6	45,60	
	None	Mo-MuLV clone 1387	48	0.18, 0.23	46,48	−
II	3.0-kbp fragment	F-MuLV clone 57	14	0.66, 0.71	NT	+
			21	2.6, 2.2	63,67	
	None	F-MuLV clone 57	21	0.28, 0.24	47,46	−
	3.0-kbp fragment	Mo-MuLV clone 1387	14	1.7, 1.4	NT	+
			21	2.2, 4.9	66,55	
	None	Mo-MuLV clone 1387	21	0.22, 0.24	47,48	−

[a] The characteristics of disease were monitored in intravenously injected 6- to 8-week-old NIH Swiss mice. NT = not tested

[b] The values indicated are from individual mice

clones were obtained. One clone was found to produce virus which induced the SFFV disease after injection into adult mice. These cells were labeled with ^{35}S-methionine and the extract of these cells was analyzed for gp52 by immune precipitation. Two other cell clones, derived from the same experiment, which were not producing SFFV were labeled as controls. Gp52 was detected in the SFFV-positive cell clone only. This gp52 could be precipitated by an antiserum specific for MCF viral envelope determinants which are present on the gp52, but not by normal nonimmune serum. It has the same antigenic properties and sodium dodecyl sulfate-polyacrylamide gel migration pattern as the gp52 expressed in normal rat kidney cells nonproductively infected with actual SFFV$_{LS}$ (Ruscetti et al. 1979) and is clearly not expressed by cells transfected with the helper Mo-MuLV DNA alone. The gp52 was also expressed in cells from diseased spleens of mice infected with the virus progeny of the fibroblasts cotransfected with the fragment of SFFV DNA and F-MuLV DNA.

G. Conclusions

In summary, we have shown that the genome of SFFV contains sequences homologous to the helper virus F-MuLV and sequences non-homologous to F-MuLV. These latter sequences which are unrelated to F-MuLV are related to envelope gene sequences of dualtropic MuLVs. These structural analyses indicate that SFFV$_{LS}$ is a deletion mutant of a dualtropic Friend MCF virus. Using a molecularly cloned subgenomic fragment of SFFV$_{LS}$ proviral DNA, we have shown that sequences present in the 3′ half of the SFFV genome are responsible for the SFFV-induced erythroproliferative disease. These 3′ sequences contain the dualtropic MuLV *env* gene related sequences and encode the SFFV-specified gp52 *env* gene related protein. Although it is possible that other sequences closely linked to those encoding gp52 are required for the SFFV biologic activity, such as the terminally redundant sequences, the results are consistent with the hypothesis that the gp52 plays a role in initiation of the erythroproliferation.

References

Axelrad AA, Steeves RA (1964) Virology 24:513–518 – Barbacid M, Troxler DH, Scolnick EM, Aaronson SA (1978) J Virol 27:826–830 – Bernstein A, Mak TW, Stephenson JR (1977) Cell 12:287–294 – Bernstein A, Gamble C, Penrose D,

Mak TW (1979) Proc Natl Acad Sci USA 76:4455–4459 – Coffin JM, Billeter MA (1976) J Mol Biol 100:293–318 – Dawson PJ, Tacke RB, Fieldsteel AH (1968) Br J Cancer 22:569–576 – Dresler S, Ruta M, Murray MJ, Kabat D (1979) J Virol 30:564–575 – Duesberg PH (1980) Cold Spring Harbor Symp Quant Biol 44:13–29 – Evans LH, Duesberg PH, Troxler DH, Scolnick EM (1979) J Virol 31:133–146 – Evans LH, Nunn M, Duesberg PH, Troxler DH, Scolnick EM (1980) Cold Spring Harbor Symp Quant Biol 44:823–835 – Faller DV, Hopkins N (1978) Virology 90:265–273 – Gilboa E, Goff S, Shields A, Yoshimura F, Mitra S, Baltimore D (1979) Cell 16:863–874 – Hager GL, Chang EH, Chan WH, Garon CF, Israel MA, Martin MA, Scolnick EM, Lowy DR (1979) J Virol 31:795–809 – Hirt B (1967) J Mol Biol 26:365–369 – Hsu TW, Sabran JL, Mark GE, Guntaka RV, Taylor JM (1978) J Virol 28:810–818 – Lilly F, Steeves RA (1973) Virology 55:363–370 – Linemeyer DL, Ruscetti SK, Menke JG, Scolnick EM (1980) J Virol 35:710–721 – Mak TW, Penrose D, Gamble C, Bernstein A (1978) Virology 87:73–80 – Oliff AI, Hager GL, Chang EH, Scolnick EM, Chan HW, Lowy DR (1980) J Virol 33:475–486 – PRL IB, McNab A, Harrison PR, Ostertag W (1978) Nature 272:456–458 – Rawson KE, Parr IB (1970) Int J Cancer 5:96–102 – Rommelaere J, Faller DV, Hopkins N (1978) Proc Natl Acad Sci USA 75:495–499 – Ruscetti SK, Linemeyer D, Feild J, Troxler D, Scolnick EM (1979) J Virol 30:787–798 – Ruscetti SK, Troxler D, Linemeyer D, Scolnick EM (1980) J Virol 33:140–151 – Shih TY, Weeks MO, Troxler D, Coffin JM, Scolnick EM (1978) J Virol 26:71–83 – Steeves RA, Eckner RJ, Bennett M, Mirand EA, Trudel PJ (1971) J Natl Cancer Inst 46:1209–1217 – Troxler DH, Boyars JK, Parks WP, Scolnick EM (1977a) J Virol 22:361–372 – Troxler DH, Lowy D, Howk R, Young H, Scolnick EM (1977b) Proc Natl Acad Sci USA 74:4671–4675 – Troxler DH, Parks WP, Vass WC, Scolnick EM (1977c) Virology 76:602–615 – Troxler DH, Yuan E, Linemeyer D, Ruscetti S, Scolnick EM (1978) J Exp Med 148:639–653 – Troxler DH, Ruscetti SK, Scolnick EM (1980) Biochem Biophys Acta 605:305–324 – Wang LH, Duesberg PH, Beemon K, Vogt PK (1975) J Virol 16:1051–1070

Haematology and Blood Transfusion Vol. 26
Modern Trends in Human Leukemia IV
Edited by Neth, Gallo, Graf, Mannweiler, Winkler
© Springer-Verlag Berlin Heidelberg 1981

Enhancing Effect of Murine Leukemia Virus on Fibroblast Transformation by Normal BALB/C Mouse DNA Fragments

K. J. van den Berg, V. Krump-Konvalinkova, and P. Bentvelzen

A. Introduction

Several rapidly transforming RNA tumor viruses contain inserts of cellular genetic material. These inserts seem to constitute the so-called *onc* genes of these viruses (Stephenson et al. 1979). The question arises whether during the recombination process leading to the generation of highly oncogenic viruses the cellular sequences become altered in such a way that they will cause malignant transformation. This would then be compatible with simplistic somatic mutation theories of nonviral carcinogenesis. Alternatively, with the virus acting as a vector, the insertion of normal cellular sequences involved in control of growth and/or differentiation into other sites of the host genome may lead to overproduction of certain gene products and eventually to malignant transformation. This transposition phenomenon may have important implications for models of nonviral carcinogenesis.

B. Transformation by Normal Cell DNA

Recently Cooper et al. (1980) reported that mechanically fragmented normal cellular DNA isolated from avian or mammalian cell lines could transform NIH/3T3 cells, albeit at a low frequency. Secondary transfections with DNA isolated from the transformed cells proved to be highly efficient.

During our study on transfection with the integrated provirus of Abelson murine leukemia virus (A-MuLV) utilizing the calciumtechnique of Graham and van der Eb (1973), we observed independently of Cooper et al. in control experiments that mechanically fragmented DNA isolated from the thymus of normal BALB/c mice could transform NIH/3T3 as well as BALB/3T3 cells. In contrast to the foci of transformed cells induced by the A-MuLV provirus which appear within 2 weeks, those induced by normal DNA were first observed after 4 weeks, corresponding with six subcultures of the recipient cell.

The DNA specificity can be concluded from Table 1 in which treatment of the DNA preparation with DNase abrogated fully the transforming capacity, while RNase or pronase did not. Neither calf thymus nor *E.coli* DNA induced foci of transformed cells.

Since DNA isolated from thymus, spleen, or liver had equal transforming capacity (see Table 2), the transforming sequences seem to be an integral part of the BALB/c genome. As DNA isolated from germfree BALB/c mice of a colony established 20 years ago is similarly transforming, this property cannot be due to recent infection of the germ line with an oncogenic virus.

C. Characterization of Transformed Cell Lines

A battery of cell lines were developed from foci of transformants induced by normal BALB/c DNA fragments. No reverse transcriptase activity could be detected in any of the cell lines, indicating that transformation occurred in the absence of replicating retroviruses.

The cells grew well in soft agar, indicating anchorage independence. Upon intraperitoneal inoculation into newborn athymic BALB/ nude mice, all of six tested cell lines were oncogenic. After subcutaneous injection of 10^6 cells into 3-week-old BALB/c five of six lines produced fibrosarcomas within 3 weeks.

Table 1. Transformation of 3T3 cells by normal BALB/c DNA

	Recipient cells			
	BALB/3T3		NIH/3T3	
	Fraction trans- formed cultures	Average No. foci/dish	Fraction trans- formed cultures	Average No. foci/dish
BALB/c thymus DNA 50 $\mu g \cdot ml^{-1}$	16/16	15	16/16	4
Ibid, treated with pronase[a]	8/8	4	7/8	1.5
BALB/c thymus DNA 50 $\mu g \cdot ml^{-1}$ RNase[a]	8/8	2	8/8	6
BALB/c thymus DNA 50 $\mu g \cdot ml^{-1}$ DNase[a]	0/8	0	0/8	0
BALB/c thymus DNA 50 $\mu g \cdot ml^{-1}$ heat denatured[b]	3/8	· 0.5	3/8	0.5
Calf thymus DNA, 50 $\mu g \cdot ml^{-1}$	0/8	0	0/8	0
E. coli DNA, 50 $mg \cdot \mu l^{-1}$	0/8	0	0/8	0

[a] 1 h at 37°C
[b] 5 min at 100°C, then quickly placed in ice

So far, no transforming virus could be rescued after infection with the Moloney strain of MuLV (Mo-MuLV) in contrast to cells transformed by A-MuLV proviral DNA. A hyperimmune antiserum, raised in C57BL against syngeneic A-MuLV induced lymphoma cells and absorbed with syngeneic Mo-MuLV lymphoma cells, reacted with two of seven testet cell lines transformed by normal DNA in the cytoplasmic immunofluorescence test. The antiserum reacted with a variety of A-MuLV transformed cells but not with NIH/3T3 cells infected with Mo-MuLV.

D. Enhancement of Transformation by Preinfection with Leukemia Virus

The efficiency of transformation of normal cell DNA is rather low. Since the nontransforming murine leukemia viruses make cells susceptible to the action of various carcinogenic chemicals (Huebner and Gilden 1972), we studied the influence of preinfection with MuLV-strains in this system. After incubation of NIH/3T3 cells, infected with either Rauscher or Moloney-MuLV, with normal cell DNA fragments, foci could be detected within 2 weeks after a single passage. The transformation frequency could be as high as 1 focus forming unit per 1 ug DNA (see Table 3), which would be comparable to the results obtained with the A-MuLV provirus. A linear

dose-response relationship was found in this system (Fig. 1), indicating that incorporation of a single DNA fragment would be sufficient for neoplastic conversion. Quite remarkable is that a minimal quantity of DNA is needed for transformation to occur.

E. Discussion

It is unlikely that the transforming capacity of normal cell DNA is due to sheer mutagenicity, since mouse DNA sequences homologous to the src gene of Moloney murine sarcoma virus cannot transform fibroblasts (Oskarsson et al. 1980). Our data and those of Cooper et al. (1980) support the notion that the cellular

Table 2. Effect of origin of BALB/c DNA on transforming activity[a]

Source of DNA		Recipient cells (Fraction transformed cultures)	
		BALB/3T3	NIH/3T3
Thymus	50 ug · ml^{-1}	16/16	16/16
	25 ug · ml^{-1}	8/8	N.D.
Spleen	50 ug · ml^{-1}	8/8	N.D.
	25 ug · ml^{-1}	8/8	2/8
Liver	50 ug · ml^{-1}	4/4	N.D.

[a] N.D. = not done

Table 3. Effect of preinfection with murine leukemia virus on early transformation by normal BALB/c DNA

Recipient cells	Treatment	Fraction transformed cultures at 2 weeks	Average no. foci/dish	Average transformation freq. ($\times 10^6$/ug DNA/cel)
NIH/3T3	BALB/c liver DNA[a]	0/33	0	0
	E. coli DNA	0/33	0	0
	transfection buffer	0/33	0	0
NIH/3T3-R-MuLV[b]	BALB/c liver DNA	3/3	4	2
	E. coli DNA	0/3	0	0
	transfection buffer	0/3	0	0
NIH/3T3-Mo-MuLV[c]	BALB/c liver DNA	33/33	18	7
	E. coli DNA	0/33	0	0
	transfection buffer	0/33	0	0

[a] 25 ug·ml^{-1}
[b] NIH/3T3 infected with Rauscher murine leukemia virus 4 days before transfection
[c] NIH/3T3-cloned after having been productively infected with Moloney murine leukemia virus

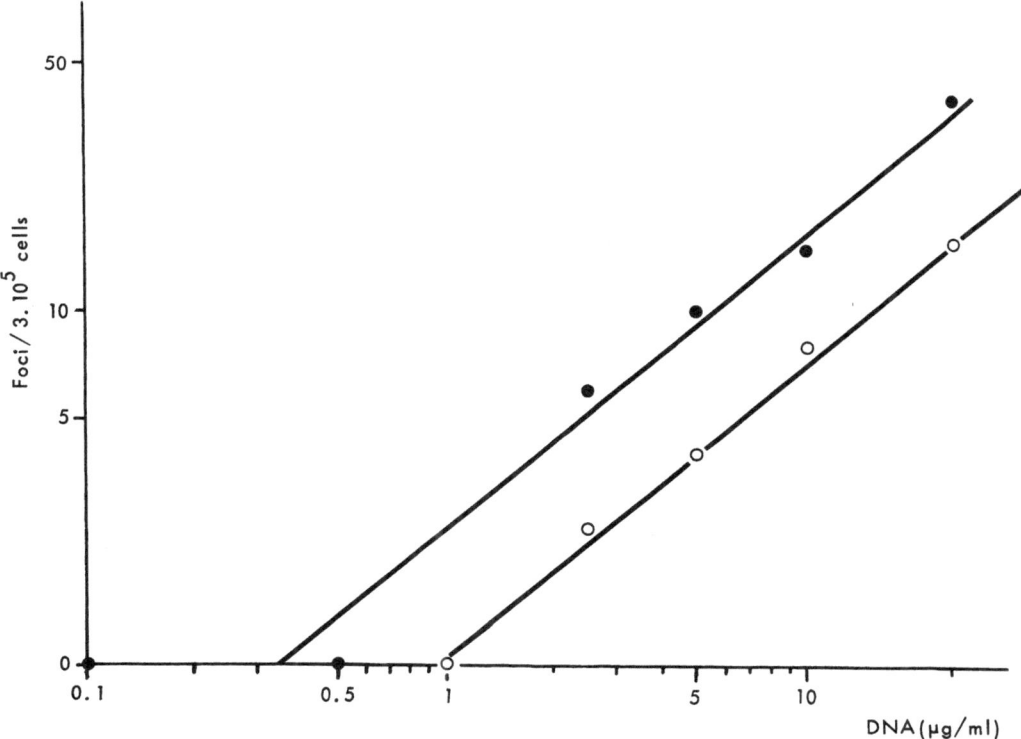

Fig. 1. Kinetics of transformation of NIH/3T3 cells infected with Mo-MuLV by fragmented normal BALB/c DNA

inserts in the genome of rapidly transforming viruses have not been perturbated. They suggest that transposition of certain cellular genes may result in oncogenic transformation. It has been hypothesized that this was due to abrogation of negative control by neighboring genes (Van Bekkum 1975). Alternatively, and more likely, it may be due to the insertion of the cellular genes close to the active promotor sequences. The latter hypothesis would explain the low efficiency of primary transfections and the better transforming rate of secondary ones.

The immunofluorescence staining of some of the transformed lines with an antiserum presumably directed against the *onc* gene of A-MuLV suggest that in these cases the homologous gene might have been incorporated at a different site resulting in transformation. Several other cellular *onc* genes must have been involved in the generation of the other transformed cell lines.

The enhancing effect of murine leukemia virus may be due to the induction of a semitransformed state of the 3T3 cells by MuLV, which would explain the single-hit transformation by normal cellular DNA fragments. Another hypothesis, which we favor at the moment, is that MuLV provides highly active promotor sequences. This is supported by the finding that the complete provirus of Moloney murine sarcoma virus, which contains leukemia virus derived promotors, is not enhanced in its transforming capacity by preinfection of recipient cells with MuLV (Anderson et al. 1979).

Acknowledgments

This investigation was supported in part by the Koningin Wilhelmina Fonds of the Netherlands Cancer Organization. Mr. R. H. van Leersum and Mr. D. S. Luyt are thanked for technical assistance.

References

Anderson P, Goldfarb MP, Weiberg RA (1979) A defined subgenomic fragment of in vitro synthesized moloney sarcoma virus DNA can induce cell transformation upon transfection. Cell 16:63–75 – Cooper GM, Okenquist S, Silverman L (1980) Transforming activity of DNA of chemically transformed and normal cells. Nature 284:418–421 – Graham FL, van der Eb AJ (1973) A new technique for the assay of infectivity of human adenovirus 5 DNA. Virology 52:456–467 – Huebner RJ, Gilden RV (1972) Inherited RNA viral genomes (virogenes and oncogenes) in the etiology of cancer. In: Emmelot P, Bentvelzen P (eds) RNA viruses and host genome in oncogenesis. North-Holland, Amsterdam, pp 197–21g – Oskarsson M, McClements WL, Blair PG, Maizel JV, van de Woude GF (1980) Properties of a normal mouse cell DNA sequence (sarc) homologous to the src sequence of Moloney sarcoma virus. Science 207:1222–1224 – Stephenson JR, Khan AS, van de Ven WJN, Reynolds FH Jr (1979) Type C retroviruses as vectors for cloning cellular genes with probable transforming function. J Natl Cancer Inst 63:1111–1119 – Van Bekkum DW (1975) Mechanisms of radiation carcinogenesis. In: Nygaard OF, Adler HI, Sinclair WK (eds) Radiation research biomedical, chemical and physical perspectives. Academic Press, New York, pp 886–894

Haematology and Blood Transfusion Vol. 26
Modern Trends in Human Leukemia IV
Edited by Neth, Gallo, Graf, Mannweiler, Winkler
© Springer-Verlag Berlin Heidelberg 1981

Role of Viruses in the Etiology of Naturally Occurring Feline Leukemia

M. Essex, C. K. Grant, S. M. Cotter, and W. D. Hardy, Jr.

A. Introduction

The search to determine if retroviruses cause human leukemia has now been underway for at least 15 years. However, the number of investigators who have conducted direct studies with human materials has been small. By contrast, major emphasis has been given to the study of retrovirus-induced tumors of inbred mice and chickens as models for understanding leukemia of man. At the same time only a limited amount of attention has ben given to the study of the agents that are known to cause leukemia in cats and cattle. Having evolved under natural circumstances in outbred species, the feline and bovine retroviruses would appear to be important agents for study. Presumably information derived about potential mechanisms of leukemogenesis in these species would be applicable to many of the questions one might pose about the etiology of human leukemia. In this context we describe recent findings on the biology and natural history of the feline retroviruses and the diseases they cause.

B. Epidemiology

Several forms of leukemia and lymphoma are caused by the feline leukemia viruses (FeLV). These include (a) thymic lymphoma, which is a T-cell neoplasm that originates in the mediastinal cavity; (b) alimentary lymphoma, which is a B cell disease that originates in the gut wall; (c) multicentric lymphoma, which presumably arises in the lymph nodes and is usually a T-cell tumor; (d) acute lymphoblastic leukemia, which originates in the bone marrow and/or blood; (e) various forms of myeloid leuke-

mias; and (f) certain miscellaneous localized lymphomas such as those that occur in the skin or the central nervous system. FeLV also causes aplastic anemia (Mackey et al. 1975), a disease which may be caused by similar imbalances in bone marrow cell populations. Additionally, because FeLV is immunosuppressive, a wide range of infectious diseases that are normally controlled by the immune response may occur more frequently in FeLV-infected animals (Essex et al. 1975a). Another group of feline retraviruses that are closely related to FeLV, the feline sarcoma viruses (FeSV), cause fibrosarcomas. The viruses designated as FeLVs are replication competent and they usually cause no visible pathology in cultured cells. The FeSVs are replication defective and they transform cultured fibroblasts.

The various morphologic forms of feline leukemia and lymphoma occur at different rates in different geographic areas (Essex 1975), an observation that suggests an association between a given form of disease and specific strains of virus. Although FeLVs have been categorized into subgroups by interference (Sarma and Log 1973) or serum antibody neutralization (Russell and Jarrett 1978) and into "strains" by T 1 oligonucleotide fingerprinting (Rosenberg et al. 1980), no association between given morphologic forms of naturally occurring disease and specific strains of subgroups has yet been recognized. One laboratory-passaged strain of FeLV has been shown to induce the thymic form of lymphoma in a consistent manner (Hoover et al. 1976).

Large clusters of feline leukemia and lymphoma were occasionally observed in pet cat populations (Cotter et al. 1973). Since such clusters usually occurred among outbred populations, it seemed likely that the virus causing the disease was transmitted in a contagious manner. This was confirmed as serologic evidence developed to show that healthy household associates of leukemic animals were very likely to be either infected with FeLV (Hardy et al. 1973) or harboring high levels of antibodies of FeLV (Stephenson et al. 1977a) or to FOCMA, the feline oncornavirus-associated cell membrane antigen (Essex et al. 1975b). Subsequently, it was shown that specific pathogen-free tracer cats introduced into cluster environments soon became viremic themselves with FeLV (Essex et al. 1977). Conversely, the removal of infected cats from such environments prevented the occurrence of future FeLV infections and disease development (Hardy et al. 1976).

The induction period for development of leukemia or lymphoma in cats that become infected with FeLV is prolonged and variable. In one series of 18 cats followed under natural conditions this interval varied from 3 months to 52 months and the mean interval was about 18 months (Francis et al. 1979b). Another issue that confuses the association between FeLV and development of neoplasia is the small proportion of exposed animals that actually develop leukemia or lymphoma. Most cats that become infected rid themselves of FeLV due to an active and efficient immune response to the virus envelope glycoproteins (Essex 1980). Of the majority of animals that do not become persistently viremic, at least some experience transient viremia (Grant et al. 1980). Whether or not all animals that become infected experience viremia is unknown. Even among the 2%–5% of the infected animals that become persistently viremic, most do not develop leukemia. About one-fourth or one-third of these chronically viremic cats get leukemia, while the others develop such diseases as infectious peritonitis, septicemia, and glomerulonephritis (Francis et al. 1980). As mentioned above, this is in part due to the immunosuppressive potential of FeLV and in part because these other diseases have shorter induction periods.

In leukemia cluster households, where cats are maintained under abnormally crowded conditions, the pattern of disease development becomes shifted (Francis et al. 1980). All of the cats are then exposed to FeLV, half or more become persistently viremic, and up to half may eventually die of leukemia or the immu-

nosuppression-related diseases. This increase in the rate of persistent viremia in such environments is due in large part to the fact that the cats first become exposed to FeLV at a very young age. Presumably higher concentrations of FeLV are also received at the time of exposure. Both factors should substantially increase the chances that persistent viremia and tumor development will occur.

Persistently viremic cats regularly release infectious FeLV in saliva (Francis et al. 1977). The amount of virus they produce ranges from 10^3 to 10^6 infectious units/ml. The virus is reasonably stable for long periods, if it is in a cool and moist environment (Francis et al. 1979c). Healthy, persistently viremic cats may excrete even higher levels than leukemic cats (Francis et al. 1979b). Since the former substantially outnumber the latter in most populations at any given period of time, it is obviously the healthy cats that represent the major link for transmission and maintenance of the agent in the population. As a result it would be impossible to control the disease only by eliminating leukemic or sick animals. By contrast, the elimination of all persistently infected animals from closed populations is effective in preventing disease development (Hardy et al. 1976).

About one-third or one-half of the cases of feline leukemia and lymphoma occur in nonviremic cats (Francis et al. 1979a; Hardy et al. 1980). In some geographic areas certain morphologic forms, especially the alimentary lymphoma, were more likely to occur in nonviremic cats. However, a significant portion of all major forms have been observed in nonviremic animals.

Recently, it was demonstrated that healthy cats that become exposed to FeLV in endemic environments have an increased risk for the development of the "virus-negative" (VN) form of lymphoma. In fact, the increase in relative risk for development of the VN form of lymphoma rises to same proportion (40-fold) as the risk for development of virus-positive feline leukemia following known exposure to FeLV (Hardy et al. 1980). This strongly suggests that FeLV plays an important role in the etiology of VN leukemia. We recently proposed an "immunoselection hypothesis" to postulate one possible mechanism by which such an event might occur (Essex 1980). Since human leukemias occur in individuals that do not harbor replicating viruses, an understanding of the role that FeLV may play in the etiology of VN feline leukemia may be important.

C. Immune Response

The FeLV particles contain seven distinct proteins designated p15c, p12, p30, p10, p15e, gp70, and reverse transcriptase. All seven have been shown to be immunogenic in cats under natural conditions of exposure (Essex 1980), and several of the proteins have more than one antigenic determinant. The major protein that serves as a target for virus neutralizing antibodies is gp70, although it seems likely that p15e could serve a similar function because of its localization in the backbone of the virion envelope. Although the proteins of the *gag* gene, i.e., p15c, p12, p30, and p10, occur at internal sites in the virus particles, they are expressed at the surface of virus-producing cells (Essex et al. 1978). Many cats that become naturally exposed to FeLV develop high levels of antibodies to such proteins as p30 (Stephenson et al. 1977a). Whether or not this response plays any role in the lysis of virus-producing cells in vivo remains to be determined.

Another antigen or antigen complex associated with FeLV is FOCMA, but only in the sense that it is found on lymphoma cells and/or leukemia cells (Essex et al. 1978; Hardy et al. 1977). In fact, it is not present in either virus-producing, phenotypically normal cells or in FeLV particles. It is present in fibroblasts that are transformed by FeSV (Sliski et al. 1977) and in FeSV particles that have been rescued by a helper other than FeLV (Sherr et al. 1978).

The immune response to FOCMA is correlated with protection against development of leukemia and lymphoma (Essex et al. 1975b) as well as against the development and progression of FeSV-induced fibrosarcomas (Essex et al. 1971) and melanomas (Niederkorn et al. 1980). Antibodies to FOCMA have been identified by membrane immunofluorescence (Essex et al. 1971), by ^{51}Cr release (Grant et al. 1977), and by radioimmunoassay (Snyder et al. 1980). Lymphoma cells can be effectively lysed with antibodies in the presence of complement (Grant et al. 1977). The lysis occurs slowly, requiring up to 20 h, and works most efficiently with cat complement. The pattern of occurrence of the lytic antibodies coincides almost perfectly with the disease associated pattern first described by membrane immunofluorescence (Essex et al. 1971; Grant et al. 1978), and allows for the possibility that such antibodies may function by complement-mediated lysis in vivo. If such a mechanism is important in vivo, depressions of complement levels might also allow immunogenic tumors to evade an otherwise effective antibody response (Grant et al. 1979). Such antibodies can also be used therapeutically to cause the regression of FeSV-induced fibrosarcomas (Noronha et al. 1980) and prevent early relapse of lymphomas after drug-induced remission (Cotter et al. 1980).

D. Tumor and Transformation Specific Antigens

Attempts to detect specific molecular species of antigens that react with typical high-titered FOCMA-type antisera from healthy »regressor" type cats led to the recognition of two general classes of molecules. The first, which was found initially on FeSV-transformed mink nonproducer fibroblasts, was a polyprotein that contained the 5' portions of the gag gene products (p15, p12, and parts of p30) covalently linked to a molecule of 60,000–70,000 daltons which presumably harbored the FOCMA determinants (Stephenson et al. 1977b). Such gag-x polyproteins have now been described for several oncogenic retroviruses and the possibility that the "x" portion of this molecule contains determinants that would be analagous to FOCMA has been considered. In the feline system two classes of gag x proteins have been found that represent the three partially characterized isolates of FeSV (Porzig et al. 1979). One class of gag-x protein contained shared antigenic cross-reactivity in the "x" portion for the Gardner-Arnstein and Snyder-Theilen viruses. The second reacts with cells transformed by the McDonough strain of FeSV and contains little if any cross-reactivity with cells transformed by the Gardner and/or Snyder strains of FeSV. These results appear analogous to those obtained by nucleic acid hybridization concerning the detection of suspected "src" sequences in fibroblasts transformed by the same three strains of FeSV (Frankel et al. 1979).

The second general class of proteins that

contains antigens which react with FOCMA-type antisera are those molecules of 65,000–70,000 daltons that have been detected in the membranes of lymphoma cells and FeSV-transformed nonproducer fibroblasts (Snyder et al. 1978; Worley and Essex 1980). Antiserum made in rabbits to the 65,000-dalton protein purified from FeSV-transformed cells could be used to precipitate an analogous 68,000-dalton protein in the membrane of cultured feline lymphoma cells. Cat antisera containing FOCMA antibodies also precipitate both the 65,000-dalton protein of transformed mink cells and the 68,000-dalton protein of lymphoid cells (Worley and Essex 1980). Earlier, Snyder et al. (1978) found that the ^{125}I-lactoperoxidase technique revealed a 70,000-dalton protein in membranes of feline lymphoma cells which reacted with FOCMA antisera (Chen et al. 1980). This 70,000-dalton protein may be the same as the 68,000-dalton protein described above.

Cats which were repeatedly immunized with their own cells that had been transformed in culture with FeSV developed high titers of antibodies to the appropriate gag-x protein. Although such sera usually contain antibodies to the virion structural proteins, they also contain antibodies to the "x" specific portion of the molecule. Thus, hyperimmune cat sera which initially reacted with the 85,000-dalton gag-x protein characteristic of the ST strain of FeSV still immunoprecipitate the same molecule after the removal of all antibodies to viral proteins by passage of the serum sample over an immunoadsorbent column (Chen et al. 1980).

The 85,000-dalton gag x polyprotein is expressed in FeSV-transformed cat cells as well as mink cells and in FeSV-transformed cells that replicate helper FeLV as well as nonproducers. This gag x protein is expressed in primary cultures of explanted FeSV-induced fibrosarcomas, suggesting that the protein may play a role in vivo as well as in transformation in vitro. Cultured explanted cells from FeSV-induced melanomas also contain the same protein, suggesting that the gag x type gene products may be expressed concordinately with malignant phenotype even in tumors originating from different embryonic germ cell layers. The latter observation suggests that at least some "x" type genes may have a pleiotropic effect and is compatible with the concept that the same or related FOCMA-type sequence may cause malignant alterations in both stromal cells and various lymphoid and hematopoietic cells (Chen et al. 1980). Several types of spontaneous tumors that were not associated with FeLV or FeSV were also checked for FOCMA and gag x type antigens and all were negative. Similarly, cat and mink cells that were transformed with agents other than FeSV did not contain these proteins.

Acknowledgments

Research done in the laboratories of the authors was supported by U.S. National Cancer Institute grants CA-13885, CA-18216, CA-16599, CA-18488, and CA-08748, contracts CB-64001 and CP-81004, and grant DT-32 from the American Cancer Society. C.K.G. is a Scholar of the Leukemia Society of America.

References

Chen AP, Essex M, Mikami T, Albert D, Niederkorn JY, Shadduck JP (1980) The expression of transformation-related proteins in cat cells. In: Hardy WD Jr, Essex M, McClelland J (eds) Feline leukemia and sarcoma viruses. Elsevier, New York pp 441–456 – Cotter SM, Gilmore CE, Rollins C (1973) Multiple cases of feline leukemia and feline infectious peritonitis in a household. J Am Vet Med Assoc 162:1054–1058 – Cotter SM, Essex M, McLane MF, Grant CK, Hardy WD Jr (1980) Passive immunotherapy in naturally occurring feline mediastinal lymphoma. In: Hardy WD Jr, Essex M, McClelland J (eds) Feline leukemia and sarcoma viruses. Elsevier, New York pp 219–226 – Essex M (1975) Horizontally and vertically transmitted oncornaviruses of cats. Adv Cancer Res 21:175–248 – Essex M (1980) Feline leukemia and sarcoma viruses. In: Klein G (ed) Viral oncology. Raven, New York, pp 205–229 – Essex M, Klein G, Snyder SP, Harrold JB (1971) Feline sarcoma virus (FSV) induced tumors: correlations between humoral antibody and tumor regression. Nature 233:195–196 – Essex M, Hardy WD Jr, Cotter SM, Jakowski RM, Sliski A (1975a) Naturally occurring persistent feline oncornavirus infections in the absence of disease. Infect Immun 11:470–475 – Essex M, Sliski A, Cotter SM, Jakowski RM, Hardy WD Jr (1975b) Immunosurveillance of naturally occurring feline leukemia. Science 190:790–792 – Essex M, Cotter SM, Sliski AH, Hardy WD Jr, Stephenson JR, Aaronson SA, Jarrett O (1977) Horizontal transmission of feline leukemia virus under natural conditions in a feline leukemia cluster household. Int J Cancer 19:90–96 – Essex M, Sliski AH, Hardy

WD Jr, de Noronha F, Cotter SM (1978) Feline oncornavirus associated cell membrane antigen: a tumor specific cell surface marker. In: Bentvelzen P, Hilgers J, Yohn DS (eds) Advances in comparative leukemia research 1977. Elsevier/North Holland Biomedical Press, Amsterdam, pp 337–340 – Francis DP, Essex M, Hardy WD Jr (1977) Excretion of feline leukemia virus by naturally infected pet cats. Nature 269:252–254 – Francis DP, Cotter SM, Hardy WD Jr, Essex M (1979a) Comparison of virus-positive and virus-negative cases of feline leukemia and lymphoma. Cancer Res 39:3866–3870 – Francis DP, Essex M, Cotter SM, Jakowski RM, Hardy WD Jr (1979b) Feline leukemia virus infections: the significance of chronic viremia. Leuk Res 3:435–441 – Francis DP, Essex M, Gayzagian D (1979c) Feline leukemia virus: survival under home and laboratory conditions. J Clin Microbiol 9:154–156 – Francis DP, Essex M, Jakowski RM, Cotter SM, Lerer TJ, Hardy WD Jr (1980) Feline lymphoma: descriptive epidemiology of a virally-induced malignancy in a closed cat population. Am J Epidemiol 111:337–346 – Frankel AE, Gilbert JH, Porzig KJ, Scolnick EM, Aaronson SA (1979) Nature and distribution of feline sarcoma virus nucleotide sequences. J Virol 30:821–827 – Grant CK, De Boer DJ, Essex M, Worley MB, Higgins J (1977) Antibodies from healthy cats exposed to feline leukemia virus lyse feline lymphoma cells slowly with cat complement. J Immunol 119:401–406 – Grant CK, Essex M, Pedersen NC, Hardy WD Jr, Cotter SM, Theilen GH (1978) Cat complement and cat antisera lyse feline lymphoblastoid cells: Correlation of lysis with detection of antibodies to FOCMA. J Natl Cancer Inst 60:161–166 – Grant CK, Ramaika C, Madewell BR, Pickard DK, Essex M (1979) Complement and tumor antibody levels in cats, and changes associated with natural feline leukemia virus infection and malignant disease. Cancer Res 39:75–81 – Grant CK, Essex M, Gardner MB, Hardy WD Jr (1980) Natural feline leukemia virus infection and the immune response of cats of different ages. Cancer Res 40:825–829 – Hardy WD Jr, Old LJ, Hess PW, Essex M, Cotter SM (1973) Horizontal transmission of feline leukemia virus in cats. Nature 244:266–269 – Hardy WD Jr, McClelland AJ, Zuckerman EE, Hess PW, Essex M, Cotter SM, MacEwen EG, Hayes AA (1976) Prevention of the infectious spread of the feline leukemia virus in pet cats. Nature 263:326–328 – Hardy WD Jr, Zuckerman EE, MacEwen EG, Hayes AA, Essex M (1977) A feline leukemia and sarcoma virus induced tumor specific antigen. Nature 270:249–251 – Hardy WD Jr, Zuckerman EE, McClelland AJ, Snyder HW Jr, Essex M, Francis DP (1980) The immunology and epidemiology of FeLV nonproducer feline lymphosarcoma. Cold Spring Harbor Conf Cell Prolif 7:677–697 – Hoover EA, Olsen RG, Hardy WD Jr, Schaller JP, Mathes LE (1976) Feline leukemia virus infecton: age-related variation in response of cats to experimental infection. J Natl Cancer Inst 57:365–370 – Mackey L, Jarrett W, Jarrett O, Laird H (1975) Anemia associated with feline leukemia virus infection in cats. J Natl Cancer Inst 54:209–218 – Niederkorn JY, Shadduck JA, Albert D, Essex M (1980) FOCMA antibodies in cats with FeSV-induced ocular melanomas. In: Hardy WD Jr, Essex M, McClelland J (eds) Feline leukemia and sarcoma viruses. Elsevier, New York pp 181–186 – Noronha F de, Grant CK, Essex M, Bolognesi DP (to be published) Passive immune serotherapy protects cats from disseminated FeSV-induced fibrosarcomas. In: Hardy WD Jr, Essex M, McClelland J (eds) Feline leukemia and sarcoma viruses. Elsevier/North Holland, New York – Porzig KJ, Barbacid M, Aaronson SA (1979) Biological properties and translational products of three independent isolates of feline sarcoma virus. Virology 92:91–107 – Rosenberg ZF, Pedersen FS, Haseltine WA (1980) Comparative analysis of the genome of feline leukemia viruses. J Virol 35:542–546 – Russell PH, Jarrett O (1978) The occurrence of feline leukemia virus neutralizing antibodies in cats. Int J Cancer 22:351–357 – Sarma PS, Log T (1973) Subgroup classification of feline leukemia and sarcoma viruses by viral interference and neutralization tests. Virology 54:160–170 – Sherr CJ, Sen A, Todaro GJ, Sliski AH, Essex M (1978) Pseudotypes of feline sarcoma virus contain an 85,000 dalton protein with feline oncornavirus-associated cell membrane antigen (FOCMA) activity. Proc Natl Acad Sci USA 75:1505–1509 – Sliski AH, Essex M, Meyer C, Todaro GJ (1977) Feline oncornavirus associated cell membrane antigen (FOCMA): expression on feline sarcoma virus transformed nonproducer mink cells. Science 196:1336–1339 – Snyder HW Jr, Hardy WD Jr, Zuckerman EE, Fleissner E (1978) Characterization of a tumour-specific antigen on the surface of feline lymphosarcoma cells. Nature 175:656–657 – Snyder HW Jr, Phillips KJ, Hardy WD Jr, Zuckerman EE, Essex M, Sliski AH, Rhim J (1980) Isolation and characterization of proteins carrying the feline oncornavirus-associated cell membrane antigen (FOCMA). Cold Spring Harbor Symp Quant Biol 44:878–899 – Stephenson JR, Essex M, Hino S, Aaronson SA, Hardy WD Jr (1977a) Feline oncornavirus-associated cell membrane antigen. VII. Relationship between FOCMA and virion glycoprotein gp70. Proc Natl Acad Sci USA 74:1219–1223 – Stephenson JR, Khan AS, Sliski AH, Essex M (1977b) Feline oncornavirus-associated cell membrane antigen (FOCMA): identification of an immunologically cross-reactive feline sarcoma virus coded protein. Proc Natl Acad Sci USA 74:5608–5612 – Worley M, Essex M (1980) Identification of membrane proteins associated with transformation-related antigens shared by feline lymphoma cells and feline sarcoma virus transformed fibroblasts. In: Hardy WD Jr, Essex M, McClelland J (eds) Feline leukemia and sarcoma viruses. Elsevier, New York pp 431–440

487

Haematology and Blood Transfusion Vol. 26
Modern Trends in Human Leukemia IV
Edited by Neth, Gallo, Graf, Mannweiler, Winkler
© Springer-Verlag Berlin Heidelberg 1981

Relationship of the Feline Oncornavirus Associated Cell Membrane Antigen to a Feline Sarcoma Virus Encoded Polyprotein

H. W. Snyder Jr., M. Dutta-Choudhury, and W. D. Hardy Jr.

A. Introduction

The feline oncornavirus associated cell membrane antigen (FOCMA) is expressed on the membranes of cells transformed by infection with the feline leukemia virus (FOCMA-L) or feline sarcoma virus (FOCMA-S) (Hardy et al. 1977; Essex et al. 1977). Expression of FOCMA is transformation-specific and not dependent upon concomitant expression of antigens associated with feline leukemia virus (FeLV) or the endogenous virus RD114 (reviewed in Snyder et al., to be published a). In the natural environment FOCMA is the target for an effective immunosurveillance response: complement-dependent lytic antibodies directed to FOCMA reverse or prevent tumor development (Essex et al. 1975; Grant et al. 1977). FOCMA-L has been isolated from feline lymphosarcoma (LSA) cell membranes and has been shown to reside on a 70,000 dalton protein which is neither glycosylated nor phosphorylated (Snyder et al. 1978, to be published a). The nature of FOCMA-S is a subject of intense investigation at the present time.

The observation that FOCMA is induced on FeSV-transformed nonproducer fibroblasts of nonfeline as well as feline origin has been interpreted as evidence that FOCMA-S may actually be encoded by FeSV (Essex et al. 1979). Present evidence suggests that in the derivation of the defective FeSV genome sequences from the *pol* and the 3' end of the *gag* and *env* genes were deleted and the *gag-pol* deletion was substituted with cat cellular DNA sequences which contain information for transformation (Frankel et al. 1979; Sherr et al. 1980). The translation products of FeSV genomes in nonproducer fibroblasts are "fusion" proteins comprised of covalently linked FeLV p15, p12, a portion of p30, and nonstructural ("x") components of differing sizes depending on the particular strain of FeSV (Khan and Stephenson 1977; Sherr et al. 1978a; Barbacid et al. 1980; Van de Ven et al. 1980; Ruscetti et al., to be published). These proteins have generally been referred to as "gag-x" polyproteins. The question of FOCMA association with the "x" portion of these fusion proteins is addressed below.

B. Results

We have previously reported the isolation of 70,000 dalton proteins from lysates of feline LSA cells by immunoaffinity chromatography on a column of Sepharose containing bound IgG from cat anti-FOCMA serum (Snyder et al., to be published a; Fig. 1A). Using the same affinity column we isolated a similarly sized protein from lysates of mink cells transformed by the Gardner-Arnstein strain of FeSV (GA-FeSV) (Fig. 1, B). This result was unanticipated since published evidence suggested an association between FOCMA and the much larger (95,000 daltons) gag-x fusion protein in these cells (Stephenson et al. 1977; Sherr et al. 1978a, b; Snyder et al. 1978). In addition to the p70 it was possible to isolate the Ga-FeSV fusion protein (termed P95^{gag-x}) from the transformed mink cells by virtue of its binding to anti-FeLV antibodies on a different affinity column (Fig. 1, C).

These purified proteins as well as those directly immunoprecipitated from detergent-lysed cultured cells were analyzed for (1) associated FeLV antigens by radioimmunopre-

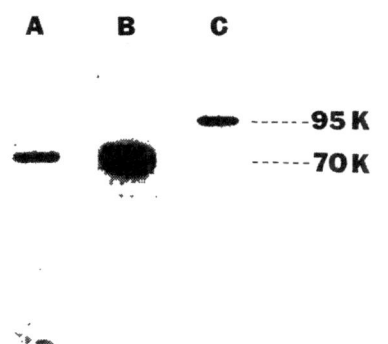

```
A    B    C

          ⟶ ------95K
  ⟶       ●   ------70K
```

Fig. 1. SDS polyacrylamide gel electrophoresis of *(A)* FOCMA-L molecules purified by immunoaffinity chromatography of a feline LSA (FeLV nonproducer) over a column of Sepharose containing bound IgG from cat FOCMA serum, *(B)* FOCMA-S molecules purified over the same column from a lysate of GA-FeSV mink cells (64F3C17 cells), and *(C)* P95^{gag-x} molecules purified on an anti-FeLV IgG immunoaffinity column from a lysate of 64F3C17 cells. Aliquots of material binding to the columns and eluted with 4 M MgCl$_2$ were radioiodinated and subjected to electrophoresis in a 5%–20% acrylamide slab gel and visualized by autoradiography.

cipitation with specific antisera to individual proteins, (2) glycosylation and phosphorylation (Snyder et al., to be published a), (3) similarities in peptides generated by partial digestion with *S. aureus* V8 protease or chymotrypsin (Snyder et al., to be published b), (4) associated protein kinase activity (Collett and Erikson 1978; Sen and Todaro 1979;

Snyder et al., to be published b), and (5) associated glucose binding and/or transport-stimulating activity (Lee and Lipmann 1977). In terms of this preliminary characterization (Table 1) the purified p70 molecules from LSA cells and GA-FeSV-transformed mink fibroblasts were indistinguishable. However, the gag-x polyprotein was distinguishable by its labeling with ^{32}P-orthophosphate, its association with a protein kinase activity, and its precipitability with antibodies in a hyperimmune antiserum to FeLV structural proteins but not with antibodies in a well-characterized cat-derived natural FOCMA serum.

C. Discussion

Previously, two independent investigators showed that absorption of certain cat FOCMA sera with FeLV structural proteins did not diminish immunoflourescent antibody reactivity for FOCMA-S on FeSV-transformed mink cells, while absorption with partially-purified gag-x polyproteins was effective (Stephenson et al. 1977; Sherr et al. 1978a). This was the most direct evidence for a link between FOCMA and the "x" portion of the FeSV polyprotein. Indirect supportive evidence came from an experiment wherein hyperimmune rabbit antibody to FeSV gag-x-containing pseudotype virions, made specific for "x" by absorption with helper virus proteins, stained the surface of FL 74 LSA cells (Sherr et al. 1978b). Khan et al. (1978) showed that many FeLV-absorbed cat FOCMA sera were capa-

Table 1. Comparison of proteins induced in cells transformed by FeLV and FeSV

	FOCMA-L p70	GA-FeSV	
		gag-x	p70
Cell localization	Plasma membrane	Plasma membrane	Plasma membrane
Molecular weight	65–70K	95K	65–70K
Associated FeLV Ag	None	p15p12(p30)	None
Protease digest maps	Similar	?	Similar
Phosphorylation	−	+	−
Glycosylation	−	−	−
Associated protein Kinase activity	No	Yes	No
Associated glucose Binding activity	No	?	No
Associated glucose transport stimulating activity	No	?	No

ble of reacting in sensitive radioimmunoprecipitation assays with a highly purified gag-x protein probe. However, the fact that not all such sera displayed this reactivity was the first suggestion that there may not be complete concordance between recognition of FOCMA and recognition of "x". Recent experiments by Barbacid et al. (1980) and Ruscetti et al. (to be published) as well as those described in the present report are consistent with this lack of complete concordance. While we have not ruled out the possibility that the p70 molecule we have isolated from GA-FeSV-transformed mink cells is a breakdown product of unstable $P95^{gag-x}$, for the present p70 appears to be a good alternate candidate for a FOCMA-bearing protein in these cells. By extrapolation from all of the available evidence one might speculate that FOCMA, as defined in terms of a tumor regression-correlated cat antibody reaction with the surface of FL74 LSA cells, may actually be a family of antigens, not all of which cross react with FeSV polyprotein antigens.

Acknowledgments

This research was supported by grants CA-16599 and CA-24357 and by NCI core grant CA-08748 from the National Institute of Health. The work was carried out while H.W.S., Jr. was a Special Fellow of the Leukemia Society of America.

References

Barbacid M, Lauver AV, Devare SG (1980) Biochemical and immunological characterization of polyproteins coded for by the McDonough, Gardner-Arnstein, and Snyder-Theilen strains of feline sarcoma virus. J Virol 33:196–207 – Collett MS, Erikson RL (1978) Protein kinase activity associated with the avian sarcoma virus src gene product. Proc Natl Acad Sci USA 75:2021–2024 – Essex M, Sliski A, Cotter SM, Jakowski RM, Hardy WD Jr (1975) Immunosurveillance of naturally occurring feline leukemia. Science 190:790–792 – Essex M, Cotter SM, Stephenson JR, Aaronson SA, Hardy WD Jr (1977) Leukemia, lymphoma, and fibrosarcoma of cats as models for similar diseases of man. Cold Spring Harbor Conf Cell Prolif 4:1197–1214 – Essex M, Sliski AH, Worley M, Grant CK, Snyder HW Jr, Hardy WD Jr, Chen LB (to be published) Significance of the feline oncornavirus-associated cell membrane antigen (FOCMA) in the natural history of feline leukemia. Cold Spring Harbor Conf Cell Prolif 7 – Frankel AE, Gilbert JH, Porzig KJ, Scolnick EM, Aaronson SA (1979) Nature and distribution of feline sarcoma virus nucleotide sequences. J Virol 30:821–827 – Grant CK, DeBoer DJ, Essex M, Worley MB, Higgins J (1977) Antibodies from healthy cats exposed to feline leukemia virus lyse feline lymphoma cells slowly with cat complement. J Immunol 119:401–406 – Hardy WD Jr, Zuckerman EE, MacEwen EG, Hayes AA, Essex M (1977) A feline leukemia and sarcoma virus induced tumour specific antigen. Nature 270:249–251 – Khan AS, Stephenson JR (1977) Feline leukemia virus: biochemical and immunological characterization of gag gene-coded structural proteins. J Virol 23:599–607 – Khan AS, Deobagkar DN, Stephenson JR (1978) Isolation and characterization of a feline sarcoma virus-coded precursor polyprotein: competition immunoassay of nonstructural components. J Biol Chem 253:8894–8901 – Lee SG, Lipmann F (1977) Isolation from normal and Rous sarcoma virus-transformed chicken fibroblasts of a factor that binds glucose and stimulates its transport. Proc Natl Acad Sci USA 74:163–166 – Ruscetti SK, Donner L, Sherr CJ (to be published) A model for FOCMA expression in cells transformed by feline leukemia and sarcoma viruses. In: Fields B, Jaenisch R, Fox CF (eds) ICN-UCLA symposia on molecular and cellular biology, Vol 18. Academic Press, New York – Sen A, Todaro GJ (1979) A murine sarcoma virus-associated protein kinase: interaction with actin and microtubular protein. Cell 17:347–356 – Sherr CJ, Sen A, Todaro GJ, Sliski A, Essex M (1978a) Feline sarcoma virus particles contain a phosphorylated polyprotein (pp85) with p15, p12 and FOCMA antigens. Proc Natl Acad Sci USA 75:1505–1509 – Sherr CJ, Todaro GJ, Sliski A, Essex M (1978b) Characterization of a feline sarcoma virus-coded antigen (FOCMA-S) by radioimmunoassay. Proc Natl Acad Sci USA 75:4489–4493 – Sherr CJ, Fedele LA, Oskarsson M, Maizel J, Vande Woude G (1980) Molecular cloning of Snyder-Theilen feline leukemia and sarcoma viruses: comparative studies of feline sarcoma virus with its natural helper virus and with Moloney sarcoma virus. J Virol 34:200–212 – Snyder HW Jr, Hardy WD Jr, Zuckerman EE, Fleissner E (1978) Characterization of a tumour-specific antigen on the surface of feline lymphosarcoma cells. Nature 275:656–658 – Snyder HW Jr, Phillips KJ, Hardy WD Jr, Zuckerman EE, Essex M, Sliski AH, Rhim J (to be published a) Isolation and characterization of proteins carrying the feline oncornavirus-associated cell membrane antigen (FOCMA). Cold Spring Harbor Symp Quant Biol 44 – Snyder HW Jr, Phillips KJ, Dutta-Choudhury M, Hardy WD Jr, Zuckerman EE (to be published b) Biochemical and serological aspects of proteins induced in cells transformed by FeLV and FeSV. In: Hardy WD Jr, Essex M, McClelland AJ (eds) Feline leukemia virus. Elsevier, New York – Stephenson JR, Khan

AS, Sliski AH, Essex M (1977) Feline oncornavirus-associated cell membrane antigen (FOCMA): identification of an immunologically cross-reactive feline sarcoma virus-coded protein. Proc Natl Acad Sci USA 74:5608–5612 – Van de Ven WJM, Khan AS, Reynolds FH Jr, Mason KT, Stephenson JR (1980) Translational products encoded by newly acquired sequences of independently derived feline sarcoma virus isolates are structurally related. J Virol 33:1034–1045

Haematology and Blood Transfusion Vol. 26
Modern Trends in Human Leukemia IV
Edited by Neth, Gallo, Graf, Mannweiler, Winkler
© Springer-Verlag Berlin Heidelberg 1981

Feline Leukemia Virus Nonproducer Lymphosarcomas of Cats as a Model for the Etiology of Human Leukemias

W. D. Hardy Jr., A. J. McClelland, E. E. Zuckerman, H. W. Snyder Jr., E. G. MacEwen, D. Francis, and M. Essex

A. Introduction

It is now thought that most human and animal tumors are caused by environmental factors such as chemical pollutants. However, a small number of animal tumors are known to be caused by viruses. The most common oncogenic viruses are the RNA-containing oncoviruses which are usually contagious and cause lymphoid tumors or sarcomas in young animals. Most of the tumors caused by oncoviruses in animals are viral producers, that is, the causative oncovirus is expressed and can be readily detected in the tumor tissue (Hardy 1978). However, some of the lymphosarcomas (LSA) of pet cats that are caused by the feline leukemia virus (FeLV) exhibit no evidence of FeLV infection even though, as will be clear from the data presented below, FeLV appears to be the etiologic agent for these viral nonproducer (NP) LSAs (Francis et al. 1979; Hardy et al. 1980).

Oncoviruses are found in many vertebrate species and it is thus likely that a human oncovirus exists. There is a high incidence of leukemia among children and, in view of the common occurrence of oncovirus induced lymphoid tumors of young animals, it is probable that some of these childhood leukemias are virally induced. However, at present there is no proof for the existence of a human oncogenic virus and it is possible that, like feline NP LSA, human leukemia is a viral NP tumor. FeLV is spread contagiously among cats and is unique among the mammalian oncoviruses in that it induces a naturally occurring NP LSA (Hardy et al. 1977). FeLV is therefore a potentially valuable model for studying how oncoviruses induce virus negative lymphoid tumors such as human leukemia.

B. Results

I. Immunology of Feline Lymphosarcoma

In order to determine the occurrence of NP feline LSA, we tested 507 cats with LSA for FeLV by the immunofluorescent antibody (IFA) test, which detects FeLV proteins in the cytoplasm of infected cells and indicates persistent infection (Hardy et al. 1973a) In addition, some cats were tested for FeLV by immunodiffusion, tissue culture isolation, and radioimmunoassay (Hardy et al. 1973b; Snyder et al. 1978). We found that 360 (71%) of the cats had FeLV positive LSAs whereas the remaining 147 cats (29%) had NP LSAs. No FeLV proteins nor infectious virus could be detected in the NP LSAs by any of the methods used. However, the FeLV induced tumor specific feline oncornavirus-associated cell membrane antigen (FOCMA) was detected on the surface of both NP and FeLV positive (producer) LSA cells by the viable cell immunofluorescent antibody test (Essex et al. 1971; Hardy et al. 1977). Since no evidence of FeLV expression could be found in feline NP LSA cells, even though they expressed the FeLV induced non-viral antigen FOCMA, it was not certain that FeLV was the etiologic agent for feline NP LSA.

II. Epidemiology of Feline Lymphosarcoma

In an attempt to determine epidemiologically if FeLV was the etiologic agent of feline NP LSA, we observed 1612 FeLV-exposed and -unexposed cats for the development of LSA. All cats were tested for FeLV by the IFA test (Hardy et al. 1973a). The control group of 1074 cats lived in 96 households and had never been exposed to FeLV. These FeLV uninfected cats were observed for a total of 3225 cat observation years (average: 3 years/cat) and during this period none of these cats developed LSA. The remaining 538 cats lived in 23 households and had been exposed to FeLV at some time in their lives. Of these 538 cats, 389 were found to be FeLV uninfected and 149 were found to be persistently infected. The exposed cats were observed for a total of 2334 cat observation years (average: 4.4 years/cat) and during this period 41 cats developed LSA – 30 cats developed FeLV positive LSA and 11 developed NP LSA. The difference in the occurrence of NP LSA among the FeLV-exposed and -unexposed cats was found to be highly significant ($P<0.001$) by the Chi Square Test. Thus, there appears to be a comparable epidemiologic association in pet cats between FeLV exposure and the occurrence of both FeLV positive and NP LSA. This exposure association, together with the finding that FOCMA is expressed on NP LSA cells, suggests that FeLV is the etiologic agent of feline LSAs regardless of their FeLV status.

C. Discussion

The mechanism by which RNA and DNA containing viruses induce tumors is not fully understood. However, it is known that both classes of viruses are oncogenic by virtue of their ability to integrate their genome into the genome of the host cell. The DNA viruses can insert their DNA directly into the host cell genome, but the oncoviruses must first make a complementary DNA copy of their viral RNA. Little is known about how the integrated viral genome induces cellular transformation and nothing is known about the mechanism by which FeLV induces NP LSA. However, several mechanisms are possible (Gallo et al. 1977). For example, FeLV may recombine with endogenous oncovirus or cellular genes and form a replication-defective leukemogenic virus. Alternatively, the FeLV genome may integrate into the host cell genome in an unstable manner and transform the cell before being lost by deletion. It is also possible that only a fragment of the FeLV genome becomes integrated into the genome of the host cell and that this fragment contains enough information to induce transformation, but not enough for viral production. Yet another possibility is that FeLV infects nonlymphoid cells and cau-

ses these cells to produce an abnormal growth factor that results in the uncontrolled proliferation of lymphocytes and, ultimately, in NP LSA.

Feline NP LSA is the only known example of a naturally occurring, virally induced, NP LSA in animals and may therefore be a useful model for elucidating the mechanism of oncovirus transformation. Viruses cause cancer in amphibians, fish, fowl, rodents, cats, cattle, and subhuman primates, and if humans were to be exempt from such a general biological phenomenon, it would be a circumstance unparalleled in the history of parasitism. In fact, evidence is accumulating that some human cancers are virally induced. For example, Burkitt's lymphoma, nasopharyngeal carcinoma, cervical cancer, and Kaposki's sarcoma are thought to be caused by Herpesviruses, which are able to remain latent in their host for many years (De-Thé 1977). Recently, the occurrence of hepatitis B virus antigens have been associated with the development of hepatocellular carcinomas in people. Most of these tumors possess the hepatitis viral antigens, but like the feline NP LSA, about 25% to 30% are antigen negative tumors (Goudeau et al. 1979). Although no oncoviruses have been proven to be associated with human leukemia, an oncovirus with properties quite distinct from those of any animal oncovirus has recently been isolated from the tumor tissue of a human with mycosis fungoides (Poiesz et al., to be published). It is thus also possible that an oncovirus causes human NP leukemias even though no oncogenic virus has been isolated from these tumors. If that is indeed found to be the case, feline NP LSA may be an important model for studying how these NP human leukemias are induced and how they might be prevented.

Acknowledgements

We thank R. Markovich, T. Paino and H. Perry for technical assistance. This work was supported by grants CA-16599, CA-08748, CA-24357, CA-19072, CA-13885, CA-18216, CB-64001 and CP-81004 from the National Cancer Institute and grants from the Cancer Research Institute and the National Branches of the American Cancer Society.

References

De-Thé G (1977) Viruses as causes of some human tumors? Results and prospectives of the epidemiologic approach. In: Hiatt HH, Watson JD, Winsten JA (eds) Origins of human cancer. Cold Spring Harbor Laboratory, Cold Spring Harbor, pp 1113–1131 – Essex M, Klein G, Snyder SP, Harrold JB (1971) Correlation between humoral antibody and regression of tumours induced by feline sarcoma virus. Nature 233:195–196 – Francis DP, Cotter SM, Hardy WD Jr, Essex M (1979) Comparison of virus-positive and virus-negative cases of feline leukemia and lymphoma. Cancer Res 39:3866–3870 – Gallo RC, Saxinger WC, Gallagher RE, Gillespie DH, Aulakh GS, Wong-Staal F (1977) Some ideas on the origin of leukemia in man and recent evidence for the presence of type-C viral related information. In: Hiatt HH, Watson JD, Winsten JA (eds) Origins of human cancer. Cold Spring Harbor Laboratory, Cold Spring Harbor, pp 1253–1285 – Goudeau A, Maupas P, Coursaget P, Drucker J, Chiron JP, Denis F, Diop Mar I (1979) Hepatitis B virus antigens in human primary hepatocellular carcinoma tissues. Int J Cancer 24:421–429 – Hardy WD Jr (1978) Epidemiology of primary neoplasms of lymphoid tissues of animals. In: Twomey JJ, Good RA (eds) The immunopathology of lymphoreticular neoplasms. Plenum, New York, pp 129–180 – Hardy WD Jr, Hirshaut Y, Hess P (1973a) Detection of the feline leukemia virus and other mammalian oncornaviruses by immunofluorescence. In: Dutcher RM, Chieco-Bianchi L (eds) Unifying concepts of leukemia. S. Karger, Basel, pp 778–799 – Hardy WD Jr, Old LJ, Hess PW, Essex M, Cotter S (1973b) Horizontal transmission of feline leukaemia virus. Nature 244:266–269 – Hardy WD Jr, Zuckerman EE, MacEwen EG, Hayes AA, Essex M (1977) A feline leukaemia virus- and sarcoma virus-induced tumour-specific antigen. Nature 270:249–251 – Hardy WD Jr, McClelland AJ, Zuckerman EE, Snyder HW Jr, MacEwen EG, Francis DP, Essex M (1980) The immunology and epidemiology of feline leukemia virus non-producer lymphosarcomas. In: Essex M, Todaro GJ, zur Hausen H (eds) Viruses in naturally occurring cancer. Cold Spring Harbor Laboratory, Cold Spring Harbor pp 677–697 – Poiesz, BJ, Ruscetti F, Gazdar AF, Bunn PA, Minna JD, Gallo RC (to be published) Isolation of type-C retrovirus particles from cultured and fresh lymphocytes of a patient with cutaneous T cell lymphoma. Proc Natl Acad Sci USA – Snyder HW Jr, Hardy WD Jr, Zuckerman EE, Fleissner E (1978) Characterization of a tumour-specific antigen on the surface of feline lymphosarcoma cells. Nature 275:656–658

Haematology and Blood Transfusion Vol. 26
Modern Trends in Human Leukemia IV
Edited by Neth, Gallo, Graf, Mannweiler, Winkler
© Springer-Verlag Berlin Heidelberg 1981

Genomic Integration of Bovine Leukemia Provirus and Lack of Viral RNA Expression in the Target Cells of Cattle with Different Responses to BLV Infection

R. Kettmann, G. Marbaix, M. Mammerickx, and A. Burny

A. Introduction

Enzootic bovine leukosis (EBL) is a contagious lymphoproliferative disease whose etiological agent is a retrovirus, the bovine leukemia virus (BLV). EBL is a complex disease. Soon after infection a strong humoral antibody response develops and persists for the animal's entire life. Such BLV-infected cattle can remain asymptomatic virus carriers for many years. They can also at a given time develop persistent lymphocytosis (PL) characterized by a permanent large number of peripheral lymphocytes. A variable but always significant percentage of PL animals develop lymphoid tumors, the terminal tumor phase of EBL. The remnant tumor cases develop suddenly in BLV carriers without any previous hematologic disorder. In general, the fate of BLV-infected animals is variable and depends upon several factors, including age, genetic make-up, environmental factors, and immunologic surveillance (see Burny et al. 1980 for a review).

In the present investigation we studied BLV integration sites in DNA preparations from target tissues of BLV-infected animals and viral RNA expression in the same cells. DNA was digested by bacterial restriction endonucleases and submitted to electrophoresis in agarose gels. After transfer to nitrocellulose paper, the DNA fragments were annealed to a specific BLV (^{32}P) cDNA probe. Genomic DNA fragments containing viral information appear after autoradiographic development as individual bands and sometimes as smears.

The results of our study allow comparison of BLV provirus integration and viral RNA expression in *leucocytes* of animals showing different responses to BLV infection, namely, in asymptomatic BLV carriers (Ab$^+$ änimals), animals in PL (PL$^+$ animals), and tumor cases (T$^+$ animals). Our major findings are: (1) No BLV proviral sequences are detected in Ab$^+$ cases by the technique used; (2) Circulating leucocytes of PL animals accomodate BLV provirus at many possible sites; (3) Lymphocytes infected by BLV and found in EBL tumors constitute monoclonal populations of cells carrying one copy of the proviral genome which is integrated at one genomic site; and (4) In the vast majority of cases studied, no viral RNA expression was detectable in the lymphoid tumor cells or circulating leucocytes of affected animals.

B. Results and Discussion

I. Viral DNA Content of BLV-Infected Cells

As shown in Fig. 1, no EcoRI fragment containing viral information was detected in the DNA samples from Ab$^+$ animals (animals no. 19, 33, and 34). The weak hybridization band of 5.0×10^6 which was common to the control DNA and all the other bovine DNAs tested corresponded to ribosomal DNA (Kettmann et al. 1979). Since no hybridization occurred with leucocyte DNA from Ab$^+$ animals, and taking account of the sensitivity of the method, we can conclude that less than 5% of the total leucocyte population can harbor the provirus. It should be noted here that EcoRI cleaves once at one kilobase distance from the 3' end of the BLV unintegrated provirus with a mol.wt. of 6.0×10^6 (Kettmann, unpublished results). Previously, we have reported that 25% to 40% of total leucocytes of animals in PL harbor BLV proviral sequences (Kettmann et al. 1980).

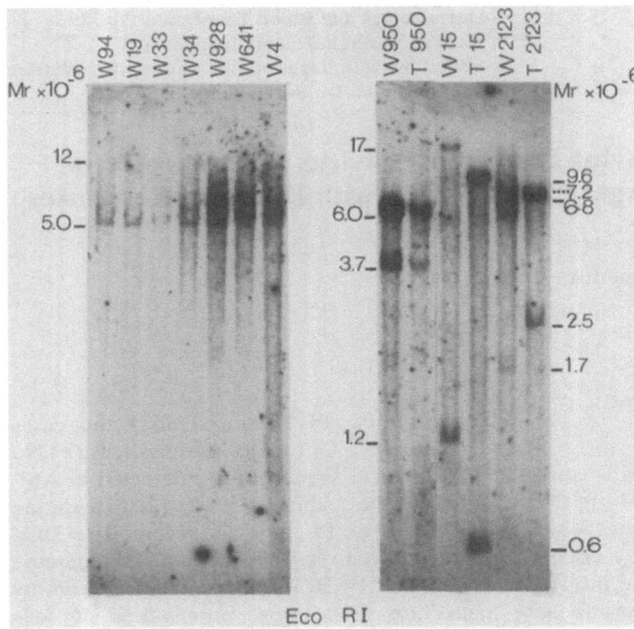

Fig. 1. Hybridization patterns of BLV (^{32}P) cDNA on DNA restriction fragments from circulating leucocytes *(W)* and tumors *(T)* of BLV-infected animals. DNAs (20 μg) of W19, W33, and W34 (Ab$^+$ animals), of W928, W641, and W4 (PL$^+$ animals), of W950, T950, W15, T15, W2123, and T2123 (T$^+$ animals), and of W94 (an Ab$^-$ animal) were exhaustively digested by EcoRI before electrophoresis on a 0.8% agarose gel, and then transferred, hybridized, and detected by autoradiography (see Kettmann et al. 1980). Autoradiographs are shown

Here we show that less than 5% of total leucocytes of Ab$^+$ animals can carry the provirus. Taken together these results demonstrate that *PL is not an amplification of a pre-existing situation found in AB$^+$ animals.*

The pattern of proviral integration in the circulating leucocytes of animals carrying lymph node tumors (animals no. 950 and 15) was completely different from that described above in that a number of well-defined provirus-positive bands were present in the EcoRI digests. These fragments had mol.wts. of 6.0×10^6 and 3.7×10^6 for animal 950 DNA and 17×10^6 and 1.2×10^6 for animal 15 DNA. These results imply that in contrast to the multiplicity of integration sites found in the DNA from circulating leucocytes from animals in PL, only a very limited number of sites accomodate BLV provirus in the DNA of circulating leucocytes from tumor bearing animals. The EcoRI pattern obtained for the circulating leucocytes of animals 2123 was more complex and reminiscent of that obtained with leucocyte DNAs from animals in PL.

In animal 950 the same restriction pattern was found for the circulating leucocyte DNA and a tumorous lymph node. These results showed that the same BLV-infected clone was present in both affected tissues. In contrast, for animals No. 15 and 2123 two different patterns were found in the circulating leucocyte DNA and in a tumor DNA of the same animal, thus showing that in these animals two clones of BLV-infected leucocytes were detected.

II. Viral RNA Content of BLV-Infected Cells

Using liquid hybridization techniques and BLV (^{3}H) cDNA as a probe, we looked for viral RNA sequences in various total RNAs samples from BLV-infected cells. Genomic 35S RNA and total RNA from the virus-producing cells were used as positive controls. The results of Table 1 clearly showed that in all cases tested but one (leucocytes of animal 15) transcription of the integrated viral genome did not occur or occurred at a very low level. Our data are, however, still compatible with either one of the following possibilities: (1) lymph node tumor cells and circulating lymphocytes of PL$^+$ or T$^+$ animals express at a low rate a very small region of the BLV genome; or (2) a small percentage of BLV-carrying cells express the entirely or in part the viral information at a low rate. In situ hybridization experiments are being performed to solve this problem.

Animal number[a]	Tissue	Percentage of hybridization	Crt × 10^{-3}	Number of viral copies[b]
94	Leucocytes	7.4%	61	0[c]
33	Leucocytes	8.6%	25	<1
34	Leucocytes	5.8%	38	<1
928	Leucocytes	7.2%	36	<1
4	Leucocytes	6.3%	34	<1
950	Leucocytes	7.0%	40	<1
	Tumor cells	6.9%	39	<1
2123	Leucocytes	7.9%	45	<1
	Tumor cells	7.1%	33	<1
15	Leucocytes	16.0%	32	1 to 2
	Spleen cells	7.8%	37	<1
	Tumor cells	7.0%	18	<1

Table 1. Viral RNA content of circulating leucocytes and tumor cells

[a] Animal 94 is normal; animals 33 and 34 are Ab[+]; animals 928 and 4 are PL[+]; animals 950, 2123 and 15 are tumor[+]

[b] Estimations were made from hybridization experiments using increasing dilutions of BLV 35S genomic RNA and assuming a cellular RNA content of 10 pg. FLK cells were shown to contain 30 copies of the BLV RNA genome

[c] Hybridization reactions run in the same conditions with E. coli total RNA showed a background level of 7.1% at a Crt value of 60×10^3

Acknowledgements

The authors warmly thank Y. Cleuter for her excellent technical assistance. This work was supported by the Fonds Cancérologique de la Caisse Générale d'Epargne et de Retraite, Belgium. R.K. is Chargé de Recherches and G.M. is Maître de Recherches of the Fonds National Belge de la Recherche Scientifique.

References

Burny A, Bruck C, Chantrenne H, Cleuter Y, Dekegel D, Ghysdael J, Kettmann R, Leclercq M, Leunen J, Mammerickx M, Portetelle D (1980) Bovine leukemia virus: Molecular biology and epidemiology. In: Klein G (ed) Viral oncology. Raven, New York, pp 231–289 – Kettmann R, Meunier-Rotival M, Cortadas J, Cuny G, Ghysdael J, Mammerickx M, Burny A, Bernardi G (1979) Integration of bovine leukemia virus DNA in the bovine genome. Proc Natl Acad Sci USA 76:4822–4826 – Kettmann R, Cleuter Y, Mammerickx M, Meunier-Rotival M, Bernardi G, Burny A, Chantrenne H (1980) Genomic integration of bovine leukemia provirus: Comparison of persistent lymphocytosis with lymph node tumor form of enzootic bovine leukosis. Proc Natl Acad Sci USA 77:2577–2581

497

Haematology and Blood Transfusion Vol. 26
Modern Trends in Human Leukemia IV
Edited by Neth, Gallo, Graf, Mannweiler, Winkler
© Springer-Verlag Berlin Heidelberg 1981

Natural Antibodies to BLV gp51 Are Reactive Against the Carbohydrate Moiety of the Glycoprotein

D. Portetelle, C. Bruck, M. Mammerickx, and A. Burny

A. Introduction

Infection of animals (cattle, sheep, goats, pigs, rabbits, etc.) with bovine leukemia virus (BLV), the etiological agent of enzootic bovine leukosis, induces a rapid and strong humoral antibody response directed against all structural proteins of the virus (Burny et al. 1980). This humoral reaction does not arrest BLV multiplication in the infected host; surprisingly enough, anti-gp51 antibody titer increases steadily and inexorably until the animal's fatal outcome in the tumor phase of the disease. Failure of the immune system to eliminate an established BLV infection does not prove, however, that adequate vaccination of animals at risk would be unseccessful. From recent experiments by Mammerickx et al. (to be published), we know that passive antibody provided to sheep by colostrum feeding prevented BLV take, irrespective of the route of virus administration. The latter observations reinforced our decision to thoroughly investigate the antigenic site of BLV gp51 exposed at the cell membrane of virus producing cells and recognized as target by sera exhibiting strong cytolytic activity towards these cells (Portetelle et al. 1978, to be published).

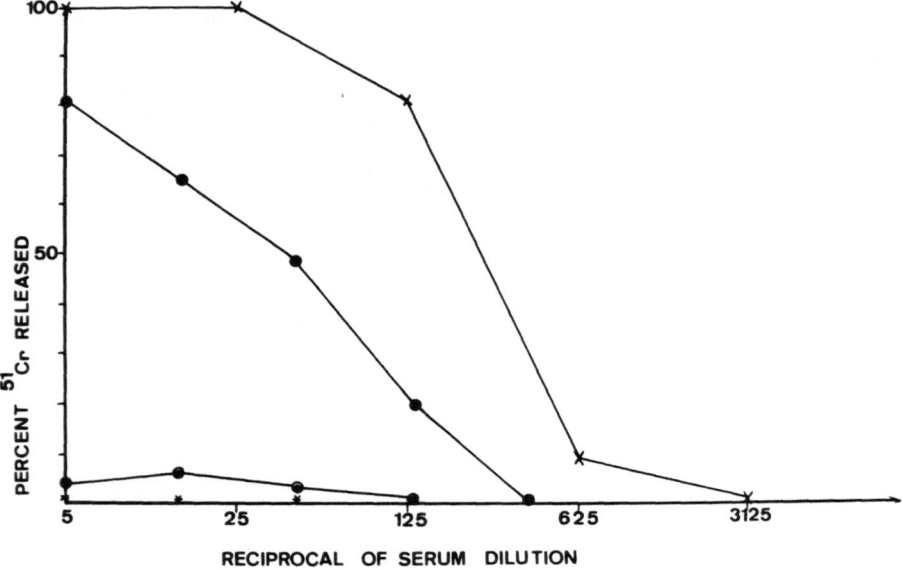

Fig. 1. Susceptibility of FLK-BLV cells to lysis by bovine serum 67 (X—X), bovine serum 351628 (●——●), normal bovine serum (*——*), and rabbit serum 167 (◉——◉). ^{51}Cr labeled FLK-BLV cells were incubated with dilutions of the serum to be tested and with a 1:8 final dilution of rabbit complement

The series of experiments summarized here showed that cytotoxic antibodies present in BLV-infected animals were mostly directed against the carbohydrate part of the gp51 molecule. On the contrary, monospecific immune sera prepared in the rabbit by injection of purified BLV gp51 are directed against determinants of the polypeptide backbone of the antigen.

B. Sera

Sera 2146 and 2152 were prepared in the rabbit by injection of BLV-infected bovine lymphocytes. Sera 67 and 82 were from cattle in the tumor phase of enzootic bovine leukosis. Serum 3162 was from a animal in persistent lymphocytosis and serum 351628 from an asymptomatic BLV carrier. Rabbit serum 167 was raised by injection of purified BLV gp51.

C. Results

Complement-dependent antibody-mediated immune cytolysis was previously shown to recognize mostly, if not solely, gp51 as the target molecular structure (Portetelle et al. 1978). Data presented in Fig. 1 illustrate the striking difference between natural sera (serum 67 X——X and serum 351628 ●—●) and rabbit serum 167 (◉——◉) prepared against purified gp51.

To confirm that cytolytic and noncytolytic antibodies recognized separate sites on the gp51 molecule, a competition radioimmunoassay was performed between bovine serum 67 and rabbit sera 2146 (Fig. 2).

Advantage was also taken of a solid phase radioimmunoassay. The results obtained indicated that: (1) natural sera and rabbit serum 167 reacted with different antigenic regions of gp51, and (2) the antigenic site recognized by natural sera was most probably unique (Fig. 3).

Importance of the carbohydrate moiety of gp51 was finally assessed by glycosidase treatment of ^{125}I-labeled antigen followed by addition of a variety of antisera (Fig. 4). Sera 2152, 3162, and 67 behaved similarly: removal of the carbohydrate moiety of the antigen resulted in almost complete loss of reactivity with the three sera. The behavior of serum 167 was strikingly different. Glycosidase digestion

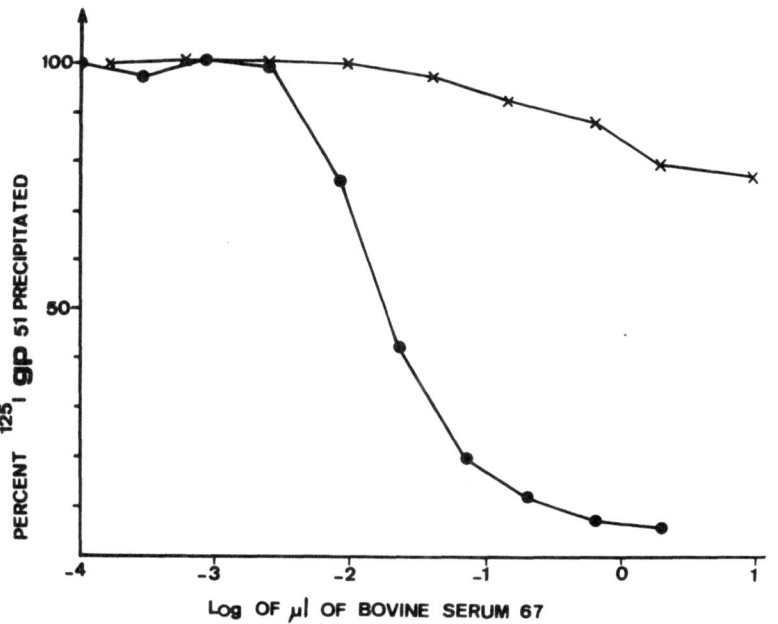

Fig. 2. Competition by bovine serum 67 of the immune precipitation of ^{125}I gp51 by rabbit sera 167 (X——X) and 2146 (●—●). Labeled antigen (0.5 ng) and a limiting rabbit antibody dilution (1/40.000 for serum 167; 1/75,000 for serum 2146) were incubated with increasing amounts of bovine serum 67. After a 72 h incubation, anti-rabbit Ig coated cellulose was added to adsorb immune complexes involving rabbit antibody. Pelleted and washed immunosorbent was counted in a γ counter

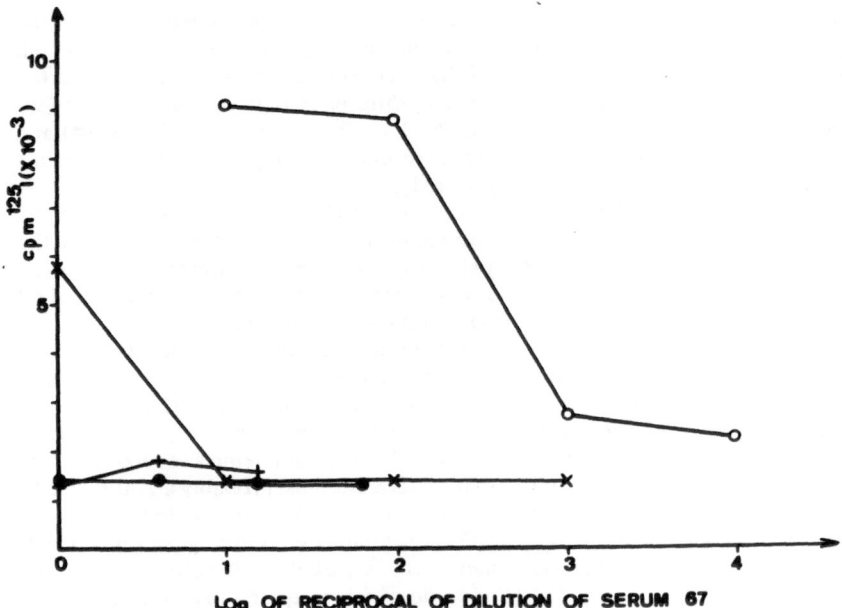

Fig. 3. Solid phase radioimmunoassay. Reagents were added to the wells in the following order: (1) Ig82-gp51-serum 67-^{125}I gp51 (X——X), (2) Ig82-gp51-normal bovine serum-^{125}I gp51 (●——●), (3) Ig rabbit 167-gp51-serum 67-^{125}I gp51 (○——○), and (4) Ig rabbit 167-gp51-normal bovine serum-^{125}I gp51 (+——+). At each step an excess reagent was added, incubation was performed, and nonadsorbed excess protein was washed away. After completion of the last step, the wells were separately counted in a γ counter

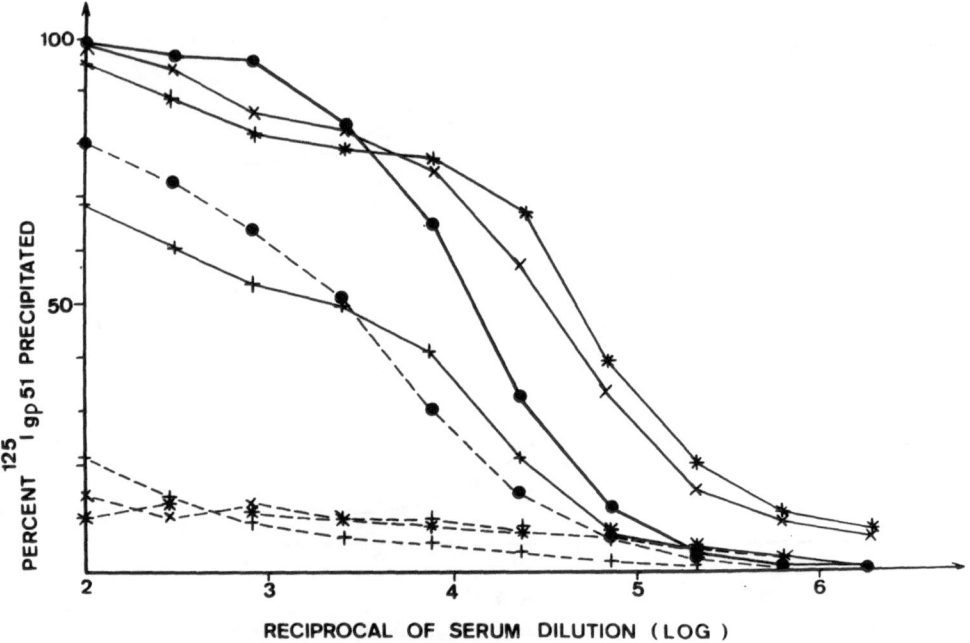

Fig. 4. Effect of glycosidase digestion of ^{125}I gp51 on direct radioimmunoassay with sera of different origins. Precipitation curves obtained with sera from rabbit 167 (●——●), cow 3162 (X——X), cow 67 (*——*), and rabbit 2152 (+——+) are taken as controls. The precipitation curves obtained with the same sera after glycosidase treatment of the antigen are depicted as interrupted lines

lowered maximal precipitability of gp51 by only 20%. Consequently, apparent antibody titer was also slightly lowered.

That the polypeptide backbone of gp 51 was the target for serum 167 reactivity was later demonstrated by protease treatment of the antigen (data not shown). Finally, SDS-PAGE analysis of native and glycosidase-treated BLV gp51 showed that the enzyme treatment reduced the apparent molecular weight from 51,000 to about 30,000 (Portetelle et al., to be published).

D. Conclusion

In conclusion, a probably unique carbohydrate antigenic site belonging to BLV envelope gp51 is strongly immunogenic for naturally infected animals or for rabbits injected with BLV lymphocytes. On the other hand, when purified gp51 is used as immunogen, it induces synthesis of antibodies directed to the protein skeleton of the glycoprotein antigen. From a very practical point of view it follows that purified BLV gp51 should not be used as a vaccinal preparation against BLV infection. Results very similar to those reported here have been obtained by Schmerr et al. (1980), personal communication).

References

Burny A, Bruck C, Chantrenne H, Cleuter Y, Dekegel D, Ghysdael J, Kettmann R, Leclercq M, Leunen J, Mammerickx M, Portetelle D (1980) Bovine leukemia virus: Molecular biology and epidemiology. In: Klein G (ed) Viral oncology. Raven, New York, pp 231–289 – Mammerickx M, Portetelle D, Burny A, Leunen (to be published) Detection by immunodiffusion- and radioimmunoassay-tests of antibodies to bovine leukemia virus antigens in sera of experimentally infected sheep and cattle. Zentralbl Veterinaermed [B] 27 – Portetelle D, Bruck C, Burny A, Dekegel D, Mammerickx M, Urbain J (1978) Detection of complement-dependent lytic antibodies in sera from Bovine Leukemia Virus-infected animals. Ann Rech Vet 9:667–674 – Portetelle D, Bruck C, Mammerickx M, Burny A (to be published) In animals infected by bovine leukemia virus (BLV), antibodies to envelope glycoprotein gp51 are directed against the carbohydrate moiety. Virology

Haematology and Blood Transfusion Vol. 26
Modern Trends in Human Leukemia IV
Edited by Neth, Gallo, Graf, Mannweiler, Winkler
© Springer-Verlag Berlin Heidelberg 1981

Regulation of Human T-Cell Proliferation: T-Cell Growth Factor and Isolation of a New Class of Type-C Retroviruses from Human T-Cells

R. C. Gallo, B. J. Poiesz, and F. W. Ruscetti

A. Summary

The discovery, characterization, and purification of human T-cell growth factor (TCGF) has led to the establishment of continuously growing T-lymphoblast cell lines from normal people and from patients with certain T-cell neoplasias. In contrast to normal T-cells, neoplastic mature T-cells respond directly to TCGF, requiring no prior lectin or antigen in vitro activation. The transformed T-cell lines have phenotypic characteristics consistent with the neoplastic cells of their disease of origin. A novel retrovirus, human T-cell lymphoma-leukemia virus (HTLV), has been isolated from the fresh and cultured cells of two of these patients. Subsequent characterization of this virus has shown that it is not significantly related to any known animal retrovirus, is not an endogenous (genetically transmitted) virus of man, and so far has been associated only with fresh or cultured T-cells from patients with T-cell neoplasia. These results suggest that HTLV infected some mature T-cells of some people and that it might be involved in some neoplasias involving these cells.

B. Introduction

There are various clinical presentations of T-lymphocytic neoplasia in man, including approximately 25% of both childhood and adult acute lymphatic leukemia (Brouet et al. 1975b), rare cases of chronic lymphatic leukemia (Brouet et al. 1975a), and hairy cell leukemia (Saxon et al. 1978), a minority of cases of diffuse non-Hodgkin's lymphoma (a majority of cases in childhood diffuse poorly differentiated lymphoma) (Gajl-Peczalska et al. 1975; Jaffe et al. 1975), and all patients with cutaneous T-cell lymphomas (mycosis fungoides, Sezary syndrome, and nodular papulosis) (Lutzner et al. 1975). Although the Epstein-Barr virus (EBV), a DNA virus of the herpes group, is implicated in some aspect of Burkitt's lymphoma, a B-cell disease (De-The 1980), the etiology of all the T-cell neoplasias is, as of yet, obscure. RNA tumor viruses have been shown to be the etiologic agent of lymphomas and leukemias in several animal species, including chickens, mice, cats, cows, and gibbon apes (Cockerell 1976; Gallo 1976; Gallo and Reitz 1976; Gallo et al. 1975; Haran-Ghera 1980; Klein 1980). In several instances these leukemias involve T-cells. When bovine leukemia virus (BLV), a causative agent of B-cell leukemia and lymphoma of cows, is injected into sheep, lymphoid leukemia and lymphoma, including a cutaneous form, occur which to our knowledge have not been subclassified (Olson 1979). It would seem reasonable then to survey human T-cell malignancies for the presence of retroviruses. Since several animal RNA tumor viruses (Klein 1980) and cells of the putative human retroviruses isolated to date (Bronson et al. 1979; Gallagher and Gallo 1975; Kaplan et al. 1977; Nooter et al. 1975; Panem et al. 1975) have required the establishment of continuously growing cell lines from the disease of origin or cocultivation of these cells with previously established cell lines, the ability to grow malignant T-cells in long-term culture could facilitate the isolation of retroviruses from these diseased states. We have, therefore, been interested in developing these and other cellular systems.

Although there are many immunologic and cytochemical differences between mature human T- and B-lymphocytes, human T-cells are primarily distinguished by their participation in cell mediated immunity and possession of receptors for sheep red blood cells. The elaboration of immunoglobulins and presence of receptors for EBV are most characteristic of human B-cells. T-cell differentiation is characterized by the successive gain or loss of certain cell surface markers and cytoplasmic enzymes which precede or coincide with the development of immunologic functions (Gupta and Good 1980). The best defined examples are: terminal deoxynucleotidyl transferase, a marker for immature or pre-T-cells; rosette formation with sheep red blood cells, a characteristic of more mature cells; and human T-cell antigens recognized by certain monoclonal antibodies on both immature and mature T-cells. In previous studies from this laboratory "activated" (by lectins) lymphoblasts from either peripheral blood or bone marrow from normal human donors were grown continuously with TCGF. Examination of these cells showed that over 90% were E-rosette positive and that all were karyotypically normal and negative for terminal transferase, EBV, and surface immunoglobulins (Morgan et al. 1976), indicating that these cells were T-lymphoblasts of relative maturity. Hence, in our initial attempts to develop cell lines from patients with T-cell neoplasias, we chose clinical subpopulations which represent a more mature form of disease, namely, the cutaneous T-cell lymphomas and leukemias and E-rosette positive T-cell ALL (Gupta and Good 1980). In this report we have summarized our recent results with TCGF, the various T-cell systems, and the isolation of a new type-C retrovirus released from growing T-cells from some of these T-cell neoplasias.

C. Growth of Thymus-Derived (T) lymphocytes

Lymphocyte reactions are complex and involve interactions between subsets of T- and B-lymphocytes and accessory adherent cells. Understanding of the regulation of the immune response has recently advanced considerably with the development of new culture methodologies (Morgan et al. 1976; Ruscetti et al. 1977) for the long-term growth of human T-cells. Using these methods, animal and human T-cells from numerous lymphoid or-

gans have been maintained in continuous culture for 1–3 years, provided that they were supplemented every 3–5 days with conditioned media from lectin-stimulated mononuclear cells. Subsequent studies have shown that the agent responsible for this growth promotion is indeed a lymphokine, designated T-cell growth factor (TCGF) (Ruscetti and Gallo 1981; Smith, to be published). Thus, for the first time continuously growing clones of lymphocytes, capable of unlimited expansion in culture while retaining functional specificity and responsiveness to normal humoral regulation, were developed (Schreier et al., to be published; Smith, to be published). These cloned T-cells will be essential reagents in studies to better define the T-cell proliferative responses.

The method used in our laboratory for culturing human T-cells is as follows: Leucocyte-enriched cell populations are seeded at $2-5 \times 10^5$ cells/ml suspended in tissue culture medium containing 15% heat-inactivated fetal calf serum and 20% conditioned media from PHA-stimulated leucocytes and incubated at 37°C. The cells reach their saturation density $(1-2 \times 10^6$ cells/ml) in 4–5 days. It is critical that the cells are subcultured and refed with fresh Ly-CM-containing media for continued cell growth. The morphologic and functional characteristics of these cultured cells are characteristic of mature T-lymphocytes (Table 1). These cells were over 90% positive for the sheep red blood cell receptor, a test specific for T-cells, and were sensitive to human anti-T-cell sera. As a test of T-cell-specific function, they responded to, but were unable to stimulate, allogeneic cells in one-way mixed leucocyte

Table 1. Some characteristics of purified human TCGF

Nature of molecule	Protein
Size	About 13,000 daltons
pI	6.8
Glycosyl moiety	None detected
Target cell	Activated T-lymphocyte
Mode of action	Unknown
Cell of origin	Probably a subset of activated T-lymphocytes distinct from the target T-cell
Stability	Very labile unless stored in albumin or PEG

cultures. These cells did not contain detectable levels of terminal deoxynucleotidyl transferase, an enzyme marker for immature lymphoid cells. The population of growing cells appears to be purely T-cells, since there were no markers for other types of leucocytes. In particular, surface markers for B-lymphoblastoid cells were not detectable, including tests for surface and intracellular immunoglobulin, EBV-receptors, and B-cell-specific complement receptors. These cells could be distinguished from permanently transformed lymphoblastoid cell lines by their: (1) dependence for growth upon the continuous presence of TCGF, (2) lack of detectable EBV and surface immunoglobulins, and (3) exhibition of immunologic reactivities not associated with transformed lymphoblastoid cells. Nevertheless, in the constant presence of TCGF we have no evidence that the lifetime of these cells is finite.

D. The Functional Significance of TCGF

Human TCGF has been substantially purified (Mier and Gallo, 1980) and its biochemical characteristics are summarized in Table 1. The central observation concerning the control of T-cell proliferation was made using this partially purified TCGF. This was the realization that the proliferative stimulus is provided by TCGF rather than the lectin or antigen which in themselves are mitogenic only in situations where they stimulate the release of TCGF. The fact that TCGF is depleted by proliferating T-cells (Bonnard et al. 1979; Smith et al. 1980) explains the finite nature of lectin-stimulated T-cell responses and the apparent infinite proliferative capacity of T-cells continuously supplemented with TCGF.

The T-cell proliferative response and acquisition of effector cell function depends upon interactions between at least three cell types as illustrated by the model in Fig. 1. The addition of antigen or lectin to a mixed population of these cell types results in a cellular activation which is characteristic for each cell. An activated adherent cell, most likely the macrophage, processes the antigen/lectin and releases a soluble product termed lymphocyte activating factor (LAF) (Oppenheim et al. 1979). This activity is not in itself a proliferative stimulus but it appears to stimulate the production and/or release of TCGF (Larsson et al. 1980;

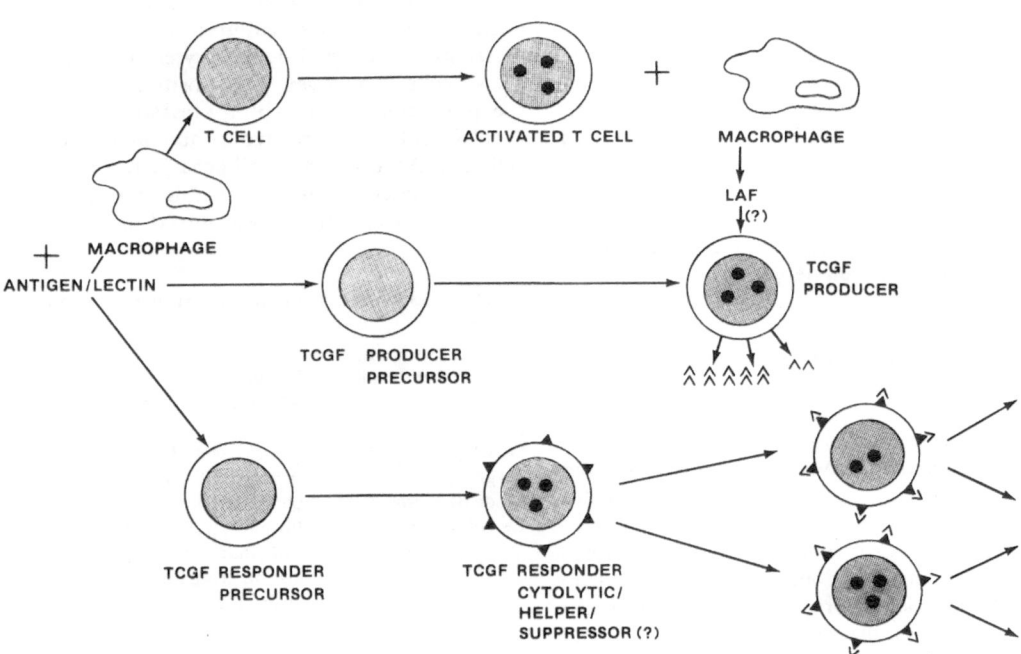

Fig. 1. A model for the action of purified T-cell growth factor in regulating T-cell proliferation

Smith et al. 1980). The actual mechanism of action of LAF remains obscure. However, once the T-cells are activated and TCGF is present, the T-cells will proliferate in the absence of antigen, adherent cells, or adherent cell products. Several observations suggest that the TCGF producing-cell is a mature T-cell that is activated by antigen and stimulated by LAF to release TCGF. Highly purified T-cells produce TCGF when provided with these signals (Smith et al. 1980). TCGF production requires the maturational influence of the thymus (Gillis et al. 1979). Cloned T helper cells can produce TCGF in vitro (Smith, to be published). It is not clear whether under normal circumstances the TCGF producer T-cell can respond to TCGF. All the T-cell lines reported to date have required the addition of exogenous TCGF for continuous proliferation in the absence of other cells. No normal T-cell lines capable of making enough growth factor to be independent of added T-cells have been found. If the same subset of helper T-cells have the ability both to make and respond to TCGF, then it may be possible to select self-replicating helper T-cell lines. Our current views on the regulation of T-cell proliferation by TCGF is illustrated in Fig. 1.

An initial result of antigen/lectin binding to the TCGF responder cell population, whether they are cytotoxic, suppressor, or helper in nature, is the acquisition of a TCGF responsive state. This responsiveness appears to be a direct result of the development of TCGF-specific membrane recpetors (Bonnard et al. 1979; Smith et al. 1979). Freshly isolated T-cells will neither bind nor proliferate in response to TCGF, but the addition of antigen/lectin to these T-cells will allow absorption of and proliferation in response to TCGF. The results indicate that the specificity of T-cells is restricted by the antigen that activated the cell but that the proliferate stimulus is provided by TCGF which itself has no antigenic specificity (Schreier and Tees 1980).

The discovery that T-cell clonal expansion is dependent upon TCGF and is mediated through a specific receptor suggests that derangements in the immune system seen in immunodeficiency and neoplastic states can be explained by alterations in the release of or response to TCGF. In addition, agonists and antagonists of the immune system may well function by affecting TCGF production or function.

E. Establishment and Characterization of Cell Lines from Patients with T-Cell Neoplasias Using Purified TCGF

A few non-B lymphoblastoid cell lines (e.g., Molt 4, 8402, CCRF-CEM) have been established from patients with ALL. Generally, these cell lines are terminal deoxynucleotidyl transferase (TdT) positive, which as noted earlier is a marker for immature lymphoblasts usually but not necessarily restricted to the T-lymphoid lineage. These cell lines either have no or a small percentage of E-rosette-positive cells (Nilsson and Ponten 1975), and they neither produce TCGF nor respond to it (our unpublished observations). We assayed some malignant T-cells, particularly those of mature T-cell origin, for their capacity to maintain responsiveness to TCGF.

As previously discussed, purified TCGF does not stimulate the growth of freshly isolated normal T-cells. If the malignant T-cells were activated during the process of transformation, these cells could then be selectively grown by treatment with the purified TCGF. In fact, this was observed. Long-term growth of T-cells from tissue samples from six of six patients with cutaneous T-cell lymphoma (CTCL) and six of six patients selected as having acute lymphocytic leukemia of a T-cell origin was achieved by using partially purified mitogen-free TCGF (Poiesz et al. 1980a). All these fresh samples began to proliferate after 24–48 h and were in continuous culture for at least 4 months. Some have been maintained in culture for over a year. These cell lines remained E-rosette positive, TdT negative, and negative for B-cell markers, typing them as mature T-cells. The CTCL, ALL, and normal cultured T-cells can be distinguished from one another by cytochemical procedures. All the CTCL cell lines (and only those lines) were strongly positive for nonspecific esterase, utilizing assay conditions which only stain monocytes. The presence of markers for both T-cell and monocytoid characteristics on these CTCL-cultured cells is puzzling but probably means they are neoplastic T-cells with aberrant properties. Normal cultured T-cells exhibited a mild granular cytoplasmic staining for acid phosphatase which is typical of freshly isolated T-cells. The majority of the cultured ALL cells showed a strong concentration of the staining pattern in the Golgi region of the cells which has been reported to be a strong indication of malignant T-cells in fresh ALL samples (Catousky et al. 1978; Schwarce 1975). Also, in one case, CTCL-3, the fresh and cultured cells had metaphases which showed the same karotypic abnormalities. Also, in one case, CTCL-2, the cells became independent of added TCGF for continuous growth after ten passages in culture. The morphology of the cultured cells was of interest and very similar to cells of the primary neoplasias. For instance cultured CTCL cells contained many giant multinucleated cells often surrounded by many mono- or binucleated smaller cells, the nuclei of which were often convoluted (see Fig. 2) (Poiesz et al. 1980a). The independent growth of CTCL-2, the abnormal karyotype of CTCL-3, the *direct* response to TCGF, the cytochemistry patterns of the cell lines as consistent with studies performed on fresh

samples from patients with CTCL and ALL (Catousky et al. 1978; Schwarce 1975), and perhaps most evidently, the abnormal morphology of the cells strongly indicate that the cell lines represent the neoplastic cell populations. We think these cell systems will be useful for (1) comparative studies between normal and neoplastic T-cells, (2) possible predictive value in patients in remission by utilizing the direct response of transformed T-cells to TCGF as an indication of the presence of residual neoplastic cells, and (3) providing malignant T-cells for biochemical and virological studies relating to etiology. Their properties are summarized in Table 2.

It has been proposed that TCGF is a second signal for sustained growth of previously activated normal T-lymphocytes (Ruscetti and Gallo 1981). Presumably, antigen or mitogen

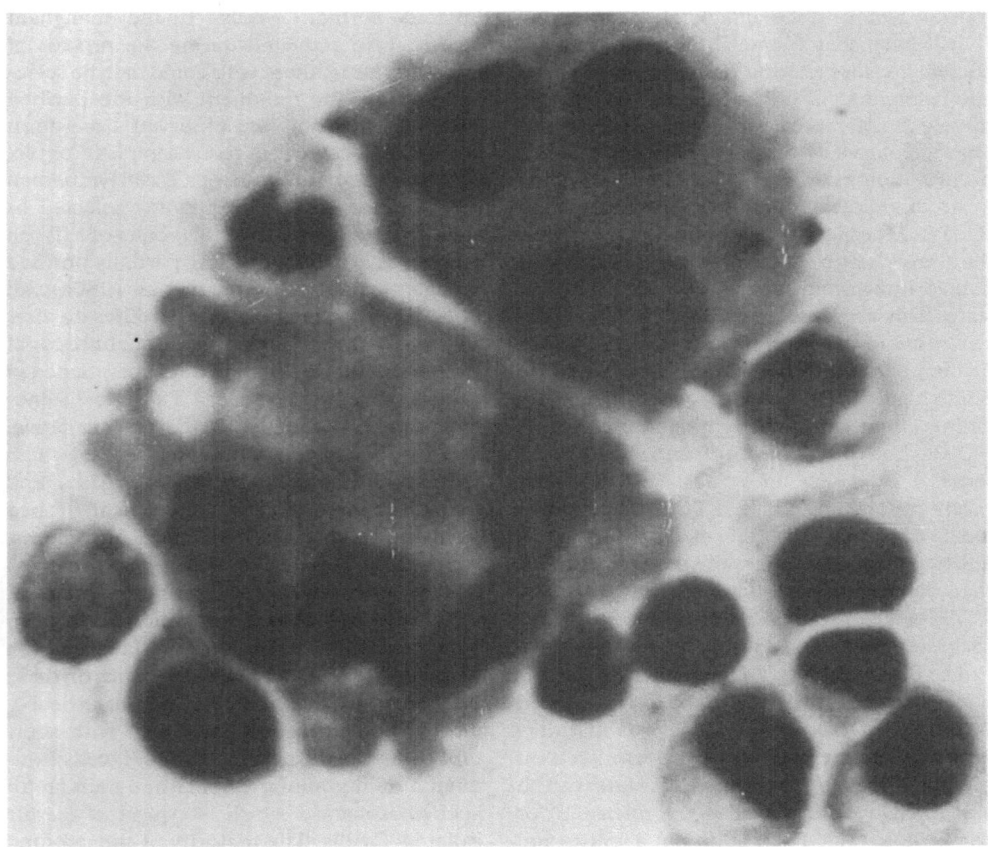

Fig. 2. Light microscopic appearance of cultured cutaneous T-cell lymphoma cells. Cytocentrifuge preparation of cultured CTCL-2 cells, illustrating the varying size and nuclear number of cultured CTCL cells Wright-Giemsa stain. x1800

Table 2. Comparative properties of continuously cultured human T-cells

Source of cells	Requirements of growth			Morphology	TdT	EBV, IgG	E-, Rosette	Acid phosphatase	Nonspecific esterase	Chromosomes
	No additions	TCGF Alone	TCGF and PHA initia.							
Normal	−	−	+	Normal lymphoblasts	−	−	+	+ Mild granular cytoplasmic	−	Normal diploid
ALL[a]	− (rarely +)	+	+	Homogenous lymphoblasts – sometimes with multiple nucleoli in nucleus	+	−	+	++ Concentrated in Golgi region	−	Variable and like primary cells
CTCL[b]	− (rarely +)	+	+	Heterogenous giant multinucleated cells and other smaller lymphoblasts mono- or binucleated; some with convoluted nuclei	−	−	+	+++ Diffuse intense reaction	Diffuse intense reaction in a few cells; majority – small paranuclear cytoplasmic granule	Variable and like primary cells

[a] ALL is acute lymphoblastic leukemia. The cells were from peripheral blood of untreated patients with T-cell disease
[b] CTCL is cutaneous T-cell lymphoma or leukemia. Cells were from blood or lymph nodes

stimulation induces cell membrane alterations to produce or expose a receptor(s) for TCGF. Neoplastic T-cells may have such a receptor(s) on their cell surface at all times, thereby explaining the ability to grow T-cells from CTCL and ALL samples with pp-TCGF without prior mitogen stimulation. This could be due to either chronic stimulation by some ill-defined antigen or cellular membrane changes which lead to exposure of a receptor or its synthesis de novo. If TCGF plays a role in the in vivo regulation of T-cell replication, as seems most probably, the above model may explain a growth advantage of malignant lymphocytes over normal T-cells.

F. Some of the Cultured Mature T Cells from Patients with T-Cell Leukemias-Lymphomas Release Retroviruses

Retrovirus particles were observed budding from fresh and cultured cells from two patients, each with a clinical variant of a cutaneous T-cell lymphoma (Poiesz et al. 1980b, and to be published). These viruses were subsequently isolated and characterized (see below). Patient C.R. was a 28-year-old male with Stage IV mycosis fungoides and patient M.B. was a 64-year-old female with the leukemic phase of Sezary syndrome. Abnormal T-lymphoblast cell lines were derived from both these patients using TCGF. The cell lines, HUT102 (Gazdar et al. 1980; Poiesz et al. 1980a) and CTCL-3 were established 1 year apart from the right inguinal lymph node and peripheral blood of patient C.R. Another cell line, CTCL-2, was derived from a leukemic peripheral blood sample from patient M.B. (Poiesz et al. 1980). HUT102 and CTCL-2 cells are now grown independent of added TCGF, but CTCL-3 still requires it. Morphologically typical (Schidlovsky 1977) type-C budding, immature, and mature virus particles have been observed on electron micrographs of cell pellets from all three of these cell lines and fresh peripheral blood lymphocytes from patient C.R. (Fig. 3).

Initially, virus production from HUT102 cells required prior induction iododeoxyuridine (IDUR) but spontaneously became a constitutive producer of virus at a later passage, whereas CTCL-3 cells have always been con-

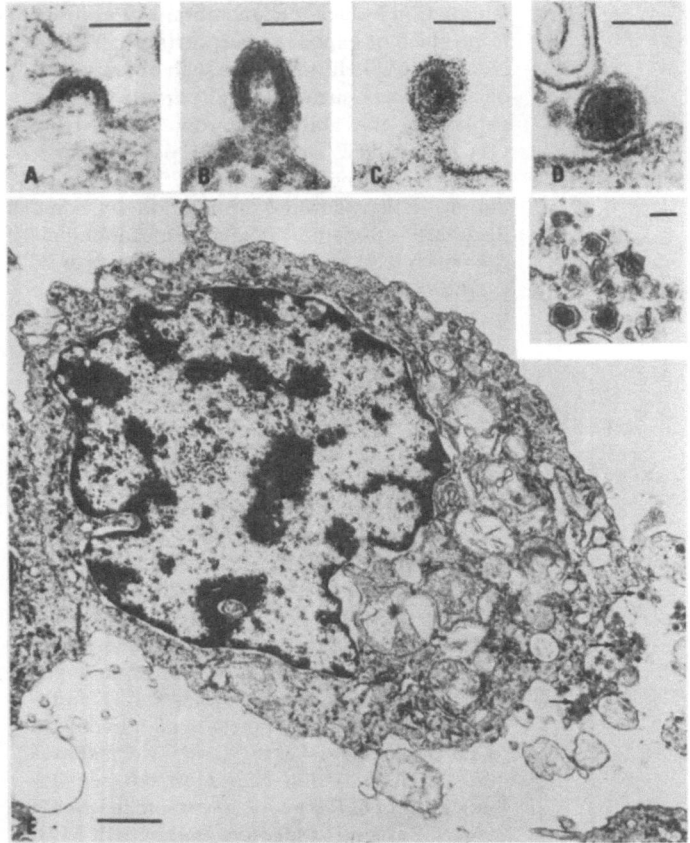

Fig. 3. Thin-section electron micrographs of budding HTLV$_{CR}$ particles seen in pelleted HUT 102 cells. **A** Early viral bud. **B** Late viral bud with nearly completed nucleoid. **C** »Immature" extracellular virus particle *(top)* with incomplete condensation of the nucleoid. **D** »Mature" extracellular virus particles with condensed, centrally located nucleoid surrounded by an outer membrane separated by an electron lucent area. **E** HUT 102 cell 72 h after IDUR induction. Many mature particles are found in the extracellular space in clumps associated with cellular debris *(inset)*. The *bar lines* in A–D and inset equal 100 nm. The *bar line* in E equals 1000 nm

stitutive producers. CTCL-2 cells have always required IDUR induction of virus. Typical of a retrovirus, the HTLV isolates band at a density of 1.16 gm/ml in continuous sucrose gradients (Poiesz et al. 1980, and to be published), contain 70S RNA (Reitz et al., to be published) and are associated with a DNA polymerase which prefers the template primers poly rA.oligo dT and poly rC.oligo dG over poly dA.oligo dT. Purified DNA polymerase from HTLV$_{CR}$ has shown the same results with the above template primer and has been demonstrated to catalyze transcription of purified simian sarcoma virus (SSV) 70S RNA and human mRNA (Rho et al., to be published).

These are all characteristics of a viral reverse transcriptase (RT) (Sarngadharan et al. 1978). The molecular weight of purified HTLV RT is about 95,000. The enzyme shows preference for Mg^{++} as its divalent cation, especially with the template-primer, poly rC.oligo dG (Kalyanaraman et al., to be published). This combination of morphologic and biochemical characteristics are atypical for most known animal viruses; HTLV does not easily fit into a clear type C, B, or D pattern. Rather, it is suggestive of those viruses which are difficult to classify, e.g., BLV (Olson 1979) or the particle-associated RT-like activity found in some fresh human placentas (Nelson et al. 1978).

The major protein bands of disrupted purified $HTLV_{CR}$ and $HTLV_{MB}$ particles as determined by SDS polyacrylamide gel electrophoresis are identical and have mol. wts. of approximately 81,000 (p81), 52,000 (p52), 42,000 (p42), 24,000 (p24), 18,000 (p18), 12,000 (p12), and 10,000 (p10) (Reitz et al., to be published; Rho et al., to be published). These proteins are consistent in size and number with that expected of a retrovirus (August et al. 1974). These same proteins bands are identified when HUT102 cells are grown in H^3-leucine and the subsequently isolated and purified $HTLV_{CR}$ particles are disrupted and examined by SDS PAGE. Hence, they represent either viral or cellular proteins rather than a contaminant from the fetal calf serum in which the cells are grown.

Several proteins, p81, p24 and p18 are labeled with I^{125} only after disruption of $HTLV_{CR}$ particles with detergent and, therefore, probably are viral core proteins (Kalyanaraman et al., to be published). We think p24 is the major structural core p30 of HTLV because of its relative quantity, molecular weight, elution profile on phosphocellulose (Kalyanaraman et al., to be published and see below), and co-purification with viral cores.

G. The HTLV Isolates Are Retroviruses and They Are a New Retrovirus Class

As is evident from the above discussion the HTLV isolates can be categorized as retroviruses because they have retrovirus morphology and mode of budding from cell membranes, a density of 1.16 g/ml by sucrose gradient analysis, and contain 70S RNA, structural proteins analogous to retrovirus proteins, and a DNA polymerase. There are four independent cell sources from two different patients which release HTLV; all were grown in culture in the presence of TCGF. Two of these cell lines (HUT-102 and CTCL-2) have become TCGF independent, apparently because they produce their own TCGF. These two cell lines are producers of HTLV.

The characterization of the HTLV DNA polymerase clearly indicates that it is a RT. Prior to its purification HTLV RT catalyzes an endogenous DNA synthesis. The cDNA product can be isolated and purified. It completely (>90%) hybridizes back to purified HTLV 70S RNA (see Reitz et al. in this book). Purified HTLV RT catalyzes transcription of purified viral 70S RNA (or mRNAs) in reconstituted reactions (Reitz et al., to be published). Purified HTL RT utilizes poly rC.oligo dG and poly rA.oligo dT, but not poly dA.oligo dT (Rho et al., to be published) – characteristics of a retrovirus RT (Gallo and Reitz 1976); Gallo et al. 1975; Sarngadharan et al. 1978). Purified HTLV RT is about 95,000 daltons, shows preference for Mg^{++} for its divalent cation, and of all synthetic template primers, utilizes poly rC.oligo dG most efficiently (Rho et al., to be published). As noted above these characteristics mimic the difficult-to-classify retroviruses, i.e., those not clearly type C, D, or B, e.g., (BLV).

Several analyses of HTLV have been completed. All of these results show that HTLV is not closely related to previously isolated animal retroviruses. These results are summarized here.

I. Reverse transcriptase

As noted above, HTLV RT has been purified. We (Rho et al., to be published) have compared purified HTLV to other RTs purified from animal retroviruses for immunologic relatedness. We have described these types of assays previously at these meetings in other comparative studies (Gallo 1976; Gallo 1979). Briefly, we have made antibodies to RTs from many animal retroviruses by inoculating goats or rats with the purified RT (Mondal et al. 1975; Smith et al. 1975; Todaro and Gallo 1973). The hyperimmune sera are obtained, and in most cases they strongly neutralize the DNA polymerase activity of the homologous RT. These antisera also generally show cross reactions which are in keeping with the known relatedness of lack of relatedness of different retroviruses as determined by other types of comparisons. Sometimes neutralization of polymerase activity of the homologous enzyme is not obtained. In these cases, however, a positive and specific binding of the antibody to the RT can be demonstrated (Robert-Guroff and Gallo 1977; 1979). When these tests were made with RT from HTLV no detectable cross reactons was found with any of the antisera to animal retroviruses (Poiesz et al. 1980b; Rho et al., to be published). These results are summarized in Table 3.

Table 3. Lack of detectable relatedness of purified reverse transcriptase of HTLV to reverse transcriptase of several animal retroviruses[a]

Anti-RT IgG[b]	Amount of Anti-RT IgG required for >50% inhibition of RT activity of:	
	Homologous RT[c] (µg)	HTLV RT (µg)
SSAV	10–15	>>150
GaLV	10–15	>>150
BaEV	10–15	>>150
FeLV	5–10	>>150
RD114	10–15	>>150
R-MuLV	5–10	>>150
MPMV	10–15	>>150
SMV	20–25	>>150
MMTV	20–25	>>150
BoLV	15–20	>>150
AMV	5–10	>>150

[a] Assays were carried out by determining the percentage neutralization of DNA polymerases (Reverse transcriptases) by different amounts of hyperimmune sera. The hyperimmune sera were prepared by inoculation of rats or goats with the various reverse transcriptases. Controls were with buffer alone or with nonimmune sera. Preincubations of antibodies and polymerases were for 3 h at 4° followed by polymerase assays which were carried out with standard conditions and 20 mM Mg^{++} and poly rC.oligo dG or 0.05 mM Mn^{++} and poly rA.oligo dT

[b] Anti-RT IgG refer to the hyperimmune sera made against RT from the viruses listed in the table

[c] Homologous RT refers to the RT the antibody was made against

II. Core Protein p24

The major internal protein of HTLV has a molecular weight of 24,000 (Kalyanaraman et al., to be published). This protein is analogous to the major core protein (p24 to p30) of animal retroviruses. The evidence that HTLV p24 is a viral protein of HTLV and not a cellular or serum protein contaminating the virion preparations is as follows:

1. The p24 is the major protein associated with HTLV;
2. p24 copurifies with HTLV cores and increases as virus titer is increased;
3. p24 has the same biochemical behavior as animal retrovirus core proteins (p24 to p30), e.g., size and characteristics of elution from phosphocellulose columns; and

4. p24 is readily detectable in the neoplastic human T-cells producing HTLV but not in normal human cells, including normal growing human T-cells.

These observations are all reported in detail elsewhere (Kalyanaraman et al., to be published).

The p24 of HTLV is not significantly related to proteins of animal retroviruses. The evidence for this is summarized here. Hyperimmune serum was obtained against p24 of HTLV (Kalyanaraman et al., to be published). This antibody precipitates I^{125}-labeled HTLV p24 but not significantly proteins of animal retroviruses. Conversely, antibodies to p24–p30 of various animal retroviruses do not significantly precipitate HTLV I^{125}-p24. Competition radioimmune assays were next employed. None of the tested animal retroviruses p24–p30 competed in precipitation of HTLV I^{125}-p24 by HTLV p24 antisera, while cold HTLV competed completely. Conversely, HTLV p24 did not compete in various homologous radioimmune precipitation assays using I^{125} p24–p30 of animal retroviruses and their corresponding antisera. For example, whereas 10 to 100 µg of unlabeled p30 from SSAV, BaEV, or MuLV-Rauscher competed 50% of the precipitation of their I^{125}-p30 by the corresponding antisera, unlabeled HTLV p24 did not compete. Finally, p30 of certain retroviruses are known to contain interspecies determinants. These cross reactions can be detected by heterologous competitive radioimmune assays, i.e., by using I^{125} p30 of one virus and antisera to p30 of another (related) virus. These assays show, for example, that p30 of some mammalian retroviruses are closely related (reviewed in Aaronson and Stephenson 1976). We have confirmed the reported relatedness of some of the Type-C mammalian retroviruses, and we have shown that HTLV p24 does not compete in these assays. These results are reported in detail elsewhere (Kalyanaraman et al., to be published), and a list of the animal retroviruses tested for lack of p24–p30 relatedness to HTLV p24 is presented in Table 4.

III. Nucleotide Sequences

The relatedness of HTLV nucleotide sequences to those of animal retroviruses was examined by several approaches. These results show a very slight but reproducible homology between HTLV and sequences from viruses of the

Table 4. HTLV p24 is distinct from p24-p30 of the animal retroviruses listed here[a]

Primate Type-C
  SSV(SSAV) (woolly monkey virus)
  GaLV (gibbon ape leukemia virus)
  BaEV (baboon endogenous virus)
  OMC-1 (owl monkey virus)
Primate Type-D
  MPMV (Mason Pfizer monkey virus)
  SMRV (squirrel monkey retrovirus)
Feline Type-C
  FeLV (feline leukemia virus)
  RD114 (endogenous feline virus)
Murine Type-C
  $MuLV_R$ (murine leukemia virus, Rauscher Strain)
Murine Type-B
  MMTV (mouse mammary tumor virus)
Miscellaneous Type-C and Unclassified
  BLV (bovine leukemia virus)
  GPV (guinea pig virus)
  DKV (deer kidney virus)
  VRV (viper virus)

[a] Details are reported elsewhere (Kalyanaraman et al., to be published)

SSV(SSAV)-GaLV primate type-C oncogenic infectious virus group (about 10% to 15% above background) and no detectable homology to other animal retroviruses. Several approaches were used. They included tests of homology between:

1. ^{3}H-cDNA of HTLV and 70S RNA of various animal viruses;
2. ^{3}H-cDNA of HTLV and DNA from cells infected by various viruses and, therefore, containing DNA proviruses;
3. ^{3}H-cDNA of HTLV and DNA from tissues of animals containing multiple copies of endogenous genetically transmitted virogenes;
4. I^{125}-70S RNA of HTLV and DNA from infected cells and DNA from animal tissues containing endogenous virogenes;
5. ^{3}H-cDNA of animal retroviruses and 70S RNA from HTLV; and
6. ^{3}H-cDNA of animal retroviruses and DNA and RNA from cells (HUT-102) infected by and producing HTLV.

These results were uniform in showing that the HTLV isolates are related to each other but not significantly related to known animal retroviruses. The results are summarized by Reitz et al. elsewhere in this book and will be published in detail elsewhere (Reitz et al. 1981).

IV. Attempts to Transmit HTLV to Other Cells

In vitro and in vivo experiments are in progress to determine whether HTLV can infect certain cell types or effect their growth. So far HTLV have not been transmitted to any of several cell types from different animals including humans. The results to date suggest that either the HTLV isolates are in some way defective or that cell receptors for them are unusual and yet to be found. The two suggestions are not mutually exclusive.

H. HTLV is Not an Endogenous Wide-Spread (Germ-Line) Transmitted Virus of Humans

Many animal retroviruses are endogenous to a given species, that is, their genomes are present in the DNA of all tissues of most and in some cases possibly all members of a species. They are not generally infectious to the species but are transmitted in the germ line in a Mendelian genetic manner. These retroviruses are often nononcogenic in contrast to BLV, GaLV, FeLV, AMV, etc. which cause leukemias and lymphomas by some kind of infection. We do not know how HTLV is transmitted. It is possible that it is endogenous and vertically transmitted in the germ line of select families[1]. However, we can conclude that it is not a widespread endogenous genetically transmitted virus of humans because ^{3}H-cDNA and I^{125}-70S RNA of HTLV does not hybridize to DNA purified from normal human tissues. Over 30 samples were examined and none contained detectable HTLV sequences under conditions that would readily detect one copy per haploid genome. These results are also summarized by Reitz et al. elsewhere in this book and will be reported in detail in a separate publication (Reitz et al., to be published).

---

[1] *Note added in proof:* New results have shown that sequences of HTLV can not be found in cultured normal B-cells from patient C. R. Therefore, this virus in the neoplastic T-cells must be acquired not genetically transmitted

I. HTLV Was Present in the Primary (Uncultured) Fresh Cells

There is now substantial evidence that HTLV was present in the primary tissues or leukemic blood cells of some of the patients we have had the opportunity to study. The evidence summarized here is as follows.

1. HTLV nucleotide sequences were found in the DNA of the fresh leukemic cells of patient M.B., the patient with Sezary leukemia from which cell line CTCL-2 was established (Poiesz et al., to be published). As noted earlier, CTCL-2 releases virus (called HTLV$_{MB}$) very similar to the first isolate of HTLV (Poiesz et al., to be published).
2. HTLV nucleotide sequences were found in the DNA of uncultured leukemic cells of a 16 yr. old young man with T-cell ALL. Some of these results are summarized by Reitz et al. in this book and published in detail elsewhere (Reitz et al. 1981).
3. Extracts of the fresh leukemic cells of patient M.B. competed for the radioimmune precipitation of I^{125} HTLV-p24 by its homologous antisera, suggesting that HTLV p24 was in the fresh leukemic cells of patient M.B. (Poiesz et al., to be published) and
4. Antigens detected by HTLV antibodies and antibodies reactive with HTLV proteins have been found in some other patients by M. Robert-Guroff and L. Posner in our laboratory.

We have not yet found HTLV, antigens, or HTLV nucleic acids in normal cells or in cells or tissues derived from patients with myeloid leukemias, B-cell leukemias, or carcinomas. Our evidence to date then associates HTLV only with neoplastic and relatively mature T-cells of some patients. Therefore, our working hypothesis is that HTLV is an unusual infection of humans with a very specific target cell.

J. Conclusions

HTLV are novel retroviruses which are found in some human mature T-cell lymphomas and leukemias. We think they are an unusual infection with very specific target cells. They may act on those subsets of T-cells which are able to produce TCGF. This interaction might allow for abnormal TCGF release which in turn leads to abnormal proliferation, a model similar to the proposed model made previously at these meetings (Gallo 1979). A wide epidemiological survey by more than one sensitive technique is now needed to further understand the possible role of this virus in human disease.

References

Aaronson SA, Stephenson JR (1976) Endogenous type-C RNA viruses of mammalian cells. Biochim Biophys Acta 458:323–354 – August JJ, Bolognesi DP, Fleessner I, Gilden RV, Nowinski RC (1974) A proposed nomenclature for the virion proteins of oncogenic RNA viruses. Virology 60:595–605 – Bonnard GD, Yasaka K, Jacobson D (1979) Lectin-activated T-cell growth factor-induced proliferation: Absorption of T-cell growth factor by activated T-cells. J Immunol 123:2704–2709 – Bronson SL, Fraley EE, Fogh J, Kalter SS (1979) Induction of retroviral particles in human testicular tumor (Tera-1) cell cultures. An electron microscopic study. J Natl Cancer Inst 63:337–339 – Brouet JC, Flandrin G, Sasportes M, Preud-Homme JL, Seligmann M (1975a) Chronic lymphocytic leukemia of T-cell origin, immunological evaluation in eleven patients. Lancet 2:890–893 – Brouet JC, Preud'Homme JL, Seligmann M (1975b) The use of band T membrane markers in the classification of human leukemias with special reference to acute lymphocytic leukemia. Blood Cells 1:81–90 – Catousky D, Cheschi M, Greaves MF (1978) Acid-phosphatase reaction in acute lymphoblastic leukemia. Lancet 1:749–751 – Cockerell GL (1976) Characterization of feline T and B lymphocytes and identification of experimentally induced T cell neoplasias in the cat. J Natl Cancer Inst 57:907–914 – De-The' G (1980) Epstein-Barr virus in human diseases: Infectious mononucleosis, Burkitt's lymphoma and nasopharyngeal carcinoma. In: Klein G (ed) Viral oncology. Raven, New York, pp 769–798 – Gajl-Peczalska K, Bloomfield CD, Sosein H (1975) Analysis of blood and lymph nodes in 87 patients. Am J Med 59:674–685 – Gallagher RE, Gallo RC (1975) Type-C RNA tumor virus isolated from cultured human acute myelogenous leukemia cells. Science 187:350–353 – Gallo RC (1976) RNA tumor viruses and leukemia: Evaluation of present results supporting their presence in human leukemias. In: Neth R, Gallo RC, Mannweiler K, Moloney WC (eds) Modern trends in human leukemia II. Lehmanns, Germany, pp 431–450 – Gallo RC (1979) Cellular and virological studies directed to the pathogenesis of the human myelogenous leukemias. (The First Frederick-Stohlman memorial lecture) In: Neth R, Gallo RC, Hofschneider PH, Mannweiler K (eds) Modern trends in human leukemia III. Springer, Berlin Heidelberg New

York, pp 7–24 – Gallo RC, Reitz MS (1976) Molecular probes for tumor viruses in human cancer. Int Rev Exp Pathol 16:1–58 – Gallo RC, Gallagher RE, Miller NR, Mondal H, Saxinger WC, Mayer RJ, Smith RG, Gillespie DH (1975) Relationships between components in primate RNA tumor viruses and in the cytoplasm of human leukemic cells: Implications to leukemogenesis. Cold Spring Harbor Symp Quant Biol 39:933–961 – Gazdar AF, Carney DN, Bunn PA, Russell EF, Jaffe ES, Schechter GP, Guccion JG (1980) Mitogen requirements for the in vitro propagation of cutaneous T cell lymphomas. Blood 55:409–417 – Gillis S, Baker PE, Union NA, Smith KA (1979) The in vitro generation and sustained culture of nude mouse cytolytic T-lymphocytes. J Exp Med 149:1460–1466 – Gupta S, Good RA (1980) Markers of human lymphocyte subpopulations in primary immunodeficiency and lymphoproliferate disorders. Semin Hematol 17:1–29 – Guroff MR, Gallo RC (1977) Serological analysis of cellular and viral DNA polymerases by an antiserum to DNA polymerase μ of human lymphoblasts. Biochemistry 16:2874–2880 – Guroff MR, Gallo RC (1979) Type-specific binding antibody to baboon endogenous virus (M7) reverse transcriptase. J Gen Virol 43:1–6 – Haran-Ghera N (1980) Pathogenesis of murine leukemia. In: Klein G (ed) Viral oncology. Raven, New York, pp 161–185 – Jaffe ES, Shevach EM, Sussman EH (1975) Membrane receptor sites for the identification of lymphoreticular cells in benign and malignant conditions. Br J Cancer 31:107–120 (Suppl) – Kalyanaraman VS, Sarngadharan MG, Poiesz B, Ruscetti FW, Gallo RC (to be published) Immunological properties of a type-C retrovirus isolated from cultured human T-lymphoma cells and comparison to other mammalian retroviruses. – Kaplan HS, Goodenow RS, Epstein AL, Gartner S, Decleve A, Rosenthal PN (1977) Isolation of type-C RNA virus from an established human histiocytic lymphoma cell line. Proc Natl Acad Sci USA 74:2564–2568 – Klein G (1980) Viral Oncology. Raven, New York – Larsson EL, Iscove NN, Coutinko A (1980) Two distinct factors are required for induction of T-cell growth. Nature 283:664–666 – Lutzner M, Edelson R, Schein P, Green I, Kirkpatrick C, Ahmd A (1975) Cutaneous T-cell lymphomas: The Sezary syndrome, mycosis fungoides and related disorders. Ann Intern Med 83:534–552 – Mier JW, Gallo RC (1980) Purification and some characteristics of human T-cell growth factor (TCGF) from PHA-stimulated lymphocyte conditioned media. Proc Natl Acad Sci USA 77:6134–6138 – Mondal H, Gallagher RE, Gallo RC (1975) RNA-directed DNA polymerase from human leukemic blood cells and from primate type-C virus producing cells: High and low molecular weight forms with variant biochemical and immunological properties. Proc Natl Acad Sci USA 72:1194–1198 – Morgan DA, Ruscetti FW, Gallo RC (1976) Selective in vitro growth of T-lymphocytes from normal human bone marrows.

Science 193:1007–1008 – Nelson J, Yeong J, Levy J (1978) Normal human placentas contain RNA-directed DNA polymerase activity like that in viruses. Proc Natl Acad Sci USA 75:6263–6267 – Nilsson K, Ponten J (1975) Classification and biologic nature of established human hematopoietic cell lines. Int J Cancer 15:321–341 – Nooter K, Aarssen AM, Bentvelzen P, d'Groot FG (1975) Isolation of an infectious C-type oncornavirus from human leukemic bone marrow cells. Nature 256:595–597 – Olson C (1979) Progress for control of bovine leukosis. Practitioner 14:115–120 – Oppenheim JJ, Mizel SB, Meltzer MS (1979) Biological effects of lymphocyte and macrophage-derived mitogenic "amplication" factors. In: Cohen S, Peck E, Oppenheim JJ (eds) Biology of the Lymphokines. Academic, New York, pp 291–323 – Panem S, Prochownik EV, Reale FR, Kirsten WH (1975) Isolation of C-type virions from a normal human fibroblast strain. Science 189:297–299 – Poiesz BJ, Ruscetti FW, Gazdar AF, Bunn PA, Minna JD, Gallo RC (to be published a) Isolation of type-C retrovirus particles from cultured and fresh lymphocytes of a patient with cutaneous T-cell lymphoma. Proc Natl Acad Sci USA – Poiesz BJ, Ruscetti FW, Mier JW, Woods AM, Gallo RC (1980) T cell lines established from human T-lymphocytic neoplasias by direct response to T-cell growth factor. Proc Natl Acad Sci USA 77:6815–6819 – Poiesz BJ, Ruscetti FW, Reitz MS, Kalyanaraman VS, Gallo RC (1980) Evidence for nucleic acids and antigens of a new type-C retrovirus (HTLV) in primary ulcultured cells of a patient with Sezary T-cell leukemia and isolation of the virus. Proc Natl Acad Sci USA 77:7415–7419 – Reitz MS JR, Poiesz BJ, Ruscetti FW, Gallo RC (1981) Characterization and distribution of nucleic acid sequences of a novel type-C retrovirus isolated from neoplastic human T-lymphocytes. Proc Natl Acad Sci USA 78:1887–1891 – Rho HM, Poiesz B, Ruscetti FW, Gallo RC (to be published) Characterization of the reverse transcriptase from a new retrovirus (HTLV) produced by a human cutaneous T-cell lymphoma cell line. – Ruscetti FW, Gallo RC (1981) Human T-lymphocyte growth factor: Regulation of growth and function of T-lymphocytes. Blood (Ed. Review) 57:379–394 – Ruscetti FW, Morgan DA, Gallo RC (1977) Functional and morphological characterization of human T cells continuously grown in vitro. J Immunol 119:131–138 – Sarngadharan MG, Robert-Guroff M, Gallo RC (1978) DNA polymerases of normal and neoplastic mammalian cells. Biochim Biophys Acta 516:419–487 – Saxon A, Stevens RH, Golde DW (1978) T-lymphocytic variant of hairy cell leukemia. Ann Intern Med 88:323–326 – Schidlovsky G (1977) Structure of RNA tumor viruses. In: Gallo RC (ed) Recent advances in cancer research: Cell biology, molecular biology and tumor virology, Vol I. CRC, Cleveland Ohio, pp 189–245 – Schreier MH, Tees R (1980) Clonal induction of helper T cells: Conversion of specific signals into nonspecific signals. Int Arch Allergy Appl Immunol 61:227–231 – Schreier MH, Iscove NN, Tees R, Aardon L, von Boehmer H (to be published) Clones of killer and helper T cells: Growth requirements, specificity and retention of functions in long-term culture. Immunol Rev – Schwarce WW (1975) T cell origin of acid-phosphatase positive lymphoblasts. Lancet 2:1264–1266 – Smith KA (to be published) T-cell growth factor. Immunol Rev – Smith RG, Abrell JW, Lewis BJ, Gallo RC (1975) Serological analysis of human deoxyribonucleic acid polymerases. J Biol Chem 250:1702–1709 – Smith KA, Lachman LB, Oppenheim JJ, Favata MF (1980) The functional relationship of the interleukemias. J Exp Med 151:1551–1555 – Todaro GJ, Gallo RC (1973) Immunological relationship of DNA polymerase from human acute leukaemia cells and primate and mouse leukaemia virus reverse transcriptase. Nature 244:206–209

Haematology and Blood Transfusion Vol. 26
Modern Trends in Human Leukemia IV
Edited by Neth, Gallo, Graf, Mannweiler, Winkler
© Springer-Verlag Berlin Heidelberg 1981

Characterization by Nucleic Acid Hybridization of HTLV, a Novel Retrovirus from Human Neoplastic T-Lymphocytes

M. S. Reitz, jr., B. J. Poiesz, F. W. Ruscetti, and R. C. Gallo

Recently this laboratory reported the isolation of a retrovirus from a patient with cutaneous T-cell lymphoma (mycosis fungoides) (Poiesz et al., to be published). Several different tissue specimens from this patient were positive for virus production, including malignant lymph node tissue and peripheral blood samples. In addition, a similar or identical virus was also isolated from a patient with cutaneous T-cell leukemia (Sezary leukemia) Gallo, see this volume). The virus displayed all the properties of a type-C retrovirus, including virus budding, viral type reverse transcriptase, and poly(A)-containing 70S RNA. We have prepared cDNA and 70S RNA from this virus, called HTLV, and used these as probes to determine: (1) the degree of relatedness to other viruses, (2) whether or not HTLV is a human endogenous virus, and (3) whether related sequences could be found in other human tissues.

HTLV cDNA hybridizes 90% to its own 70S RNA with a $Crt_{1/2}$ of 0.15, which is similar to the kinetics of hybridization of other type-C viral cDNAs to their homologous 70S RNAs. HTLV cDNA hybridizes to cytoplasmic RNA from HUT 102 (the T-cell line producing the first HTLV isolate) with a $Crt_{1/2}$ of 50–60, which is indicative of a viral RNA content of about 0.2% by weight. HTLV cDNA hybridizes to HUT 102 cell DNA with a $Cot_{1/2}$ of 900–1000 compared with a $Cot_{1/2}$ for cell unique DNA of 2200, indicating that the provirus is present at about 2–3 copies per haploid genome.

The HTLV cDNA does not hybridize significantly to 70S RNA of a wide variety of retroviruses, including murine and feline leukemia and sarcoma viruses, baboon endogenous virus, Mason-Pfizer virus, squirrel monkey retrovirus, bovine leukemia virus, RD 114

endogenous cat virus, murine mammary tumor virus, or avian myeloblastosis virus (Table 1). Very low levels of hybridization (5%–10%) are achieved with 70S from woolly monkey virus and gibbon ape leukemia virus. In reciprocal experiments no hybridization was ob-

Table 1. Lack of relatedness of HTLV to other retroviruses[a]

Viral 70S RNA from	% Hybridization of HTLV ^{3}H-cDNA
HTLV	90
SSV/SSAV	16
GaLV$_H$	13
MuLV	9
MuSV	9
FeLV	8
FeSV	7
BaEV	7
M-PMV	3
SMRV	6
BLV	11
MMTV	8
AMV	4
RD114	3

[a] HTLV ^{3}H-cDNA was hybridized to 1 µg of the indicated 70S viral RNA to a Crt ≥2, then assayed for hybridization by S1 nuclease digestion. Values are not normalized or corrected for t=0 values. AMV, avian myeloblastosis virus; SSV, simian sarcoma virus; SSAV, simian sarcoma associated virus; GaLV$_H$, gibbon ape leukemia virus, Hall's Island strain; MuLV, murine leukemia virus; MuSV, murine sarcoma virus; FeLV, feline leukemia virus; FeSV, Feline sarcoma virus; BaEV, baboon endogenous virus; M-PMV, Mason-Pfizer monkey virus; SMRV, squirrel monkey retrovirus; BLV, bovine leukemia virus; MMTV, murine mammary tumor virus

Table 2. Distribution of HTLV-related sequences in human DNA

DNA-from	No. samples tested	No. samples:		
		Negative	Intermediate	Positive
1. Cultured CTCL, lines[a]	3	1	0	2
2. Myelogenous leukemia lines	3	3	0	0
3. Fresh CTCL (Sezary) peripheral blood	2	1	0	1
4. Autopsy tissue, M. fungoides	1	1	0	0
5. Fresh peripheral blood, ALL	3	1	1	1
6. Fresh peripheral blood, CLL	6	6	0	0
7. Fresh peripheral blood, AML	5	5	0	0
8. Fresh peripheral blood, CML	7	7	0	0
9. Burkitt tumor	2	2	0	0
10. Normal autopsy tissue	10	9	1	0

[a] HTLV ^{3}H-cDNA was hybridized to 600 μg of DNA from the indicated tissues in 0.4 M NaCl (65°), then assayed by digestion with S1 nuclease. Negative indicates >20% of the homologous hybridization, intermediate indicates 20%–40% of the homologous hybridization. Positive samples gave 50%–80% of the homologous hybridization. One of the two positive CTCL lines is HUT 102. CTLC, continuous T-cell line; ALL, acute lymphocytic leukemia; CLL, chronic lymphocytic leukemia; AML, acute myelogenous leukemia; CML, chronic myelogenous leukemia

served to HUT 102 cytoplasmic RNA or cell DNA with cDNA from the above animal viruses, i.e., only cDNA from HTLV hybridized to the nucleic acids from the human T-cell lymphoma cell line. No hybridization was observed to the proviral DNA of a number of species harboring endogenous retroviruses, including langur, owl monkey, baboon, squirrel monkey, colobus, macaque, cat, rat, mouse, guinea pig, and hamster. Therefore, HTLV is not related to any of the endogenous retroviruses of these species.

Although HTLV hybridizes to DNA and cytoplasmic RNA from HUT 102, the infected HTLV-producing cell line, no hybridization is obtained with DNA or RNA from normal human peripheral blood T-lymphocytes, stimulated in short-term culture (72 h) with phytohemagglutinin (PHA) or with DNA from a number of non-neoplastic autopsy tissues or peripheral blood samples from patients with acute myelogenous leukemia (AML), chronic myelogenous leukemia (CML), or chronic lymphocytic leukemia (CLL) (Table 2). DNA from one out of three acute lymphocytic leukemias (ALL) and one out of two fresh (uncultured) Sezary syndrome peripheral blood samples hybridized a significant (20%–25% compared to 40% for the homologous DNA) amount of HTLV cDNA. The positive ALL was a T-cell ALL.

A T-cell line was established from the positive Sezary T-cell leukemia sample, and a second isolate of type-C virus was obtained (Poiesz et al., unpublished work). HTLV cDNA hybridizes to DNA and cytoplasmic RNA from the cell line (CTCL-2) producing the second virus to about the same extent as do the homologous DNA and RNA. The Tm of the hybrid formed with HTLV cDNA and CTCL-2 RNA is identical to the homologous. Virus from CTCL-2 was used to prepare cDNA. This cDNA hybridized to HTLV 70S RNA but not to AMV 70S RNA. The above data indicates that the virus from CTCL-2 is closely related to HTLV.

Detailed descriptions of these viruses and their isolation are presented elsewhere in this symposium (Gallo). It would appear from the data above that HTLV is a novel retrovirus isolate not related to previously described retroviruses to a significant extent and that it is not an endogenous human virus. It appears instead to be an acquired virus which has infected some humans, and the preliminary data suggests that it is specifically associated with T-cell lymphomas and leukemias of a mature cell type. Studies are underway to further explore the role of HTLV in these diseases.

Reference

Poiesz BJ, Ruscetti FW, Mier JW, Woods AM, Gallo RC (to be published) Proc Natl Acad Sci USA

Haematology and Blood Transfusion Vol. 26
Modern Trends in Human Leukemia IV
Edited by Neth, Gallo, Graf, Mannweiler, Winkler
© Springer-Verlag Berlin Heidelberg 1981

Different Frequency Classes of Sequences in Heterogeneous Nuclear RNA of Normal Promyelocytes and Lymphoblasts and of Leukemic Blast Cells of Circulating Blood and of the HL60 Line

U. Torelli, G. Torelli, F. Narni, A. Donelli, S. Ferrari, G. Franchini, and B. Calabretta

A number of studies have led to the conclusion that each differentiated cell nucleus includes not only all of the genes ever utilized in the organism but also transcripts of most of these genes. A direct implication is that both the quantitative and qualitative structure of cytoplasmic messenger RNA populations are controlled posttranscriptionally. The control process would function by determining the fraction from 0 to 100% of the potential mRNA precursors from each gene that survive and that are processed and transferred to the cytoplasm (Davidson et al. 1977). Only for those few mRNAs which are represented at very high concentration in the cell, such as the globin mRNA in reticulocytes, has evidence been presented that regulation may occur at the transcription level (Tobin et al. 1978).

By studying the kinetics of DNA-RNA hybridization RNA sequence classes with different abundance may be detected in hnRNA, provided that critical conditions are maintained (Melli et al. 1971; Vogelstein and Gillespie 1977). We have determined the relative representation of sequence classes with different abundance in the heterogeneous nuclear RNA of two types of normal cells, i.e; lymphoblasts and promyelocytes, and three types of acute leukemia cells, i.e., acute lymphocytic leukemia (ALL), acute myelocytic leukemia (AML) blast cells from circulating blood, and HL60 promyelocytic cells.

A. Materials and Methods

Normal lymphoblasts were obtained by stimulating circulating blood lymphocytes with PHA for 48 h. Normal promyelocytes were obtained by fractionating normal bone marrow cells on albumin gradients.

ALL and AML blast cells were obtained from the circulating blood of untreated patients. HL60 cells were studied in the logarithmic phase of growth. RNA was labeled by incubating the cells for at least 3 h with ^{3}H-uridine and extracted several times with phenol and chlorophorm-isoamyl alcohol. After sedimentation in a preparative sucrose gradient, fractions corresponding to S values >50 were pooled and used in the hybridization reaction with human normal DNA. The reaction was carried out in 70% formamide and the DNA/RNA ratio was at least 5×10^3. DNA was sheared at an average length of fragments of 700 nucleotides.

B. Results

The results of two hybridization experiments, one with hnRNA from normal promyelocytes and one with hnRNA from HL60 cells, are given in Fig. 1. The values plotted as solid lines are derived from a least squares computer analysis. The results of this analysis carried out in all the experiments performed with both normal and leukemic cells are given in Table 1. They indicate the presence in the hnRNA of normal cells of three kinetic classes of sequences, whereas in the hnRNA of leukemic cells the analysis shows only two second order components, roughly corresponding, as far as the rate of hybridization is concerned, to the first and second class of sequences revealed by the analysis in the hnRNA of normal cells.

C. Discussion and Conclusions

The results of our experiments show that the hnRNA of normal hemopoietic cells includes a class of sequences with very low abundance which is absent in leukemic cells. In fact,

517

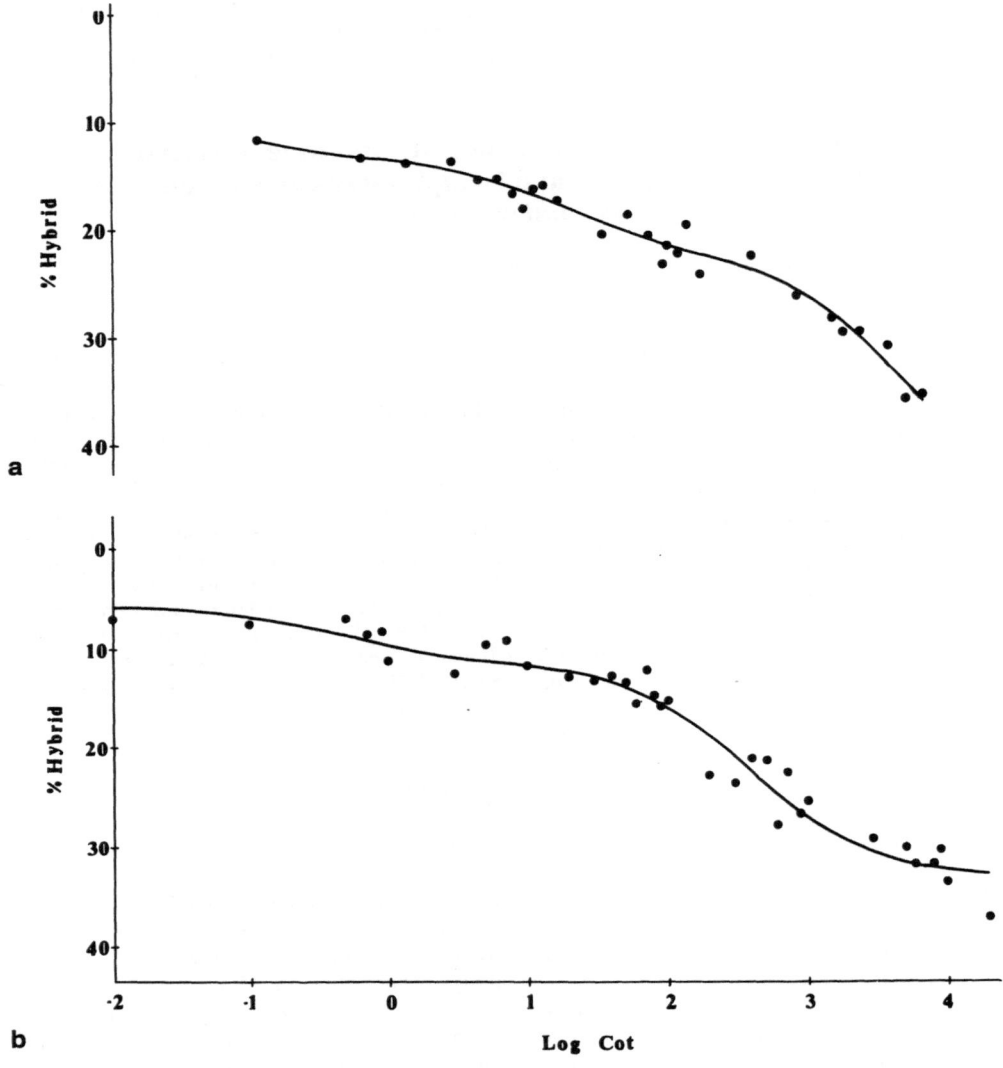

Fig. 1. Kinetics of hybridization to human DNA of hnRNA isolated from normal human promyelocytes **(a)** and HL60 leukemic cells **(b).** The hnRNA fractions >50S were obtained as described in the text. The length of DNA fragments was 700 nucleotides in both the experiments and the DNA/RNA ratio was 5×10^3

although the comparison with DNA reassociation values (Torelli et al. 1979) is only approximate, the main component in hnRNA of normal cells is formed by sequences appearing probably at levels of one or a very few copies per cell. The computer analysis does not show the presence of this component in the early transcript of the leukemic cells. The largest kinetic class of sequences of the hnRNA of these cells is formed by sequences more frequent than that forming the main kinetic class in hnRNA of normal cells. The main difficulty in making a conclusion is the failure to achieve complete hybridization of hnRNA. This failure has been already observed by several authors (Melli et al. 1971; Kline et al. 1974; Spradling et al. 1974) who have reported maximal proportions of hybridization of

Table 1. Kinetic parameters derived from the least squares computer analysis applied to the hybridization values obtained with hnRNA from normal and leukemic cells

Cell Type	First component			Second component			Third component		
	%	K	$Cot_{1/2}$	%	K	$Cot_{1/2}$	%	K	$Cot_{1/2}$
Normal promyelocytes	7.3	3.66125	0.273	9.4	0.00992	100	26.8	0.00004	24870
Normal promyelocytes	5.7	1.97528	0.534	11.2	0.00759	120	29.5	0.00004	25125
Normal lymphoblasts	5.1	0.60000	1.666	9.7	0.00473	211	28.8	0.00004	23192
Normal lymphoblasts	4.4	0.76000	1.403	14.0	0.00863	180	29.6	0.00006	17808
ALL	4.6	3.55457	0.280	29.0	0.00317	315			
AML 1	10.7	0.59314	1.68	30.7	0.00211	474			
AML 2	10.6	0.52518	1.90	38.9	0.00206	484			
HL60	5.9	0.43278	2.30	25.2	0.00180	554			
HL60	5.3	2.09849	0.47	24.6	0.00261	382			

hnRNA from different cell types ranging from 40% to 60%. Whereas some of them (Kline et al. 1974) assume that the hnRNA which fails to hybridize belongs exclusively to the low frequency class of sequences, other authors (Spradling et al. 1974) believe that the incomplete hybridization of RNA in vast DNA excess may affect all classes of sequences equally. Whatever interpretation finally proves to be correct, our results indicate that at least part of the hnRNA of leukemic cells is characterized by a sequence frequency higher than that of hnRNA of normal cells.

Acknowledgments

This research was supported by a grant from the National Research Council PFCCN contract no. 79.0068.396.

References

Davidson EH, Klein WH, Britten RJ (1977) Sequence organization in animal DNA and a speculation on hnRNA as a coordinate regulatory transcript. Dev Biol 55:69 – Kline WH, Murphy W, Attardi G, Britten RJ, Davidson EH (1974) Distribution of repetitive and non repetitive sequence transcripts in HeLa mRNA. Proc Natl Acad Sci USA 71:1785 – Melli M, Whitefield DC, Rao KV, Richardson M, Bishop JO (1971) DNA-RNA hybridization in vast DNA excess. Nature New Biol 231:8 – Spradling A, Penman S, Campo MS, Bishop JD (1974) Repetition on hnRNA as a coordinate regulatory transcript. nuclear and cytoplasmic messenger RNA of mammalian cells. Cell 3:23 – Tobin AJ, Selvig SE, Lasky L (1978) RNA synthesis in avian erythroid cells. Dev Biol 67:11 – Torelli G, Cadossi R, Ferrari S, Narni F, Ferrari S, Montagnani G, Torelli U, Bosi P (1979) Reassociation kinetics of the DNA of human acute leukemia cells Biochim Biophys Acta 561:301 – Vogelstein B, Gillespie D (1977) RNA-DNA hybridization in solution without reannealing. Biochem Biophys Res Commun 75:1127

Haematology and Blood Transfusion Vol. 26
Modern Trends in Human Leukemia IV
Edited by Neth, Gallo, Graf, Mannweiler, Winkler
© Springer-Verlag Berlin Heidelberg 1981

Characterization of Antigens in SSV Nonproducer Cells

H.-J. Thiel, T. Matthews, E. Broughton, A. Butchko, and D. Bolognesi

A. Summary

An autologous antiserum against simian sarcoma virus (SSV) nonproducer cells (SSV-NP
cells) was characterized by radioimmunoprecipitation. It reacts specifically with two different molecules in SSV-NP cells, a SSV transformation-specific glycoprotein (SSV TrS-gp)
and p65, which probably represents a modified
gag-precursor.

B. Introduction

The SSV complex [SSV(SSAV)] contains a replication defective transforming virus (SSV) as
well as an associated helper virus (SSAV). This
mixture of transforming pseudotype
SSV(SSAV) and helper virus was originally
isolated from a spontaneous fibrosarcoma of
a New World primate, the woolly monkey
(Theilen et al. 1971). While SSAV has been
quite well characterized (Aaronson et al.
1976; Benveniste et al. 1977; Deinhardt et al.
1978), relatively little is known about the
replication defective transforming virus,
SSV (Aaronson et al. 1975; Bergholz et al.
1977).

In an attempt to identify putative transformation specific information coded for by SSV,
we isolated goat cells nonproductively transformed by SSV(SSV-NP) and inoculated these
several times as live cells into the same goat
from which they originated. The resulting
hyperimmune serum (SSV-NP serum) was
reacted in radioimmunoprecipitation against
different transformed and nontransformed cell
lines.

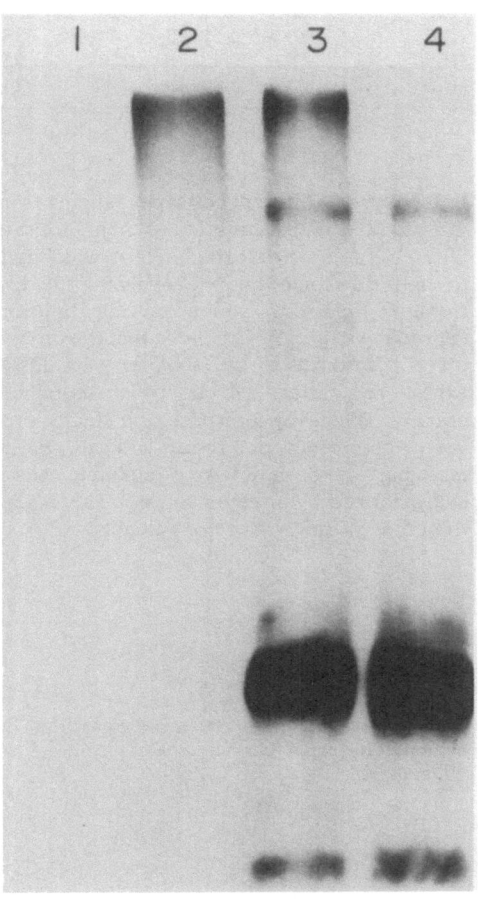

Fig. 1. Immunoprecipitation of SSV TrS-gp from
tissue culture supernatants of NRK SSV-NP cells
analyzed on a 5% SDS gel. Cells were labeled by
a 7 h pulse followed by a 14 h chase: ^{3}H-glucosamine
label with preimmune serum *(Lane 1)* and SSV-NP
serum *(Lane 2)*. ^{35}S-cysteine label with SSV-NP
serum *(Lane 3)* and preimmune serum *(Lane 4)*

C. Results

I. A Simian Sarcoma Virus Transformation-Specific Glycoprotein (SSV TrS-gp) in SSV-transformed cells

After labeling SSV-NP cells with ^{3}H-glucosamine and ^{35}S-cysteine using a 7 h pulse followed by a 14 h chase, the respective tissue culture supernatants were immunoprecipitated with SSV-NP serum (Fig. 1). The reactive molecule labels with glucosamine as well as cysteine and is therefore considered to represent a glycoprotein. On a 5% SDS-gel it migrates only a few millimeters into the separating gel. In addition, tissue culture supernatants from a variety of cell lines were labeled with ^{3}H-glucosamine and immunoprecipitated with SSV-NP serum. The ability of the immune serum to precipitate ^{3}H-glucosamine label from tissue culture supernatants is depicted in Fig. 2 in comparison to preimmune serum. The following tissue culture supernatants and respective cell extracts did not react in RIP assays: SSAV-infected normal cells (autologous goat fibroblasts, NRK cells), Gib-bon ape lymphoma virus (GALV) infected cells, NRK cells transformed by Kirsten sarcoma virus (KiSV) or Moloney sarcoma virus (MoSV), mink cells transformed by the Snyder-Theilen strain of FeSV (MSTF), and transformed mouse cell lines (Moloney S^+L^-, Harvey sarcoma virus-NP, methylcholanthrene – MCA transformed cells). In contrast, a strongly positive RIP reaction was found with the tissue culture supernatant of SSV-transformed cells from three different species including goat (Go), rat (NRK), and marmoset (HF) cells. This reactivity was found only with the SSV-NP serum. Other sera tested, including anti-SSAV p30, gp70, and anti disrupted SSV(SSAV), did not specifically precipitate glucosamine label from supernatants of SSV-transformed NP cells. This apparent SSV specificity was further tested by passing the serum over an SSAV immunoadsorbent column. This step did not diminish its reactivity with the ^{3}H-glucosamine labeled supernatant and the corresponding eluate was not reactive.

To characterize this molecule further, different radioactive compounds were used for metabolic labeling of SSV-NP cells. While the

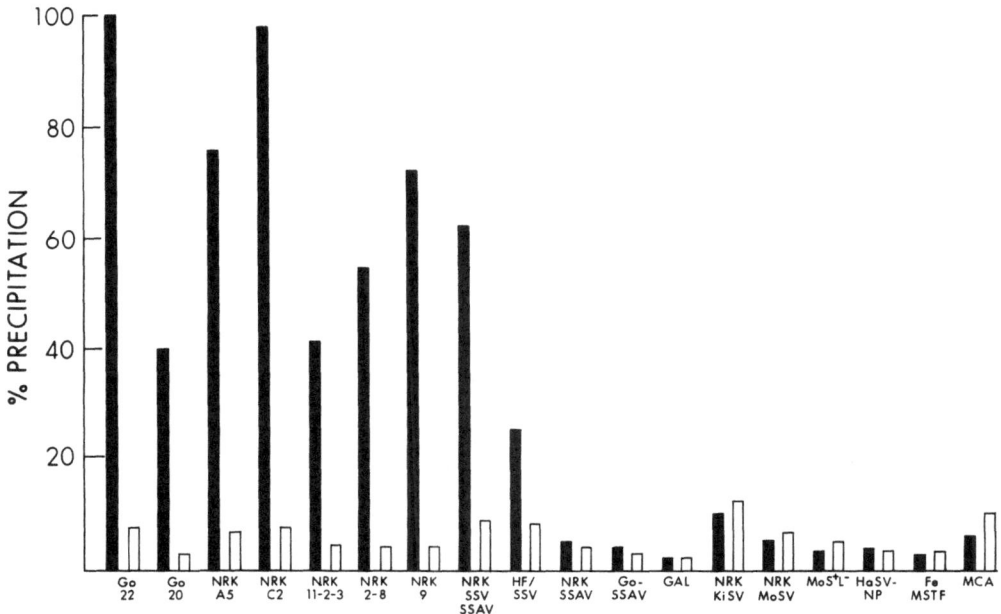

Fig. 2. Precipitated ^{3}H-glucosamine label from tissue culture supernatants of different cell lines. Cells were labeled with ^{3}H-glucosamine for a 7 h pulse followed by a 14 h chase. Each tissue culture supernatant was membrane filtered, extracted, and incubated with 1 µl of serum. The 100% value is taken as the counts precipitated from goat clone 22 with SSV-NP serum. Clone 22 and 20 are goat SSV-NP clones; *A5, C2, 11-2-3, 2-8* and *9* are NRK SSV-NP clones. *solid bars*, SSV-NP serum; *open bars*, preimmune goat serum

SSV TrS-gp labeled effectively with ³H-galactose, it did not incorporate mannose, fucose, or phosphate. On the other hand, various protein precursors were only poorly incorporated. This material may thus represent a glycoprotein, but one belonging to a class in which the carbohydrate is the overwhelmingly dominant component. Because of the large complement of sugar, molecular size estimation of this material by SDS Polyacrylamide gel electrophoresis (PAGE) is difficult. We therefore examined the immune precipitate by gel filtration on a Sepharose 6B column in the presence of 6M guanidine hydrochloride (not shown). Using cold FLV as standard, a single radioactive peak was found corresponding to the void volumn of the column. This indicates a molecular weight of at least 200,000 daltons.

II. Precipitation of p65 from SSV-NP Cells

The reactivity of the SSV-NP serum was examined through immunoprecipitation analyses of ³H-leucine labeled cell extracts. Figure 3 shows the reaction products with NRK SSV-NP cells (Lane 2) subsequent to analysis by SDS-PAGE. The only component which is specifically precipitated in comparison to the same cell extract reacted with the respective preimmune serum is a 65,000 mol. wt. protein (p65). Further serological analysis of p65 indicated that this molecule possesses SSAV p12, p30, and probably p15 determinants. To determine the relationship of p65 to the SSAV gag-precursor, peptide analyses on these molecules were performed (Fig. 4) as described by Cleveland et al. (1976). While these maps show a considerable degree of homology, there is also at least one clear difference with each proteolytic enzyme tested.

D. Discussion

Our study was aimed at the preparation and characterization of an autologous antiserum against SSV-NP cells. Serum from this immunization was assayed by RIP against various SSV-NP cells and found to have specific reactivity for a 65,000 dalton polypeptide (p65) and a glycoprotein (SSV TrS-gp). Serological data and peptide analyses indicate that p65 probably represents a modified gag-precursor and not a gag-gene related transformation specific fusion protein.

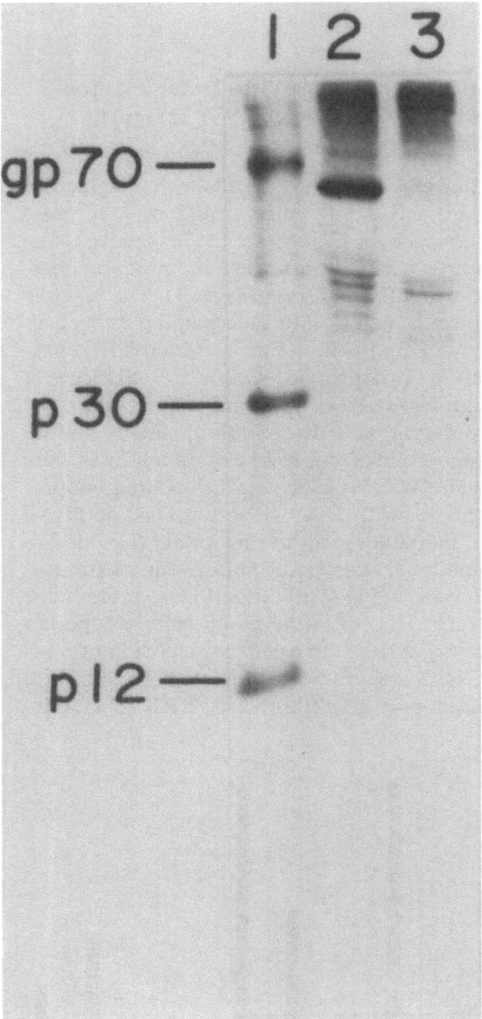

Fig. 3. Immunoprecipitation of p65 from NRK SSV-NP cells. Cells were pulse labeled with ³H-leucine for 7 h, extracted, and 5×10^6 cpm incubated with 1 µl of serum. The molecular weight markers on this 12% slab gel are ³H-leucine labeled FLV structural proteins *(Lane 1)*. SSV-NP cells with SSV-NP serum *(Lane 2)*, and SSV-NP cells with preimmune goat serum *(Lane 3)*

The autologous goat serum recognizes an additional component which represents a rather unique glycoprotein (SSV TrS-gp). This molecule appears to be present in all SSV transformed cells tested, including goat, rat, and marmoset cells. It appears to be a large glycoprotein (at least 200,000 daltons) which possesses a fairly small protein backbone. Preliminary results indicate that the protein moiety is important for the integrity of the

molecule on a 5% SDS gel as well as for its antigenicity (unpublished).

The SSV TrS-gp is probably coded for by SSV, because it was demonstrated in cells from three different species transformed by SSV and not by other transforming viruses. Our studies indicate that the SSV TrS-gp is easily shed or secreted by the transformed cell, and since the goat was immunized with live autologous transformed cells, the SSV TrS-gp might serve as an important target antigen for tumor cell recognition in vivo. Elucidation of the role of this glycoprotein in transformation by SSV awaits its purification and characterization.

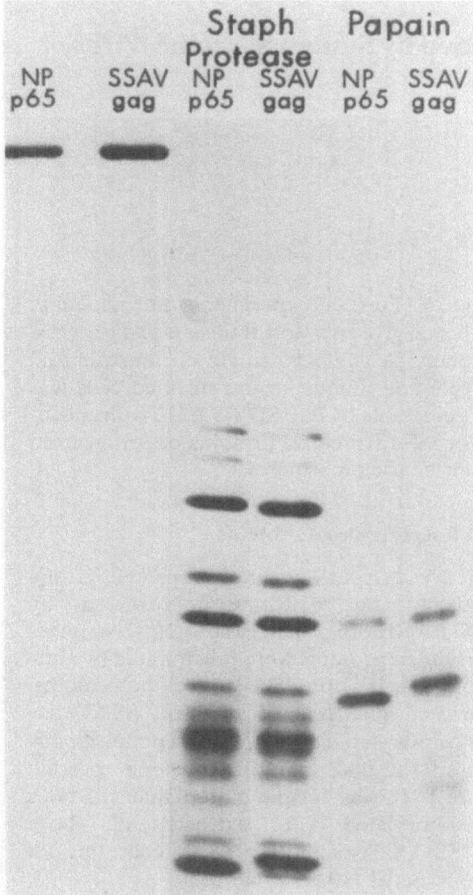

Fig. 4. After immune precipitation of ³H-leucine labeled p65 from SSV-NP cells and the gag-precursor from SSAV infected cells, the precipitates were electrophoresed on a preparative SDS gel and the respective bands cut from the gel. The slices were applied to a second SDS gel (15%) and electrophoresed in the presence of either no enzyme, Staphylococcus aureus protease (5 µg), or papain (40 ng) as described (Cleveland et al. 1976)

References

Aaronson SA, Stephenson, JR, Hino S, Tronick SR (1975) Differential expression of helper viral structural polypeptides in cells transformed by clonal isolates of woolly monkey sarcoma virus. J Virol 16:1117–1123 – Aaronson SA, Stephenson JR, Tronick SR, Hino S (1976) Immunological analysis of structural polypeptides of woolly monkey – gibbon ape type-C viruses. In: Clemmesen J, Yohn DS (eds) Comparative leukemia research, vol 43. Karger, Basel, pp 102–109 – Benveniste RE, Callahan R, Sherr CJ, Chapman V, Todaro GJ (1977) Two distinct endogenous type C viruses isolated from the Asian rodent Mus cervicolor: Conservation of virogene sequences in related rodent species. J Virol 21:849–862 – Bergholz CM, Wolfe LG, Deinhardt F (1977) Establishment of simian sarcoma virus, type 1 (SSV-1)-transformed non-producer marmoset cell lines. Int J Cancer 20:104–111 – Cleveland DW, Fischer SG Kirschner MW, Laemmli UK (1976) Peptide mapping by limited proteolysis in sodium dodecyl sulfate and analysis by gel electrophoresis. J Biol Chem 252:1102–1106 – Deinhardt F, Bergholz C, Hunsmann G, Schneider J, Thiel HJ, Beug H, Schäfer W (1978) Studies of simian sarcoma and simian sarcoma-associated virus. I Analysis of viral structural proteins, and preparation and characterization of antiserum specific for viral envelope components. Z Naturforsch [C] 33:969–980 – Theilen GH, Gould D, Fowler M, Dungworth DL (1971) C-type virus in tumor tissue of a woolly monkey (Lagothrix spp.) with fibrosarcoma. J Natl Cancer Inst 47:881–889

Haematology and Blood Transfusion Vol. 26
Modern Trends in Human Leukemia IV
Edited by Neth, Gallo, Graf, Mannweiler, Winkler
© Springer-Verlag Berlin Heidelberg 1981

Viral Gene Expression in Cells Transformed by Simian Sarcoma Virus, an Infectious Primate Type C Retrovirus

C. M. Bergholz

A. Introduction

Simian sarcoma virus (SSV) is a replication-defective transforming virus isolated in the presence of excess nontransforming associated virus (SSAV) from a spontaneous sarcoma of a woolly monkey. Previous studies have shown that the structural proteins of SSV(SSAV) are similar to the corresponding components of murine leukemia virus (MuLV). Studies reported here focus on viral gene expression in SSV-transformed virus producing marmoset monkey cells [HF/SSV(SSAV)] and SSV-transformed nonproducer marmoset cell lines (HF/SSV-NP).

I. Precursor Polypeptides in Virus Producing Cells

Antiserum specific for SSV(SSAV) p30 (kindly provided by Dr. H. J. Thiel) and another specific for SSAV envelope proteins were reacted with ^{35}S-methionine-labeled extracts of HF/SSV(SSAV) cells. Normal HF and HF/SSAV cells were tested in parallel. Analysis of radioimmunoprecipitates (RIP) by SDS-PAGE and fluorography demonstrated that anti-SSAV p30 precipitated predominantly polypeptides of approximately 30,000 and 60,000–62,000 daltons and, in addition, polypeptides of approximately 72,000 and 52,000 daltons (Fig. 1). Results of pulse-chase experiments indicated that the 60,000 dalton protein (pr60gag) is processed to yield p30, the major viral core protein (Fig. 1). Using antiserum specific for gp70 and p15E/p12E large amounts of an 82,000 dalton polypeptide were precipitated, and results of pulse-chase experiments indicated that it is an envelope precursor protein processed to yield p15E and p12E

(Fig. 2). Further experiments are aimed at analyzing glycosylation of the *env* and *gag* gene products. A *gag* polyprotein or nonstructural polypeptide unique to transformed cells was not detectable by RIP SDS-PAGE with antisera for viral structural proteins or serum from tumor bearing marmosets.

II. Phosphorylated Proteins

Two virus-specific phosphoproteins, the pr60gag and p12, were revealed by SDS-PAGE of ^{32}P-labeled proteins. No phosphorylated proteins were precipitated by antiserum specific for SSAV envelope proteins, providing further evidence that SSAV has a phosphorylated core p12 and a nonphosphorylated 12,000 dalton envelope protein (p12E). It was further noted that IgG was phosphorylated in extracts of both HF/SSV(SSAV) and HF/SSAV cells, but not in extracts of HF/SSV-NP cells.

III. SSV Gene Expression

Establishment of HF/SSV-NP cells has been described previously (Bergholz et al. 1977). Presence of the SSV genome was demonstrated by rescue of transforming virus following superinfection with SSAV, GALV, or MuLV. Expression of the SSAV-related sequences by the SSV provirus was investigated by reacting an SSAV cDNA with increasing concentrations of RNA extracted from two HF/SSV-NP cell lines. The results (Fig. 3) indicated that SSAV-related sequences were transcribed but represented a smaller proportion of the total cell RNA relative to virus producing cells. Comparison of maximum levels of hybridization indicated that less of the SSAV genome is represented in the SSV transcripts relative to RNA in SSAV-infected cells.

Virus-specific protein synthesis in five HF/SSV-NP cell lines was investigated by RIP and SDS PAGE. No viral polypeptides were precipitated by antiserum specific for SSAV envelope proteins. Anti-SSAV p30 and antiserum to Tween-ether disrupted virus detected one SSAV-related protein, pr60 gag, in only

one cell line (HF/SSV-NP VE). The pr60 gag apparently is not processed to yield p30 or lower molecular weight structural proteins, suggesting that a helper virus gene function may be required for processing. The failure to detect virus-specific proteins in cell lines

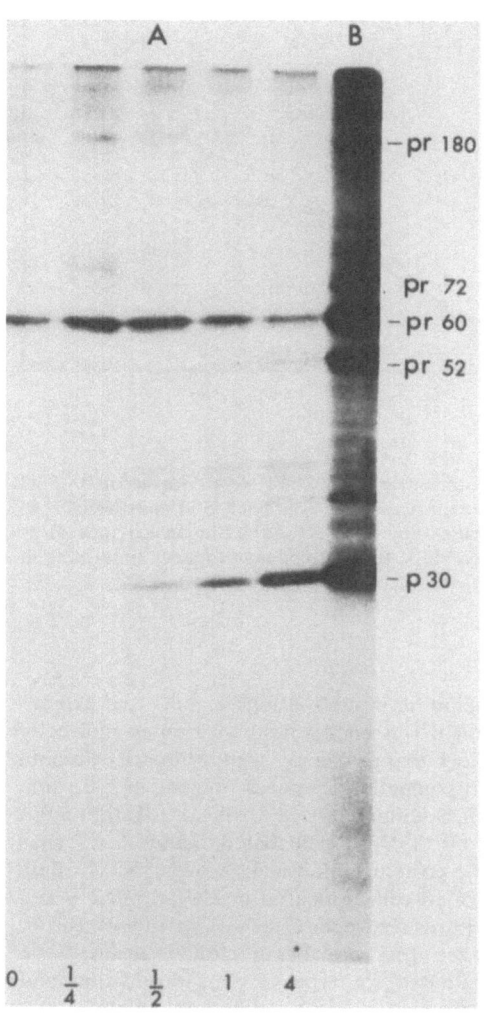

Fig. 1. Autoradiogram of 12% SDS-PAGE resolving ^{35}S-methionine-labeled proteins precipitated from HF/SSV(SSAV) cell extracts by anti-p30 serum. *A,* cells were pulse-labeled with 100 μci/ml ^{35}S-methionine for 15 min and were chased for 0, 1/4, 1/2, 1, and 4 hr before lysis. *B,* cells labeled for 4 h, then lysed

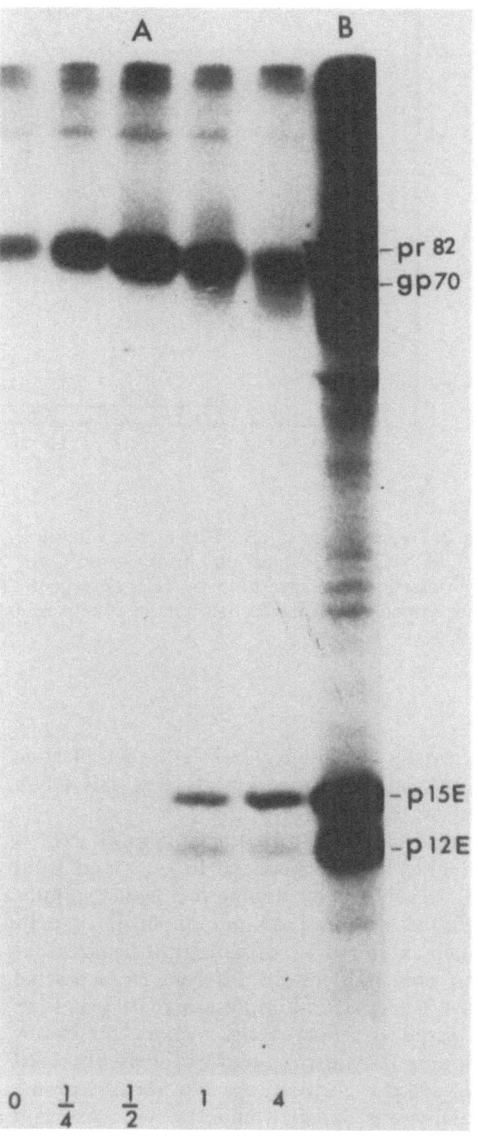

Fig. 2. Autoradiogram of 12% SDS-PAGE resolving ^{35}S-methionine-labeled proteins precipitated from HF/SSV(SSAV) cell extracts by antiserum for SSAV envelope proteins performed as described in Fig. 1

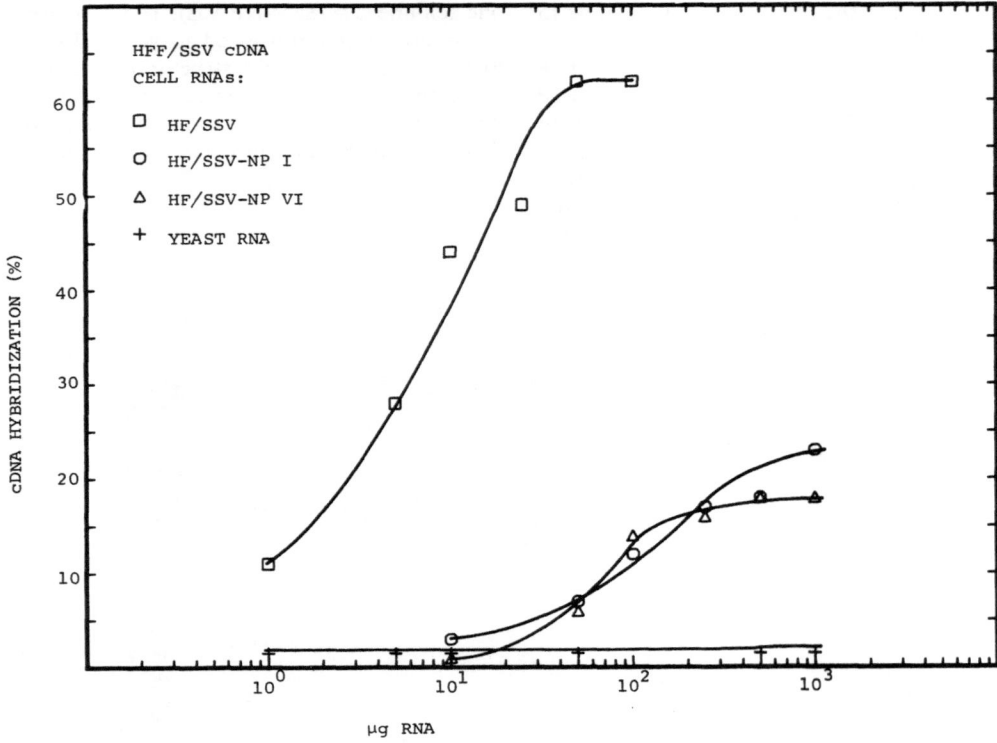

Fig. 3. Hybridization of SSAV ³H-cDNA with increasing concentrations of cell RNA performed in 2X SSC (0.3 M NaCl, 0.03M sodium citrate) at 66°C for 20 hr. Each reaction contained 500 cpm ³H-cDNA. Hybridization was measured by resistance to S1 nuclease digestion. *HF/SSV*, Simian sarcoma virus transformed producing marmoset monkey cells; *HF/SSF-NP*, SSV-transformed nonproducer marmoset cell lines

shown to contain SSAV-related cytoplasmic RNA suggests that translation of this RNA may be restricted.

It is of interest that HF/SSV-NP VE is a highly transformed cell line derived from HF/SSV-NP V by cloning foci which spontaneously appeared on a monolayer of cells which exhibited a morphology of transformation only moderately different from normal cells. Reverse transcriptase activity was later detected in supernatant media and a few budding C-type virus particles were observed by electron microscopy. No focus forming activity was detected and efforts to transmit virus to other cell lines were unsuccessful. The possibility that HF/SSV-NP VE cells are producing an endogenous marmoset virus is being investigated. As no viral structural proteins are detected in HF/SSV-NP V cells, these

preliminary observations suggest that expression of an endogenous virus may indirectly affect expression or translation of sarcoma virus genetic sequences present in the same cell. Sodium butyrate, BrdU, or IdU treatment of HF/SSV-NP cells failed to alter SSAV-specific protein synthesis. However, foci of transformed cells appeared in HF/SSV-NP V cell cultures six weeks after treatment with BrdU. These foci are being cloned and will be evaluated for type C virus production and expression of SSAV-related polypeptides.

Reference

Bergholz CM, Wolfe LG, Deinhardt F (1977) Establishment of simian sarcoma, type 1 (SSV-1)-transformed nonproducer marmoset cell lines. Int J Cancer 58:104–111

Haematology and Blood Transfusion Vol. 26
Modern Trends in Human Leukemia IV
Edited by Neth, Gallo, Graf, Mannweiler, Winkler
© Springer-Verlag Berlin Heidelberg 1981

Cell Fusion as a Tool for the Detection of Viral Footprints in Childhood Leukemia

J. Jore, R. Dubbes, J. Coolen, and K. Nooter

A. Introduction

In our studies on a possible role of type C oncoviruses in human leukemia we applied the technique of cocultivation of human bone marrow with an animal indicator cell line. Dog thymus A7573 cells were cocultivated with human bone marrow samples from normal individuals, leukemic patients, and nonleukemic patients. By means of the indirect cytoplasmic immunofluorescence assay (IFA), antigens which crossreacted with the major internal protein (p30) of the woolly monkey (simian) sarcoma leukemia virus (SiSV) complex could be detected (Nooter et al. 1979). In the case of childhood leukemia, five out of nine cocultures showed virus-related IFA staining.

It was hypothesized that the expression of antigens in the cocultivated A7573 cells is the result of an infectious type C virus originating from the leukemic bone marrow cells. In that case it may be expected that cell fusion instead of cocultivation would facilitate the transfer of a putative human virus to the indicator cells. We describe here our preliminary results of fusion experiments of human leukemic bone marrow with animal cell lines.

B. Materials and Methods

I. Cell Fusion

Cell fusion was essentially as described by Hales (1977). Normally, eight million nucleated bone marrow cells were mixed with two million indicator cells (either fetal dog thymus A7573 cells or rabbit cornea SIRC cells), pelleted, and fused. After fusion the cells were seeded in a 75 cm² Falcon. The cultures were transferred every 5 days. At each passage cells were grown on microscope slides for the fluorescence test.

II. Patient Information

Nucleated cells from bone marrow aspirates from leukemic children were obtained by sedimentation in 1% (v/v) methylcellulose in culture medium.

III. Immunofluorescence Assay

Indirect cytoplasmic immunofluorescence assays (IFA) were carried out on aceton-fixed cells as has been described previously (Nooter 1979). For IFA 50 µl of a suspension of freshly trypsinized cells ($10^5 \cdot ml^{-1}$) were transferred into wells of Teflon-coated microscope slides. The cells were incubated at 37°C for 20 h in a humidified CO_2 incubator. Thereafter the cells were fixed in aceton.

IV. Antisera

The IgG fractions of antisera were prepared according to Joustra and Lundgren (1970). The characteristics of the antisera used have been described previously (Nooter et al. 1979).

C. Results

Seven bone marrow samples from leukemic children were fused with A7573 cells and two, selected at random, with SIRC cells. The fused cultures were screened periodically for the presence of viral antigens with the IFA, using antiviral antisera directed at the major internal polypeptide [with a mol. wt. of 30,000 (p30)] of a murine type C virus (R-MuLV) and a primate type C virus (SiSV). One to five weeks after fusion antigens appeared in seven of nine cultures which predominantly reacted in the IFA with the SiSV antiserum (Table 1). The presence of antigens is a transient phenomenon: after 2 to 3 months of propagation the cultures were negative in the IFA.

	Antisera[a]	
	RA-SiSV-p30	RA-R-MuLV-p30
cultures[b]		
Af 91277	40	10
Af 10278	−	−
Af 51278	−	−
Af 81277	80	20
Af 10179	80	<10
Af 14879	80	20
Af 24779	40	10
Sf 23779	80	<10
Sf 14879	40–80	20
Virus positive control cultures		
REF + SiSV[c]	320–640	20–40
BALB/3T3 + R-MuLV[d]	40–80	160–320
Virus negative control cultures		
REF		
BALB/3T3, A7573		
SIRC, A204[e], NC37[f]	●—●10	●—●10

Table 1. Immunofluorescence end point titers

[a] Results are expressed as end point titers, presenting the reciprocal of the highest antiserum dilution with which virus-specific cytoplasmic fluorescence was still observed RA-SiSV-p30: rabbit anti-SiSV-p30; RA-R-MuLV-p30: rabbit anti-Rauscher-MuLV-p30

[b] Af and Sf cultures are fused cell cultures of A7573 and SIRC cells and leukemic bone marrow

[c] Rat embryonic fibroblasts (REF) infected with SiSV

[d] Mouse cells infected with R-MuLV

[e] Human rhabdomyosarcoma cell line

[f] Human lymphoblastoid cell line

The fused cultures have been monitored for several months for the production of extracellular reverse transcriptase. None gave positive results.

Finally, three of the fusion experiments were repeated with a HGPRT mutant of A7573 developed in our laboratory. This offered the possibility of selection for hybrid cells by growing the fused cells in so-called HAT medium (Szybalski et al. 1962). This selection did not result in higher IFA titers (they were the same or slightly lower) nor did it lead to reverse transcriptase production.

D. Discussion

The presence of type C oncovirus footprints in human mesenchymal tumors is a rather infrequent finding (for a recent review, see Nooter 1979). These observations include studies on virus polymerase, nucleic acid homology, virus antigens, antiviral antibodies, and virus isolation. The apparent low frequency of isolation of putative human retroviruses strongly suggests that these viruses are not ubiquitous in the human population. On the other hand, restricted virus expression and/or replication defectiveness could play a role as well. Subsequently, methods which facilitate virus transmission by intensive cell-to-cell contact, e.g., cell fusion in combination with sensitive detection methods, could be appropriate in studies on presumptive human viruses. In our studies described here two mammalian cell lines were fused with human bone marrow. Antigens of a possible viral origin were detected in some of these fused cultures by means of the IFA. These preliminary results show that the frequency of antigen positive cultures is comparable with the frequency found in previous cocultivation experiments (Nooter et al. 1979). However, it looks like that cell fusion is superior to cocultivation in that it speeds up the appearance of antigens with cell passage number (1 to 5 weeks after fusion compared to 1 to 2 months after starting cocultivation). However, our cell fusion procedure never led to overt virus production. This means that the exact nature of this possible virus-related antigen has still to be determined.

Acknowledgments

Drs. H. Behrendt, G. van Zanen and G. Wagemaker are thanked for providing the human bone marrow samples. This work was partly supported by a grant from the Dutch Organization for the Fight against Cancer, "the Queen Wilhelmina Fund".

References

Hales A (1977) A procedure for the fusion of cells in suspension by means of polyethylene glycol. Somatic Cell Genet 3:227–230 – Joustra M, Lundgren H (1970) Preparation of freeze-dried monomeric and immunochemically IgG by a rapid and reproducible technique. In: Peeter H (ed) Protides of the biological fluid. Pergamon Oxford, p 511 – Nooter K (1979) Studies on the role of RNA tumour viruses in human leukaemia. Thesis, University of Leiden, pp 38–40 – Nooter K, Coolen J, Dubbes R, Zurcher C, Koch G, Bentvelzen P (1979) Type C virus antigen detection in co-cultures of human leukaemic bone marrow and dog cells. J Gen Virol 45:711–721 – Szybalski W, Szybalska EH, Ragni G (1962) Genetic studies with human cell lines. Natl Cancer Inst Monogr 7:75

Haematology and Blood Transfusion Vol. 26
Modern Trends in Human Leukemia IV
Edited by Neth, Gallo, Graf, Mannweiler, Winkler
© Springer-Verlag Berlin Heidelberg 1981

ELISA for the Detection of Antigens Cross-Reacting with Primate C-Type Viral Proteins (p30, gp70) in Human Leukemic Sera*

R. Hehlmann, H. Schetters, and V. Erfle

A number of methods have been applied in the past to the serologic identification and characterization of C-type viral proteins. The most specific and most sensitive system used has been the competition radioimmunoassay (RIA). This assay detects group specific as well as interspecies activity of the major viral proteins (Parks and Scolnick 1972; Strand and August 1973). Disadvantages of this assay include the necessity of radioactive isotopes, false positive results from contaminating proteases, and the limited stability of the radioactively labeled reagents.

Recently, the enzyme immunoassay (EIA) technique has been developed (Engvall and Carlsson 1976). This technique has also proved to be highly specific and sensitive in detecting antigens and antibodies in a variety of systems (Voller et al. 1976). It avoids the biohazards of radioactivity and is simple and cheap. A further advantage is the stability of the coupled reagents. Low cost and simplicity of the EIA technique allow the screening of large numbers of samples.

We report here the application of the enzyme linked immunosorbent assay (ELISA) to the detection and quantification of the core protein p30 of the murine leukemia viruses (MuLV), the baboon endogenous virus (BaEV), and the simian sarcomavirus (SiSV) and of the envelope glycoprotein gp70 of SiSV. We further report attempts to detect with this technique the presence in human leukemic sera of antigens cross-reacting with primate viral structural proteins.

A. Methods and Materials

I. Antigens

MuLV p30, BaEV p30, and SiSV p30 were purified by a two step electrofocusing procedure (Schetters et al. 1980). Homogeneity of the purified viral proteins was demonstrated by SDS gel electrophoresis. SiSV gp70 was the gift of Dr. R. Gallo, NCI.

II. Antibodies

Antibodies against viral p30 proteins were prepared from immunized rabbits. The specificity of the antisera was controlled by precipitation of disrupted virus and subsequent gel electrophoretic analysis of the precipitated proteins. The activities of the sera were directed almost exclusively against the respective p30s. Antiserum against SiSV gp 70 as the gift of Dr. R. Gallo, NCI. IgG was purified as described (Schetters et al. 1980).

III. Coupling Procedure of Peroxidase to IgG

In essence the procedure of Nakane and Kawaoi (1974) as modified by Mesa-Tejada et al. (1978) was followed which involves blocking of the amino groups of the peroxidase with phenylisocyanate, introduction of aldehyde groups with Na-periodate, and formation of a Schiff's base with the IgG by incubation of the IgG with the activated peroxidase.

IV. ELISA Procedure

In essence, the procedure as described by Schetters et al. (1980) was followed. Microtiter plates were coated with 200 µl per well of 5–10 µg IgG/ml 50 mM carbonate-bicarbonate buffer, pH 9.6, at 37° for 2 h. After washing, the antigen of interest was added

---

* Conducted, in part, as study of the Süddeutsche Hämoblastosegruppe (SHG).

in phosphate buffered saline (Dulbecco's PBS) containing 5% normal rabbit serum, 5% aprotirin (Trasylol), 0.1 mM thimerosal, and 0.1% tween 20, and plates were incubated at 4° overnight. After extensive washing the peroxidase-coupled IgG was added and incubated at 37° for 2 hours. After washing 200 μl of substrate solution (20 mg o-phenylenediamine · 2HCl and 0.005% H_2O_2 per 50 ml substrate buffer) were added, and the colour reaction was followed photometrically with a Titertek-Multiscan (Flow) at 450 nm. Backgrounds generally ranged from 0.02 to 0.1 A_{450}.

V. Glycosidase Treatment

The procedure as described by Ohno et al. (1979) was followed and adapted to the ELISA technique. The glycoprotein was bound to microtiter plates under standard conditions. The glycoprotein-coated plates were washed, and 200 μl of a glycosidase mixture (Miles, Frankfurt) was added at a concentration of 100 μg/ml in 50 mM citrate buffer, pH 4.0, containing 100 μg BSA/ml. The plates were incubated at 37°C overnight, washed, and then used under standard conditions. The efficacy of the glycosidase treatment was controlled by gel electrophoresis of radioactively labeled glycoproteins with and without glycosidase treatment on parallel gels.

B. Results

I. Detection and Quantification of p30

The ELISA test system was standardized and optimized with purified viral antigens of three viral systems: p30 of MuLV, p30 of SiSV, and p30 of BaEV. Figure 1 depicts representative standard concentration curves with the three viral p30s. As can be seen, p30 is detected specifically and sensitively down to quantities of 0.01 to 0.5 ng per 200 μl reaction volume in all three systems tested. For better comparison of different tests, maximal absorbance of the reaction was designated 100% representing A_{450} values ranging from 0.7 to 1.7. Fetal calf serum, normal goat and rabbit sera, extracts of uninfected cells of the cell lines in which the viruses were grown, viral glycoprotein, and human lipoprotein did not react. The reaction was abolished by pronase digestion, but not by extraction with ether or digestion with nucleases.

The ELISA was successfully applied to the detection and quantification of p30 in tissue culture cells, in tumor tissue, and in sera (Schettler et al. 1980). Parallel determinations

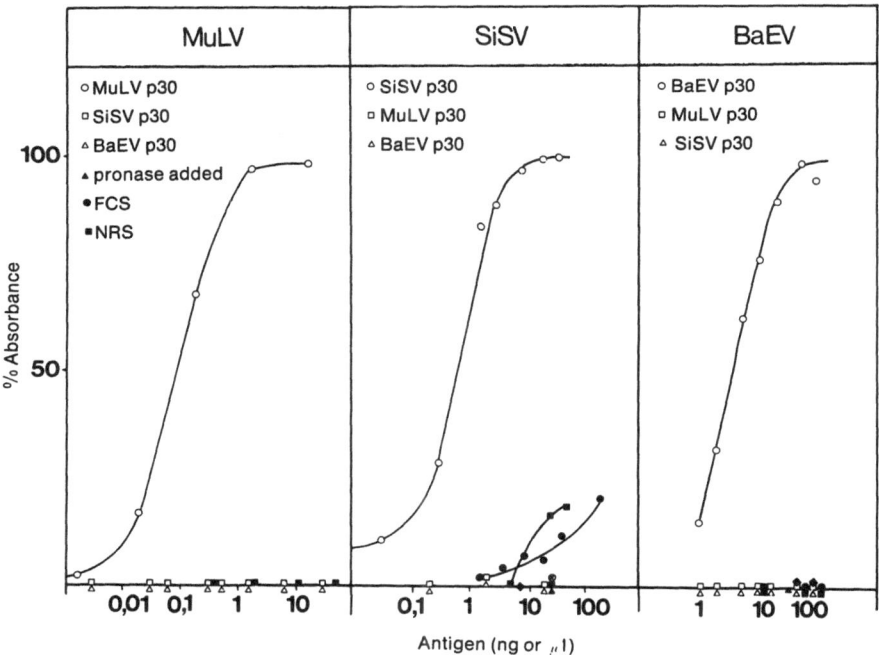

Fig. 1. ELISA standard concentration curves with purified homologous p30 from MuLV, SiSV, and BaEV

by competition RIA yielded virtually identical results (data not shown).

II. Detection and Quantification of gp 70

The ELISA technique was applied to the viral glycoprotein SiSV gp70 in a similar way as described for p30 (Schetters et al., in press). Figure 2 depicts a representative standard concentration curve similar to those observed with p30. Sensitivity and specificity were comparable to those obtained with the RIA. Fetal calf serum, normal rabbit serum, normal goat serum, extracts of uninfected cells, and components of normal human sera did not react. To exclude unspecific reactions with the carbohydrate moieties of glycoproteins the reactivity of the anti-SiSV gp70 antisera with the carbohydrate and protein moieties of SiSV gp70 was determined. For this purpose the reactivity of anti gp70 IgG with gp70 antigen was determined before and after treatment with a mixture of different glycosidases. The reactivity with gp70 was not changed by treatment with glycosidases. It therefore is concluded that the protein part and not the sugar part of the glycoprotein is recognized by the antiserum.

III. Detection in Human Leukemic Sera of Antigens Cross Reacting with SiSV p30 and with BaEV p30

The ELISA technique was then applied to the search in human leukemic sera for the presence of antigens reactive with antisera against BaEV p30 and SiSV p30 (Hehlmann et al., to be published). Proteins reacting with antibodies against p30 of BaEV and SiSV were specifically detected in leukemic sera, but not, or at very low levels only, in sera from non-leukemic patients or from healthy laboratory workers (Fig. 3). The reaction was abolished by pronase treatment and by preabsorption of the antiserum with insolubilized positive human sera (done for anti-BaEV p30). Cross-reacting antigens were detected with anti-SiSV p30 IgG in 15 out of 49 leukemic sera (30.6%) and with anti-BaEV-p30 IgG in 19 out of 48 leukemic sera (39.6%) (Fig. 3). Reactivity was also detected in some normal sera, but this reactivity was little above background and considerably less than that detected in leukemic sera as can be seen from Fig. 3. Attempts to confirm these data by competition RIA were successful only in a small number of cases (data not shown), and the nature of these antigens is therefore presently under investigation.

IV. A. Detection in Human Sera of Antigens Cross-Reacting with SiSV gp70

We then examined with the ELISA technique human sera for the presence of antigens cross-reacting with the viral envelope glycoprotein of SiSV. Cross-reacting antigens were detected in human leukemic sera, but similar reactions were obtained with a number of normal human sera (H. Schetters, V. Erfle, R.

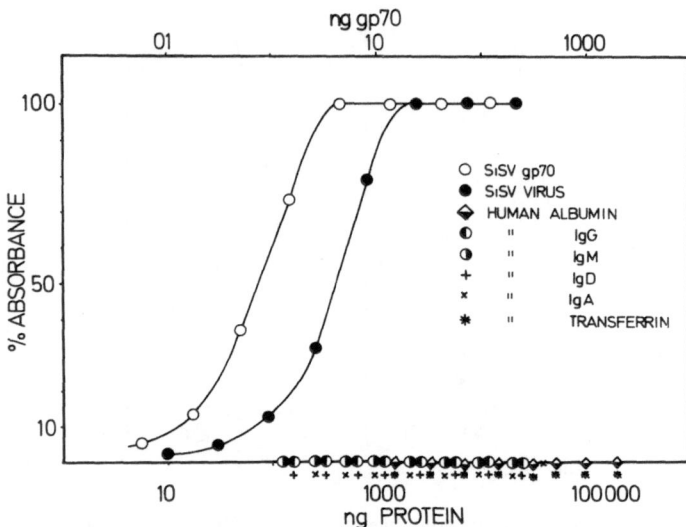

Fig. 2. ELISA standard concentration curve with purified SiSV gp70

ELISA-ANTI-BaEV p30 IgG   ELISA-ANTI-SSV p30 IgG

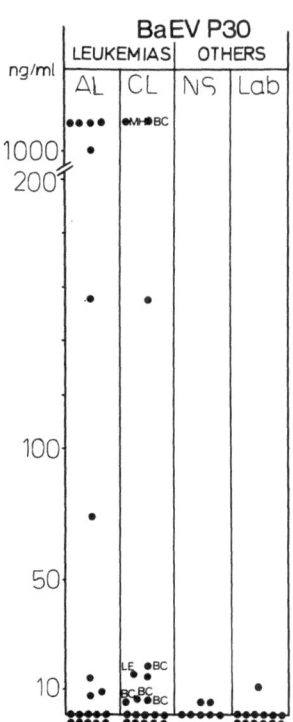 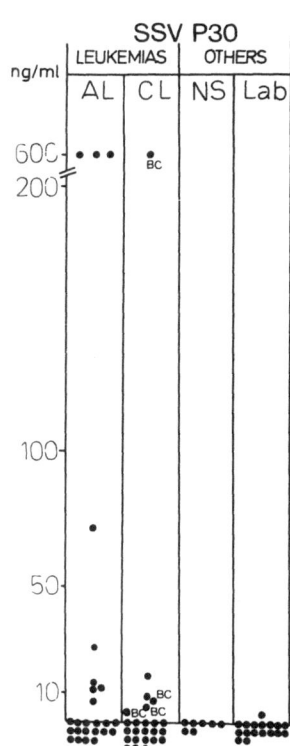

Fig. 3. Detection in human leukemic sera of antigens reactive with antisera against SiSV p30 and BaEV p30 by ELISA. AL=acute leucemias, CL=chronic leucemias, NS=normal sera, Lab=sera of laboratory workers, BL=CML blast crisis

Hehlmann, manuscript in preparation). The reactions were not due to recognition of carbohydrate moieties as demonstrated by prior treatment with glycosidases. Absorption experiments to increase specificity and to diminish possible unspecific reactivities are under way.

In order to examine a possible physiological or prognostic role of antigens cross-reacting with SiSV gp70 for human disease, we examined the sera from 23 patients with chronic myelogenous leukemia (CML) in blast crisis for cross-reacting antigens, antibodies, and immune complexes and correlated the presence and absence of these parameters with survival (Hehlmann et al., in manuscript). As can be seen in Fig. 4, about half of the sera are positive for one or more structures cross-reacting with SiSV gp70, whereas the other half is negative. Clinical data are available on 16 of the 23 patients. Of these 16 patients those patients with cross-reacting antigens or antibodies (nine patients) had a median survival after

the diagnosis of blast crisis of 2.5 months, whereas those patients negative for SiSV gp70 (seven patients) had a median survival of 7.4 months. This difference of survival in both groups is significant (P<0.005, Fisher test). The nature of the cross-reacting antigens is under further investigation. A summary of the results with human sera for which more than one cross-reacting antigen has been determined is presented in Table 1.

C. Discussion

We conclude from our studies that the ELISA technique can specifically and quantitatively detect retroviral proteins in cells, in tumor tissue, and in sera. Since the ELISA is a binding assay and no competition is involved, we would expect a somewhat broader specificity of the ELISA than of a competition assay with respect to interspecies reactivity. However,

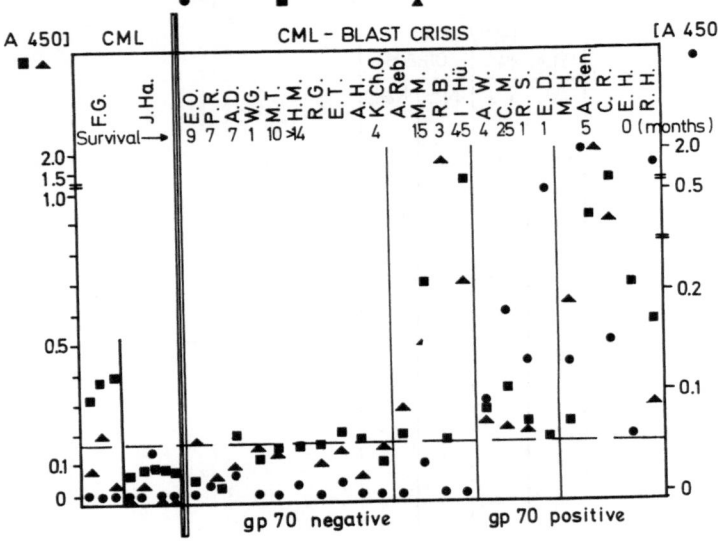

Fig. 4. Detection of antigens reactive with antiserum against SiSV gp70 in sera of patients with CML blast crisis by ELISA

Table 1. Cross-reacting antigens in human leukemias

Leukemias		Cross-reacting with SiSV		With BaEV p30 (ng equivalent/ml)
		p30	gp70	
AML	Mee.	>600 (72)	0 (2.2)	0
	Sut.	>600	16.5	>1840
	Scha.	8.5	0	1040
	Schm.	12.4 (13.2)	8 (6.8)	N.D.
	Mi.	0	0	8
AMML	Wi.	>600	0	>1840 (×2)
	Kli.	30	4.3	16
	W.-C.	80 (9.6/0)	0 (1.8/0)	>1840 (78/9.6)
	Mai.	14	0	170
ALL	Gic.	14	0.55	0
CML-BC	A.W.	15	0.8	>1840
	A.Ren.	>600	37	>1840
	J.Hü.	0	0	4.8
	E.O.	6.8	0	18.4
	C.R.	5.6	1.2	6.8
	M.H.	0	0.9	0
	P.R.	0	0	6.4
	M.M.	0	0.5	6
CML	J.Ha.	14 (8.4/18/6.4/10)	0 (0/0/5.6/0)	0
CLL	Pas.	0	0	168
Sézary	Kast.	8.8	0	N.D.
	Kö.	6.0/0	10.0/4.4	N.D.
Paraproteinemia	Scheit.	130	6	N.D.

although interspecies reactivity has been detected with the ELISA in some cases, it has not been demonstrated so regularly by ELISA as by competition RIA. It has not yet been determined whether this peculiarity is a property of the ELISA test itself or a consequence of our non-denaturing purification procedure of the proteins tested (electrofocusing, no SDS).

The detection with the ELISA-technique of antigens cross-reacting with primate C-type viral proteins in human leukemias is consistent with the earlier detection of viral structures (reverse transcriptase, RNA, virus-like particles, C-type viruses) in human leukemic cells with other methods (Gallo et al. 1975; Hehlmann 1976; Gallo et al. in this volume), although previous reports on antigens cross-reacting with viral structural proteins have been sporadic and not convincing (Sherr and Todaro 1975) and have been challenged (Stephenson and Aaronson 1976). Reports on the presence of anti-p30 antibodies in human sera (Herbrink et al. 1980) and of anti-reverse transcriptase antibodies on the surface of leukocytes from patients with AML and CML blast crisis (Jacquemin et al. 1978) have to be judged cautiously because of the known existence of heterophil antibodies (Barbacid et al. 1980; Kurth and Mikschy 1978; Snyder and Fleissner 1980).

The failure to reproduce the human ELISA results with human sera with the RIA competition technique points to the possibility that some unrelated but cross-reacting antigens have been detected. Alternatively, the ELISA binding assay might recognize p30-related antigens of low avidity not detected by the more stringent RIA competition assay. To decide on these alternatives the nature of the detected antigens is under further investigation.

The observation that the presence of cross-reacting antigens is associated with leukemia or with shorter survival suggests that regardless of their etiologic role, these antigens might be of prognostic use.

Acknowledgments

The technical assistance of E. Jatho and S. Ireland is acknowledged. This work was supported by the Deutsche Forschungsgemeinschaft (SFB 51) and by Euratom (contract 218-76-1 BIAD).

References

Barbacid M, Bolognesi D, Aaaronson SA (1980) Humans have antibodies capable of recognizing oncoviral glycoproteins: Demonstration that these antibodies are formed in response to cellular modification of glycoproteins rather than as consequence of exposure to virus. Proc Natl Acad Sci USA 77:1617–1621 – Engvall E, Carlsson HE (1976) Enzyme-linked immunosorbent assay, ELISA. Immuno enzymatic techniques. Elsevier/North-Holland, Amsterdam Oxford, pp 135–147 – Gallo RC, Gallagher RE, Miller NR, Mondal H, Saxinger WC, Mayer RJ, Smith RG, Gillespie DH (1975) Relationships between components in primate RNA tumor viruses and in the cytoplasm of human leukemic cells: Implications to leukemogenesis. Cold Spring Harbor Symp Quant Biol 933–961 – Hehlmann R (1976) RNA tumorviruses and human cancer. Curr Top Microbiol Immunol 73:141–215 – Hehlmann R, Schetters H, Erfle V (to be published) ELISA detects antigens in human leukemic sera that cross-react with primate C-type viral p30-proteins – Herbrink P, Moen JET, Brouwer J, Warnaar SO (1980) Detection of antibodies cross-reactive with type-C RNA tumor viral p30 protein in human sera and exudate fluids. Cancer Res. 40:166–173 – Jacquemin PC, Saxinger C, Gallo RC (1978) Surface antibodies of human myelogenous leukemia leukocytes reactive with specific type-C viral reverse transcriptases. Nature 276:230–236 – Kurth R, Mikschy U (1978) Human antibodies reactive with purified envelope antigens of primate type-C tumor viruses. Proc Natl Acad Sci USA 75:5692–5696 – Mesa-Tejada R, Keydar I, Ramanarayanan M, Ohno T, Fenoglio C, Spiegelman S (1978) Immunohistochemical detection of a cross-reacting virus antigen in mouse mammary tumors and human breast carcinomas. J Histochem Cytochem 26:532–541 – Nakane PK, Kowaoi A (1974) Peroxidase-labelled antibody, a new method of conjugation. J Histochem Cytochem 22:1084–1091 – Ohno T, Mesa-Tejada R, Keydar I, Ramanarayanan M, Bausch J, Spiegelman S (1979) The human breast carcinoma antigen is immunologically related to the polypeptide of the group-specific glycoprotein of the mouse mammary tumor virus. Proc Natl Acad Sci USA 76:2460–2464 – Parks WP, Scolnick EM (1972) Radioimmunoassay of mammalian type-C viral proteins: Interspecies antigenic reactivities of the major internal polypeptide. Proc Natl Acad Sci USA 69:1766–1770 – Schetters H, Hehlmann R, Erfle V, Ramanarayanan M (1980) The detection and quantification of C-type viral proteins in tissues and sera with an enzyme immunoassay. Infect Immun 29:972 – Schetters H, Hehlmann R, Erfle V (1981) ELISA for the detection and quantification of C-type viral glycoprotein (gp70) using antibodies that recognize the protein moieties of the glycoprotein J Virological Methods, in press – Sherr CJ, Todaro GJ (1975) Primate type-C virus p30 antigen in cells from humans with acute leukemia. Science 187:855–857 – Snyder HW Jr, Fleissner E (1980) Specificity of human antibodies to oncovirus glycoproteins: Recognition of antigen by natural antibodies directed against carbohydrate structures. Proc Natl Acad Sci USA 77:1622–1626 – Stephenson JR, Aaronson SA (1976) Search for antigens and antibodies cross-reactive with type C viruses of the woolly monkey and gibbon ape in animal models and in humans. Proc Natl Acad Sci USA 73:1725–1729 – Strand M, August JT (1973) Structural proteins of oncogenic ribonucleic acid viruses interspec II, a new interspecies antigen. J Biol Chem 248:5627–5633 – Voller A, Bidwell DE, Bartlett A (1976) Enzyme immunoassays in diagnostic medicine. Bull WHO 53:55–65

Haematology and Blood Transfusion Vol. 26
Modern Trends in Human Leukemia IV
Edited by Neth, Gallo, Graf, Mannweiler, Winkler
© Springer-Verlag Berlin Heidelberg 1981

Radiation-Induced Murine Leukemias and Endogenous Retroviruses: The Time Course of Viral Expression

V. Erfle, R. Hehlmann, H. Schetters, J. Schmidt, and A. Luz

A. Introduction

Ionizing radiation is well known to be a potent inducer of leukemias in animals and man (for review see UNSCEAR report 19). The mouse has been most frequently chosen to elucidate the factors and mechanisms necessary for leukemia development by irradiation. In the mouse the association of radiation-induced lymphoblastic leukemias with retroviruses has been detected which has led to the concept of an etiologic involvement of endogenous retroviruses in the induction of this disease. This concept implies the activation by radiation of endogenous, genetically inherited retrovirus sequences which acquire oncogenic properties and then transform their specific target cells (Kaplan 1977). This concept has been supported by the isolation of leukemogenic viruses from radiation-induced lymphoblastic leukemias (Gross 1958; Lieberman and Kaplan 1959). But recent work from several laboratories has brought contradicting results. At the moment there is no sufficient experimental evidence to decide whether endogenous retroviruses play a major role in the induction of radiation-induced leukemias.

Our approach to this problem was the evaluation of the time course of retrovirus expression and of the tissue distribution of viral expression. For this purpose the content of viruses and of viral proteins was determined in spleen, bone marrow, thymus, and lymph nodes of irradiated C57Bl/6 mice from the time of irradiation to the time of tumor development. We report here the radiation-induced changes of viral expression prior to and at the time of appearance of lymphoblastic leukemia and discuss their possible contribution to tumor development.

B. Materials and Methods

I. Leukemia Induction

Specific pathogen-free female C57Bl/6 mice of our own colony have been submitted at 4 weeks of age to 4×175 rads whole-body irradiation in weekly intervals (Caesium 137 source, 30 rads/min). Separate groups of irradiated and control animals were observed daily for gross signs of leukemia.

II. Tissue Preparation

Irradiated and control mice were sacrificed monthly. Spleen, thymus, bone marrow, and inguinal and mesenteric lymph nodes were aseptically removed. Single cell preparations for cocultivation studies have been prepared with one part of the tissue samples. The remaining part was homogenized and then frozen at $-70°C$ for the determination of viral proteins.

III. Virus Assays

Single cell suspensions of 1×10^6 cells were cocultivated with indicator cells [C3H 10 T 1/2 for N-tropic ecotropic virus and mink lung cells (CCL 64) for xenotropic virus] which had been seeded 24 h earlier in 5 cm culture dishes at a cell number of 2×10^5. Virus growth was tested after the first and the fifth passage by immunoperoxidase staining with antimurine leukemia virus (MuLV), anti-p30-serum (Nexø 1977), and by the XC plaque test. MuLV p30 content was determined by the ELISA technique according to Schetters et al. (1980).

IV. Viral Antibodies

The antibodies against eco- and xenotropic MuLV have been determined by the ELISA method with sucrose density gradient purified viruses as antigen.

C. Results

The fractionated whole-body irradiation of our C57Bl/6 mice with a dose of 4×175 rads resulted in a total incidence of lymphoblastic leukemia of 34% (17/50) within 12 months after irradiation. The first tumor appeared in month 5 and the majority of the animals came down with leukemia in month 6, 7, and 8.

The expression of endogenous retroviruses in the leukemia latency period has been evaluated by testing the appearance of infectious ecotropic virus (which infects mouse cells), of infectious xenotropic virus (which does not infect mouse cells), and of the major viral core protein p30 in spleen, thymus, bone marrow and lymph nodes. Ecotropic virus could be isolated very rarely. Only one or two animals per month in the irradiated and the control groups were found to express ecotropic virus in one of the organs tested. The majority of the isolations occurred in months 6 to 9, and there were no major differences between the treated mice and the controls during the time of observation. In contrast, xenotropic viruses could be isolated in much higher frequency and most frequently in irradiated animals. In some months all animals in the irradiated group were found to harbour xenotropic virus in bone marrow and spleen. The peak of xenotropic virus expression was during the time period from month 5 to 10. More animals in the irradiated groups than in the control groups showed the occurence of xenotropic virus in spleen (45% to 28%), thymus (21% to 4%), and bone marrow (52% to 24%).

Xenotropic virus yield in lymph nodes was equally low in irradiated and control animals (7% to 7%). The data on infectious virus expression in the time from months 5–10 are shown in Table 1.

Virus expression in the leukemic animals was without a regular pattern. One animal out of eight was found to have ecotropic and xenotropic virus in all of the four organs tested, two animals expressed xenotropic virus in all organs, and one mouse was found to have ecotropic virus only in the spleen. In four leukemic animals no infectious retroviruses could be detected.

With increasing age the control animals developed increasing antibody titers against ecotropic and xenotropic virus. The mean antibody titers in the irradiated animals followed the same pattern except in the 2 months after the last whole-body irradiation. In these 2 months, the irradiated mice exhibited markedly higher antibody titers than the control animals. In the 1st month after the last irradiation all irradiated animals showed higher antibody titers than the control mice, whereas in the following month some of the treated mice had titers like the controls (Fig. 1).

The viral p30 protein content in spleen, thymus, bone marrow, and lymph nodes did not exhibit major differences between irradiated and control animals during the observation period. The mean p30 values rose from initially 5–10 ng/mg protein in month 1 and 2 to values of about 200 ng/mg protein in spleen, thymus, and bone marrow and 500 ng/mg in lymph nodes in month 6 and 7. Thereafter the p30 content declined in treated and untreated animals to less than 100 ng/mg protein in month 9 and 10. A significant difference of p30 content has been observed between thymus of leukemic animals (mean value 210 ng/mg

Table 1. Expression of infectious retroviruses during months 5–10 (age) in C57Bl/6 mice after whole-body irradiation

	Ecotropic				Xenotropic			
	Spleen	Thymus	Bone marrow	Lymph-nodes	Spleen	Thymus	Bone marrow	Lymph-nodes
Irradiated	19%	8%	12%	12%	45%	21%	52%	7%
Animals	5/26 [a]	2/26	3/25	3/25	13/29	6/29	15/29[b]	2/28
Controls	16%	4%	4%	20%	28%	4%	24%	7%
	4/25	1/25	1/25	5/25	8/29	1/25	7/29[b]	2/29

[a] Number of animals expressing virus/number of animals tested
[b] $p < 0.05$

538

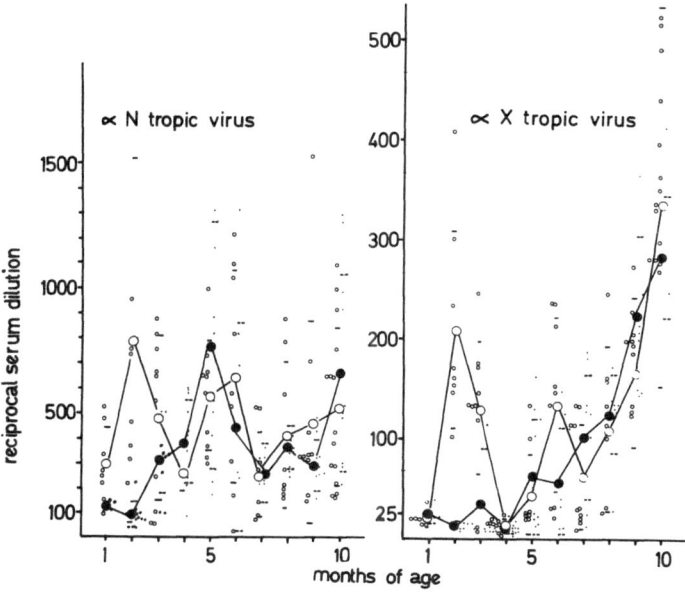

Fig. 1. Antiviral antibodies against ecotropic and xenotropic endogenous retrovirus in C57B1/6 mice after whole-body irradiation. The mean antibody titer of 10 animals per month together with the single values is indicated. O, irradiated animals; ●, control animals

protein) and that of age-matched control animals (mean value 30 ng/mg protein).

D. Discussion

Our main findings in favor of radiation-induced changes of retrovirus expression in irradiated mice are (1) the early increase of antiecotropic and antixenotropic virus antibody titers and (2) the increased expression of xenotropic virus in spleen, thymus, and bone marrow later on during the time of leukemia appearance. Our results do not indicate a major role for ecotropic viruses in the development of radiation-induced murine leukemias (Ellis et al. 1980; Haas 1977; Sankar-Mistry and Jolicoeur 1980). This is consistent with the fact that radiation-induced leukemias can also be induced in mouse strains such as the NZB mouse which do not harbor the genome for the production of infectious ecotropic MuLV (Harvey et al. 1979).

Our results may suggest some function of xenotropic viruses in the process of radiation-induced murine leukemogenesis. However, since xenotropic murine retroviruses normally do not infect mouse cells, an induction of lymphoblastic leucemia in these mice via an activation of infectious xenotropic viruses seems not to be a plausible mechanism. Also the

infection of mouse thymocytes with xenotropic viruses by coinfection with ecotropic virus (Declève et al. 1977) appears to be unlikely because of the lack of expression of ecotropic virus in these mice.

One possible conclusion would be that endogenous retroviruses are not involved in the induction of murine radiation-induced leukemias. An alternative would be that these viruses take part in the disease in the following way: Endogenous retroviruses are discussed to have a physiologic role in differentiation and in the immune system (McGrath and Weissman 1978; Moroni and Schumann 1977). Changes in cell surface structures of lymphocytes may disturbe the complex cell to cell interactions which regulate normal lymphocyte kinetics. The appearance of humoral antibodies against such (viral) cell surface structures could be a factor in the disturbance of normal regulation. The induction of antiviral antibodies by radiation might be a first step toward unlimited growth, since all the irradiated animals developed antibodies, whereas only 34% of the animals became leukemic.

Such antibody-mediated effects can be demonstrated by the induction of leukemia in thymectomized AKR mice by antibodies against leukemic cells reactive also with retrovirus antigens (Kohn et al. 1977). Experiments defining the biologic activity of the radiation-induced antibodies as well as experiments evaluating different viral parameters in time course experiments with individual animals exposed to radiation doses that induce about 50% leukemia incidence should throw more light on this problem.

Acknowledgments

This work was performed in association with EU-RATOM (Contract No. 218-76-1 BIO D) and was supported in part by the Deutsche Forschungsgemeinschaft (SFB 51). The expert technical assistance of Ms. S. Schulte-Overberg, S. Hartnagel, E. Jatho, L. Ireland, E. de Fries, and L. Strubel is gratefully acknowledged.

References

Declève A, Lieberman M, Ihle JH, Kaplan HS (1977) Biological and serological characterization of the C-type RNA viruses isolated from the C57Bl/Ka strains of mice. III. Characterization of the isolates and their interactions in vitro and in vivo. In: Duplan JF (ed) Radiation-induced leukemogenesis and related viruses. Elsevier/North Holland Biomedical Press, Amsterdam Oxford New York, pp 247–264 – Ellis RW, Stockert E, Fleissner E (1980) Association of endogenous retroviruses with radiation-induced leukemias of BALB/c mice. J Virol 33:652–660 – Gross L (1958) Attempt to recover filterable agent from X-ray-induced leukemia. Acta Haematol (Basel) 19:353–361 – Haas M (1977) Transient virus expression during murine leukemia induction by X-irradiation. J Natl Cancer Inst 58:251 – Harvey JJ, Tuffrey M, Holmes HC, East J (1979) Absence of ecotropic or recombinant murine leukaemia virus in preleukaemic and leukaemic X-irradiated NZB mice. Int J Cancer 24:373–376 – Kaplan HS (1977) Interaction between radiation and viruses in the induction of murine thymic lymphomas and lymphatic leukemias. In: Duplan JF (ed) Radiation-induced leukemogenesis and related viruses. Elsevier/North Holland Biomedical Press, Amsterdam Oxford New York, pp 1–18 – Kohn RR, Scoitto CG, Hensse S (1977) Age-dependent leukemia produced in thymectomized AKR mice by antiserum to leukemic cells. Exp Gerontol 13:181–187 – Lieberman M, Kaplan HS (1959) Leukemogenic activity of filtrates from radiation-induced lymphoid tumors of mice. Science 130:387–388 – McGrath MS, Weissman IL (1978) In: Clarkson B, Marks P, Till J (eds) Normal and neoplastic hematopoietic cell differentiation. Cold Spring Harbor Laboratory, Cold Spring Harbor, pp 577–589 – Moroni C, Schumann G (1977) Are endogenous C-type viruses involved in the immune system? Nature 269:600–601 – Nexø BA (1977) A plaque assay for murine leukemia virus using enzymecoupled antibodies. Virology 77:849–852 – Sankar-Mistry P, Jolicoeur P (1980) Frequent isolation of ecotropic murine leukemia virus after X-ray irradiation of C57Bl/6 mice and establishment of producer lymphoid cell lines from radiation-induced lymphomas. J Virol 35:270–275 – Schetters H, Hehlmann R, Erfle V, Ramanarayanan M (1980) The detection and quantification of C-type viral proteins in tissues and sera with an enzyme immunoassay. Infect Immun 29:972–980

Haematology and Blood Transfusion Vol. 26
Modern Trends in Human Leukemia IV
Edited by Neth, Gallo, Graf, Mannweiler, Winkler
© Springer-Verlag Berlin Heidelberg 1981

Retrovirus Particle Production in Three of Four Human Teratocarcinoma Cell Lines

J. Löwer, R. Löwer, J. Stegmann, H. Frank, and R. Kurth

A. Introduction

In spite of a long and intensive search, human retroviruses have not yet been demonstrated unambiguously (for review see Pimentel 1979). The electron microscopic detection of retrovirus particles in human term placentas by Kalter and others (Kalter et al. 1973; Vernon et al. 1974) represents at present the most convincing piece of evidence that human oncornaviruses may exist. As our attempts to isolate these viruses from placentas or to cultivate placentas in vitro have not succeeded, tumors containing tissues histologically similar to that of the placenta were investigated for virus expression. Among other tumors, teratocarcinomas from males and choriocarcinomas from females were studied. In contrast to choriocarcinomas, most of the teratocarcinomas can be induced to produce retrovirus particles in tissue culture.

B. Methods and Results

Specimens of human testicular teratocarcinomas were taken immediately after extirpation, cut into small pieces, and incubated at 35° C in Dulbecco's modified Eagle's minimal essential medium supplemented with nonessential amino acids, 20% heat-inactivated fetal calf serum, 10% tryptose phosphate boullion, and antibiotics. Within a few weeks, fibroblasts and epithelial cells grew out as monolayers. Thereafter, the epithelial cells began to form domes and free-floating vesicles, which could be aspirated and subcultivated to obtain cell cultures free of fibroblasts. Two of the cell lines established in this manner at Tübingen are designated GH and HL. The two other human teratocarcinoma cell lines, Tera-1 and Tera-2, were kindly donated by J. Fogh (New York), who had established these lines from pulmonary metastases in 1970 and 1971, respectively (Fogh and Trempe 1975).

The initial search for retrovirus particle expression in Tera-1 and Tera-2 cells by electron microscopy revealed only a single particle with an equivocal morphology of retroviruses in a Tera-1 culture. This result parallels the essentially negative findings of Fogh and others (Bronson et al. 1979; Fogh and Trempe 1975). After treatment of the cultures with iododeoxyuridine (IUdR, 20 μg/m1), dexamethasone (DXM, 10^{-6}M), and dimethylsulfoxide (DMSO, 1%) for 24 h, retrovirus particles could be easily detected in three of the four teratocarcinoma cell lines investigated (Fig. 1 and Table 1). All other human cell cultures, including choriocarcinomas, seminomas, fibroblasts, melanomas etc., remained virus negative even after the induction regime.

The observed particles resemble C-type retroviruses but share a unique morphologic feature with viruses found budding from the syncytiotrophoblast of human term placentas (Dalton et al. 1974) in that their core appears adjacent to the virus envelope without the usual intermittent space seen with C-type virus particles. Similar morphologic observations have been made by Bronson using human teratocarcinoma cell cultures (Bronson et al. 1978, 1979). The missing electron lucent space between envelope and nucleocapsid may either be a property of the budding particles or may be the result of cellular influences on the budding process. We have never seen a single "mature" particle with a condensed core in all teratocarcinoma cell cultures investigated.

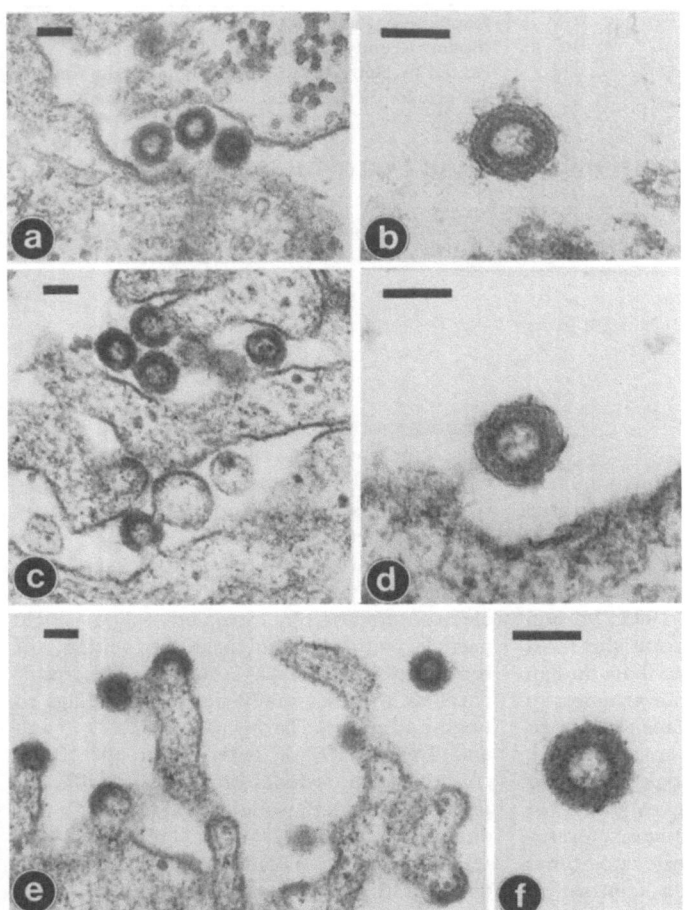

Fig. 1a–f. Retrovirus particles produced by teratocarcinoma cells after induction. **a** and **b** Tera-1 cells; **c** and **d** GH cells; **e** and **f** HL cells. The *bars* represent 100 nm

Table 1. Effects of in vitro virus induction treatment of human teratocarcinoma cultures

Tumor	Morphology		Beta-HCG synthesis (m IU/ml)[a]		Virus production	
	Before induction	After induction	Before induction	After induction	Before induction	After induction
Tera-1	Monolayer	Domes, vesicles	0.7	25.6	+[b]	+ +
Tera-2	Monolayer	Monolayer	2.2	3.0	−	−
GH	Domes, vesicles	Domes, vesicles	10.8	21.2	+	+ + +
HL	Domes, vesicles	Domes, vesicles	52.3	100.2	−	+

[a] m IU/ml = Milli international units/ml. Background ≤ 5 mIU/ml
[b] Arbitrary judgement from electron microscopical observations

After the induction treatment not only a striking increase in virus production but also an alteration in cell morphology can be recognized. While uninduced cultures of Tera-1 show a monolayer of homogeneous cells, after induction several cell types arise within a matter of 3 to 4 days and dome and vesicle formation can be seen. The GH and HL cells, already selected for dome and vesicle formation, exhibit only limited morphologic alterations. In contrast, Tera-2 cells cannot be induced by chemical means to initiate virus production and cellular differentiation (see Table 1).

In the differentiated tumor cell populations the proportion of cells producing virus-like particles as judged by electron microscopy varies from a few in HL to over 10% in Tera-1 to almost 100% in GH cultures. The latter cell line, subcultivated only by transferring vesicles to new culture flasks, exhibits in any case a low spontaneous production of retrovirus particles. Thus it appears likely that virus replication is permitted only in a specific cell type of the differentiating culture.

In placentas it is the syncytiotrophoblast cell layer from which retrovirus particles can occasionally be seen budding (Kalter et al. 1973; Vernon et al. 1974). Syncytiotrophoblasts at the same time produce human chorionic gonadotropin (HCG) (Morisada et al. 1972). As a first step in determining the type of the virus-producing cell, we tested the secretion of HCG into the culture medium before and after the induction procedure (Table 1). While in Tera-1, GH, and HL cells HCG production after induction is significantly increased, this hormone is not detectable in the supernatant of Tera-2 cell cultures. Induction or enhancement of virus synthesis is thus paralleled by induction of HCG production. The alteration in hormone release may well reflect cellular differentiation, but it is not possible at present to claim that in analogy to the findings in human placentas, it is a trophoblastic or at least a HCG-secreting cell that is permissive for virus replication.

Attempts to further characterize the human teratocarcinoma derived viruses have so far been unsuccessful. Firstly, we were not able to demonstrate unambiguously reverse transcriptase (RT) activity either in uninduced or induced cultures. Transient small peaks of RT activity (Kurth et al. 1980) are observed but are difficult to interpret. The difficulty in detecting RT activity in the supernatant of teratocarcinoma cell cultures has also been reported by Bronson et al. (1978). Secondly, the teratocarcinoma viruses have not yet been demonstrated to be infectious. Cultivations between induced teratocarcinoma cells and a number of uninfected indicator cell lines did not yield replicating virus even after repeated cocultivations and passages for over 20 weeks. The indicator cells were derived from dog thymus (8155), bat lung (Tb-1-Lu), marmoset fibroblasts (HF), tupeia embryo kidney (TEK), mink lung (C58), and feline embryo fibroblasts (FEF), as well as from human cells (rhabdomyosarcoma RD, amnion cells AV-3).

C. Discussion

Whereas in uninduced human teratocarcinoma cells expression of retrovirus particles is a rare event (Bronson et al. 1978, 1979; Kurth et al. 1980), the production of such particles in three out of four teratocarcinoma cell lines can easily be demonstrated after treatment with IUdR, DXM, and DMSO. Individual tumor lines may also produce virus particles spontaneously.

The human teratocarcinoma derived particles differ morphologically from mammalian type-C viruses by the lack of a clear electron lucent space between core and envelope. In this regard they resemble the particles observed in human term placentas. The lack of easily demonstrable RT activity and infectivity as well as the absence of "mature" particles with condensed cores is also reminiscent of a number of retrovirus mutants (e.g., murine leukemia virus murants ts3 and ts24) (Witte and Baltimore 1978). These mutants are characterized by a defect in viral precursor protein processing. It is as yet largely unknown to what extent viral or host cell proteases contribute to the specific cleavage of virus precursor proteins to yield mature and infectious particles.

Therefore, the question cannot yet be decided whether the human teratocarcinoma-derived viruses posses an intrinsic genetic defect or whether the host cell is lacking a factor which is necessary for an appropriate processing of viral structural components. The latter possibility is somewhat favored by the recent findings of Gautsch (1980) that murine teratocarcinoma cells lack a factor needed to support the replication of infecting murine leukemia (Teich et al. 1977) and papova (Swartzendruber and Lehman 1975) viruses.

References

Bronson DL, Ritzi DM, Fraley EE, Dalton AJ (1978) Morphologic evidence for retrovirus production by epithelial cells derived from a human testicular tumor metastasis. J Natl Cancer Inst 60:1305–1308 – Bronson DL, Fraley EE, Fogh J, Kalter SS (1979) Induction of retrovirus particles in human testicular tumor (Tera-1) cell cultures: an electron microscopic study. J Natl Cancer Inst 63:337–339 – Dalton AJ, Hellman A, Kalter SS, Helmke RJ (1974) Ultrastructural comparison of placental virus with several type-C oncogenic viruses. J Natl Cancer Inst 52:1379–1381 – Fogh J, Trempe G (1975) New human tumor cell lines. In: Fogh I (ed) Human tumor cells in vitro. Plenum, New York, pp 115–159 – Gautsch JW (1980) Embryonal carcinoma stem cells lack a function required for virus replication. Nature 285:110–112 – Kalter SS, Helmke RJ, Heberling RL, Panigel M, Fowler AK, Strickland JE, Hellman A (1973) C-type particles in normal human placentas. J Natl Cancer Inst 50:1081–1084 – Kurth R, Löwer R, Löwer J, Harzmann R, Pfeiffer R, Schmidt CG, Fogh J, Frank H (1980) Oncornavirus synthesis in human teratocarcinoma cultures and an increased antiviral immune reactivity in corresponding patients. In: Todaro G, Essex M, zur Hausen H (eds) Viruses in naturally occurring cancers. Cold Spring Harbor Laboratory, New York pp 835–846 – Morisada M, Yamaguchi H, Lizuka R (1972) Toxic action of anti-h.c.g. antibody to human trophoblasts. Int J Fertil 17:65–71 – Pimentel E (1979) Human oncovirology. Biochim Biophys Acta 560:169–216 – Swartzendruber DE, Lehman JM (1975) Neoplastic differentiation: Interaction of simian virus 40 and Polyoma virus with murine teratocarcinoma cells in vitro. J Cell Physiol 85:179–188 – Teich NM, Weiss RA, Martin GR, Lowy DR (1977) Virus infection of murine teratocarcinoma stem cell lines. Cell 12:973–982 – Vernon ML, McMahon JM, Hackett JJ (1974) Additional evidence of type-C particles in human placentas. J Natl Cancer Inst 52:987–989 – Witte ON, Baltimore D (1978) Relationship of retrovirus Polyprotein cleavages to to virion maturation studied with temperature-sensitive murine leukemia virus mutants. J Virol 26:750–761

General Summary

Haematology and Blood Transfusion Vol. 26
Modern Trends in Human Leukemia IV
Edited by Neth, Gallo, Graf, Mannweiler, Winkler
© Springer-Verlag Berlin Heidelberg 1981

General Summary

F. Deinhardt

During the last few days we have met for the fourth time here in Wilsede to discuss *Modern Trends in Human Leukemia*. The title itself is rather a misnomer because there are no modern trends in leukemia, a disease which does not change from year to year; our present day civilization probably influences profoundly leukemia's incidence and course but this aspect found no place in our deliberations. It is our approach to understanding the pathogenicity of leukemia, lymphoma, and related diseases which changes, and I will reflect briefly on this.

The clinical papers have been summarized by Dr. Frey and discussed by Dr. M. Feldman. Dr. Frey's statement that "antibody – drug complexes" might be one of the future approaches to chemotherapy of leukemia and related diseases was particularly interesting and reminded me of Albert Coon's early studies on the combination of antitumor antibodies with chemicals, mostly dyes, with the goal of concentrating cytostatic or cytotoxic substances in tumors. This idea did not work then but it brought about the development of the fluorescent antibody techniques. Maybe today the time has come when the combination of more highly specific antibodies, i.e., monoclonal antibodies, with more potent chemotherapeutics would be successful.

During the other sessions of the conference I looked for indications of trends, for those "red threads" which may be a guide for future work. In the virology section the long arguments of the past on the specificity of molecular hybridization and the stringency needed for obtaining significant results have disappeared, and in comparison to past conferences, there were few reports on virus isolations or detection of viral antigens or antibodies in man. The

retroviruses supposedly isolated from man, all of which shared genetic information with nonhuman primate viruses, received relatively little attention, but the riddle of these isolations has not been solved nor has the question whether they were all laboratory contaminations been answered. Much more work is needed before further discussion of these agents would be fruitful, but most of these isolates can probably be declassified from their human status, and the significance of the indirect evidence for human retroviruses by demonstration in man of antigens or antibodies which were related or identical to simian viruses is at least questionable. Even so, as I am tempted to announce that "The king is dead", Dr. Gallo is proclaiming "Long live the king" as he presented us with a new candidate for a human leukemia virus, a report which is certain to stimulate a new wave of research in this area.

In contrast, we heard a great deal (perhaps too much and in too much technical detail) about *gag, env, pol, onc, sarc, leuk,* and other genes of animal and particularly avian retroviruses, their characteristic gene products, and their functions. The relevance of these studies of experimental, artificially produced diseases created under laboratory conditions for the natural genesis of leukemia is questionable. Nevertheless, dissection of the genomes of these retroviruses with endonucleases and the cloning of specific parts of the genomes in bacterial plasmids with subsequent evaluation of the function of the various regions of the genes and of the gene products, both in in vitro translation systems and in their normal eukaryotic target cells, may improve our understanding of the basic mechanisms of cell transformation in vitro and possibly also of tumor induction in vivo by the RNA retroviruses. It is still a major puzzle that similar or identical genomes can induce quite different malignancies, as observed for example in the induction of tumors as different as fibrosarcomas, melanomas, and glioblastomas by a single strain of Rous sarcoma virus, and that the same malignancy can be initiated by different viral genomes. I am sure that the pathogenicity of these diseases will be understood much better during the coming years, although this understanding will be achieved not only by analysis of the genomes down to the last base pair but more by examination of the total process of transformation, i.e., the virus, the route of infection, the type and physiologic state of the infected cells, and the response of the total organism to the emergence of transformed cell clones.

There was relatively little discussion of DNA tumor viruses, except for an overview of the structure of the primate lymphotropic herpesviruses and discussions of the pathogenesis of Epstein – Barr virus (EBV) infections. The pathogenic events leading from primary lymphoproliferative EBV infections to complete recovery with a lifelong carrier state and the development later of monoclonal malignancies or an immediate progression of an acute monucleosis into a malignant fatal lymphoproliferative disease are particularly interesting and deserve intensive study. The report of lytic activity of EBV is important for two reasons: it allows better study in vitro of EBV and it may explain the infection of epithelial cells in vivo. Of importance also is the demonstration of EBV genomes in normal parotic cells which may answer the old question of where EBV multiplies during the long periods of oral excretion.

On reflecting generally on the viral studies I want to repeat a caution sounded often before: We must not ignore the fact that some of our virus models, and I am referring particularly to the avian and murine retroviruses, are highly artificial, using inbred selected animals and laboratory-propagated and perhaps laboratory-created viruses, whose relevance to naturally occurring disease is at least in part questionable, although their value for a basic understanding of cell function and regulation is undisputed. Studies in outbred animal populations, such as cats and cattle, may be more comparable to real life. Particularly intriguing is the situation of "virus-free" cat leukemias in which the virus might have acted as a "hit and run" villain, leaving either only a small part of itself behind or changing only the genes responsible for cell regulatory mechanisms without a need for persistence of any part of the viral genome, a mechanism which has also been considered for the transformation of cells by some DNA viruses, particularly the herpesviruses.

In yesterday's sessions we heard about very exciting developments in cell biology and immunology. The differentiation of the cells of the hematopoietic and the immune systems into many highly specialized cell subpopulations has been analyzed in detail, thus allowing a much finer and detailed analysis of the immune mechanisms which play a role in the emergence of tumors and the defense of the organism against them. Use of monoclonal antibodies has almost revolutionized this field, and it will be most interesting to study not only the physiologic and immunologic functions and antigenic identities of the various cell types but also their susceptibility to exogenous viral infection, to activation of endogenous viral genes, and to chemical or physical carcinogens. The development of cell culture techniques and separation of various cell populations have progressed rapidly and already have improved our understanding of normal differentiation and of regulatory disturbances leading to malignant transformation, although this is another area in which we must remember that isolated cells in vitro may behave quite differently from cells in the intact organism with its multiple cell interactions and regulatory mechanisms, to which we should add Dr. Moore's newly defined "oncgene"-mediated "pericrine" controls as well as still unidentified influences. The report of thymic nurse cells within which differentiation of other cells seems to occur is an intriguing observation, the general significance of which needs further exploration. In addition the nude thymusless, the spleenless, and the very special mice lacking both of these organs are now joined by the "beige mouse," a strain which is deficient for natural killer cells and which will permit a further dissection of the immune defenses against tumor development. The new perspective of the various, specific chromosomal aberrations in different diseases should stimulate further research to relate specific chromosomal to specific pathologic changes, and in this respect the studies on the X-linked lymphoproliferative syndrome (Duncan's disease) which is associated with immunodeficiency, multiclonal lymphoproliferation, and finally lymphoma or lymphosarcoma are particular interesting. Better tools will be needed for a finer analysis of the human genetic material before we can understand the genetic influences on leukemias and lymphomas, as our current methods of chromosomal analysis are at best very crude. Another significant observation was the identification of Ia antigens on various tumor cells and the implication that they have not only immunologic functions but also play some role in differentiation and cell regulation.

In closing, it must be said that we are still far from understanding the pathogenicity of leukemia, lymphoma, and related diseases but that our knowledge has rapidly increased and will continne to do so with the help of modern molecular, virologic, and immunologic techniques developed during the last years. I must, however, remind you that in the clinical arena the battle against leukemia needs a better exchange and co-ordination between clinicians, immunologists, molecular biologists, geneticists, and virologists. Only then can our potential be realized.

Subject Index

Abelson leukemia virus 7, 384, 467
– – –, bone marrow cultures 272
– – –, target cells 468
Adipocytes 278
ADP Ribosylation 225
Adriamycin see also chemotherapy
– in AML 39, 46, 54
Agar colony technique 237, 251
ALL see also leukemia
–, cellmembran antigen in 326
–, CFU-C in 239, 243, 246, 251, 256
–, natural killer cells 351
–, relaps in 95, 114
–, treatment of 77, 79, 88, 91, 100, 108
Alpha-naphthylacetate-esterase in blood cells 268
– in bone marrow cultures 277, 291
– in Reed-Sternberg cells 12
– in T- cell lines 505
AML
–, antiserum 334
–, cellmembran antigen in 332
–, CFU-C in 239, 243, 246, 251
–, continuous cell line of 517
–, CSF in 239, 243
–, immunotherapy in 39, 55
–, meningeal leukemia in 51
–, remission of 40, 55
–, surface immunglobulins in 340
–, treatment of 38, 54
ANLL
–, treatment with low dose cytosine arabinoside 59
–, natural killer cells in 351
Anthracycline, treatment with 38, 45
Antibodies
–, for GvHD supression in bone marrow transplantation 126, 132
–, idiotypic 343, 368
–, monoclonal 548
–, secreting cells, viral expression in 365
–, to BLV 498
–, to FLV 485, 492
–, to FOCMA 484, 488, 492
–, to HLA 300, 310
–, to mouse brain 306
–, to T cells 124

Antigen
–, common ALL (c ALL) 265, 326
–, C-typ viral proteins in human leukemia 527, 530
–, human leucocyte 309
–, leukemic 332
–, T- cell 266
–, transformation specific 485, 521
–, tumor 378, 485
Anti-idiotypic immunity 343, 368
– –, progressiv tumor growth stimulated by 371
Asparaginase see also chemotherapy
–, treatment with 54
Ataxia telangiectasia, chromosom 14 anomalia in 5, 181
Avian
–, erythroblastosis virus (AEV) 417
–, gene products of 397
–, leukosis viruses 417, 432, 439, 445, 452
–, myeloblastosis genom 429
–, myelocytomatosis virus 418
–, sarcoma virus 397, 405, 409
–, target cells for 419
–, transformation of hematopoietic cells by 418
–, transforming gen product of 397

Bacterial binding to lymphocytes 356
– –, to leukemic cells 358
BALB/c mouse 479
B-cells see lymphocytes and lymphoma
BFM study group 87
BFUE 301
Blast colony forming cells, recloning of 248
B-lymphocytes 179, 191, 314
–, differentiation 318
–, lymphoma 3, 191, 315, 439
Bone-marrow
–, culture 243, 246, 252, 255
– –, continuous 272, 276, 289
–, transplantation 132, 136
– –, treatment with ATCG in 133
Bovine leukemia 495, 498
– –, antibody response to 499
– –, genom of 496

Bovine leukemia
– –, proteins of 499
– –, provirus of 495
– –, virus 495, 498
Bromodeoxyuridine, effect on endogeneous retrovirus production 365
Burkitt lymphoma 3
– –, chromosomal changes in 4, 31, 179, 192

Carcinogen 5, 9, 393
Cat leukemia see FLV
Cell culture 276, see also cell lines
Cell differentiation 548
– –, block of 215
– –, cellmembran antigens in 265, 296, 311
– –, expression of lysozyme gene in 177
– –, glycophorin A in 305
– –, induction of 216
– –, of leukemic cells 261, 265, 268
– –, viral expression in 366
Cell fusion 527
– –, induced by EBV 193
Cell hybrids, production of monoclonal antibodies in 294
Cell line
– –, DAUDI 180
– –, HL-60 215
– –, Hodgkin 232
–, human Teratocarcinom 541
– –, K 562 339
– –, leukemia lymphoma 323
– –, metastasing tumor 378
– –, murine myelomonocytic (WEHI-3) 238
– – –, Ragi 182
– – –, Reh 265
– – –, T-cell neoplasias 505
– – –, U-937 215
– – –, WEHI-3 238, 273
Cell-mediated immunity in X-linked lymphoproliferative syndrome 207
Cell membrane see cell surface
Cell surface antigen
– – –, bacteria as markers for 355
– – – in ALL 265
– – – in AML 334
– – – in bloodcell differentiation 215, 265, 301, 305, 310, 340
– – – in leukemia 340
– – –, monoclonal antibodies against 294, 310
– – –, receptor in leukemogenesis 360
Cell transformation 397
CFU
– –C 239, 277, 291, 305
– –E 301
– –GEMM 247
– –GM
– –, inhibition by Ferritin 244
– – – by LIA 243
– –S 305

Chemoimmunotherapy of AML 39, 140
Chemotherapy
–, combination 39, 45, 53, 79, 88, 91, 100, 108, 116, 122, 547
–, cytoreduction under 73
–, drug sensitivity in 55
– – in vitro test for 56
–, for relaps 95, 112
Childrens Cancer study group 77, 84
Chromosomes abnormalities
– – in atraxia telangiectasia 181
– – in Burkitt lymphoma 180
– – in leukemia 27, 161
– – in lymphoreticularneoplasias 5, 161
– – in human malignancies 160, 162
– – in malignant transformation 151
– and myeloid differentiation 8
– and viral onc genes 392
–, banding technique 151
–, flow sorting 156
–, gene mapping of 156
–, nucleolar organizing region of 152
Clonal, origin of tumor 447
Cloning cells 294
–, molecular 474
CML, chromosom abberation in 164
–, diffusions chamber culture in 262
CNS-leukemia 104
–, prophylaxis of 95, 122
Cocultivation 527
Common ALL antigen 296
– – – in bone marrow cells 299, 326
– – – in serum of leukemia patients 330
– – –, preparation of 296, 326
Computer tomography after intra theleal therapy 105
Contignity theory in Hodgkin's disease 15
Corticosteroids in bone marrow cultures 278, 291
Cox regression analysis 80, 90
CSF 237
–, independent colony forming cells 272
–, production in WEHI-3 cells 238
C-type virus see viral and virus
Cyclophosphamide see chemotherapy
Cytochemistry in ALL 268
– in plasma clot cultures 255
– in T-cell lines 505
Cytosine arabinosid see chemotherapy
– –, treatment of ANLL with low dose 59
Cytotoxity 346, 351, see also T-cells

DAUDI cell line 180
Daunorubicine see chemotherapy
Diffusion chamber, differentiation of leukemic cells in 62, 262, 265
Dihydrofolate reductase gene 167, 171
– – –, transformation of human HCT-8 cells by 171
Dimethylbenz(a)anthrancene, T-cell leukemia induced by 5

Dimethylsulfoxide (DMSO), differention of human leukemic cells by 215, 268
DNA fragments 479, 496
– –, expression 201
– –, mediated gene transfer 171
– –, methylation and gene
–, RNA hybridization 515, 517
–, tumor virus 447, 497, 548
–, viral 197, 383, 497
Double minutes 153

EBNA 3, 184
ELISA 530
Epigenetic, controll in tumorgenicity 8
Episomes, viral DNA in 198
Epstein-Barr virus 3, 179, 207, 548
– –, antibodies against 192, 208
– –, Buskitt lymphoma 3, 179, 191
– –, cell fusion with 193
– –, genom 191
– –, infected cells 192
– –, mononucleosis infectiosa 4, 179, 191, 207
– –, nasopharyngeal carcinoma 179, 191
– –, receptor 180
– –, Virus Capsid Antigen of 192
– –, X-linked malignant lymphoma 207
Erythrocyte ghosts, loaded with EBNA 185
– –, used for microinjection 143, 185
– –, used for therapy 143

FeLV/FeSV 384, 483, 488, 492
– –, anti-sera 492
– –, viral nonproducer 492
Flow cytometry of chromosomes 156
FOCMA 484, 488, 492
–, immune response to 485, 490, 492
Friend leukemia virus in haemopoiesis 272, 472
Fujinami sarcoma virus 389
Fusion injection technique 143

Gag see also gene
–, gene 386
– - x polyproteins 485, 488
Gene
–, aev 389
–, amplification 153
–, amv 430
–, carcino 5, 9, 393
–, DHFR- 172
–, drug resistance 167
–, EBV see EBV
–, env 386, 455
–, episomal viral 197
–, expression and DNA methylation 201
–, fev 389

–, gag 386
– -globin 157
–, insertion 167
–, integration 172
–, lysozyme 175
–, mal 460
–, mcv 389
–, mos 460
–, onc 386, 455, 482
–, pol 386, 455
–, retrovirus 383
–, src 385
–, transforming 168, 171, 383, 441
Genetic, control in tumorigenicity 8
–, elements 152
–, influence on myelopoiesis 237
–, of leukemogenesis 432
–, structures of viruses 386
–, traits 152
Genom see also gene
–, AMV 430
–, BALB/c 479
–, SFFV 472
–, virus 433
Glycophorin A 300, 338
– – in erythroid differentiation 301, 340
– – in leukemic cells 340
– –, structur 238
Graft versus host disease 124, 137, 140
– – – –, pretreatment with antisera 124
– – – –, suppression of 124
Growth-control of T-cell 363, 504
– –, T-lymphomas 363, 504
– -factor dependent blood cell lines 273
– -inhibition by monoclonal antibodies 364
–, U₃ region for 433

Hematopoietic
–, differentiation 325
– – and virus 272
– –, glycophorin A in 339
–, progenitors 246
–, regulation of 272
–, target cells 417
Herpes virus 197
– –, DNA-sequences in lymphoid tumor cell lines 198
Heterogeneous nuclear RNA 517
– – – in leukemia 518
HLA-ABC in erythropoetic cells 301
– -DR in leukemic cells 300
– – in erythropoetic cells 301, 340
–, monoclonal antibodies against 300, 310
HL60-promyelocytic cells 517
Hodgkin's disease 11
– –, immunological defect in 16
– –, long term cultures of 229
Homogeneously staining regiones 153
Human T-cell lymphoma leukemia virus (HTLV) 509

Human T- cell
−−, characterization by nucleic acid hybridization 515
Hybrid cells 181
Hyperthermia, treatment with 146

Ia-antigen 297
−, expression on Hodgkin cell lines 213
−−, U-937 cell-surface 219
− in lymphoid cell differentiation 180
Idiotypic-antibodies 343
Immune response
−−, against antigen loaded erythrocytes ghost 144
−− in Hodgkin's disease 17
−− in X-linked lymphoproliferative syndrome 210
−−, to FOCMA 485
Immune system
−−, adaption to tumor cells 378
−−, cloning cells of 294
−−, idiotypic compartments 343
−−, network concept of 343
Immunotherapy of AML 39, 54
−, nonspecific 343
Initiation factor in protein synthesis 147
Insertion of genes 167
Interferon, activated lymphocytes 346
−, effect of translation 148
−, treatment of leukemia 63
Iron, apoferritin in Hodgkin's disease 20
−, binding proteins 20, 244
−, ferritin inhibition activity on CFU-MG 244
Isoenzyme in lymphomas 222

Karyotype 151
− in leukemia 27
− in nasopharyngeal carcinomas 195
Killer cells 346, 351
−−, isolation by bacteria binding 358

Lactoferrin, inhibition of CSF production by 244
Lectin induced cell killing 362
Leukemia
−, ADP-ribosylation in 226
−, associated inhibitory activity (LIA) 242
−, bovine 495
−, cell markers in 355
−, CFU-C in 243, 246, 252, 255
−, chromosom abnormalities in 27, 161
−, CNS 104
−, cytoreduction 73
−, diffusion chamber culture in 62, 262, 265
−, feline 483
−, genetic factors 237
−, hn RNA in 517
−, human, oncoviruses in 502, 527, 530

−, infections 483, 495, 512
−, interferron treatment of 63
− in vitro induction of 272
−, killer cells in 351
−, meningeal 51, 81
−, network concept in 343
−, prognostic factor in 78, 89
−, radiation induced 537
−, T-cell 5, 70, 90, 506
−, terminale deoxynucleotidyl transferase in 69
−, treatment of 2, 22, 53, 79, 88, 91, 100, 108, 116
−, treatment with bone marrow transplantation 132, 136, 140
−−, with high dose thymidin 73
−, viruses 390, 409, 455
−, virus negative 492
Leukemic cell
−−, antigens, related to C-typ viruses see viral and virus
−−, cALL-antigen expression in see commonALL-antigen
−−, differentiation of, in culture 62, 262, 265, 268
−−, drug sensitivity of 55
−−, killer cells against 348
−−, lines see cell lines
−−, surface marker of 298, 355
Leukemogenesis, mechanism of 272
−, genetics of 432
−, promoter insertion model for 444
−, retrovirus in 445, 512
−, U_3-region in 435
Long terminal repeat 458, 460
LPS see also lectin
−, stimulated lymphocyt cultures 366
Lymphangiogram in Hodgkin's disease 16
Lymphocytes see also B- and T-lymphocytes
−, antiidiotypic 343
−, bacteria binding to 355
−, T- 343
Lymphomas
−, cell lines 198, 323, 377, 505
−, histological types of 318
−, immunological subtypes of 315
−, isoenzymes in 222
−, pathogenesis of 372
−, T-cell 502
−, TDT-activities in 69
Lymphoreticular neoplasias 14q$^+$ markers in 4, 31
Lymphotoxicity 345
Lysozyme gene 175
−−, expression in macrophages 176
−−− in Oviduct 176

Macrophage, expression of lysozyme gene in 176
−, isoenzyme in 222
−, regulation of myelopoiesis by 238
−, synthesis of CSF- and PGE by 239
Meningeal leukemia 51
Methotrexate see also chemotherapy

Methotrexate
–, intermediate dose of 99
–, resistant dihydrofolate reductase 167
–, treatment with 47
Methylation of DNA 201
–, of viral DNA 199
Methylnitrosourea, induction of leukemia in culture 273
Microinjection, intracellular 143
Moloney murine sarcoma virus (MSV), cloned fragments 462
Monoclonal antibodies 179, 294, 296, 309, 360, 548
– –, against hemopoietic precursor cells 296, 310
– –, OKT 297, 311
Mononucleosis infectiousa, EBV in 4, 179, 191
– –, killer cells in 347
Murine leukemia virus, fibroblast transformation 479
– – –, surface receptors for 360, 363
Mutation in malignancy 163
Mycosis fungoides 502, 515
Myeloid differention, expression of lysozyme gene in 177
– –, dysplasia 34
– – –, chromosome determinants in 8
– – –, TDT in 76
Myeloperoxidase 256
– in bone marrow cultures 277, 291
– in plasma clot cultures 256
Myelopoiesis, genetic and oncogenic influences 237
–, inhibition of 238
–, regulation of 241

Nasopharyngeal carcinoma 179
– –, EBV in 192
– –, karyotypes of 195
Natural killing 345
– –, cells 351
Nephroblastomas, virus induced 452
Network concept 343
Nude mice, Hodgkin cell lines in 232

OKT series of monoclonal 297, 311
Oncgen 387, see also gene
–, designs 390
Oncogenetic influences on myelopoiesis 237
Oncorna virus in human leukemia 502, 527
Osteosarcoma, virus induced 452

Papovavirus 3
–, B-lymphotropic 204
Philadelphia chromosome in leukemia 27, 164
Phosphoproteins 524
–, gag related 389
Phosphorylation 397

–, gag related 389
– in protein synthesis 148, 414
–, of initial factor 147
–, phosphoproteins 524
Plasma clot cultures 255
pp60^{src} 397, 402, 405, 411
Precursor polypeptides 524
Prednisolone, treatment with 47
Preleukemia, histopathology of 34
–, induction in bone marrow culture 274
–, ph^1-chromosom in 37
Prognostic factors in leukemia 78, 82, 90, 112, 118, 121
Promoter, insertion model for leukemogenesis 444
–, tumor 201
Prostaglandines, effect of leukemia cell differentiation 270
–, inhibition of CFU-C proliferation by 238
–, production of 239
Protein kinase 398, 402, 405, 414
– –, of the HS-HL system 147
– – in leukemic cells 225
Protein synthesis, control of 414
–, inhibition by HS, HL-heme 148
– –, by interferon-ds RNA 148
–, initiation factor in 146, 414
Provirus, moloney sarcoma (-mos) 460

Radiation, induced murine leukemia 538
Raji-cell line 182
Recombinants of viruses 435, 457
Read-Sternberg cell 12, 229
– –, cytochemistry of 13, 232
Relaps in childhood leukemia 94, 101, 114, 121
–, CNS 81, 101, 119, 121
– in T-cell leukemia 122
–, leukemic 94
–, testicular 81, 114, 119, 121
–, therapy of 95, 112
Remission in AML 40, 47, 140
– – –, after bone marrow transplantation 140
–, cause of death in 109
–, CFU-C in 252, 256
– in childhood leukemia 81, 90, 96, 103, 111, 117, 122
– in T-cell leukemia 122
Restriction analysis 430
– –, of SFFV-DNA 475
– –, of tumor DNA 441, 446, 496
Retrovirus 383, 547
–, endogenes 537
–, genes in thymic nurse cells 374
– in human teratocarcinoma cell lines 541
Reverse transcriptase in thymic epithelial cells 374
– – in human T-cell leukemia virus 509
– – in thymic epithelial cells 374
Risk index in leukemia 82, 89, 101, 118
RNA, heterogeneous 517

RNA
–, of tumor virus 439
Rous sarcoma virus 383, 402

Sarcoma virus 384, see also virus
Sezary syndrome 502
Simian sarcoma virus 409, 520, 524
–––, non producer cells 520, 524
–––, p30 positiv immunreaction in human leukemia
    528, 530
–––, protein 411
–––, transformation specific glycoprotein 521
6-Mercaptopurine see chemotherapy
6-Thioguanine see also chemotherapy
–, treatment in AML 54
Src-gene 385, 402
Suppressor cell in Hodgkin's disease 19
Surface markers in Hodgkin cell lines 231
–– in leukemia lymphoma cell lines 324, 456
–– in U-937 cells 218
Susceptibility theory of Hodgkin's disease 15

Target cells for AEV 419
––, for transformation 455, 468
––, hemopoietic 417
T-cell
–, alloreactive 320
–, antigen 297, 311
–, anti-human globulin against 129
–, clones see hybridomas
–, culture 301, 507
–, cytotoxic 321, 343, 346, 377
–, differention 372
–, growth factor 70, 294, 320, 343, 503
–, helper 294, 320
–, hybridomas 294, 320, 360
– in Hodgkin disease 19
–, leukemia 5, 70, 90, 122, 505, 515
–, line 505
–, to HLA-antigenes 311
–, triosomy in 15
Teratocarcinoma 8
–, retrovirus in human 541
Terminal deocynucleotidyl transterase in leukemia
    68, 296
– and response to therapy 71
– in lymphomas 69
– in normal tissues 296
– in T-cell differentiation 311, 503
Thymic, lymphomas 360
–, nurse cells 372
––, expression of retroviral determinants in 374
Thymidin, high dose therapy in leukemia 75
Transfection, with subgenomic DNA fragments 462
Transformation
–, chromosomes in see chromosomes
–, of bone marrow cells 168

–, of fibroblasts 479
–, of human HCI-8 cells 171
–, specific antigens 485, 521
–, subgenomic fragments induced 461, 476
–, target cells for 455, 467
–, virus induced 384, 417
Transforming gene 168, 171, 383, 441
––, activity of cloned MSV fragments 462
––, products 397
––, proteins 391
Translation of viral RNA 389
–––, limited by interferon 148
––––, by hyperthermia 148
Translocation 151
–, for ph[1]-chromosomes 28
– in CMC 164
– in myeloblastic leukemia 30
Transplantation of bone marrow 132, 136, 140
––––, prevention of GvHD by T-cell anti sera 132
– in leukemia 132, 136, 140
Transposable genetic elements 152
Treatment see also chemotherapy and leukemia
–, of ALL 79, 88, 91, 100, 108, 116
–, of AML (ANLL) 2, 22, 53
–, of T-cell leukemia 122
–, with drug loaded erythrocyts ghosts 143
–, with immunotherapy 139, 343
–, with transplantation 132, 136
Trisomy 7 in lymphoma cell lines 180
–, 15 in T-cell leukemogenesis 6
Tumor cell
––, associated transplantation antigens 377
––, clonal origin 447
––, evolution 9
––, growth, stimulated by anti-idiotypic lymphocy-
    tes 368
––, immunoadaption of 378
––, metastasis 368, 377
––, specific DNA 446
Tupaia, bone marrow cultures 281
12-Tetra-decanoyl-phorbol-13-acetate (TPA), dif-
    ferentiation of human leukemic cells by 315

U_3-region in growth 433
– in leukemogenesis 435
U-937 cell line 215

VAPA[10] treatment of AML with 45
Vincristine see also chemotherapy
–, treatment with in AML 39, 47, 54
Viral see also virus
–, antigens 184, 230
–– in human leukemia 527, 530
–– in humoral immune response 485, 492
–, DNA 198
––, restriction analysis of 441, 446, 496
–, expression in differentiating lymphocytes 366

Viral
−, genes 462 see also gene
−, genome 197, 433, 444
−, proteins in human leukemia 527, 530
−, RNA 439, 515, 517
−−, translation of 148
Virus see also viral
−, AEV 384, 418
−, AMV 418
−, avian tumor 386
−, endogen 435, 537
−−, expression in lymphocytes 366
−, exogen 435
−, HTLV 507, 515

−, MC 29, 384, 409, 418
−, sarcoma 384
−, SFFV 472

Waldeyer's ring, EBV-linked carcinoma in 192
WEHI-3 cell line 238, 273

X-linked lymphoproliferative syndrom 207
−−−, EBV infection in 207
−−−, immunopathology of 210

Haematology and Blood Transfusion

Supplement volumes to the journal „Blut"

Editors: H. Heimpel, D. Huhn, G. Ruhenstroth-Bauer, W. Stich

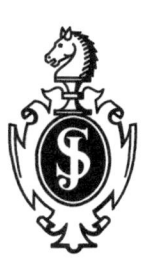

Springer-Verlag
Berlin
Heidelberg
New York

Aplastic Anemia

Pathophysiology and Approaches to Therapy
International Symposium on Aplastic Anemia
July 19–22, 1978, Schloß Reisensburg
Editors: H. Heimpel, E. C. Gordon-Smith, W. Heit, B. Kubanek
1979. 81 figures, 71 tables. XIII, 292 pages (Volume 24)
ISBN 3-540-09772-4

Immunobiology of Bone Marrow Transplantation

International Seminar, March 8–10, 1979, Neuherberg/München
Editors: S. Thierfelder, H. Rodt, H. J. Kolb
1980. 123 figures, 123 tables. XV, 430 pages (Volume 25)
ISBN 3-540-09405-9

Immunological Diagnosis of Leukemias and Lymphomas

International Symposium of the Institut für Hämatologie, GSF, October 28–30, 1976, Neuherberg/München
Editors: S. Thierfelder, H. Rodt, E. Thiel
1977. 98 figures, 2 in color, 101 tables. X, 387 pages (Volume 20)
ISBN 3-540-08216-6

Modern Trends in Human Leukemia II

Biological, Immunological, Therapeutical and Virological Aspects
Editors: R. Neth, R. C. Gallo, K. Mannweiler, W. C. Moloney
1976. 150 figures, 141 tables. XI, 576 pages. (Volume 19)
ISBN 3-540-79785-8

Modern Trends in Human Leukemia III

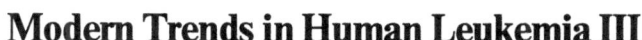

Newest Results in Clinical and Biological Research
9th Scientific Meeting of „Gesellschaft Deutscher Naturforscher und Ärzte"
Together with the "Deutsche Gesellschaft für Hämatologie"
Wilsede, June 19–23, 1978
Editors: R. Neth, R. C. Gallo, P.-H. Hofschneider, K. Mannweiler
1979. 171 figures, 128 tables. XXII, 599 pages. (Volume 23)
ISBN 3-540-08999-3

Automation in Hematology

What to Measure and Why
Editors: D. W. Ross, G. Brecher, M. C. Bessis
1980. 106 figures, 45 tables. VIII, 338 pages
(Monograph edition of the international journal *Blood Cells,*
Vol. 6, 2–3) ISBN 3-540-10225-6

J. C. Cawley, G. F. Burns, F. G. J. Hayhoe

Hairy-Cell Leukemia

1980. 64 figures, 4 tables. IX, 123 pages
(Recent Results in Cancer Research, Vol. 72)
ISBN 3-540-09920-4

Fundamentals of Immunology

By O. G. Bier, W. Dias Da Silva, D. Götze, I. Mota
Revised for the English edition by D. Götze
1981. 168 figures, approx. 73 tables. Approx. 460 pages
ISBN 3-540-90529-4

Immunodiagnosis and Immunotherapy of Malignant Tumors

Relevance to Surgery
Editors: H.-D. Flad, C. Herfarth, M. Betzler
1979. 101 figures, 109 tables. X, 329 pages
ISBN 3-540-09161-0

Immunostimulation

Editors: L. Chedid, P. A. Miescher, H. J. Mueller-Eberhard
1980. 44 figures, 39 tables. VIII, 236 pages
(Monograph edition of the international journal *Springer Series in Immunopathology,* Vol. 2, 1–2) ISBN 3-540-10354-6

K. Lennert

Histopathology of Non-Hodgkin's Lymphomas

(Based on the Kiel-Classification)
In collaboration with H. Stein
Translation from the German by M. Soehring, A. G. Stansfeld
1981. 68 figures (some in color), 5 tables. Approx. 130 pages
ISBN 3-540-10445-3

Preleukemia

Editors: F. Schmalzl, K.-P. Hellriegel
1979, 64 figures, 56 tables. XII, 194 pages
ISBN 3-540-09698-1

Strategies in Clinical Hematology

Editors: R. Gross, K. P. Hellriegel
1979. 22 figures, 33 tables. X, 140 pages
(Recent Results in Cancer Research, Vol. 69)
ISBN 3-540-09578-0

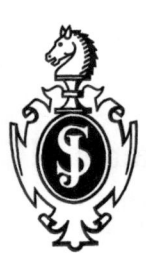

Springer-Verlag
Berlin
Heidelberg
New York